PEDIATRIC DENTISTRY

Associate Editors

Paul S. Casamassimo, D.D.S., M.S.

Professor and Chairman
Department of Pediatric Dentistry
College of Dentistry
Ohio State University
Columbus, Ohio

Henry W. Fields, Jr., D.D.S., M.S., M.S.D.

Professor and Dean
College of Dentistry
Ohio State University
Columbus, Ohio

Dennis J. McTigue, D.D.S., M.S.

Professor and Associate Dean for Academic
  Affairs
Department of Pediatric Dentistry
Ohio State University College of Dentistry
Columbus, Ohio

Arthur Nowak, D.M.D., M.A.

Professor
Departments of Pediatric Dentistry and
  Pediatrics
Colleges of Dentistry and Medicine
University of Iowa
Iowa City, Iowa

PEDIATRIC DENTISTRY

Infancy Through Adolescence

Third Edition

Senior Editor

J.R. Pinkham, D.D.S., M.S.

Professor and Head
Department of Pediatric Dentistry
University of Iowa College of Dentistry
Iowa City, Iowa

W.B. SAUNDERS COMPANY

An Imprint of Elsevier Science
Philadelphia London New York St. Louis Sydney Toronto

W.B. SAUNDERS COMPANY
An Imprint of Elsevier Science

The Curtis Center
Independence Square West
Philadelphia, Pennsylvania 19106

Library of Congress Cataloging-in-Publication Data

Pinkham, J. R.
Pediatric Dentistry: infancy through adolescence / J. R. Pinkham, Paul S. Casamassimo, Henry J. Fields, Jr., Dennis J. McTigue, Arthur J. Nowak

p.   cm.

ISBN 0–7216–8238–3

1. Pedodontics.   I. Pinkham, J. R.

RK55.C5P448   1999

617.6′45—dc21

DNLM/DLC   99-24326

PEDIATRIC DENTISTRY: INFANCY THROUGH ADOLESCENCE   ISBN 0–7216–8238–3

Printed in the United States of America.

Last digit is the print number: 9   8   7   6   5   4   3

Contributors

Steven M. Adair, D.D.S, M.S.
Chairman and Director of Advanced Education, Department of Pediatric Dentistry, Medical College of Georgia, Augusta, Georgia
Conception to Age Three: The Dynamics of Change: Epidemiology and Mechanisms of Dental Disease; Oral Habits; Adolescence: The Dynamics of Change: Epidemiology and Mechanisms of Dental Disease

Jay A. Anderson, D.D.S., M.S.
Private Practice of Anesthesiology; Active Staff, Tuomey Regional Medical Center, Sumter, South Carolina
Pain and Anxiety Control (Part I: Pain Perception Control); Pain and Anxiety Control (Part II: Pain Reaction Control—Conscious Sedation); Medical Emergencies

Gary K. Belanger, D.D.S.
Associate Professor and Chairman, Pediatric Dentistry, University of Colorado School of Dentistry, Denver, Colorado
Pulp Therapy for Young Permanent Teeth

Paul S. Casamassimo, D.D.S., M.S.
Professor and Chairman, Department of Pediatric Dentistry, College of Dentistry, Ohio State University, Columbus, Ohio; Chief of Dentistry, Columbus Children's Hospital, Columbus, Ohio
The Primary Dentition Years: Three to Six Years: Examination, Diagnosis, and Treatment Planning; The Transitional Years: Six to Twelve Years: Examination, Diagnosis, and Treatment Planning; Adolescence: Examination, Diagnosis, and Treatment Planning for General and Orthodontic Problems

John R. Christensen, D.D.S., M.S., M.S.
Adjunct Clinical Professor in Pediatric Dentistry and Orthodontics, School of Dentistry at the University of North Carolina, Chapel Hill, North Carolina

The Primary Dentition Years: Three to Six Years: Examination, Diagnosis, and Treatment Planning; Space Maintenance in the Primary Dentition; Oral Habits; Orthodontic Treatment in the Primary Dentition; The Transitional Years: Six to Twelve Years: Examination, Diagnosis, and Treatment Planning; Treatment Planning and Treatment of Orthodontic Problems; Adolescence: Examination, Diagnosis, and Treatment Planning for General and Orthodontic Problems

James Crall, D.D.S., Sc.D.
Head, Department of Pediatric Dentistry, University of Connecticut, School of Dental Medicine, Farmington, Connecticut; Director, Department of Dentistry, Connecticut Children's Medical Center, Hartford, Connecticut
Conception to Age Three: Prevention of Dental Disease; The Primary Dentition Years: Three to Six Years: Prevention of Dental Disease; The Transitional Years: Six to Twelve Years: Prevention of Dental Disease; Adolescence: Prevention of Dental Disease

Mary A. Curtis, M.D.
Associate Professor of Pediatrics, Director of Clinical Genetics, University of Arkansas for Medical Sciences, Little Rock, Arkansas
Congenital Genetic Disorders and Syndromes

Diane C. Dilley, D.D.S.
Associate Professor of Pediatric Dentistry and Predoctoral Program Director, University of North Carolina, Chapel Hill, North Carolina; Associate Professor, UNC Hospitals, Department of Pediatric Dentistry, Chapel Hill, North Carolina
Pain and Anxiety Control (Part I: Pain Perception Control); Pain and Anxiety Control (Part II: Pain Reaction Control—Conscious Sedation)

Kevin James Donly, D.D.S., M.S.
Professor, Department of Pediatric Dentistry,
Dental School, University of Texas Health
Science Center at San Antonio, San Antonio,
Texas; Postgraduate Director, Pediatric Dentistry,
Santa Rosa Children's Hospital, San Antonio,
Texas
Dental Materials

C. O. Dummett, Jr., D.D.S., M.S.D., M.Ed.
Professor and Coordinator, Postgraduate
Pediatric Dentistry, Louisiana State University
School of Dentistry, New Orleans, Louisiana;
Chief, Pediatric Dentistry Section, Charity
Hospital of New Orleans, New Orleans,
Louisiana
Anomalies of the Developing Dentition

Henry W. Fields, Jr., D.D.S., M.S., M.S.D.
Dean and Professor of Orthodontics, College of
Dentistry, Ohio State University, Columbus,
Ohio; Chair, Department of Dentistry, Ohio
State University Hospital, Columbus, Ohio;
Attending, Children's Hospital, Columbus, Ohio
*Examination, Diagnosis, and Treatment
Planning; Space Maintenance in the Primary
Dentition; Oral Habits; Orthodontic Treatment
in the Primary Dentition; The Transitional
Years: Six to Twelve Years: Examination,
Diagnosis, and Treatment Planning; Treatment
Planning and Treatment of Orthodontic
Problems; Adolescence: Examination,
Diagnosis, and Treatment Planning for
General and Orthodontic Problems*

Catherine M. Flaitz, D.D.S., M.S.
Professor, Division of Oral and Maxillofacial
Pathology, Department of Pediatric Dentistry,
University of Texas–Houston Dental Branch,
Houston, Texas; Consultant, Texas Children's
Hospital, Houston, Texas
*Oral Pathologic Conditions and Soft Tissue
Anomalies; The Acid-Etch Technique in Caries
Prevention: Pit and Fissure Sealants and
Preventive Restorations*

Anna B. Fuks, C.D.
Professor of Pediatric Dentistry and Coordinator
of Post-Graduate Courses, Hebrew University,
Hadassah School of Dental Medicine,
Department of Pediatric Dentistry; Pediatric
Dentistry Consultant, Cleft Palate Team,
Hadassah Hospital, Jerusalem, Israel
Pulp Therapy for the Primary Dentition

C. A. Full, B.S., D.D.S., M.S.
Professor Emeritus, University of Iowa College
of Dentistry, Iowa City, Iowa

*Conception to Age Three: The Dynamics of
Change: Dental Changes; The Primary
Dentition Years: Three to Six Years: Dental
Changes; The Transitional Years: Six to Twelve
Years: Dental Changes; Adolescence: The
Dynamics of Change: Dental Changes*

Stephen Goepferd, D.D.S., M.S.
Professor, Department of Pediatric Dentistry,
University of Iowa College of Dentistry, Iowa
City, Iowa; Director, Division of Pediatric
Dentistry, Department of Hospital Dentistry,
University of Iowa Hospitals and Clinics, Iowa
City, Iowa
Examination of the Infant and Toddler

Ann L. Griffen, D.D.S., M.S.
Associate Professor, Department of Pediatric
Dentistry, College of Dentistry, Ohio State
University, Columbus, Ohio; Attending,
Children's Hospital, Columbus, Ohio
*Periodontal Problems in Children and
Adolescents*

M. John Hicks, D.D.S., M.S., Ph.D., M.D.
Associate Professor, Department of Pathology,
Baylor College of Medicine, Houston, Texas;
Adjunct Professor, Department of Pediatric
Dentistry, University of Texas–Houston Health
Science Center, Dental Branch, Houston, Texas;
Attending Pathologist and Director of Surgical
and Ultrastructural Pathology, Department of
Pathology, Texas Childrens Hospital, Houston,
Texas
*The Acid-Etch Technique in Caries Prevention:
Pit and Fissure Sealants and Preventive
Restorations*

M. J. Kanellis, D.D.S., M.S.
Associate Professor, Department of Pediatric
Dentistry, University of Iowa College of
Dentistry, Iowa City, Iowa; Staff, University of
Iowa Hospitals and Clinics, Iowa City, Iowa
*Dental Public Health Issues in Pediatric
Dentistry; Conception to Age Three: The
Dynamics of Change: Disease Risk Factors of
the Infant and Toddler*

Wilma A. Lim, M.D.
Clinical Associate Professor, School of Medicine,
University of North Carolina at Chapel Hill,
Chapel Hill, North Carolina; Clinical Associate
Professor, Division of Pediatric Infectious
Diseases, Department of Pediatrics, University
of North Carolina Hospitals, Chapel Hill, North
Carolina
Antimicrobials in Pediatric Dentistry

Dianne M. McBrien, M.D.
Assistant Professor of Clinical Pediatrics,
University of Iowa Hospitals and Clinics, Iowa
City, Iowa
Topics in Pediatric Physiology

Dennis J. McTigue, D.D.S., M.S.
Professor and Associate Dean for Academic
Affairs, College of Dentistry, Ohio State
University, Columbus, Ohio; Attending,
Children's Hospital, Columbus, Ohio
*Introduction to Dental Trauma: Managing
Traumatic Injuries in the Primary Dentition;
Managing Traumatic Injuries in the Young
Permanent Dentition*

R. Denny Montgomery, D.D.S.
Clinical Assistant Professor, Section of Oral and
Maxillofacial Surgery, Ohio State University,
College of Dentistry, Columbus, Ohio; Attending
Staff, Children's Hospital and Riverside Hospital,
Columbus, Ohio
Local Anesthesia and Oral Surgery in Children

Arthur Nowak, D.M.D., M.A.
University of Iowa Colleges of Dentistry and
Medicine, Departments of Pediatric Dentistry
and Pediatrics, Iowa City, Iowa; Department of
Hospital Dentistry, University of Iowa Hospitals
and Clinics, Iowa City, Iowa
*Conception to Age Three: Prevention of Dental
Disease; The Primary Dentition Years: Three to
Six Years: Prevention of Dental Disease; The
Transitional Years: Six to Twelve Years:
Prevention of Dental Disease; Adolescence:
Prevention of Dental Disease*

J. R. Pinkham, B.S., D.D.S., M.S.
Professor and Head, Department of Pediatric
Dentistry, University of Iowa College of
Dentistry, Iowa City, Iowa; Staff, University of
Iowa Hospitals and Clinics, Iowa City, Iowa
*The Practical Importance of Pediatric
Dentistry; Conception to Age Three: The
Dynamics of Change: Body; Cognitive Changes;
Emotional Changes; Social Changes; The
Primary Dentition Years: Three to Six Years:
The Dynamics of Change: Body; Cognitive
Changes; Emotional Changes; Patient
Management; The Transitional Years: Six to
Twelve Years: The Dynamics of Change: Body;
Cognitive Changes; Emotional Changes;
Adolescence: The Dynamics of Change: Body;
Cognitive Changes; Social Changes*

Dennis N. Ranalli, D.D.S., M.D.S.
Professor and Chairman, Department of
Pediatric Dentistry, University of Pittsburgh,
School of Dental Medicine, Pittsburgh,
Pennsylvania; Consultant, Sports Medicine
Program, and Member, Sports Medicine
Performance Team, Department of Athletics,
University of Pittsburgh, Pittsburgh,
Pennsylvania
Sports Dentistry and Mouth Protection

John W. Reinhardt, D.D.S., M.S., M.P.H.
Professor and Head, Department of Operative
Dentistry, University of Iowa College of
Dentistry, Iowa City, Iowa
*Esthetic Restorative Dentistry for the
Adolescent*

Michael W. Roberts, D.D.S., M.Sc.D.
Associate Professor and Chair, Department of
Pediatric Dentistry, School of Dentistry,
University of North Carolina at Chapel Hill,
Chapel Hill, North Carolina; Chair, Division of
Pediatric Dentistry, Department of Dentistry,
University of North Carolina Hospitals, Chapel
Hill, North Carolina
Antimicrobials in Pediatric Dentistry

Adriana Segura, D.D.S., M.S.
Associate Professor, Department of Pediatric
Dentistry, Dental School, University of Texas
Health Science Center at San Antonio, San
Antonio, Texas; Santa Rosa Children's Hospital,
San Antonio, Texas
Dental Materials

Andrew Sonis, B.A., D.M.D.
Associate Clinical Professor of Pediatric
Dentistry, Harvard School of Dental Medicine,
Boston, Massachusetts; Associate in Dentistry,
Children's Hospital, Boston, Massachusetts;
Associate in Surgery, Brigham and Women's
Hospital, Boston, Massachusetts
*Diseases and Oral Manifestations of Systemic
Disease*

William F. Vann, Jr., D.M.D., M.S., Ph.D.
Professor and Graduate Program Director,
Pediatric Dentistry, University of North Carolina
School of Dentistry, Chapel Hill, North Carolina;
Professor and Graduate Program Director, UNC
Hospitals, Department of Pediatric Dentistry,
Chapel Hill, North Carolina
*Pain and Anxiety Control (Part I: Pain
Perception Control); Pain and Anxiety Control
(Part II: Pain Reaction Control—Conscious
Sedation)*

Kaaren G. Vargas, D.D.S., Ph.D.
Assistant Professor, Department of Pediatric
Dentistry, University of Iowa College of
Dentistry, Iowa City, Iowa
Medical Emergencies

Marcos A. Vargas, D.D.S., M.S.
Associate Professor, Department of Operative
Dentistry, University of Iowa College of
Dentistry, Iowa City, Iowa
*Esthetic Restorative Dentistry for the
Adolescent*

William F. Waggoner, D.D.S., M.S.
Private Practice, Pediatric Dental Care
*Restorative Dentistry for the Primary
Dentition*

Jerry Walker, D.D.S., M.A.
Professor, Department of Pediatric Dentistry,
University of Iowa College of Dentistry, Iowa
City, Iowa; Staff Dentist, University of Iowa
Hospital and Clinics, Iowa City, Iowa
*Conception to Age Three: The Dynamics of
Change: Craniofacial Changes; The Primary
Dentition Years: Three to Six Years:
Craniofacial Changes; The Transitional Years:
Six to Twelve Years: The Dynamics of Change:
Craniofacial Changes; Adolescence: The
Dynamics of Change: Craniofacial Changes*

Stephen Wilson, D.M.D., M.A., Ph.D.
Professor, Section of Pediatric Dentistry, College
of Dentistry, Ohio State University, Columbus,
Ohio; Director, Pediatric Dentistry Residency
Program, Columbus Childrens Hospital,
Columbus, Ohio
*Nonpharmacologic Issues in Pain Perception
and Control; Pain and Anxiety Control (Part I:
Pain Perception Control); Pain and Anxiety
Control (Part II: Pain Reaction
Control—Conscious Sedation); Local
Anesthesia and Oral Surgery in Children*

Orientation to the Text

Pediatric Dentistry: Infancy Through Adolescence is divided into a section of introductory chapters and four major age-related sections. The introductory chapters deal with basic information and themes pertinent to dentistry for children at virtually all ages. Eleven chapters are included in this division of the book.

In inspecting the information covered in the introductory chapters of this book, a student will readily see that much of this information has been, or probably will be, covered in other aspects of his or her dental school's curriculum. However, because of the uniqueness of children, their physiologic differences from adults, and other age-related issues, no textbook on pediatric dentistry would be complete without a discussion of the topics covered in this section of the textbook.

The four remaining sections of the textbook divide childhood into four age groups and address each of these age groups according to the changes the child experiences physically, cognitively, emotionally, and socially; the epidemiology of dental diseases; examination requirements; prevention needs; and possible treatment considerations. These four age groups are as follows:

- Conception to age three
- The primary dentition years: Three to six years
- The transitional years: Six to twelve years
- Adolescence

The division of the textbook according to these age groups was a deliberate decision. The editors felt that a discussion of dentistry for children should be divided into logical age-related categories, since each age range has certain themes that should be emphasized. Positive feedback from many dental educators who used the first edition of this book supports the appropriateness of this conclusion.

The child from conception to age 3 historically has not been involved in professional dental supervision. In fact, until recently dentistry has never actively encouraged children of this age to be involved in professional care. Age 3 has for many years been the customary entry age of children to the dental experience. This texbook certainly does not encourage this tradition. It is deeply believed by the editors and authors that prevention programs must be started well before age 3 to ensure success. Therefore, Section I: Conception to Age Three, exists to focus on the needs of an age group that has been virtually overlooked previously.

Section II: The Primary Dentition Years: Three to Six Years deals with children with a complete primary dentition who generally are capable of going into the dental office as cooperative patients. Indeed, most of the literature on techniques useful for behavior management of children is directed to this young age group. The clinician who works with this age group needs to understand the morphology and anatomy of the primary dentition, how to preserve dental arch integrity if teeth are lost, and how to intercept malocclusions in the primary dentition. The primary dentition presents its own challenges regarding restoration and pulpal therapy. The primary dentition also serves as a template for the permanent dentition and contains many clues to the final form of the permanent dentition. Because of the management concerns related to age and the importance of maintaining an intact primary dentition, the information in this section is critical to the family dentist.

Section III: The Transitional Years: Six to Twelve Years is so labeled because between 6 and 12 years of age the majority of children shed all of their primary teeth and gain all of their permanent teeth except the third molars. With this "transition" to the permanent dentition comes the responsibility of the clinician for understanding the treatment needs of young permanent teeth. Orthodontic considerations and esthetic considerations become more and more important in this age group also. Although the prevention needs of the preschool child remain pertinent in the transitional years, the transitional years also see children taking on more and more responsibility for their own oral hygiene.

The last section, Section IV, deals with adolescence. The adolescent is also a child who is believed by many involved in dentistry for children to have been largely overlooked by the profession. The needs of the adolescent in regard to prevention and treatment planning considerations, the seriousness of dental and facial esthetics at this age, and the increasing concerns about periodontal disease certainly justify a major section in any pediatric dental textbook.

Although redundancy can have educational merit, the editors have tried to provide the least redundant textbook possible. Obviously, there are certain examination considerations and preventive issues that are pertinent to all four age groups. In such situations, relevant information is addressed again if necessary. However, as much as possible, issues are discussed once and only once at that point in a child's development at which they are first most appropriate, in the editors' judgment, to be discussed. For instance, fluoride supplementation, which certainly is pertinent for the very young child, is discussed in Section I: Conception to Age Three. It is only referred to in following sections, even though supplementation is certainly a fundamental feature of many children's prevention programs from 3 to 6 years and even in the first several years of adolescence. Using the same guideline, stainless steel crown technique is discussed in the restorative chapter of Section II: The Primary Dentition Years: Three to Six Years. This is because it is rare for dentists to treat children younger than 3 years of age restoratively but commonplace after age 3.

The following represent the locations of themes that occur in at least two of the sections:

Dynamics of change: Chapters 12, 17, 29, 36
Examination: Chapters 13, 18, 30, 37
Treatment planning: Chapters 13, 18, 30, 37
Radiographic concerns: Chapters 18, 30, 37
Prevention: Chapters 14, 19, 31, 38
Trauma: Chapters 15, 34, 39, 40
Restorative dentistry: Chapters 20, 21, 32, 39
Pulp therapy: Chapters 22, 33
Orthodontic therapy: Chapters 27, 35
Orthodontic diagnosis: Chapters 18, 30, 37
Behavior management: Chapters 6, 23

If a student is using the text as a reference and wants to find out where a certain issue or technique is covered, he or she is encouraged first to look at the table of contents, and then, if not successful there, to check the index. A quick perusal of the text should also help in orienting a student to the location of certain information.

There is a brief introduction and concluding summary to each of the four age-related divisions of this book. It is recommended that the student who is trying to gain or enhance a perspective on a dentist's responsibilities for the child of each group read these before trying to assimilate the information in any of the age-related chapters.

NOTICE

Pediatric Dentistry is an ever-changing field. Standard safety precautions must be followed, but as new research and clinical experience broaden our knowledge, changes in treatment and drug therapy become necessary or appropriate. Readers are advised to check the product information currently provided by the manufacturer of each drug to be administered to verify the recommended dose, the method and duration of administration, and contraindications. It is the responsibility of the treating dentist, relying on experience and knowledge of the patient, to determine dosages and the best treatment for the patient. Neither the publisher nor the editors assume any responsibility for any injury and/or damage to persons or property.

THE PUBLISHER

Preface

....

My co-editors—Drs. Casamassimo, Fields, McTigue, and Nowak—and I are proud to introduce the third edition of our textbook, *Pediatric Dentistry: Infancy Through Adolescence.* We appreciate W.B. Saunders' enthusiasm for this new edition. We also deeply appreciate the dental educators, dental students, and dental practitioners who bought the second edition in numbers sufficient to justify optimism about a market for a third edition. This book, whose first edition was in 1988, has been received favorably around the world. Obviously the substantial work of all contributors to this book is the reason for its success.

Readers familiar with the first and second editions will readily see that the most critical format decision imposed upon the first two editions has been retained in this edition. Specifically, this means that this edition, after initially covering some very basic information pertinent to all age levels of dentistry for children, is divided into four large sections by developmental age. Just as we maintained in the 1980s, we submit that it is even more true today, "that pediatric dentistry now approaches children of varying ages with such specificity that a book portraying the realistic differences between dentistry for various age groups is needed."

It should be pointed out that this is an expanded edition. There is a new chapter on public health issues in pediatric dentistry, and except for those chapters handling just very basic issues in dentistry for children, such as the histology of the developing teeth, almost every chapter has been modified in some form. Also, there are new contributors to the "box" information contained in various chapters. A few have been retained from the second edition because they were judged by the editors to be of high educational value. Others from the second edition have been adjusted. Finally, there are new "box" additions that were not included in the second edition.

The reader/student of this textbook should read "Orientation to the Text" before starting to study this book.

JIMMY R. PINKHAM, B.S., D.D.S., M.S.

Acknowledgments

....

The editors of the text wish to thank the following individuals for their contribution by way of "boxes" of specific information that are contained within certain chapters of this textbook

JAMES W. BAWDEN, D.D.S., M.S., Ph.D.
Alumni Distinguished Professor, Department of Pediatric Dentistry, School of Dentistry, University of North Carolina, Chapel Hill, North Carolina
Chapter 14

WILLIAM L. CHAMBERS, D.D.S., M.S.
Associate Clinical Professor, School of Dentistry, University of North Carolina, Chapel Hill, North Carolina; Active Staff, Mission-St. Joseph Hospital, Thoms Rehabilitation Hospital, Asheville, North Carolina
Chapter 40

THEODORE P. CROLL, D.D.S.
Private Practice, Pediatric Dentistry, Doylestown, Pennsylvania; Clinical Professor of Clinical Dentistry, University of Pennsylvania, Philadelphia, Pennsylvania; Adjunct Associate Professor of Pediatric Dentistry, University of Iowa College of Dentistry, Iowa City, Iowa; Clinical Professor of Pediatric Dentistry, University of Texas Health Sciences Center, Dental Branch, Houston, Texas
Chapter 20

BURTON EDELSTEIN, D.D.S., M.P.H.
Department of Oral Health Policy and Epidemiology, Harvard School of Dental Medicine, Boston, Massachusetts; Director, Children's Dental Health Project, Washington, D.C.
Chapters 17 and 24

DAVID C. JOHNSEN, D.D.S., M.S.
Professor, Department of Pediatric Dentistry, University of Iowa College of Dentistry; Dean, University of Iowa College of Dentistry, Iowa City, Iowa
Chapter 12

GEORGIA K. JOHNSON, D.D.S., M.S.
Professor and Head, Department of Periodontics, Dow Institute for Dental Research, University of Iowa College of Dentistry, Iowa City, Iowa
Chapter 37

N. SUE SEALE, D.D.S., M.S.D.
Regents Professor and Chairman, Program Director, Advanced Education Program, Baylor College of Dentistry, Dallas, Texas; Director of Dental Service, Texas Scottish Rite Hospital for Children, Dallas, Texas; Chairman, Department of Dentistry, Children's Medical Center, Dallas, Texas
Chapter 21

MARK D. SIEGAL, D.D.S., M.P.H.
Adjunct Assistant Professor, Ohio State University, Columbus, Ohio, and University of Michigan, Ann Arbor, Michigan
Chapter 11

REBECCA L. SLAYTON, D.D.S., Ph.D.
Assistant Professor, Department of Pediatric Dentistry, University of Iowa College of Dentistry, Iowa City, Iowa
Chapter 16

CHRISTOPHER A. SQUIER, Ph.D., D.Sc., F.R.C.Path.
Professor, Department of Oral Pathology, Radiology and Medicine, and Associate Dean for Research and Graduate Studies, University of Iowa College of Dentistry, Iowa City, Iowa; Consultant, Veterans Hospital Medical Center, Iowa City, Iowa
Chapter 37

NORMAN TINANOFF, D.D.S., M.S.
Professor and Chair, Department of Pediatric
Dentistry, Baltimore College of Dental Surgery,
Baltimore, Maryland
Chapter 17

H. BARRY WALDMAN, D.D.S., Ph.D., M.P.H.
Department of General Dentistry, School of
Dental Medicine, State University of New York,
Stony Brook, New York
Chapter 1

KARIN WEBER, D.D.S., M.S.
Pediatric Dentistry Department, University of
Iowa College of Dentistry, Iowa City, Iowa
Chapter 11

Contents

Introduction

The Practical Importance of Pediatric Dentistry

J.R. Pinkham

Chapter Outline

Pediatric dentistry is synonymous with dentistry for children. Pediatric dentistry exists because children have dental and orofacial problems. The genesis of dentistry for children unquestionably is allied to dental decay, pulpitis, and the inflammation and pain associated with infected pulpal tissue and suppuration in alveolar bone.

From its extraction-oriented beginnings, pediatric dentistry phased into an era of decay interception with an emphasis on diagnostic procedures and the maintenance of arch integrity in instances of tooth loss due to decay or trauma. Restorative techniques, pulpal therapy, space maintenance, and interceptive orthodontics were the main themes of this era. This era is not over. Tooth decay still exists, although its incidence is significantly less in certain areas of the United States than it was several decades ago. Therefore, these treatment techniques are covered in detail in this book.

Today, however, pediatric dentistry also emphasizes prevention. Unquestionably, the prevention of dental diseases is a primary focus of this book, and it is addressed specifically for each of the four age groups that determine the organization of this book.

HISTORICAL PERSPECTIVE

In at least one state of the United States, a major dental supplier, up until the middle 1950s, gave all new clients opening dental offices a very handsome sign that said: *No children under age 13 treated in this office.* Fortunately, such attitudes and such signs are now gone. Over the past several decades, specific educational guidelines for pediatric dentistry have been adopted and are imposed on all dental schools accredited by the American Dental Association's Commission on Accreditation. Graduates of all accredited dental schools have not only a didactic education in dentistry for children but also a clinical education. Furthermore, through the efforts of organized dentistry and other organizations and individuals interested in the oral health of children, the ignorant notion that the "baby teeth don't deserve care because you lose them anyway" has largely disappeared save for the most uninformed persons.

Indeed, at the writing of the first edition of this book in the 1980s, it was asserted that dentistry seemed to be on the brink of advocating routine "well baby" dental consultations and examinations for children younger than 3 years of age. In fact, both the American Academy of Pediatric Dentistry and the American Society of Dentistry for Children now advocate a routine dental appointment on or before the first birthday. Unquestionably, the appropriateness of this recommendation for earlier dental care is due to the quality of prevention information, treatment, and techniques available to the profession today. This recommendation parallels the change in the voices within the dental profession that for years questioned the best age for a child to enter professional supervision. When dentistry was treatment-oriented, age was a consideration because of behavioral reasons and the inability of the clinician and the child patient to communicate. For these reasons the customary age of the first dental appointment was on or after the third birthday. With the maturity of the dental profession in the area of preventive dentistry for the child patient, however, this age became far too old for the initiation of appropriate preventive services. Prevention of disease can never be started too early. The importance of dentistry's involvement with infants on or before their first birthday cannot be overstated. Despite the truth of this conclusion, addressing the needs of this age group remains a relevant challenge to the dental profession.

MILESTONES IN DENTISTRY FOR CHILDREN IN THE UNITED STATES

1900 Few children are treated in dental offices. Little or no instruction in the care of "baby teeth" is given in the 50 dental schools in the United States.

1924 First comprehensive textbook on dentistry for children is published.

1926 The Gies Report on dental education notes that only 5 of the 43 dental schools in the United States have facilities especially designed for treating children.

1927 After almost a decade of frustration in getting a group organized to promote dentistry for children, the American Society for the Promotion of Dentistry for Children is established at the meeting of the American Dental Association (ADA) in Detroit.

1932 A report of the College Committee of the American Society for the Promotion of Dentistry for Children states that in 1928, 15 dental schools provided no clinical experience with children and 22 schools had no didactic information in this area.

1935 Six graduate programs and eight postgraduate programs exist in pedodontics.

1940 The American Society for the Promotion of Dentistry for Children changes its name to the American Society of Dentistry for Children (ASDC).

1941 1941 Children's Dental Health Day is observed in Cleveland, and Children's Dental Health Week is observed in Akron, Ohio.

1942 The effectiveness of topical fluoride applications at preventing caries is described.
The Council on Dental Education recommends that all dental schools have pedodontics as part of their curriculum.

1945 First artificial water fluoridation plant is begun at Grand Rapids, Michigan.

1947 The American Academy of Pedodontics is formed. (To a large degree, the start of the Academy was prompted by the need for a more scientifically focused organization concerned with the dental health of children.)

1948 The American Board of Pedodontics, a group formulated to certify candidates in the practice of dentistry for children, is formally recognized by the Council on Dental Education of the ADA.

1949 The first full week of February is designated National Children's Dental Health Week.

1955 The acid-etch technique is described.

1960 Eighteen graduate programs and seventeen postgraduate programs in pedodontics exist.

1964 Crest becomes the first ADA-approved fluoridated toothpaste.

1974 The International Workshop on Fluorides and Dental Caries Reductions recommends that appropriate fluoride supplementation begin as soon after birth as possible. (This recommendation was later modified by authorities to start at 6 months of age.)

1981   February is designated National Children's Dental Health Month.

1983   A Consensus Development Conference held at the National Institutes of Dental Health endorses the effectiveness and usefulness of sealants.

1984   The American Academy of Pedodontics changes its name to the American Academy of Pediatric Dentistry.

1995   A new definition is adopted for the specialty of pediatric dentistry by the ADA's House of Delegates.

Pediatric dentistry is an age-defined specialty that provides both primary and comprehensive preventive and therapeutic oral health care for infants and children through adolescence, including those with special health care needs.

APPLICATION OF OTHER DISCIPLINES

Unquestionably, pediatric dentistry, as a body of knowledge and as a clinical discipline, has borrowed heavily from other aspects of dental schools' curricula and from breakthroughs in other specialty areas of dentistry. To be a complete clinician capable of handling the majority of needs of the children of any community, a dentist needs to know thoroughly preventive dentistry techniques, pulpal therapy, instrumentation and restoration of teeth, dental materials, oral surgery, preventive and interceptive orthodontics, and principles of prosthetics. In addition, to really be knowledgeable about the best needs of child patients, the dentist must know certain basics in pediatric medicine, general and oral pathology, and growth and development. A knowledge of nutrition and an understanding of both systemic and topical fluorides are essential in the development of appropriate prevention strategies for the child patient. Lastly, it is inconceivable that a person would be happy dedicating a significant amount of practice time to children without understanding their emotional and psychological needs as well as their processes of emotional change and social maturation. The child has to be managed differently than the adult and, in fact, the modes of management are extremely age-related.

Pediatric dentistry does in fact borrow a lot from other disciplines, but beyond this borrowing it is a discipline unto itself. The student who wishes to master intellectually and clinically the challenges that this age group presents must understand and be able to discern when simple transfers from one discipline can be made to the child patient and when transfers must be modified because of the age requirements or limitations that the child patient presents. The student must also understand that these requirements and limitations may vary from one age group to another.

CHALLENGES FOR PEDIATRIC DENTISTRY IN THE 21ST CENTURY

In the last two editions of this textbook this introductory chapter contained a section that addressed recent trends in dentistry for children. In the second edition, published in 1994, the following fifteen trends were highlighted:

- Preventive dentistry, including understanding the caries process as it relates to such factors as nutrition, sealants, water fluoridation, topical fluorides, fluoridated toothpastes, and home care
- Infant oral health
- Acid-etch techniques, sealants, and composite resins
- Dentistry for the disabled patient and other children with special needs
- Early orthodontic diagnosis and treatment
- More sophisticated modalities of pain and anxiety control such as sedation techniques
- Sophistication of radiographic techniques and machinery
- Expanding problem with fluorosis
- Eating disorders and their dental implications
- Smokeless tobacco use, particularly by adolescent boys
- Informed consent and risk management
- Infection control, barrier techniques, sterilization methods, and concerns about the transmission of disease from patient to clinician and from clinician to patient
- Early predisposing factors to temporomandibular joint problems in adolescents and adults
- Possible diminishing numbers of children who are generally and dreadfully afraid of dentists
- Abused and neglected children

None of these fifteen issues has gone away, but most are so much a part of the landscape of contemporary pediatric dentistry today that addressing them in this third edition as recent trends does not seem to be a substantive need. All of these themes are addressed in this textbook.

Six phenomena that will need to be addressed in the 21st century are deemed important enough to be reviewed in this introductory chapter. These are child abuse and neglect, the children of poverty, informed consent and risk management, technology, health care delivery strategies/payment strategies, and emergence of pediatric dentistry as a worldwide community.

Child Abuse and Neglect

Child abuse and child neglect are sick and ugly emotional aspects of the more general problem of family dysfunction in our society and are themes that since the 1960s have received increased attention from the legal and health science professions. By 1966, each of the 50 states had drafted legislation describing the responsibilities of professionals to report suspected abuse of children. The same laws that mandate dentists to report suspected abuse often also protect him or her from legal litigation, often brought by angry and vengeful innocent parents.

These laws also spell out the legal implications for the dentist who knowingly and willfully fails to report suspected child abuse. Although the laws vary from state to state, generally the dentist who fails to report such cases is considered guilty of a simple misdemeanor and is subject to a fine or jail sentence, usually 30 days in length. The law usually also makes the dentist civilly liable for any damages to the child caused by a failure to report abuse. In other words, litigation for damages can be conducted against the dentist for any further abuse received by the child.

If while performing an examination on a child something questionable like a bruise becomes apparent, the child should be interviewed for his or her analysis and explanation of the injury. Obviously, this approach is more effective for the older child. Next, after the examination is completed, the parents should be interviewed separately from the child to see whether the two stories correlate. If there is no correlation between the two accounts of the injury, the appropriate authorities should be informed.

Abuse can be documented because of the trauma caused by burning, slapping, hitting, choking, twisting, pulling, and pinching. Broken teeth, burns, lacerations, bruises, and broken bones alert the dentist that something may be wrong. Neglect, however, is more subtle. The dentist should look at overall hygiene as well as dental hygiene and adequate clothing. Suspicion of poor nutrition, apparent lack of medical care, and absence of previous dental care are situations that should alert the dentist to consider neglect. The dentist is responsible for taking the

same approach to neglect as to abuse; reporting of such cases is mandatory. The American Academy of Pediatric Dentistry defines dental neglect as failure of the parent or guardian to seek treatment for caries, oral infections, or oral pain or failure of the parent or guardian to follow through with treatment once he or she is informed that the aforementioned conditions exist.

Milestones in the American Recognition and Approach to Family Dysfunction and Other Cruelties to Children

19th century	House of refuge movement. This movement occurred in many major cities and enabled the state to place abandoned or neglected children somewhere safe.
1870s	Formation of the New York Society for the Prevention of Cruelty to Children. This was the first of many groups that worked in cooperation with the houses of refuge to rescue endangered children.
1899–1920	Establishment of juvenile courts. The first juvenile court was begun in Illinois in 1899. By 1920, all but three states had such courts.
1946	Medical discovery of child abuse. A paper by Caffey concludes that many long bone fractures in children could not be specifically documented as to their origin.
1957	Caffey asserts that injuries such as fractures in long bones of infants have often been deliberately inflicted.
1961	First conference is held on the battered child syndrome.
1962	Article on battered children (Kempe et al.) is published in the Journal of the American Medical Association. The concept of parental cruelty is made public. By this time, there is a movement toward doing something about this problem.
1966	All 50 states have passed laws describing the responsibilities of health science professionals in reporting suspected abuse.
1971	Fontana proposes a more global definition of the mistreatment of children. Neglect is now consid-

1974   A National Center on Child Abuse and Neglect is established by Congress to provide further leadership in improving the potential protection of children. Sexual abuse is added as a category of child abuse.

1976–1979   The number of cases of child abuse reported nationally rises 71% from 1976 to 1979, when 711,142 cases are reported (American Humane Association, 1981).

1995   The number of reported cases of child abuse continues to increase to approximately 1 million. Approximately 2000 children are estimated to die from child abuse cases each year.

1996   Nearly all states have child death review teams. Mental injury and passive exposure of children to illegal drugs are increasingly recognized as other forms of child abuse.

Children of Poverty

Even though there is delightful news about the success of dentistry in addressing the dental diseases of children and the fact that preventive dentistry is today a successful phenomenon for literally millions of children, students reading this book are urged to understand that this is not true for all children. Those children who come from the circumstances of poverty are at substantial risk for the ravages of dental decay despite all the preventive dentistry accomplishments of the last 30 years.

The children of poverty have always presented unique problems to the dental profession (Pinkham et al., 1988). First, certain forms of poverty make accessibility to dental care by poor patients difficult. Poverty also may predict a lack of knowledge about home care, prevention techniques, proper diet, and even when professional dental care should be started. The decay rates among the children of poverty are higher today than they are among more fortunate children. Unfortunately, the number of poor children continues to increase as the years go by.

The editors and contributors to this text hope that the dental profession, government agencies, and other advocacy groups for children in general and particularly children in special circumstances, such as poverty, will act responsibly to solve the growing need for a more vigorous and determined policy of health care, dental as well as medical, for these particular children.

Informed Consent and Risk Management

Informed consent is the legal issue that protects a patient's right not to be touched or in any way treated without the patient's authorization. The issue assumes that it is a right of a mentally competent adult human being to determine what, if anything, a practitioner of health sciences may do to his or her body.

There are two kinds of consent, expressed and implied. Implied consent is determined by the behavior of the patient. For instance, the patient got in the chair, opened his mouth, but said nothing. Expressed consent is written or oral. A signed written consent to treatment is the most substantial consent for protecting a dentist from litigation.

Informed consent also implies that the patient is aware of the nature of the treatment, alternatives to treatment, probable sequelae to treatment, and potential benefits and possible risks of any treatment. In other words, an "uninformed" patient is incapable of giving informed consent. A signature, if the patient is uninformed, is legally useless also.

The law assumes that minors cannot take the responsibility for giving informed consent. To avoid liability, the dentist must secure consent from the parent or the person acting *in loco parentis*. An exception to this would be the rendering of emergency care that preserves life or avoids severe compromise to the child's health when the parents cannot be located in the time available.

Obtaining informed consent can be a difficult problem for the dentist who treats children. It is not unusual for older children and adolescents to come to the dental office unaccompanied by a parent. In such cases, it is advised that only very safe, limited-risk procedures be performed.

Risk management is a broad term that describes the attitudes, processes, and techniques that a dentist and the staff can have and can do to minimize legal involvement in the circumstances that arise in the course of treating people. Obviously, in pediatric dentistry this management involves not only how the dentist and child interact but also, importantly, how the dentist and child's parents or guardians interact.

The practice of informed consent is basic to

The Evolving Present and Future of Pediatric Dentistry

H. Barry Waldman

Changing Environment and the Continued Need for Care

The overall number of children will continue to increase, and there will be demographic changes, increased numbers of special populations, and continued need for dental care.

- The next generation of children will increase by 8 million, but the number of white children will decrease while minority group children will increase (Table 1-1).
- Hispanic children, Asian American and Pacific Islander children, and immigrant children will become an increasing component of pediatric dental practices (Waldman, 1992, 1995a, 1995b).
- There are about 11 million special children (the developmentally disabled, the acutely ill, the hospitalized, and the high-risk) (Waldman, 1991).
- There are almost 20 million chronically ill children (Waldman, 1994a).
- The acquired immunodeficiency syndrome (AIDS) and drug epidemics continue to spread to children (Waldman, 1993, 1996a).
- Significant numbers of children live in single-parent families and in poverty (Waldman, 1996b).
- Although minority population children are in need of increased care (including the children of migrant farm workers), they neither receive optimal preventive care nor visit a dentist regularly (Gift and Newman, 1992; Waldman, 1994b) (Table 1-2).

TABLE 1–1. Changing Number of Children by 2020 (in Millions)

	1990	2010	2020	Percent Change 1990–2020
		<5 Years		
White	14.9	13.1	13.0	−12.8%
African American	2.8	2.8	2.9	3.5
Hispanic	2.3	2.9	3.2	39.1
Other	0.7	1.0	1.2	71.4
		5–17 Years		
White	36.5	35.3	34.7	−4.9%
African American	7.2	7.8	7.9	9.7
Hispanic	4.9	6.8	7.7	57.1
Other	1.9	2.7	3.0	57.8

From U.S. Bureau of the Census: Population projections for states, by age, sex, race and Hispanic origin: 1993-2020. Current Population Reports, Series P25-1111, 1994.

Production of Dentists

The overall dentist-to-population ratio continues to fall, and the number of pediatric dental program graduates will not be enough to maintain the current ratio of pediatric dentists in our country (Waldman, 1995c).

- There are now fewer pediatric dental programs but a gradual increase in enrollment has happened (Table 1–3). One in five trainees are foreign students, however, most of whom will not remain in this country for pediatric dental practice (American Academy of Pediatric Dentistry, 1996; American Dental Association, 1984, 1995, 1996a, 1996b).
- There is increasing interest in and numbers of applications for pediatric training programs (American Dental Association, 1996b; Waldman, 1995d).

TABLE 1–2. Results from the Third National Health and Nutrition Survey: 1988–91

Children Who Are NOT Caries-Free

	Primary Dentition 2–9 yrs	Permanent Dentition 5–17 yrs
Non-Hispanic white	34%	45%
African American	39	39
Mexican American	53	49

Decay Score Component of DMFS Age 5–17 yrs

Non-Hispanic white	14.6%
African American	37.9
Mexican American	36.4

Children with NO Sealants in Permanent Teeth Age 5–17 yrs

Non-Hispanic white	77%
African American	92
Mexican American	93

From Brown, IJ, Kaste LM, Selwitz RH, et al: Dental caries and sealant usage in U.S. children, 1988–1991. J Am Dental Assoc *127*:335–343, 1996.

TABLE 1–3. Number of Students Enrolled in First Year of Pediatric Dentistry Programs: 1983–1995

Year	First-Year Enrollment
1983	149
1985	157
1987	165
1989	168
1991	177
1993	173
1995	181

From American Dental Association, Council on Dental Education: Advanced Dental Education, 1984; American Dental Association, Survey Center: 1994/95 Survey of Predoctoral Educational Institutions, Trend Analysis, 1995; American Dental Association, Survey Center: 1995/96 Survey of Advanced Dental Education: Annual Report, 1996a; American Dental Association, Survey Center: 1995/96 Survey of Predoctoral Dental Education Institutions: Academic Programs, Enrollment and Graduates, 1996b.

A Changed Future?

The environment within which children are being raised is changing: single-parent families, mothers in the labor force with diverse arrangements for child care, continued poverty (more than one child in five), and increased incidents of child abuse and neglect (1 million cases per year) (Waldman, 1996b).

The system for the delivery of services is evolving. Health Maintenance Organizations (HMOs), Preferred Provider Organizations (PPOs), and capitation arrangements increasingly may be the future of pediatric dental practice. Will managed care (really, managed economics) change pediatric dentistry? Most assuredly! But increased numbers of children (particularly, special patient and minority population children) will require the services of pediatric dentists.

Box continued on following page

The Evolving Present and Future of Pediatric Dentistry *continued*

REFERENCES

American Academy of Pediatric Dentistry: Status of the specialty of pediatric dentistry—handout. AAPD Program Director's Symposium, Chicago, April 19–21, 1996.

American Dental Association, Council on Dental Education: Advanced Dental Education. Chicago, American Dental Association, 1984.

American Dental Association, Survey Center: 1994/95 Survey of Predoctoral Educational Institutions: Trend Analysis. Chicago, American Dental Association, 1995.

American Dental Association, Survey Center: 1995/96 Survey of Advanced Dental Education: Annual Report. Chicago, American Dental Association, 1996a.

American Dental Association, Survey Center: 1995/96 Survey of Predoctoral Dental Education Institutions: Academic Programs, Enrollment and Graduates, Vol 1. Chicago, American Dental Association, 1996b.

Brown LJ, Kaste LM, Selwitz RH, et al: Dental caries and sealant usage in U.S. children, 1988-1991. J Am Dent Assoc, *127:*335-343, 1996.

Gift HC, Newman JF: Oral health activities of U.S. children: Results of a national health interview survey. J Am Dent Assoc *123:*96-106, 1992.

U.S. Bureau of the Census: Population projections for states, by age, sex, race and Hispanic origin: 1993-2020. Current Population Reports, Series P25-1111. Washington, D.C., U.S. Government Printing Office, 1994.

Waldman HB: Almost eleven million special children. J Dent Child *58:*237-240, 1991.

Waldman HB: Hispanic children: An increasing reality in pediatric dental practice. J Dent Child *59:*221-224, 1992.

Waldman HB: Is your next pediatric patient an addict? J Dent Child *60:*136-139, 1993.

Waldman HB: Almost twenty million chronically ill children. J Dent Child *61:*129-133, 1994a.

Waldman HB: Invisible children: The children of migrant farm workers. J Dent Child *61:*218-221, 1994b.

Waldman HB: Asian American and Pacific Islander children: They will become an increasing reality in your practice. J Dent Child *62:*136-140, 1995a.

Waldman HB: Immigrant children and pediatric dental practice. J Dent Child *62:*288-294, 1995b.

Waldman HB: Planning for the children of your current pediatric dental patients. J Dent Child *62:*418-425, 1995c.

Waldman HB: Correction and update: Interest in pediatric dentistry. J Dent Child *62:*426-427, 1995d.

Waldman HB: Pediatric AIDS epidemic reflects the first half million AIDS cases in the U.S. J Dent Child *63:*89-94, 1996a.

Waldman HB: Mid-1990s profile of U.S. children and the conditions in which they live. J Dent Child *63:*285-290, 1996b.

risk management. Risk management involves issues other than those that are technically legal, however. It involves a satisfaction in communication between the clinician and the public, community, or people with whom he or she works. In the area of dentistry for children, risk management encourages open dialogue between the dentist and the people who bring children to the clinic.

Although much of risk management centers on actual treatment, in the area of pediatric dentistry behavioral management of the child and the perception of how the dentist appropriately or inappropriately reacts to the developing psyche of the child are important issues. These issues are addressed in Chapter 23.

Technology

The technologies already available and the technologies that are on the horizon will remain a constant challenge for dentists to learn in order to better be able to serve their patients. The 21st century promises new materials, changes in techniques, electronic records, further use of lasers, advanced x-ray machinery, and further use of computers. Even the World Wide Web has already affected dentistry.

Health Care Delivery Strategies/ Payment Strategies

This was not a theme in the first or second edition of this book; however, health care reform initiatives in the United States in recent years and the promise of continuing dialogue at the federal, state, and corporate levels on the issues of delivery and payment demand that a responsible education in pediatric dentistry today embrace these themes. Some of these are covered in Chapter 11.

Emergence of Pediatric Dentistry as a Worldwide Community

Children are a resource of the world. They are a promise of what our future is going to be. A healthy child is a better promise of a better world than an unhealthy child. Therefore, the dental health of any child is a concern to the world's dental community regardless of the child's nationality, ethnicity, and geographic location. Dentistry for children is now an international community with international initiatives, concerns, strategies, and cooperation.

REFERENCES

American Humane Association: National Analysis of Official Child Neglect and Abuse Reporting (1979). DHHS Publication No. (OHDS) 81-30232, revised 1981. Washington, D.C., U.S. Government Printing Office, 1981.

Caffey J: Multiple fractures in the long bones of infants suffering from chronic subdural hematoma. Am J Roentgenol 56:163, 1946.

Fontana V: The Maltreated Child: The Maltreatment Syndrome in Children. Springfield, IL, Charles C Thomas, 1971.

Kempe CH, Silverman EN, Steele BF, et al: The battered child syndrome. JAMA 181:17, 1962.

Pinkham JR, Casamassimo P, Levy S: Dentistry and the children of poverty. J Dent Child 55(1):17-23, 1988.

Chapter 2

Oral Pathologic Conditions and Soft Tissue Anomalies

Catherine M. Flaitz

The purpose of this chapter is to highlight selected oral lesions and soft tissue anomalies that occur in children. Because of the expansive nature of this topic, the more common oral diseases for this age group are emphasized. In addition, oral lesions associated with several genetic disorders and specific malignancies, which may mimic inflammatory conditions, are included to broaden the disease scope. The material is outlined in tabular form in order to make this comprehensive subject both practical and meaningful. The brief discussion for each of the lesions concisely summarizes the most important information that is relevant to pediatrics.

Each oral disease is described according to these key points: (1) the most common pediatric age group affected and the gender of children in whom the lesion is found, (2) the characteristic clinical and radiographic findings of the lesion, (3) the typical location of the lesion, (4) the pediatric significance of the lesion, (5) the treatment and prognosis of the lesion, and (6) a differential diagnosis that is relevant to this age group.

The tables are arranged according to related groups of oral lesions for the purpose of comparison. The sequential headings for each of the tables consist of the following disease categories:

- Developmental anomalies and variations of the soft tissues (Table 2-1, Fig. 2-1)
- Benign mucosal surface lesions (Table 2-2, Figs. 2-2 to 2-5)
  White lesions
  Pigmented lesions
  Red and ulcerated lesions
  Papillary lesions
- Benign exophytic submucosal lesions (Table 2-3, Fig. 2-6)
- Cysts and pseudocysts of soft tissues (Table 2-4, Fig. 2-7)
- Odontogenic cysts and neoplasms of bone (Table 2-5, Fig. 2-8)
- Benign nonodontogenic neoplasms and cysts of bone (Table 2-6, Fig. 2-9)
- Inflammatory lesions of bone (Table 2-7, Fig. 2-10)
- Malignancies of soft tissue and bone (Table 2-8)

TABLE 2–1. Developmental Anomalies and Variations of the Soft Tissues (Fig. 2–1)

Condition	Pediatric Age and Gender	Clinical Findings	Location	Pediatric Significance	Treatment and Prognosis	Differential Diagnosis
Fordyce granules	First and second decades No gender predilection	Small, yellow or white, multifocal papules; discrete or plaque-like; slightly elevated; asymptomatic	Bilateral, buccal and labial mucosa, retromolar pad and lip vermilion	60% occur under 10 years of age; there is an increase in size during puberty	No treatment necessary; may become hyperplastic	Focal keratosis Pseudomembranous candidiasis
Retrocuspid papilla	First and second decades Female predilection	Soft, pink, sessile nodule with smooth to stippled surface; usually bilateral	Lingual attached gingiva of mandibular canines	Occurs in 50% of children; regresses with age	No treatment necessary; normal anatomic structure	Traumatic fibroma Soft tissue abscess
Fissured tongue	First and second decades No gender predilection	Small furrows or grooves of varying depths on tongue; tender if inflamed	Dorsum of tongue	Polygenic or autosomal dominant trait; occurs in *Down's syndrome* and mouthbreathers; detected in 1% of children	Brush tongue daily to remove entrapped debris; may be source of halitosis	Benign migratory glossitis Lateral crenations of tongue Partial cleft tongue
Congenital labial and commissural pits	Present at birth No gender predilection	Localized depressions or fistulas; occasional mucus secretion; lip may be enlarged	Commissures of lips or mandibular vermilion; usually bilateral	Autosomal dominant trait; labial pits associated with cleft lip or palate	Surgical excision if a cosmetic problem or infection occurs	Draining mucocele Soft tissue abscess with sinus tract
Lingual thyroid	Second decade Female predilection	Nodular enlargement with a vascular or normal-appearing, smooth surface; may cause dysphagia, dysphonia or dyspnea	Midline, base of tongue; *thyroglossal tract cyst* is a variant that occurs in midline of neck	Most cases develop during puberty or pregnancy; normal thyroid tissue absent in majority of cases; hypothyroidism in 15–30%	Replacement thyroid hormone therapy or excision; neoplasias may arise in ectopic tissue	Hyperplastic lingual tonsil Hemangioma Lymphangioma Median rhomboid glossitis
Partial ankyloglossia (tongue-tie)	Present at birth No gender predilection	Short lingual frenum or anterior attachment of frenum to tip of tongue	Ventral tongue and floor of mouth	May interfere with speech and swallowing; may cause gingival recession	Infrequently, frenectomy is indicated	Complete ankyloglossia Bifed tongue

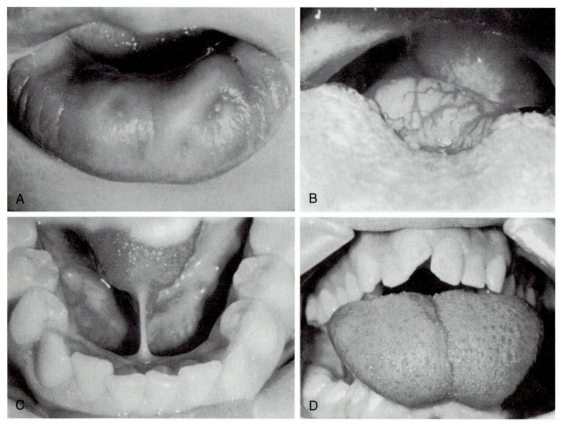

Figure 2–1. *A,* Congenital labial pits of the mandibular lip. *B,* Lingual thyroid of the posterior dorsal tongue (courtesy of Dr. G. E. Lilly, University of Iowa College of Dentistry). *C* and *D,* Partial ankyloglossia with lingual frenum attachment at the tip of the tongue *(C).* Note the restricted mobility of the tongue with extension *(D).*

TABLE 2–2. Benign Mucosal Surface Lesions

Lesion	Pediatric Age and Gender	Clinical Findings	Location	Pediatric Significance	Treatment and Prognosis	Differential Diagnosis
White Lesions (Fig. 2-2)						
Focal keratosis	First and second decades No gender predilection	Localized to diffuse, white, rough or shredded patches; does not rub off; asymptomatic	Mucosa prone to chronic irritation, especially buccal, labial mucosa, lateral tongue and gingiva	Common causes include orthodontic appliances, fractured teeth and chronic biting from factitial injury	Removal of local irritant; regresses if cause is eliminated	Leukoedema Linea alba Smokeless tobacco lesion White sponge nevus
Smokeless tobacco lesion	Second decade Male predilection	Localized or diffuse, translucent to opaque, white patches with wrinkled surface; intervening pink to red furrows; asymptomatic	Labial, buccal and vestibular mucosa; usually mandibular involvement	Lesions occur in 50% of chronic users; other problems include periodontal disease, elevation in blood pressure and dependence	Discontinuation of habit results in lesion reversal; biopsy necessary for persistent lesions; may undergo malignant transformation	Focal keratosis Leukoedema
Leukoedema	First and second decades No gender predilection	Diffuse, filmy white, wrinkled mucosa; bilateral; disappears when tissue is stretched; asymptomatic	Buccal, labial mucosa, and soft palate	More common in blacks; incidence increases with age; more pronounced in smokers	No treatment necessary; common variant of normal mucosa	Focal keratosis White sponge nevus Smokeless tobacco lesion
White sponge nevus	First and second decades No gender predilection	Diffuse, thickened, white patches with a wrinkled surface; spongy texture; asymptomatic	Widespread involvement: buccal, labial mucosa, floor of mouth and ventral tongue are most affected	Autosomal dominant trait; may be present at birth but reaches full expression during adolescence	No treatment necessary; benign condition	Leukoedema Focal keratosis Smokeless tobacco lesion
Pseudomembranous candidiasis (thrush)	First and second decades No gender predilection	Soft, creamy white plaques that wipe off, leaving a red, raw surface; burning sensation; other variants appear as red, thin patches or white adherent, rough plaques	Any mucosal site but most common on the buccal mucosa, tongue, and palate	Opportunistic infection; associated with antibiotics, diabetes, oral appliances, immunosuppresion, HIV and endocrine disease; may have diaper rash and nail involvement	Antifungal medication and proper oral hygiene; prognosis is good if reason for infection is eliminated or adequately monitored	Plaque Superficial bacterial infection Chemical burn Coated tongue

Table continued on following page

TABLE 2–2. Benign Mucosal Surface Lesions *Continued*

Lesion	Pediatric Age and Gender	Clinical Findings	Location	Pediatric Significance	Treatment and Prognosis	Differential Diagnosis
Linea alba	First and second decades No gender predilection	White smooth to shaggy line; bilateral, asymptomatic; may be scalloped	Buccal and labial mucosa adjacent to the plane of occlusion, most prominent in the molar region	May be associated with frictional irritation or sucking habit	No treatment is necessary; may spontaneously regress	Cheek-biting keratosis Leukoedema Scar formation
Benign migratory glossitis (geographic tongue)	First and second decades Female predilection	Multiple oval or circular red patches with a white, thickened border; loss of filiform papillae; pattern changes; may be tender	Dorsal and lateral borders of the tongue; may involve the ventral surface	Lesions on buccal, labial mucosa and palate are known as erythema migrans; increased incidence in atopic children	No treatment is necessary; periods of remission; may be irritated by acidic or spicy foods and beverages, toothpaste and oral rinses	Candidiasis Fissured tongue Median rhomboid glossitis Contact stomatitis
Scar formation (cicatrix)	First and second decades No gender predilection	Pale to white striae or patches with a smooth surface; cross-hatch or starburst pattern; asymptomatic	Labial, buccal mucosa, tongue, and vermilion border of lips	History of oral trauma or surgery; multiple scars may represent child abuse or self-mutilation	No treatment is necessary; significant scarring may restrict mobility of tongue and perioral opening	Focal keratosis Linea alba Fordyce granules
Pigmented Lesions (Fig. 2–3)						
Physiologic pigmentation	First and second decades No gender predilection	Diffuse gray, brown, or black patches; flat, smooth surface; symmetrical distribution; common in dark-complexioned children	Any location; attached gingiva is most common site	Antimalarial medications, oral contraceptives, minocycline, cigarette smoking and lead poisoning may cause diffuse oral pigmentation	No treatment is necessary; common variant of normal mucosa	Postinflammatory pigmentation Drug-induced pigmentation Smoker's melanosis Heavy metal pigmentation
Amalgam tattoo	First and second decades No gender predilection	Blue-gray, localized patch; irregular margins; smooth surface; radiographs may demonstrate opaque foci; asymptomatic	Gingiva, buccal and alveolar mucosa	History of amalgam restoration; graphite tattoo is usually observed on palate due to self-inflicted pencil wound	No treatment is necessary; permanent stain	Oral melanotic macule Late ecchymosis Nevus

Lesion	Age/Gender	Clinical Features	Location	Comments	Treatment	Differential Diagnosis
Oral melanotic macule (focal melanosis)	First and second decades Female predilection	Well delineated, single or multiple, flat macules; brown, black or blue in color; asymptomatic	Lips, gingiva, buccal mucosa, and palate	Most common oral pigmentation of fair-complexioned children; multiple lip macules associated with *Peutz-Jeghers syndrome*	No treatment necessary; excision if nevus cannot be excluded; no evidence of malignant transformation	Amalgam/graphite tattoo Nevus Late ecchymosis
Nevus	Second decade Female predilection	Well delineated, elevated nodule; brown, black or blue in color; some lesions are flat; asymptomatic; uncommon intraorally	Hard palate, buccal mucosa, lip, and gingiva	Congenital or acquired lesion; average 20 nevi on body; excision of oral nevus due to chronic irritation to mucosa	Excision because of potential for malignant transformation; recurrence is uncommon	Oral melanotic macule Amalgam/graphite tattoo Late ecchymosis
Petechiae, ecchymosis and hematoma	First and second decades No gender predilection	Localized to diffuse, flat to slightly elevated macules or masses; fluctuant to firm; early lesions are red; late lesions are blue-black; may be tender	Buccal mucosa, lips, lateral tongue and soft palate	Multiple lesions may be due to child abuse or bleeding disorder; palatal lesions caused by coughing, vomiting, fellatio, measles, and infectious mononucleosis	No treatment necessary; resolution of lesion within 7–14 days; may need to evaluate for systemic disease	Amalgam/graphite tattoo Oral melanotic macule Nevus Hemangioma Blood dyscrasia
Red and Ulcerated Lesions (Fig. 2–4)						
Traumatic ulcer and erosion	First and second decades No gender predilection	Usually solitary lesion; variable shape with irregular margins; shallow or deep; red or yellow pseudomembranous surface; painful	Lateral tongue, buccal mucosa, lips, palate; *Riga-Fede disease* occurs in infants on ventral tongue from rubbing against lower incisors	Most common oral ulcer; may indicate child abuse, neurologic impairment or factitial injuries when history of chronic or recurrent lesions	Symptomatic relief; removal of cause if present; heals within days or weeks; factitial lesions are a diagnostic and management problem; may cause scarring	Aphthous ulcer Secondary herpetic ulcer Contact stomatitis Mucosal burn

Table continued on following page

TABLE 2–2. Benign Mucosal Surface Lesions *Continued*

Lesion	Pediatric Age and Gender	Clinical Findings	Location	Pediatric Significance	Treatment and Prognosis	Differential Diagnosis
Aphthous ulcer	First and second decade. Female predilection	Recurrent, painful ulcers. **Minor form:** solitary, superficial oval ulcer; ≤1 cm in size; resolves in 7–10 days. **Major form:** multiple, crateriform ulcers; ≥1 cm in size; resolves in 3–6 weeks. **Herpetiform:** uncommon	All areas except attached gingiva, hard palate, and vermilion of lips; usually involves the nonkeratinized mucosa	Occurs in one third of children; unknown cause but probable immune defect; other factors include trauma, stress, allergies, nutritional deficiencies, hematologic abnormalities and hormonal changes; genetic predisposition	Symptomatic relief; topical and systemic steroids, topical amlexanox, and antimicrobial oral rinses, such as tetracycline and chlorhexidine gluconate 0.12%, may be effective; **Major form** heals with scarring	Traumatic ulcer. Secondary herpetic ulcer. Crohn's disease. Behçet's syndrome. Celiac disease. Neutropenic ulcer
Secondary herpetic ulcer	First and second decades. No gender predilection	Multiple, recurrent, small ulcers preceded by vesicles; clustered pattern; prodromal tingling or burning sensation; heals within 7–14 days	Vermilion of lips, hard palate, attached gingiva, perioral region; *Herpetic whitlow* on fingers, especially with digit sucking habit	Infectious disease due to reactivation of herpes simplex virus; triggering factors include sunburn, fever, stress, trauma and menses; occurs in one third of children	Symptomatic relief; sunscreen on lips; acyclovir for immuno-compromised children or with multiple recurrences; variable frequency of recurrence	Aphthous ulcer. Traumatic ulcer. Contact stomatitis. Angular cheilitis. Impetigo
Angular cheilitis	First and second decades. No gender predilection	Deep fissures that bleed and ulcerate; develop superficial exudative crust; dryness and burning sensation	Commissures of the mouth	Occurs with mouthbreathing, chronic licking of lips and with concurrent oral candidal infection; causative microorganisms include *Candida* species and staphylococci	Lubrication of lips; antifungal or antibiotic ointment for persistent lesions; tendency to recur; may result in scarring; recurrent lesions may require intraoral antifungal treatment	Secondary herpetic ulcer. Impetigo. Exfoliative cheilitis

Condition	Age/Gender	Clinical appearance	Location	Cause/Comments	Treatment	Differential diagnosis
Contact stomatitis	First and second decades; No gender predilection	Localized or diffuse areas of erythema, vesicles and ulcerations; associated with burning sensation and pain	Any mucosal or cutaneous site in contact with the causative allergen	Wide variety of causative allergens including food and cosmetic products, dental materials, oral hygiene products, and topical medications	Identification and elimination of allergen; patch testing may be helpful; topical steroids may reduce symptoms; lesions recur with re-exposure to allergen	Chemical/thermal burn; Aphthous ulcer; Secondary herpetic ulcers; Erythema multiforme
Erythema multiforme	Second decade; Male predilection	Widespread, red macules, vesicles, bullae and ulcers; acute onset; target lesions on skin; painful	**Oral:** lips, tongue, palate, buccal mucosa, and gingiva **Skin:** extremities, head and neck	Common precipitating factors include HSV and medications; severe variant is *Stevens-Johnson syndrome*	Identification and withdrawal of the medication; recurrences are common if triggered by HSV	Primary herpetic gingivostomatitis; Contact stomatitis; Major aphthae; Acute necrotizing ulcerative gingivitis
Primary herpetic gingivostomatitis	Usually first decade; No gender predilection	Fever, irritability, pain, lymphadenopathy, drooling, halitosis, multiple vesicles and ulcers, diffuse redness and swelling	Widespread oral and perioral involvement; gingival lesions are usually the chief complaint	Self-limiting infectious disease caused by HSV; high fever and dehydration are serious complications in children	Supportive care includes antipyretics, analgesics, palliative oral rinses, force fluids; acyclovir may be indicated; resolves in 7–10 days	Acute necrotizing ulcerative gingivitis; Erythema multiforme; Contact stomatitis
Median rhomboid glossitis	First and second decades; Male predilection	Flat or elevated, red patch; oval or diamond shape; may burn; occasionally is ulcerated	Anterior to circumvallate papillae; midline dorsum tongue; "kissing" lesion may be present on the palate	Cause is controversial; most lesions are acquired and associated with a chronic candidal infection	Antifungal treatment is usually effective	Benign migratory glossitis; Contact stomatitis; Mucosal burn; Lingual thyroid
Papillary Lesions (Fig. 2-5)						
Squamous papilloma	First and second decades; No gender predilection	Pedunculated exophytic enlargement; cauliflower or finger-like surface projections; pink to white in color; solitary lesion; soft; asymptomatic	Any oral site but palate and tongue are the most common	Most common papillary lesion of the oral mucosa; caused by the human papillomavirus	Excisional biopsy; recurrences are uncommon	Verruca vulgaris; Giant cell fibroma

Table continued on following page

TABLE 2–2. Benign Mucosal Surface Lesions *Continued*

Lesion	Pediatric Age and Gender	Clinical Findings	Location	Pediatric Significance	Treatment and Prognosis	Differential Diagnosis
Verruca vulgaris (common wart)	First and second decades No gender predilection	Similar to squamous papilloma; usually multiple, sessile lesion with white, rough surface and finger-like projections; asymptomatic	Vermilion border, labial mucosa, and tongue are common oral sites; perioral region, hands, and fingers are common skin sites	Caused by the human papillomavirus; autoinoculation from sucking on fingers and nailbiting	Excisional biopsy of oral warts; may spontaneously resolve; recurrences are common	Squamous papilloma Condyloma acuminatum Giant cell fibroma
Condyloma acuminatum (venereal wart)	Second decade No gender predilection	Sessile mass with blunted surface projections; early lesions may be flat with stippled surface; multiple, pink, soft, coalescing clusters; painless	Tongue, labial mucosa, and soft palate are the most common sites	Sexually transmitted disease; most commonly found in the anogenital region; caused by human papillomavirus; may indicate child abuse	Excisional biopsy, laser ablation; sexual partners must be treated; recurrences are common; anogenital warts may be premalignant	Focal epithelial hyperplasia Verruca vulgaris Papillary hyperplasia
Giant cell fibroma	Second decade Female predilection	Pedunculated or sessile, solitary, firm nodule with a pebbly, pale surface; slow growing; asymptomatic	Gingiva, tongue, and palate	Reactive hyperplastic lesion; not caused by the human papillomavirus	Excisional biopsy, recurrence is uncommon if the source of irritation is eliminated	Squamous papilloma Retrocuspid papilla
Papillary hyperplasia	Second decade No gender predilection	Multiple aggregates of papular or nodular enlargements; pale to red, granular surface; cobblestone appearance; usually asymptomatic	Hard palate	Caused by continual wear of palatal coverage appliance, such as orthodontic appliances; other factors include narrow palatal vault and mouth breathing; candidal infection is common	Reline or reconstruction of maxillary appliance; topical antifungal treatment; excision of persistent lesions	Condyloma acuminata Focal epithelial hyperplasia

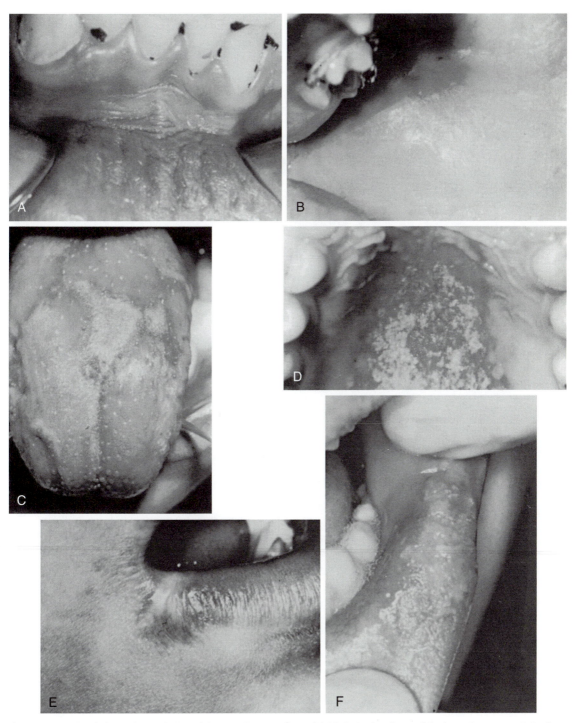

Figure 2–2. *A,* Smokeless tobacco lesion of the anterior mucobuccal fold. *B,* Leukoedema of the buccal mucosa. *C,* Benign migratory glossitis of the dorsal and lateral tongue. *D,* Pseudomembranous candidiasis of the hard palate. *E,* Scar formation of the mandibular lip resulting from a previous electrical burn. *F,* Focal keratosis of the mandibular labial mucosa from a chronic lip-biting habit.

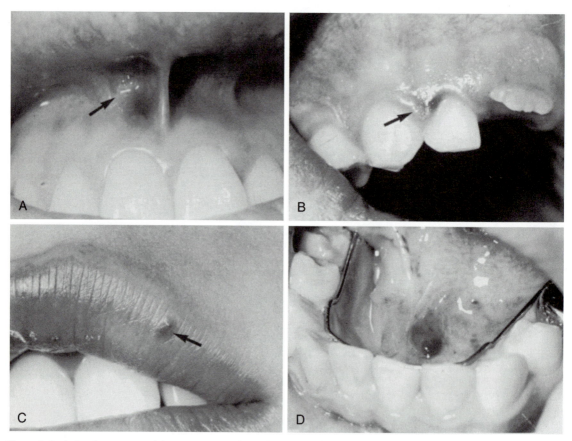

Figure 2–3. *A,* Amalgam tattoo of the anterior mucobuccal fold *(arrow). B,* Oral melanotic macule of the gingiva *(arrow). C,* Pigmented nevus of the maxillary lip *(arrow). D,* Petechiae and ecchymoses of the floor of the mouth resulting from forceful suctioning during a dental procedure.

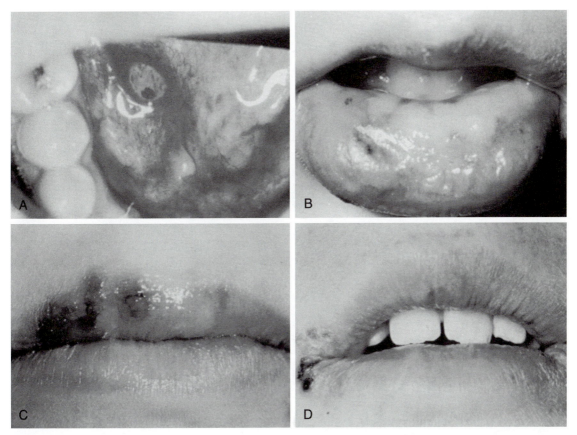

Figure 2–4. *A,* Aphthous ulcer of the floor of the mouth. *B,* Traumatic ulcer of the mandibular lip as a result of macerating the tissues after a bilateral local anesthetic injection. *C,* Recurrent herpes labialis of the maxillary lip. *D,* Angular cheilitis involving the commissure of the lips.

Illustration continued on following page

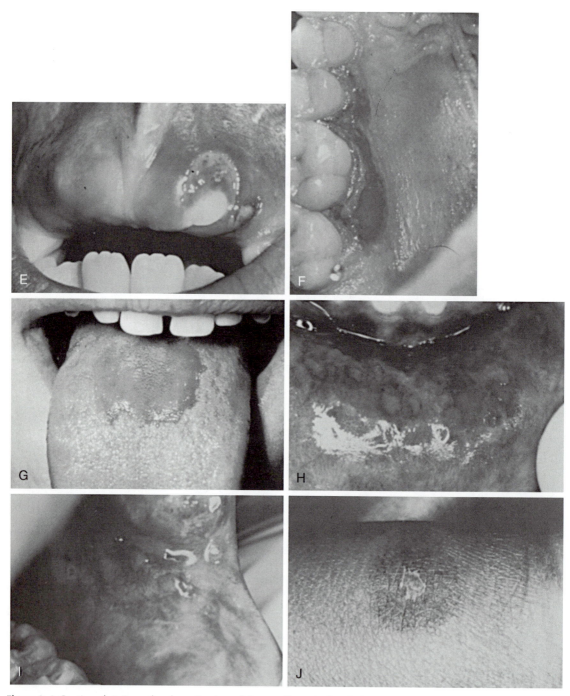

Figure 2–4 *Continued. E,* Secondary herpetic ulcer of the maxillary gingiva. *F,* Traumatic erosion of the palatal mucosa due to a thermal burn from a pizza. *G,* Median rhomboid glossitis of the dorsal tongue. *H, I,* and *J,* Erythema multiforme of the labial mucosa *(H)* and buccal mucosa *(I)* and a resolving target lesion of the skin *(J).* Widespread lesions developed after penicillin therapy for acute pericoronitis.

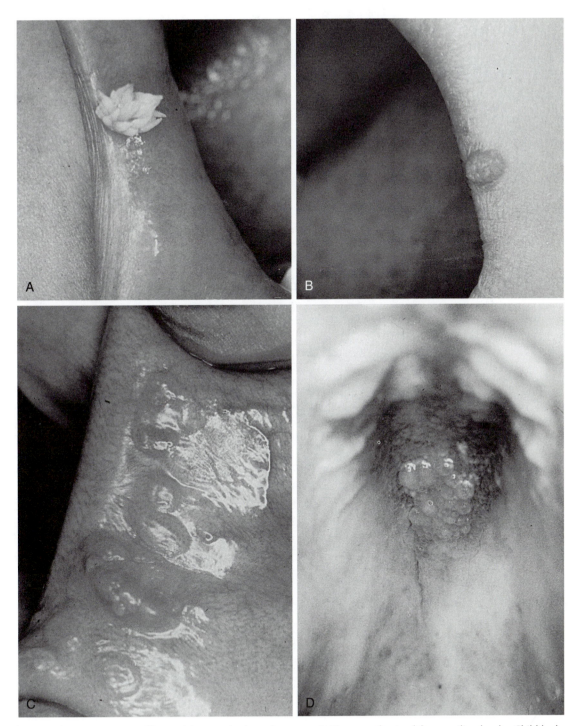

Figure 2–5. *A,* Squamous papilloma of the anterior buccal mucosa. *B,* Verruca vulgaris of the vermilion border. Child had multiple cutaneous warts on the hands. *C,* Condyloma acuminata of the buccal and labial mucosa. The child's mother had a history of venereal warts at the time of delivery. *D,* Papillary hyperplasia in a mentally handicapped teenager with a constricted palatal vault.

TABLE 2–3. Benign Exophytic Submucosal Lesions (Fig. 2–6)

Lesion	Pediatric Age and Gender	Clinical Findings	Location	Pediatric Significance	Treatment and Prognosis	Differential Diagnosis
Pyogenic granuloma	Second decade Female predilection	Localized, pedunculated or sessile nodule with a smooth, granular or ulcerated surface; red in color; bleeds freely; soft and friable; nontender	Gingiva, lips, tongue, and buccal mucosa	Reactive hyperplastic lesion due to chronic irritation; hormonal changes during puberty and pregnancy are aggravating factors	Excisional biopsy and remove source of irritation; recurs, if cause is not eliminated	Soft tissue abscess Ulcerated fibroma Peripheral giant cell granuloma Peripheral ossifying fibroma Hemangioma
Soft tissue abscess (parulis)	First and second decades No gender predilection	Localized or diffuse enlargement, with smooth, red to yellow surface; expression of purulent exudate; soft or fluctuant; sinus tract may be present; tender	Gingiva and alveolar mucosa are the most common sites	Caused by pulpal and periodontal disease or the entrapment of a foreign body; may progress rapidly to *cellulitis*; *pericoronitis* associated with erupting molars	Eliminate source of infection; may require antibiotic coverage; cyclic recurrence pattern with drainage if not properly managed	Pyogenic granuloma Retrocuspid papilla Eruption cyst Lymphoepithelial cyst
Traumatic fibroma (fibrous hyperplasia)	First and second decades No gender predilection	Localized, pedunculated or sessile nodule; pale, smooth surface; firm; limited growth potential; asymptomatic	Buccal and labial mucosa, lateral border of tongue and gingiva	Most common tumor-like lesion of the oral cavity; represents hyperplastic scar tissue	Excisional biopsy; may recur if trauma to the tissues continues	Peripheral ossifying fibroma Traumatic neuroma Giant cell fibroma Fibrosed mucocele
Peripheral ossifying fibroma	Second decade; peak incidence is 13 years old Female predilection	Localized, firm, pedunculated or sessile nodule; pale, smooth to bosselated surface; may be ulcerated; may cause erosion of alveolar bone; asymptomatic	Gingiva, anterior to first permanent molars; usually involves the interdental papilla; arises from periosteum or periodontal ligament	Reactive hyperplastic lesion; may result in delayed eruption and displacement of teeth	Excisional biopsy and removal of local irritants; recurrence rate of 16%	Pyogenic granuloma Peripheral giant cell granuloma Traumatic fibroma

Lesion	Age/Gender	Clinical Features	Location	Comments	Treatment	Differential Diagnosis
Peripheral giant cell granuloma	First and second decades; Female predilection	Localized, sessile nodule with a smooth, red to purple surface; may be ulcerated; firm; may resorb alveolar bone; asymptomatic	Gingiva, anterior to first permanent molars; arises from periosteum or periodontal ligament	Reactive hyperplastic lesion; may result in delayed eruption and displacement of teeth	Excisional biopsy and removal of local irritants; recurrence rate is 10%	Pyogenic granuloma / Peripheral ossifying fibroma / Hemangioma
Gingival fibromatosis	First and second decades; No gender predilection	Generalized firm nodular enlargements with pink to red and inflamed, smooth to stippled surfaces; affects both dentitions	Attached gingiva and alveolar mucosa	Autosomal dominant inheritance pattern; may be idiopathic; problem with delayed eruption and displacement of teeth; may be syndrome-related	Periodic gingivectomy and good oral hygiene; recurrences are common	Drug-induced gingival hyperplasia / Hormonal-induced gingival hyperplasia / Mouth breathing gingivitis / Leukemic gingival infiltrates
Hemangioma	First decade; majority detected within the first year of life; Female predilection	Localized to diffuse, red to blue lesion; may be flat, nodular or bosselated; soft and compressible; blanches; may bleed freely; 16% are multiple	Lips, tongue and buccal mucosa are the most common sites; rarely occurs in the jaws	May result in macroglossia or macrocheilia; hemorrhage from trauma is a common complication	Surgical excision, laser ablation, embolization, sclerosing agents, systemic steroids and cryotherapy; many undergo spontaneous involution; does not recur with adequate removal	Vascular malformation / Lymphangioma / Pyogenic granuloma / Peripheral giant cell granuloma / Hematoma / Mucocele or ranula
Lymphangioma	First decade; majority detected by the second year of life; No gender predilection	Localized to diffuse, red-blue to translucent enlargement with a smooth to clustered, vesicular surface; compressible and spongy; crepitus when palpated; may be multiple	Tongue, lip, buccal mucosa, floor of mouth and neck	May result in macroglossia and macrocheilia; neck lesions are called *cystic hygroma*, which may cause respiratory distress; may enlarge during upper respiratory infection, menses, or trauma	No treatment for small lesions; excision of large ones; spontaneous regression is rare; recurrences are common; may cause airway obstruction	Hemangioma / Mucocele / Plunging ranula / Cellulitis

Table continued on following page

TABLE 2–3. Benign Exophytic Submucosal Lesions *Continued*

Lesion	Pediatric Age and Gender	Clinical Findings	Location	Pediatric Significance	Treatment and Prognosis	Differential Diagnosis
Neurofibroma	Second decade No gender predilection	Localized to diffuse, solitary or multiple enlargements; nodular to pendulous shape; smooth surface; soft to firm consistency; asymptomatic	Tongue, buccal mucosa, vestibule and palate	Neurofibromatosis is autosomal dominant condition characterized by plexiform neurofibromas, café-au-lait macules, axillary freckling and other abnormalities; oral lesions in 25% of patients	Excisional biopsy, if solitary lesion. For syndrome-associated lesions, no treatment is necessary, unless a cosmetic concern or symptomatic; malignant transformation rate of 5–15% for syndrome lesions	Schwannoma Mucosal neuromas Traumatic fibroma Other benign mesenchymal and salivary gland neoplasms
Congenital epulis (gingival granular cell tumor of newborn)	Present at birth Female predilection; 90% occur in females	Localized, pedunculated to sessile, spongy nodule; smooth surface but may be ulcerated; pink to red in color	Anterior gingiva; usually maxillary; 10% are multiple	May cause feeding or respiratory problems; usually stops growing after birth	Excisional biopsy; occasional spontaneous regression; no recurrence	Pyogenic granuloma Hemangioma Neonatal alveolar lymphangioma Neuroectodermal tumor of infancy
Pleomorphic adenoma (mixed tumor)	Second decade Slight female predilection	Well circumscribed, dome-shaped enlargement with smooth pink surface; firm; slow-growing; asymptomatic, unless traumatized	**Intraoral site:** most occur in the hard or soft palate **Extraoral site:** parotid gland	Most common benign salivary gland neoplasm; mucoepidermoid carcinoma is second most common type and mimics this benign tumor	Excisional biopsy with tumor-free margins; recurrences are not uncommon; malignant transformation rate of 5% for long-term lesions	Mucoepidermoid carcinoma Neurofibroma Schwannoma Traumatic fibroma Palatal space abscess

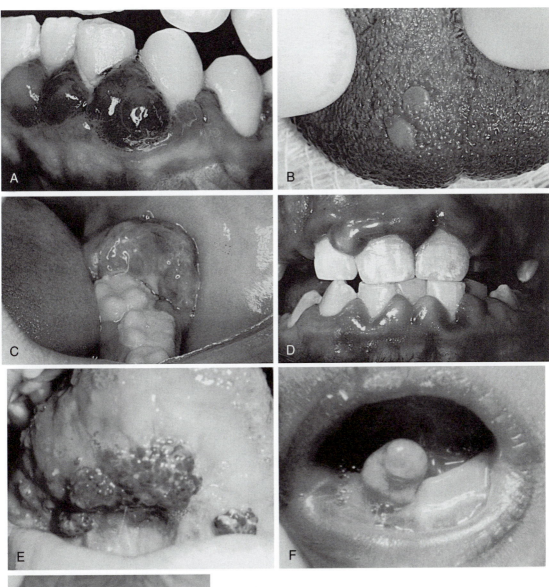

Figure 2–6. *A,* Multiple pyogenic granulomas of the mandibular gingiva in a teenager with poor oral hygiene. *B,* Traumatic fibromas of the dorsal tongue due to irritation from a palatal appliance to correct a thumb-sucking habit. *C,* Peripheral ossifying fibroma of the posterior mandibular gingiva. Note the lingual displacement of the second molar. *D,* Hereditary gingival fibromatosis in a mixed dentition. Father and a sibling demonstrated a similar pattern of gingival enlargement. *E,* Lymphangioma of the ventral tongue. *F,* Congenital epulis (congenital gingival granular cell tumor) of the mandibular alveolar ridge. *G,* Pleomorphic adenoma (mixed tumor) of the posterior hard palate.

TABLE 2-4. Cysts and Pseudocysts of Soft Tissues (Fig. 2–7)

Lesion	Pediatric Age and Gender	Clinical Findings	Location	Pediatric Significance	Treatment and Prognosis	Differential Diagnosis
Palatal and dental lamina cysts of newborn	Present at birth or neonatal period No gender predilection	Solitary or multiple, discrete papules and nodules with smooth translucent to white surface; firm; usually 1–3 mm in size; asymptomatic	**Dental lamina cysts:** alveolar ridge **Epstein's pearls:** median palatal raphe **Bohn's nodules:** lateral hard and soft palate	Found in 75% of neonates	No treatment necessary; usually slough within the first 3 months	Natal/neonatal teeth Soft tissue abscess Lymphoepithelial cyst Eruption cyst
Lymphoepithelial cyst	Second decade No gender predilection	Solitary, doughy, well-circumscribed nodule; yellow-white smooth surface with superficial vascular pattern; may enlarge and drain	Posterior lateral and ventral tongue, soft palate, tonsillar pillars and floor of mouth	Tender if irritated; related to oral lymphoid aggregates	Excisional biopsy; does not recur	Epidermoid cyst Lipoma Soft tissue abscess
Eruption cyst and hematoma	First decade No gender predilection	Localized, dome-shaped, fluctuant enlargement; translucent to bluish in color; overlying an erupting tooth; usually asymptomatic	Alveolar mucosa	May occur in either dentition; tender if inflamed; infrequently delays eruption of tooth; minimal bleeding may occur at the site	No treatment necessary; uncover tooth if symptomatic; important to exclude a hemangioma before any surgery	Hematoma Hemangioma Neonatal alveolar lymphangioma
Mucocele (mucus retention phenomenon) and ranula	First and second decades No gender predilection	Localized, compressible, fluid-filled nodule with smooth, translucent to blue surface; fluctuates in size; may be tender; periodically drains	*Mucocele* occurs in the lower labial mucosa, buccal mucosa and ventral tongue *Ranula* occurs in floor of mouth and usually involves the sublingual gland	Most common lip swelling in children; some are associated with history of trauma	Excisional biopsy with removal of adjacent lobules of minor salivary glands; marsupialization is treatment for ranula; recurrences are common with incomplete excision	Hemangioma Lymphangioma Mucoepidermoid carcinoma, low-grade

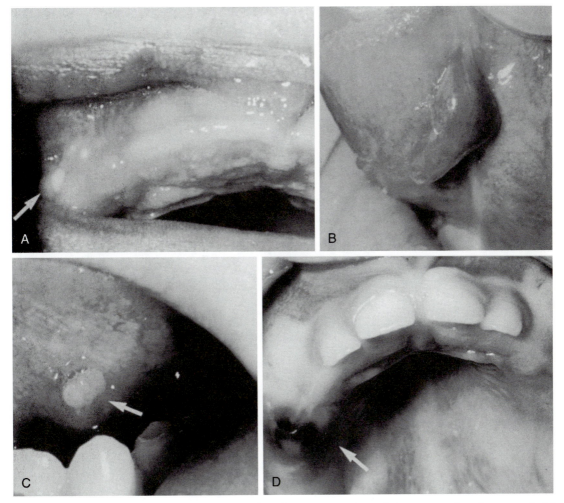

Figure 2–7. *A,* Dental lamina cyst of the maxillary alveolar ridge *(arrow). B,* Mucocele (mucus retention phenomenon) of the ventral tongue. *C,* Irritated lymphoepithelial cyst of the ventral tongue. *D,* Eruption cyst of the maxillary alveolar ridge *(arrow).*

TABLE 2–5. Odontogenic Cysts and Neoplasms of Bone (Fig. 2–8)

Lesion	Pediatric Age and Gender	Clinical and Radiographic Findings	Location	Pediatric Significance	Treatment and Prognosis	Differential Diagnosis
Dentigerous cyst	Second decade Slight male predilection	Well-defined, unilocular, radiolucency around the crown of unerupted tooth; may displace teeth; causes cortical expansion and root resorption; asymptomatic unless infected	Mandibular and maxillary third molar and canine regions	Most common intrabony cyst of jaws in children; growth may be rapid in this age group; may involve primary or supernumerary teeth	Enucleation; marsupialization if extensive; recurrence is uncommon; ameloblastomas and carcinomas rarely develop from the epithelial lining	Hyperplastic dental follicle Periapical cyst Ameloblastic fibroma Unicystic ameloblastoma Paradental cyst
Odontogenic keratocyst	Second decade Male predilection	Well-defined, unilocular or multilocular radiolucency with thin sclerotic margins; expansile; 40% associated with unerupted tooth; may cause resorption and displacement of teeth; may be painful	Posterior body and ramus of mandible; maxillary third molar region and canine region	Multiple lesions in children are consistent with *nevoid-basal cell carcinoma syndrome* and includes jaw cysts, basal cell carcinomas, palmar-plantar pits, bifed ribs, and falx cerebri	Surgical excision with osseous curettage or resection; aggressive cyst with high recurrence rate of 30%; neoplastic changes are uncommon	Dentigerous cyst Ameloblastic fibroma Odontogenic myxoma Ameloblastoma Central hemangioma Central giant cell granuloma
Calcifying odontogenic cyst (Gorlin's cyst)	Second decade No gender predilection	Well-defined, unilocular or multilocular radiolucency with variably sized opacifications; expansile; 50% associated with unerupted teeth; asymptomatic	Most develop in the incisor-canine region of the maxilla and mandible; may occur as a soft tissue lesion on the gingiva	May be associated with an odontoma in this age group	Enucleation; minimal risk of recurrence; rarely manifests an aggressive or malignant behavior	Complex odontoma Adenomatoid odontogenic tumor Ameloblastic fibro-odontoma Calcifying epithelial odontogenic tumor
Adenomatoid odontogenic tumor	Second decade; median age is 16 years old Female predilection	Well-defined, unilocular radiolucency with small opaque foci; expansile; majority associated with an unerupted tooth; may cause root divergence; asymptomatic	Anterior maxilla is most common site, especially canine region	Most lesions occur between 10 and 20 years of age; behavior is very benign; occasionally occurs as a soft tissue lesion of the gingiva	Enucleation; does not recur	Dentigerous cyst Calcifying odontogenic cyst Complex odontoma Calcifying epithelial odontogenic tumor

Lesion	Age/Gender	Radiographic Features	Location	Clinical Features	Treatment	Differential Diagnosis
Odontoma, compound and complex	First and second decades; most occur between the ages of 5 and 20 years **Compound type:** No gender predilection **Complex type:** Female predilection	Well-defined, radiopaque and radiolucent lesion, mild expansion; develop in pericoronal or radicular areas; may delay tooth eruption. **Compound type** resembles miniature teeth; **Complex type** has an amorphous opaque pattern	**Compound type:** anterior maxilla **Complex type:** posterior mandible	Most common odontogenic neoplasm; frequent cause of isolated delayed tooth eruption	Enucleation; recurrences are rare	Eruption sequestrum Ameloblastic fibro-odontoma Cementoblastoma Calcifying odontogenic cyst Adenomatoid odontogenic tumor
Ameloblastic fibroma and ameloblastic fibro-odontoma	First and second decades **Ameloblastic fibroma:** No gender predilection **Ameloblastic fibro-odontoma:** Male predilection	Well-defined, unilocular or multilocular lesion with sclerotic margins; often associated with an unerupted tooth. **Ameloblastic fibroma** is radiolucent; **Ameloblastic fibro-odontoma** is radiolucent and opaque	Mandibular molar and premolar regions	Most occur under the age of 20; rare malignant counterpart is the *ameloblastic fibrosarcoma,* which may arise de novo or from pre-existing or recurrent ameloblastic fibroma	**Ameloblastic fibroma:** Surgical excision; recurrences are common (18%); long-term follow-up is recommended **Ameloblastic fibro-odontoma:** Enucleation; recurrences are uncommon	**Ameloblastic fibroma:** Dentigerous cyst Odontogenic myxoma Central giant cell granuloma **Ameloblastic fibro-odontoma:** Developing odontoma Calcifying odontogenic cyst
Ameloblastoma	Second decade No gender predilection	Well-defined, unilocular or multilocular radiolucency with sclerotic margins; cortical perforation; expansile; slow-growing; root displacement and resorption; usually asymptomatic	Mandibular molar and ramus areas	*Unicystic ameloblastoma* is the most common variant in children and is the least aggressive; treatment is enucleation for this variant; recurrence rate of 15%	Excision with adequate osseous margins to block resection; 50–90% recur with simple curettage; rarely undergoes malignant transformation	Dentigerous cyst Odontogenic keratocyst Odontogenic myxoma Central giant cell granuloma Central hemangioma

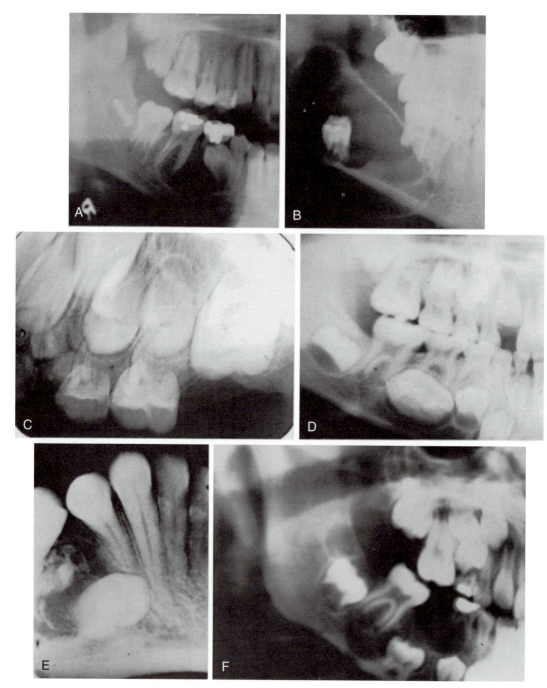

Figure 2–8. *A,* Dentigerous cyst of the posterior mandible. *B,* Ameloblastoma of the posterior mandible. *C,* Compound odontoma of the anterior maxilla. *D,* Complex odontoma of the posterior mandible. The second premolar was not present in this quadrant. *E,* Calcifying odontogenic cyst with displacement of the unerupted premolar. *F,* Ameloblastic fibroma of the posterior mandible.

TABLE 2–6. Benign Nonodontogenic Neoplasms and Cysts of Bone (Fig. 2–9)

Lesion	Pediatric Age and Gender	Clinical and Radiographic Findings	Location	Pediatric Significance	Treatment and Prognosis	Differential Diagnosis
Melanotic neuroectodermal tumor of infancy	Infancy, usually under 6 months of age No gender predilection	Rapidly expanding, bony enlargement; may exhibit blue or black pigmented surface; may be ulcerated; ill-defined radiolucency with displacement of tooth buds; floating tooth appearance	Anterior maxilla	Lesion mimics a malignancy with destructive, rapid growth rate; dental abnormalities secondary to surgical manipulation may be observed	Excisional biopsy with vigorous bony curettage; low recurrence rate; rare cases of metastasis	Neuroblastoma Rhabdomyosarcoma Langerhans cell disease Large eruption cyst
Central giant cell granuloma	Second decade Female predilection	Well defined, multilocular radiolucency with scalloped border; occasionally unilocular; expansile; displacement of teeth; root resorption is uncommon; asymptomatic	Most frequently in mandible; anterior to first molar; may cross midline	Most common, anteriorly located, multilocular, expansile radiolucency; 60% occur under the age of 20; need to rule out hyperpara-thyroidism	Surgical excision with aggressive curettage; recurrence rate as high as 13%	Odontogenic keratocyst Odontogenic myxoma Central hemangioma Aneurysmal bone cyst Ameloblastoma
Cherubism	First decade; usually obvious by 5 years of age Male predilection	Chubby face appearance; bilateral, symmetrical, painless enlargement of jaws; extensive, multiple, well defined, multilocular radiolucencies	Maxilla and mandible; in particular, the angles of mandible; all four quadrants frequently involved	Autosomal dominant inheritance; causes premature exfoliation of primary teeth; displacement of tooth buds, severe malocclusion and malformed teeth	No treatment necessary; spontaneous regression with onset of puberty; surgical recontouring may improve function and cosmetics	Nevoid basal cell carcinoma syndrome Infantile cortical hyperostosis Hyperparathyroidism
Osteoma	Second decade Male predilection	Usually solitary, well-defined, spherical radiopacity; may be expansile, resulting in marked asymmetry; slow-growing; asymptomatic	Maxilla and mandible; endosteal or periosteal presentation	Gardner's syndrome, an autosomal dominant condition, characterized by multiple osteomas, intestinal polyposis, supernumerary teeth and cutaneous lesions; malignant transformation of intestinal polyps	Excisional biopsy; does not recur	Exostosis Complex odontoma Cementoblastoma Focal sclerosing osteomyelitis

Table continued on following page

TABLE 2–6. Benign Nonodontogenic Neoplasms and Cysts of Bone *Continued*

Lesion	Pediatric Age and Gender	Clinical and Radiographic Findings	Location	Pediatric Significance	Treatment and Prognosis	Differential Diagnosis
Fibrous dysplasia	First and second decades No gender predilection	Unilateral, diffuse, fusiform enlargement; classic radiographic pattern is a ground-glass appearance; may result in displacement of teeth and delayed eruption; slow-growing and asymptomatic	Maxilla is more frequently affected than mandible; buccal cortical expansion is usually observed	Active growth phase during adolescence; may result in significant malocclusion *Albright's syndrome* includes polyostotic fibrous dysplasia, café au lait macules and endocrine abnormalities	No treatment necessary except for osseous recontouring for cosmetic and functional problems; stabilizes after completion of skeletal development; rare malignant transformation	Chronic sclerosing osteomyelitis Ossifying fibroma Osteoma Idiopathic osteosclerosis
Traumatic bone cyst (simple bone cyst)	Second decade No gender predilection	Well-defined, unilocular radiolucency with a thin, sclerotic border; scalloping between roots of teeth; 25% are expansile; teeth are vital	Posterior and anterior body of mandible and ramus; bilateral lesions are uncommon	Pseudocyst may be associated with history of previous trauma to the area; 75% of lesions occur in the second decade	Curettage and initiate bleeding; multiple lesions tend to recur	Central giant cell granuloma Dentigerous cyst Periapical cyst
Aneurysmal bone cyst	First and second decades Female predilection	Painful swelling with rapid growth; unilocular or multilocular radiolucency with ballooning distention of buccal cortex	Mandibular molar region	Blood-filled pseudocyst; pre-existing lesion may be present including central giant cell granuloma, fibrous dysplasia, and ossifying fibroma	Curettage or resection; may be associated with significant blood loss; recurrence rate as high as 50%	Ameloblastic fibroma Central giant cell granuloma Central hemangioma Dentigerous cyst Traumatic bone cyst
Ossifying fibroma (cemento-ossifying fibroma)	Second decade Female predilection	Painless swelling; circular growth pattern; well-defined, unilocular lesion with sclerotic borders; may be radiolucent, mixed or radiopaque	Premolar and molar region; usually occurs in the mandible	*Juvenile ossifying fibroma* is an aggressive variant that usually occurs in the maxilla and frequently recurs	Enucleation or resection; rarely recurs	Adenomatoid odontogenic tumor Fibrous dysplasia Osteoma Osteoblastoma

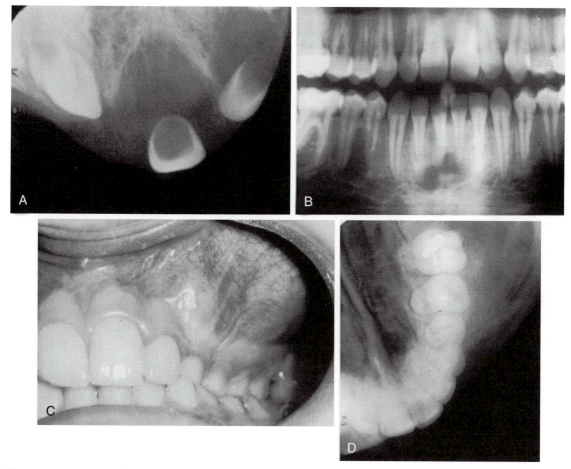

Figure 2–9. *A,* Neuroectodermal tumor of infancy of the anterior maxilla. *B,* Traumatic bone cysts of the anterior and posterior mandible. *C* and *D,* Fibrous dysplasia of the maxilla, intraoral view *(C)* and radiographic view *(D).*

TABLE 2–7. Inflammatory Lesions of Bone (Fig. 2–10)

Lesion	Pediatric Age and Gender	Clinical and Radiographic Findings	Location	Pediatric Significance	Treatment and Prognosis	Differential Diagnosis
Periapical abscess	First and second decades No gender predilection	Nonvital, mobile tooth; tender to percussion; soft tissue swelling with purulent exudate; painful; widening of periodontal ligament space or poorly defined radiolucency	Alveolus; primary dentition is most frequently affected in children	May rapidly progress to cellulitis; periapical infection of primary dentition may result in aborted development or enamel hypoplasia of the succedaneous tooth	Endodontic treatment or extraction of the nonvital tooth; antibiotic coverage, if extensive soft tissue involvement; cavernous sinus thrombosis and Ludwig's angina are life-threatening complications	Incomplete apexification of erupted tooth Periodontal abscess Periapical granuloma or cyst Langerhans cell disease
Acute osteomyelitis	First and second decades No gender predilection	Diffuse radiolucency with poorly defined margins; usually extension of periapical abscess; symptomatology includes fever, pain, swelling, lymphadenopathy, leukocytosis, and draining sinus tracts	Posterior mandible in children; anterior maxilla in infants	Although most cases of acute osteomyelitis result from odontogenic infections or jaw fractures, occasionally it is caused by bacteremia	Incision and drainage with culture and sensitivity testing; appropriate antibiotic coverage; definitive treatment of cause of infection; surgical management varies; may develop into chronic osteomyelitis	Ewing's sarcoma Burkitt's lymphoma Langerhans cell disease
Focal sclerosing osteomyelitis (condensing osteitis)	Second decade No gender predilection	Usually associated with pulpally involved tooth; localized radiopacity at root apices; margins tend to blend in with surrounding bone; asymptomatic	Mandibular first molar region is the most common site	Most common periapical radiopacity; sclerotic bone may impede eruption of succedaneous tooth	No treatment of bony lesion is necessary; surrounding teeth should be evaluated for vitality and managed according to clinical findings; may regress after treatment	Cementoblastoma Idiopathic osteosclerosis Complex odontoma Osteoma
Chronic osteomyelitis with proliferative periostitis (Garre's osteomyelitis)	First and second decades No gender predilection	Diffuse, poorly defined, mixed radiolucent and opaque lesion with a mottled appearance; expansile; cortical bone duplication with laminated or onion skin pattern; mild tenderness; usually presence of carious molar	Posterior mandible; usually involving the first permanent molar	85% of these lesions occur in children under 14 years of age; a cross-sectional, occlusal radiograph is the most diagnostic film for demonstrating this inflammatory bony lesion	Incisional biopsy of the affected bone and endodontic treatment or extraction of infected tooth; appropriate antibiotic therapy; usually expanded bone undergoes remodeling without surgical recontouring	Fibrous dysplasia Fracture callus Ewing's sarcoma Infantile cortical hyperostosis Osteosarcoma

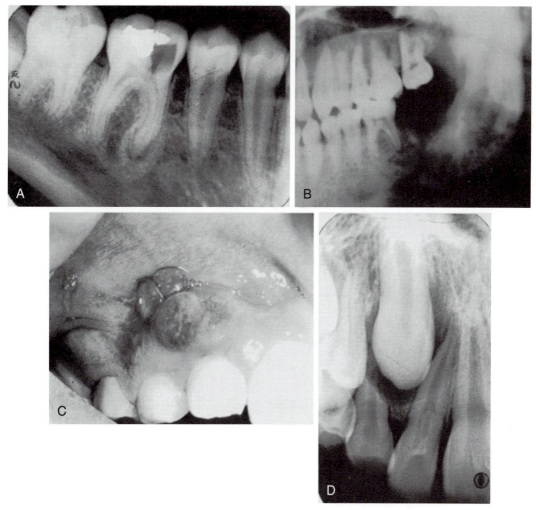

Figure 2–10. *A,* Focal sclerosing osteomyelitis involving the mesial root of a carious mandibular first molar. *B,* Chronic osteomyelitis with proliferative periostitis of the mandible. *C* and *D,* Acute periapical abscess of the maxillary lateral incisor caused by dens in dente, intraoral view *(C)* and radiographic view *(D).* Note the hyperplastic dental follicle surrounding the crown of the unerupted canine.

TABLE 2–8. Selected Malignancies of Soft Tissues and Bone

Lesion	Pediatric Age and Gender	Clinical and Radiographic Findings	Location	Pediatric Significance	Treatment and Prognosis	Differential Diagnosis
Leukemia (acute lymphoblastic leukemia [ALL] and acute myeloid leukemia [AML])	First decade Male predilection	Fatigue, easy bruising, fever, lymphoadenopathy; oral findings: palatal petechiae, gingival bleeding, ulcers, mobility of teeth, loss of lamina dura and alveolar bone; gingival enlargements in AML	Widespread mucocutaneous involvement	Represents one third of all pediatric cancers; ALL is the most common type; long-term oral complications include agenesis or aborted tooth development, and enamel hypoplasia	Chemotherapy, bone marrow transplantation; dental care in consultation with oncologist; 5-year survival rate is about 80–90% for ALL and 20–30% for AML; increased risk of a second cancer	Primary herpetic gingivostomatitis Acute necrotizing ulcerative gingivitis Infectious mononucleosis Cyclic neutropenia Chronic hyperplastic gingivitis
Langerhans cell disease (histiocytosis X)	**Disseminated form:** first decade **Localized form:** second decade Male predilection	Lymphadenopathy, rash, oral pain, gingivitis, ulcers, mobile teeth, punched-out radiolucencies with a "floating tooth" appearance; premature tooth loss	Skull, mandible, ribs and vertebrae are most often involved; jaws affected in up to 20% of cases	Reactive process versus malignancy; chronic disseminated form includes lytic bone lesions, exophthalmos, diabetes insipidus; all forms mimic periodontal disease	Chemotherapy, low-dose radiotherapy, and surgical curettage are used, depending on the form of the disease; children less than 2 years of age have the worst prognosis	Cyclic neutropenia Burkitt's lymphoma Leukemia Early-onset periodontitis Periapical abscess or granuloma
Burkitt's lymphoma	First and second decades Male predilection	Lymphadenopathy, facial swelling, tenderness, tooth mobility and extrusion; patchy loss of lamina dura, irregular radiolucencies, "floating tooth" appearance	Posterior mandible is the most common site; may involve all four quadrants; African form affects the jaws in 50–70% of the cases; American form usually involves the abdomen	The majority of jaw lesions are initially misdiagnosed as an odontogenic infection; associated with Epstein-Barr virus and chromosomal translocation	Treatment includes multiagent chemotherapy; very aggressive malignancy with a survival rate of about 40–60%	Acute osteomyelitis Langerhans cell disease Early-onset periodontitis Periapical abscess or granuloma

	Age/Sex	Clinical features	Location	Comments	Treatment	Differential diagnosis
Ewing's sarcoma	First and second decades; Male predilection	Fever, pain, leukocytosis, swelling, paresthesia, tooth mobility; irregular radiolucency; cortical perforation or expansion; may cause periosteal onion-skin or sunburst reaction	Posterior mandible; femur and pelvis are the most common sites	80% of lesions occur in children under 20 years of age; frequently mimics osteomyelitis	Multiagent chemotherapy, surgery and radiotherapy; 5-year survival rates 60–80%	Osteomyelitis Osteosarcoma Mesenchymal chondrosarcoma
Osteosarcoma (osteogenic sarcoma)	Second decade; Male predilection	Painful swelling, paresthesia, tooth mobility; radiopaque or mixed lesion with poorly defined margins; symmetrical widening of periodontal ligament space; spiky root resorption; periosteal sunburst reaction	Maxilla and mandible, posterior region; femur and tibia are the most common sites	Osteosarcomas of the jaws occur about a decade later than in long bones; the most common malignancy of bone after radiotherapy	Radical surgical resection and chemotherapy; 5-year survival rate of approximately 50–70%	Osteomyelitis Ewing's sarcoma Mesenchymal chondrosarcoma Fibrous dysplasia Osteoblastoma

REFERENCES

Farman AG, Nortje CJ, Wood RE: Oral and Maxillofacial Diagnostic Imaging. St. Louis, Mosby-Year Book, 1993.

Flaitz CM, Coleman GC: Differential diagnosis of oral enlargements in children. Pediatr Dent 17:294-300, 1995.

Hall RK: Pediatric Orofacial Medicine and Pathology. London, Chapman & Hall, 1994.

Kleinman DV, Swango PA, Pindborg JJ: Epidemiology of oral mucosal lesions in United States schoolchildren: 1986-87. Community Dent Oral Epidemiol 22:243-253, 1994.

Neville BW, Damm DD, Allen CM, Bouquot JE: Oral and Maxillofacial Pathology. Philadelphia, WB Saunders, 1996.

Neville BW, Damm DD, White DK, Waldron CA: Color Atlas of Clinical Oral Pathology. Philadelphia, Lea & Febiger, 1991.

Sedano HO, Freyre IC, de la Garza ML, et al: Clinical orodental abnormalities in Mexican children. Oral Surg Oral Med Oral Pathol 68:300-311, 1989.

Scully C, Welbury R: Color Atlas of Oral Diseases in Children and Adolescents. London, Wolfe, 1994.

Wood NK, Goaz PW: Differential Diagnosis of Oral and Maxillofacial Lesions, 5th ed. St. Louis, Mosby-Year Book, 1997.

3

Anomalies of the Developing Dentition

C. O. Dummett, Jr.

Chapter Outline

A variety of dental anomalies are associated with defects in tooth development precipitated by hereditary, systemic, traumatic, or local factors. Numerous systems have been used to classify dental anomalies, and each certainly has merit. The one used in this text categorizes them in terms of abnormalities in tooth number, size, shape, structure, and color (Stewart and Prescott, 1976). The advantage of this system is that the categories can be related to the stages of tooth development in which the respective anomalies are thought to originate. These stages of dental development are discussed in Chapter 12. The reader is also encouraged to review textbooks on dental histology, dental embryology, and oral facial genetics for more in-depth information.

ANOMALIES OF NUMBER

Alterations in tooth number result from problems during the initiation or dental lamina stage of dental development. In addition to hereditary patterns producing extra or missing teeth, physical disruption of the dental lamina, overactive dental lamina, and failure of dental lamina induction by ectomesenchyme are several examples of etiologic factors that affect tooth number (Stewart and Prescott, 1976).

Hyperdontia

Hyperdontia and *supernumerary teeth* are terms describing an excess in tooth number that

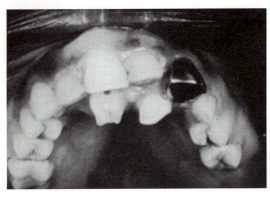

Figure 3–1. Supernumerary teeth—tuberculate morphology.

TABLE 3–1. Syndromes Demonstrating Supernumerary Teeth

Condition	Characteristics
Apert's syndrome	Scaphocephaly, craniosynostosis, bilateral syndactyly, midface hypoplasia
Cleidocranial dysplasia	Aplastic clavicles, frontal bossing, hypoplastic midface
Gardner's syndrome	Osteomas, epidermoid cysts, odontomas, intestinal polyps
Down's syndrome	Brachycephaly, mental retardation, epicanthal folds
Crouzon's disease	Craniosynostosis, exopthalmus, hypoplastic midface
Sturge-Weber syndrome	Angiomatosis and calcification of leptomeninges, seizures, portwine nevi of face
Oral-facial-digital syndrome	Hypoplastic alar cartilage, cleft tongue, clinodactyly
Hallermann-Streiff syndrome	Dyscephaly, mandibular hypoplasia, hypotrichosis

can occur in both the primary and permanent dentitions. Reports on the incidence of hyperdontia include values as high as 3%, with males being affected twice as frequently as females (Primosch, 1981). Ninety to 98% of supernumerary teeth occur in the maxilla, with the permanent dentition being more frequently affected than the primary dentition. The most common supernumerary tooth is the mesiodens, which occurs in the palatal midline and can assume a number of shapes and positions relative to the adjacent teeth. The majority tend to be located palatal to the central incisors (von Arx et al., 1992).

As reported by Primosch in 1981, supernumerary teeth are morphologically classified as either supplemental or rudimentary. Supplemental supernumerary teeth duplicate the typical anatomy of posterior and anterior teeth. Rudimentary supernumerary teeth are dysmorphic and can assume conical forms, tuberculate forms (Fig. 3–1), or shapes that duplicate molar anatomy. From a clinical standpoint, the tuberculate, or barrel-shaped, supernumeraries generate the most severe complications with respect to difficulty of removal and adverse effects on adjacent teeth, such as impaction or ectopic eruption. Additional complications associated with supernumeraries include dentigerous cyst formation, pericoronal space ossification, and crown resorption (von Arx et al., 1992). An important consideration in supernumerary tooth detection is to rule out the presence of odontoma in light of the fact that the morphology of a compound composite odontoma is similar to that of teeth.

Cleft lip and palate commonly demonstrates an excess or deficiency in the normal complement of teeth and provides a clear example of physical disruption of the dental lamina as an etiologic factor. Classic syndromes involving supernumerary teeth are summarized in Table 3-1, with *cleidocranial dysplasia* having the highest association with this dental anomaly.

Hypodontia

Hypodontia, or congenital tooth absence, is a deficiency in tooth number. Familial heredity patterns account for the largest etiologic correlation with patterns of hypodontia. Incidence reports identify a range of 1.5% to 10% excluding third molars in American populations (Maklin et al., 1979). The most frequently occurring congenitally absent permanent tooth, excluding third molars, tends to be the mandibular second bicuspid (3.4%), followed by the maxillary lateral incisor (2.2%) (Symons et al., 1993).

There is a high correlation between primary

TABLE 3–2. Syndromes Demonstrating Hypodontia

Condition	Characteristics
Ectodermal dysplasia (hypohidrotic type)	Hypotrichosis, aplasia of sweat/sebaceous glands
Chondroectodermal dysplasia	Polydactyly, mesomelic dwarfism, hidrotic ectodermal dysplasia
Achondroplasia	Short-limbed dwarfism, macrocephaly, frontal bossing
Rieger's syndrome	Iris dysplasia, midface hypoplasia, protruding umbilicus
Incontinentia pigmenti	Alopecia, pigmented macules, mental retardation
Seckel syndrome	Dwarfism, microcephaly, facial hypoplasia, low-set lobeless ears

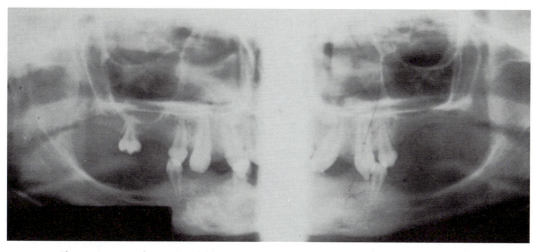

Figure 3–2. Hypodontia in a child with ectodermal dysplasia. Note atrophy of alveolar ridge.

tooth absence and permanent tooth absence (Grahanen and Granath, 1961; Whittington et al., 1996). *Ectodermal dysplasia* (ED) represents a group of classic syndromes that demonstrate oligodontia or multiple congenitally missing teeth. The most common is hypohidrotic ED, followed by hidrotic ED, ectrodactyly ED plus cleft lip and palate, Rapp-Hodgkin ED, and Robinson-type ED in descending frequency of occurrence (Fig. 3–2). Other conditions involving hypodontia are summarized in Table 3–2 as well as those demonstrating both hyperdontia and hypodontia in Table 3-3.

ANOMALIES OF SIZE

Microdontia and Macrodontia

Abnormalities in tooth size are epitomized in microdontia and macrodontia. *Hemifacial microsomia* is thought to result from a hematoma of the stapedial artery during embryologic development giving rise to a deficient nutrient supply to the affected side of the face. In addition to unilateral mandibular hypoplasia and ear malformation, less growth occurs in this less vascularized area, with smaller teeth forming as a result. Peg-shaped lateral incisors are examples of microdontia and are common in *Down's syndrome*. Other

conditions demonstrating microdontia include *ectodermal dysplasia* and *chondroectodermal dysplasia*. These size abnormalities are thought to originate during the morphodifferentiation stage of tooth development.

Facial hemihypertrophy can demonstrate comparatively larger teeth on the affected side (Fig. 3-3). Of the many factors thought to cause

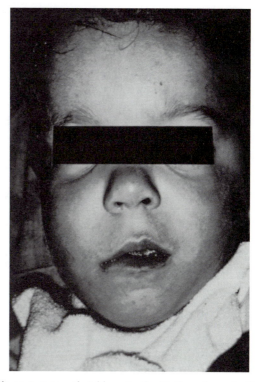

Figure 3–3. Hemifacial hypertrophy. Teeth on the patient's affected side (right) are larger in all dimensions.

TABLE 3–3. Syndromes Manifesting Both Hyperdontia and Hypodontia

....

Crouzon's disease	Oral-facial-digital syndrome I
Down's syndrome	Hallermann-Streiff syndrome

this condition, vascular and neurogenic abnormalities are considered the most likely. In addition to an increase in crown and root size, affected teeth develop more rapidly and erupt earlier than on the uninvolved side. The *otodental syndrome,* consisting of high-frequency hearing loss and globe-shaped fused molar teeth, is another condition that involves macrodontia. Isolated teeth with macrodontia can also result from twinning abnormalities that originate during the proliferation stage of tooth development. Fusion and gemination are the most common twinning abnormalities, and both include enlarged crowns.

Fusion

Fusion has an incidence of 0.5% and is more common in the primary dentition (Grahanen and Granath, 1961). The classic definition of fusion is the dentinal union of two embryologically developing teeth. Although fused teeth can contain two separate pulp chambers, many appear as large bifid crowns with one chamber, which makes them difficult to distinguish from geminated teeth.

Gemination

Gemination has a frequency of 0.5%, which is similar to that of fusion and is more common in the primary dentition. Conceptually, a geminated tooth represents an incomplete division of a single tooth bud resulting in a bifid crown with a single pulp chamber. Gemination tends to occur in a familial pattern, and its significance is similar to that of fusion in that both conditions may result in retarded eruption of the permanent successor. Clinically, fusion and gemination are usually distinguished by counting the number of teeth in the arch. If there is a deficiency in the normal complement including the bifid crown, the condition is fusion. Fusion with a supernumerary tooth must also be considered and ruled out because this would not affect the normal number of teeth.

Concrescence is a twinning anomaly involving the union of two teeth by cementum only. Its etiology is thought to be trauma or adjacent tooth malposition. Because it can occur after root development, concrescence is technically not a developmental anomaly.

ANOMALIES OF SHAPE

Abnormalities in shape originate during the morphodifferentiation stage of tooth development and are manifested as alterations in crown and root form. Modes of inheritance include both autosomal dominant and polygenic patterns.

Dens Evaginatus

Dens evaginatus is an extra cusp, usually in the central groove or ridge of a posterior tooth and in the cingulum area of the central and lateral incisors (Fig. 3–4). In incisors, these cusps appear talon-shaped and can approach the level of the incisal edge. This extra portion contains not only enamel but dentin and pulp tissue; therefore, a pulp exposure can result from radical equilibration. It occurs with a frequency of 1% to 4% and results from the evagination of inner enamel epithelium cells, which are the precursors of ameloblasts (Stewart and Prescott, 1976).

Dens in Dente

Dens in dente is a condition resulting from the invagination of the inner enamel epithelium producing the appearance of a tooth within a tooth. In 1974, Thomas reported a 7.7% prevalence, with the maxillary lateral incisors being most frequently affected. The clinical significance of this anomaly results from potential carious involvement through the communication of the invaginated portion of the lingual surface of the tooth with the outside environment. The enamel and dentin in the invaginated portion can be

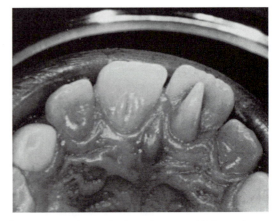

Figure 3–4. Dens evaginatis—talon cusp. All three elements of dental tissues are represented in the extra cusp.

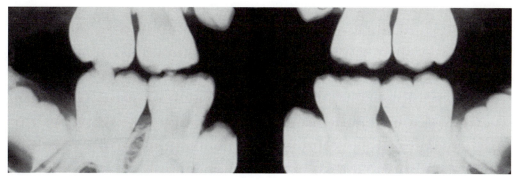

Figure 3–5. Taurodont teeth. Note that primary teeth as well as permanent teeth can be affected.

both defective and absent, allowing direct exposure of the pulp.

Taurodont

Taurodont teeth are characterized by having a significantly elongated pulp chamber with short stunted roots, resulting from the failure of the proper level of horizontal invagination of Hertwig's epithelial root sheath (Fig. 3-5). The incidence can range from 0.5% to 5% and can be classified according to the extent of the pulp chamber elongation (Mena, 1971). The conditions that classically involve taurodontism are summarized Table 3-4.

Dilaceration

Dilaceration refers to an abnormal bend of the root during its development and is thought to result from a traumatic episode,usually to the primary dentition (Fig. 3-6). In 1971, Andreason reported a dilaceration incidence of 25% in those permanent teeth with developmental disturbances secondary to primary tooth injury. Con-

genital ichthyosis, consisting of hyperkeratosis of the knees and elbows, fish-like scaly skin, and delayed tooth eruption, also includes root dilaceration as a consistent finding.

ANOMALIES OF STRUCTURE

Enamel

Tooth structure abnormalities result from disruption during the histodifferentiation, apposition, and mineralization stages of tooth development. Enamel defects are manifested as hypoplasia or hypocalcification. According to Jorgenson and Yost in 1982, they may be broadly classified as heritable defects or environmentally induced defects.

AMELOGENESIS IMPERFECTA

Amelogenesis imperfecta (AI) is a classic example of heritable enamel defects. Estimates of the incidence of this condition include 1 in 14,000 (Witkop, 1959), 1 in 8000 (Chosack et al., 1979),

TABLE 3–4. Conditions Demonstrating Taurodontism

Klinefelter's syndrome	Aspermatogenesis, mental retardation
Trichodento-osseus syndrome	Sclerotic bones, coarse gnarled hair, enamel defects
Oral-facial-digital syndrome II	Dystrophic nails, hyperplastic frenum, lobed tongue
Ectodermal dysplasia (hypohidrotic)	Hypotrichosis, aplasia of sweat/sebaceous glands
Amelogenesis imperfecta IV	Enamel hypoplasia and hypomaturation, mottled yellow teeth
Down's syndrome	Brachycephaly, mental retardation, epicanthal fold

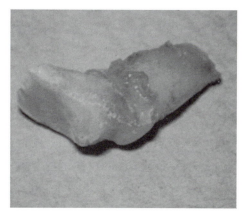

Figure 3–6. Dilacerated lateral incisor.

and 1 in 4000 (Sundell et al., 1986). Fourteen subgroup classifications of AI are listed in Table 3-5, with multiple inheritance patterns represented. It is important to remember that the sole feature that distinguishes AI from other enamel defects is its confinement to distinct patterns of inheritance and its occurrence exclusive of any syndromic, metabolic, or systemic condition (Witkop, 1988). The four major AI categories are described according to the stages of tooth development in which each is thought to occur. Further information on the subgroups can be obtained from more comprehensive resources.

Hypoplastic Type. Heritable enamel defects occurring in the histodifferentiation stage of tooth development are exemplified by the hypoplastic type of AI wherein an insufficient quantity of enamel is formed (Fig. 3-7). This is due to areas of the enamel organ that are devoid of inner enamel epithelium, causing a lack of cell differentiation into ameloblasts. Both primary and permanent dentitions are affected, and the condition is inherited predominantly as an autosomal dominant trait depending on the subgroup pattern. Affected teeth appear small with open contacts, and areas of the clinical crowns contain very thin or nonexistent enamel resulting in high sensitivity to thermal stimuli. Anterior open bite has been observed in 60% of reported cases (Rowley et al., 1982).

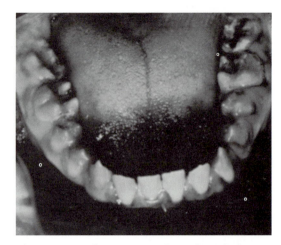

Figure 3–7. Amelogenesis imperfecta—hypoplastic type.

Hypomaturation Type. The hypomaturation type of AI is an example of an inherited defect in enamel matrix apposition and is characterized by teeth having normal enamel thickness but a low value of radiodensity and mineral content (Fig. 3-8). The problem is related to the persistence of organic content in the rod sheath resulting in poor calcification, low mineral content, and a porous surface that becomes stained.

HYPOPLASTIC/HYPOMATURATION WITH TAURODONTISM

This form of AI is an example of inherited defects in both apposition and histodifferentiation stages of enamel formation. The enamel appears mottled with a yellow-brown color and is pitted on the facial surfaces, exemplifying the features of

TABLE 3–5. Classification of Amelogenesis Imperfecta

Type I	**Hypoplastic**	
1A	Hypoplastic, pitted autosomal dominant	
1B	Hypoplastic, local autosomal dominant	
1C	Hypoplastic, local autosomal recessive	
1D	Hypoplastic, smooth autosomal dominant	
1E	Hypoplastic, smooth X-linked dominant	
1F	Hypoplastic, rough autosomal dominant	
1G	Enamel agenesis, autosomal recessive	
Type II	**Hypomaturation**	
IIA	Hypomaturation, pigmented autosomal recessive	
IIB	Hypomaturation, X-linked recessive	
IID	Snow-capped teeth, autosomal dominant?	
Type III	**Hypocalcified**	
IIIA	Autosomal dominant	
IIIB	Autosomal recessive	
Type IV	**Hypomaturation-hypoplastic with taurodontism**	
IVA	Hypomaturation-hypoplastic with taurodontism, autosomal dominant	
IVB	Hypoplastic-hypomaturation with taurodontism, autosomal dominant	

Adapted from Witkop CJ Jr: Amelogenesis imperfecta, dentingenesis imperfecta and dental dysplasia revisited: Problems in classification. J Oral Path *17*:547–558, 1988.

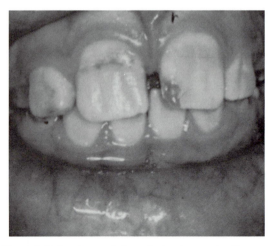

Figure 3–8. Amelogenesis imperfecta—hypomaturation type.

both hypoplasia and hypomaturation previously described. Molar teeth demonstrate taurodontism, and other components of the dentition have enlarged pulp chambers.

HYPOCALCIFICATION TYPE

The hypocalcification type of AI is an example of an inherited defect in the calcification stage of enamel formation. Quantitatively, the enamel is normal, but qualitatively the matrix is poorly calcified with a resultant fracturing of the enamel surface (Fig. 3-9). The hypocalcified enamel is soft and fragile, especially at the incisal regions, and is easily fractured, exposing the underlying dentin that produces an unesthetic appearance. Increased calculus formation and marked delay in tooth eruption are consistent findings. Anterior open-bite occurs in 60% of cases demonstrating this defect (Rowley et al., 1982).

ENVIRONMENTAL ENAMEL HYPOPLASIA

Examples of environmentally induced enamel hypoplasia can result from systemic or local causes. Examples of systemic causes producing generalized enamel hypoplasia include nutrition deficiencies, particularly in vitamins, A, C, and D as well as in calcium and phosphorous (Jorgenson and Yost, 1982). Severe infection, such as exanthematous diseases and fever-producing disorders, particularly during the first year of life, can directly affect ameloblastic activity, resulting in enamel hypoplasia. *Rubella embryopathy* has a high correlation with prenatal enamel hypoplasia in the primary dentition. *Syphilis* caused by the spirochete *Treponema pallidum* produces classic patterns of hypoplastic dysmorphic permanent teeth. The tapered and notched incisal edges of anterior teeth with screwdriver shapes are called *Hutchinson incisors,* and the crenated occlusal patterns of posterior teeth known as *mulberry molars* are classic clinical findings for prenatal syphilis infection.

Neurologic defects as exemplified in children with cerebral palsy and *Sturge-Weber syndrome* have an increased likelihood of generalized enamel hypoplasia. Children with asthma also demonstrate a higher frequency of enamel hypoplasia than do nonafflicted children. Prematurity and excess radiation exposure can disrupt ameloblastic matrix formation or subsequent mineralization and are additional causes of systemic enamel hypoplasia. A number of syndromes involve enamel hypoplasia as a consistent dental characteristic and are listed in Table 3-6.

Excess ingestion of systemic fluoride can produce generalized enamel defects. Dental fluorosis can be manifested as a defect in the calcification of the teeth in milder forms, with significant pigmentation and ameloblastic impairment in the more severe forms. Fluorosis occurs when the concentration of ingested fluoride is above 1.8 parts per million per day (Jorgenson and Yost, 1982). There is a 90% chance of some degree of dental fluorosis when the amount of ingested fluoride is greater than 6 parts per million, although the severity of morphologic defects cannot be predicted from specific quantities of infested fluoride.

LOCALIZED ENAMEL HYPOPLASIA

Causes of enamel hypoplasia affecting individual teeth include local infection, local trauma, iatrogenic surgery as occurs in cleft palate closure, and primary tooth overretention. Turner's hypoplasia is a classic example of hypoplastic defects in permanent teeth resulting from local infection or trauma to the primary precursor (Fig. 3-10).

ENAMEL HYPOCALCIFICATION

Hypocalcification defects can be directly related to faults in the mineralization of the organic ma-

TABLE 3-6. Syndromes Demonstrating Enamel Hypoplasia

Down's syndrome	Pseudo-hypoparathyroidism
Tuberous sclerosis	Trichodento-osseous
Epidermolysis bullosa	syndrome
Hurler's syndrome	Vitamin D–dependent rickets
Hunter's syndrome	Lesch-Nyhan syndrome
Treacher Collins syndrome	Fanconi's syndrome
Phenylketonuria	Sturge-Weber syndrome
	Turner's syndrome

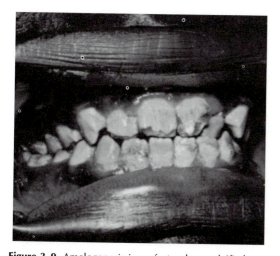

Figure 3-9. Amelogenesis imperfecta—hypocalcified type.

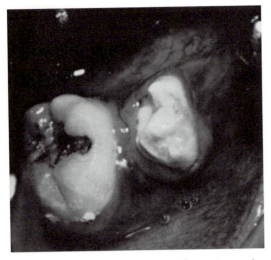

Figure 3–10. Turner's hypoplasia. Note that cementum is formed on the crown areas that are denuded of enamel.

trix in enamel formation. The same factors that cause enamel hypoplasia also cause hypocalcification. The majority of localized hypocalcific defects, as in the case of Turner's hypoplasia, are subsequent to localized infection and trauma. Excess exposure to citric acid resulting from habitual sucking on citrus fruits can produce generalized erosive hypocalcified lesions that mimic the hypocalcification type of AI.

Dentin

DENTINOGENESIS IMPERFECTA

Dentinogenesis imperfecta is an example of an inheritable dentinal defect originating during the histodifferentiation stage of tooth development (Fig. 3-11). This anomaly involves a defect of predentin matrix that results in amorphic, disorganized, and atubular circumpulpal dentin. The mantle dentin is normal, in contrast with the previously described circumpulpal dentin, which is high in organic content and contains interglobular calcification. Its frequency of occurrence is about 1 in 8000. Dentinogenesis imperfecta can be subdivided into three basic types (Shields et al., 1973).

Shields Type I occurs with osteogenesis imperfecta. An inherited defect in collagen formation results in osteoporotic brittle bones, bowing of the limbs, bitemporal bossing, and blue sclera. Primary teeth tend to be more severely affected than permanent teeth. Periapical radiolucencies, bulbous crowns, obliteration of pulp chambers, and root fractures are evident. An amber translucent tooth color is common.

Shields Type II, also known as hereditary opalescent dentin, tends to occur as a separate entity apart from osteogenesis imperfecta. In this case, both primary and permanent dentitions are equally affected and the characteristics previously described for Type I are the same. This condition is inherited as an autosomal dominant trait.

Shields Type III is rare and represents many of the features described earlier with a predominance of bell-shaped crowns, especially in the permanent dentition. Unlike Types I and II, Type III involves teeth with a shell-like appearance and multiple pulp exposures. It has occurred exclusively in a triracial isolated group in Maryland known as the Brandywine population (Shields et al., 1973). Type III has been proposed to be a different expression of the same Type II gene (Levin, 1983).

DENTIN DYSPLASIA

Dentin dysplasia represents another group of inherited dentin disorders resulting in characteristic features involving the circumpulpal dentin and root morphology. In 1973, Shields and associates proposed a classification based on characteristic patterns of dentinal dysplasia.

Shields Type I demonstrates normal primary and permanent crown morphology with an amber translucency (Fig. 3-12). The roots tend to be short and sharply constricted. Primary teeth have obliterated pulps. Both primary and permanent dentitions demonstrate multiple periapical radiolucencies and absent pulp chambers. Cascading tubule patterns are due to blockage of normal dentin tubules by calcified masses.

Shields Type II involves amber-colored primary

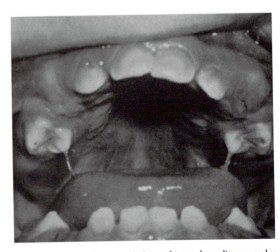

Figure 3-11. Dentinogenesis imperfecta—hereditary opalescent dentin.

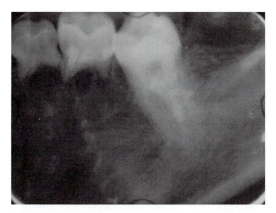

Figure 3–12. Dentinal dysplasia Type I. Note rootless primary teeth.

teeth closely resembling dentinogenesis imperfecta Types I and II. Permanent teeth appear normal but radiographically demonstrate thistle-tube shaped pulp chambers with multiple pulp stones (Fig. 3-13). No periapical radiolucencies are visible.

REGIONAL ODONTODYSPLASIA

Odontodysplasia is a condition representing a localized arrest in tooth development thought to result from a regional vascular developmental anomaly. Affected teeth have thin layers of poorly calcified enamel and dentin with large diffusely calcified pulp chambers and shortened, poorly defined roots (Crawford and Aldred, 1989) (Fig. 3-14). The teeth have a ghost-like radiographic appearance with shortened roots and shell-like crowns and are dysmorphic in overall appearance. No conclusive etiologic factor or inheritance pattern has been identified that can explain the reported cases.

Additional conditions involving dentin abnor-malities relate to systemic abnormalities that impair normal absorption and circulating serum levels of calcium and phosphorous. *Vitamin D-resistant rickets, hypoparathyroidism,* and *pseudo-hyperparathyroidism* are all conditions demonstrating characteristic dentinal abnormalities that are summarized as follows (Stewart and Prescott, 1976).

Vitamin D–Resistant Rickets

- Hypomineralized dentin
- Increased width to predentin
- Odontoblastic disorganization
- Decreased alkaline phosphatase activity in tooth germ
- Enlarged pulp and pulp horns
- No enamel defect

Hypoparathyroidism

- Tooth defects are more severe in males
- Permanent teeth are predominantly affected
- Short, wedge-shaped roots with delayed apical closure
- Interglobular calcification in dentin, especially at apices
- Enamel hypoplasia

Pseudohypoparathyroidism

- Enlarged pulp chambers
- Irregular dentinal tubules
- Small crowns and short, blunted roots
- Pitted enamel surfaces

Cementum

Developmental defects involving cementum as an exclusive entity apart from other dental structures are uncommon. It is especially difficult to identify problems in cementogenesis from dis-

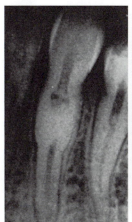
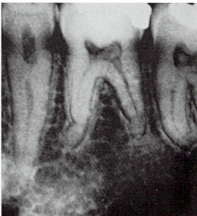

Figure 3–13. Dentinal dysplasia Type II. Note thistle-tube shape to permanent pulp chambers.

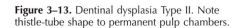

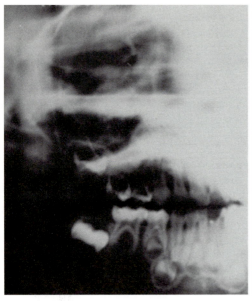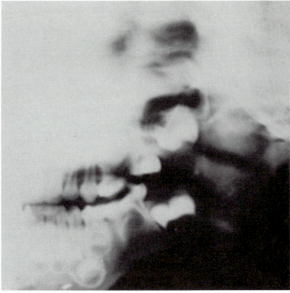

Figure 3–14. Odontodysplasia in the patient's upper left maxillary area.

eases involving the periodontal ligament. An interesting finding in Turner's hypoplasia is that in addition to coronal enamel defects of the affected permanent teeth, cementum is formed in the coronal areas denuded of enamel (Stewart and Prescott, 1976). This underscores the protective role that the reduced enamel epithelium plays on the unerupted tooth crown. Furthermore, it represents the reciprocal inductive effect of dentin that, when in direct contact with the dental follicle mesenchymal cells, causes them to differentiate into cementoblasts. Areas denuded of enamel allow this phenomenon to occur.

Histologically defective cementum occurs in three noteworthy conditions. *Epidermolysis bullosa dystrophica,* an inherited vesicular and bullous disease of the skin and mucous membranes, involves fibrous, poorly calcified acellular cementum and an overproduction of cellular cementum. Cleidocranial dysplasia also displays histologic alterations in cementum formation. Lukinmaa and associates noted that permanent teeth were devoid of cellular cementum and had partially hyperplastic acellular cementum (Lukinmaa et al., 1995).

Hypophosphatasia is a complex condition involving the failure of bone to mineralize properly, which is associated with low serum alkaline phosphatase levels. Osteoporosis, bone fragility, and premature loss of primary incisors are classic clinical features (Fig. 3-15). The latter finding is ascribed to the failure of cementum formation on the prematurely exfoliated incisors and to a decrease in cementum formation in the retained

primary teeth. The condition exerts its greatest effect prenatally and during the first year of life. Bone and dentin are affected as well as cementum, so the entity is not exclusively a cementum defect.

ANOMALIES OF COLOR

Both the primary and permanent dentitions can manifest significant color changes from extrinsic or intrinsic stains. Because of their developmental significance, only the intrinsic stains are addressed here. In 1975, Eisenberg and Bernick provided a detailed classification of the causes of tooth discolorations. Causes of intrinsic stains

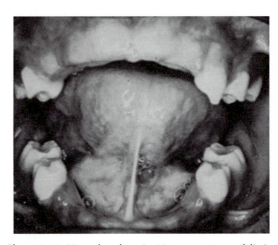

Figure 3–15. Hypophosphatasia. Note premature exfoliation of primary anterior teeth in the upper and lower areas.

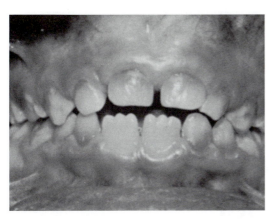

Figure 3–16. Tetracycline staining of primary and permanent dentitions. Note darker hues to the primary teeth with more diffuse yellow stain to permanent incisors.

can be due to blood-borne pigments, drug administration, and hypoplastic-hypocalcified disease states. Congenital porphyria, bile duct defects, anemias, and transfusion-reaction hemolysis are examples of blood-borne pigments.

A classic example of drug-induced intrinsic staining occurs from tetracycline antibiotics. Both dentitions can have severe discoloration from this antibiotic when given in concentrations of 21 to 26 mg/kg or greater over a period as brief as 3 days (Moffitt et al., 1974) (Fig. 3–16). Tetracycline hydrochloride has the greatest potential for staining among the tetracyclines. The agent forms an orthocalcium phosphate complex with dentin and enamel, which is then oxidized by ultraviolet light. The oxidation process results in pigments that stain the hard tissues. The critical period for initiation of primary and permanent tooth staining is that of intrauterine development through 8 years of age. Tetracycline administration must be especially avoided during this time.

Systemic and localized enamel hypoplasia can result in tooth discoloration. Many of the enamel and dentin dysplasias also result in tooth color changes as well as in the heritable anomalies of AI and dentinogenesis imperfecta. Excess fluoride overlaps both the drug-induced and hypoplastic categories of agents responsible for tooth discoloration. The more severe form of dental fluorosis can produce a range of discoloration, from opaque white spots with diffuse striations to a brown mottling.

REFERENCES

Andreason JO: The effect of traumatic injuries to primary teeth on their permanent successor. Scand J Dent Res *145:*229, 1971.

Chosack A, Edelmann E, Wisotski I, Choen T: Amelogenesis imperfecta among Israel: Jews and the description of a new type of local hypoplastic autosomal recessive amelogenesis imperfecta. Oral Surg *47:*148, 1979.

Crawford PJM, Aldred MJ: Regional odontodysplasia: A bibliography. J Oral Pathol Med *18:*251–263, 1989.

Eisenberg E, Bernick SM: Anomalies of the teeth with stains and discolorations. J Prev Dent *2:*7–20, 1975.

Grahanen H, Granath L: Numerical variations and their correlations with the permanent dentition. Odont Rev *4:*348–357, 1961.

Jorgenson RT, Yost C: Etiology of enamel dysplasias. J Pedo *6:*316–329, 1982.

Levin LS, et al: Dentinogenesis imperfecta in the Brandywine isolet (DI-III). Oral Surg Oral Med Oral Pathol *56:*267, 1983.

Lukinmaa PL, et al: Histological observations of teeth and peridental tissues in cleidocranial dysplasia imply increased activity of odontogenic epithelium and abnormal bone remodeling. J Craniofac Genet Dev Biol *15:*212, 1995.

Maklin M, Dummett CO Jr, Weinberg R: A study of oligodontia in a sample of New Orleans children. J Dent Child *46:*478, 1979.

Mena CA: Taurodontism. Oral Surg Oral Pathol Oral Med *32:*812–823, 1971.

Moffitt JM, et al: Prediction of tetracycline-induced tooth coloration. JADA *88:*547, 1974.

Primosch RE: Anterior supernumerary teeth—assessment and surgical intervention in children. J Pediatr Dent *3:*204, 1981.

Rowley C, Hill FJ, Winter IGB: An investigation of the association between anterior openbite and amelogenesis imperfecta. Am J Orthod *81:*220, 1982.

Shields ED, Bixler D, El-Kafrawy AM: A proposed classification for heritable human dentine defects with a description of a new entity. Arch Oral Biol *18:*543–553, 1973.

Stewart RE, Prescott GH: Oral Facial Genetics. St. Louis, CV Mosby, 1976.

Sundell S, Valentin J: Hereditary aspects of hereditary amelogenesis imperfecta. Community Dent Oral Epidemiol *14:*211, 1986.

Symons AL, et al: Anomalies associated with hypodontia of the permanent lateral incisor and second premolar. J Clin Pediatr Dent *17:*109, 1993.

Thomas JG: A study of dens in dente. Oral Surg Oral Pathol Oral Med *38:*653, 1974.

von Arx T, et al: Anerior supernumerary teeth: A clinical and radiographic study. Aust Dent J *37:*189, 1992.

Whittington BR, Durward CS: Survey of anomalies in primary teeth and their correlation with the permanent dentition. N Z Dent J *92:*4, 1996.

Witkop CJ Jr: Genetics in dentistry. Eugenics Q *5:*15–21, 1959.

Witkop CJ Jr: Amelogenesis imperfecta, dentinogenesis imperfecta and dentinal dysplasia revisited: Problems in classification. J Oral Pathol *17:*547–553, 1988.

Chapter **4**

Diseases and Oral Manifestations of Systemic Disease

Andrew Sonis

Chapter Outline

HERPETIC GINGIVOSTOMATITIS

Causative Agent: Herpes Simplex Virus Type I. Manifestations of the infection represent the patient's primary exposure to the virus. Herpetic gingivostomatitis is most common in young children, but it may also occur in adolescents, young adults, and immunocompromised patients.

Evaluation. Recent exposure to an infected person should be ascertained. A lack of previous history of a similar infection is important because infection with the virus imparts lifetime immunity. Viral cultures, serum antibody titers, and cytologic examination may aid in making the diagnosis.

Diagnosis. Subjective findings include a viral prodrome of malaise, arthralgia, and anorexia accompanied by fever and chills.

Objective Findings. Initially, vesicles develop on the mucosa of the lips, tongue, and gingiva, which shortly thereafter rupture into large, painful, ulcerated areas. The gingiva is edematous, erythematous, and bleeds readily upon mild provocation. The tongue may have a white coating (Fig. 4-1).

Tzanck preparation of vesicles may reveal multinucleated giant cells with inclusion bodies. Serum antibody titers obtained during the acute and convalescent period (6 weeks later) reveal a rise in the antivirus antibody levels.

Therapy

1. The disease is self-limiting, and the acute phase generally lasts 7 to 10 days. Treatment consists of bed rest, antipyretics, and analgesics to control fever and relieve pain. Palliative mouthrinses may offer some relief.

2. Encourage oral fluid intake because dehy-

dration may be a problem, particularly in the younger patient. Occasionally, intravenous fluid intake is necessary.

3. Isolate the patient from peers and siblings in an attempt to prevent spread of the disease.

4. Ulcers heal without scarring.

5. Antibiotics are contraindicated unless specific signs of secondary infection are present.

6. Steroids are contraindicated.

Case Study

A 19-month-old female is referred from her pediatrician's office with a chief complaint of decreased appetite and malaise thought to be secondary to mouth pain and fever. The pediatrician performed a cursory oral examination and noted several erupting teeth to which the child's discomfort and fever were attributed. Your examination likewise reveals several partially erupted teeth. In addition you note generalized erythematous gingiva, several ulcerated areas of the mucosa, and a coated white tongue.

Diagnosis

Primary herpetic gingivostomatitis. Although teething is frequently implicated as the etiology of low-grade fevers, diarrhea, or both, there are few supporting scientific data. Studies have demonstrated that in many children who present with teething pain, culture is positive for herpes simplex type 1.

RECURRENT HERPES SIMPLEX (HERPES LABIALIS)

Causative Agent: Herpes Simplex Type I Virus. Lesions are believed to result from reactivation of the virus lying dormant in the trigeminal ganglia in a previously infected host. Approximately 25% of affected patients experience one or more episodes per month. Activation of the virus may be related to cold, sunlight, or stress.

Evaluation. Patients generally give a previous history of similar lesions. Look for small vesicular or ulcerative lesions involving the lips at the mucocutaneous junction, at the corners of the mouth, or beneath the nose.

Diagnosis. Subjective findings often include a prodrome of itchiness or a tingly sensation preceding the development of lesions. Patients may experience mild flu-like symptoms.

Objective findings include vesicles of 2 to 4 mm in diameter located at the mucocutaneous junction of the lips, at the corners of the mouth, and beneath the nose. Vesicles subsequently rup-

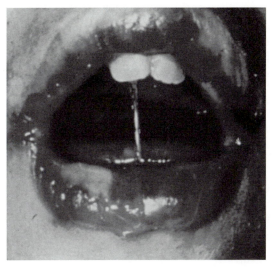

Figure 4–1. Herpetic gingivostomatitis: painful ulcerations involving the gingiva, tongue, and lips.

ture and crust over in 36 to 48 hours. Healing occurs in 7 to 10 days. Viral titers peak during the first 48 hours of infection, then taper off. Tzanck preparation of vesicles may reveal multinucleated giant cells with inclusion bodies.

Therapy. Numerous treatment modalities have been proposed for herpes labialis, but none is well substantiated. It is generally best to keep the lesions well lubricated with an emollient to promote healing. Isolate the patient from persons who are at risk for primary herpes infection. A review of several clinical trials of prophylactic or oral acyclovir for the suppression of herpes labialis by Spruance, Rea, and Thoming (1997) suggested little or no evidence that topical therapy was effective. Oral acyclovir taken prophylactically did result in a reduction in frequency of this disease, however. The best success was observed in those patients with monthly or more frequent recurrences and those with prodromal symptoms. A newly introduced topical antiviral agent, pentciclovir, has shown some promise in treatment of herpes labialis.

Ulcers heal without scarring.

HERPES ZOSTER (CHICKEN POX)

Causative Agent: Varicella-Zoster Virus. Reactivation of the virus months or years after chicken pox can occur in a dorsal spinal or cranial nerve ganglion, with spread to the appropriate cutaneous dermatome and occasionally to distant sites.

Evaluation. Recent exposure to an infected

person should be ascertained. Chicken pox occurs most commonly during winter and spring months. Although most persons with chicken pox develop life-long immunity, children who are infected early in life or experience a particularly mild or subclinical case may become re-infected.

Diagnosis

Subjective Findings. Patients may experience a mild viral prodrome of malaise, arthralgia, and anorexia accompanied by fever and chills.

Objective Findings. Lesions appear as crops of vesicles on an erythematous base; the vesicles usually begin on the trunk and spread to the extremities and face. Several stages of lesions are usually present at one time. Lesions eventually crust over and heal.

Lesions involving the oral mucosa may appear as small vesicles that subsequently rupture, leaving small ulcerations with an erythematous margin. Generally, these lesions are not very painful.

Therapy. The disease is self-limiting, and the acute phase generally lasts 7 to 10 days. Treatment consists of bed rest, antipyretics, and analgesics to control fever and relieve pain. Occasionally, antibiotics are necessary for secondary infection of the vesicles. The disease is contagious; therefore, isolation of an infected patient is recommended to prevent spread of disease to susceptible persons.

HERPANGINA

Causative Agent: Coxsackie A Virus. Herpangina is common in young children under the age of 4 years and is caused by coxsackie A virus types 2, 3, 4, 5, 6, 8, and 10.

Evaluation. Recent exposure to an infected person should be determined because disease may occur in epidemics.

Diagnosis. Subjective findings include a viral prodrome of rapid onset of fever, malaise, myalgia, runny nose, throat pain, and dysphagia. Twenty-five percent of infected persons experience vomiting and abdominal pain. The disease shows a seasonal predilection, with the highest incidence in the summer and fall.

Objective findings include multiple small, ovoid, vesicular lesions that develop on the soft palate and tonsillar pillars. The vesicles rapidly ulcerate, leaving a gray or white central area surrounded by an erythematous base (Fig. 4–2). These painful lesions usually do not involve the anterior two thirds of the mouth. Lymphadenopathy may be present. Bacterial throat cultures may be useful to rule out bacterial pharyngitis (i.e., "strep" throat).

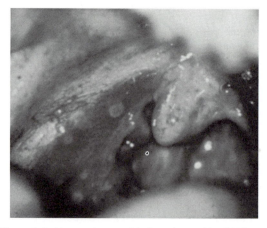

Figure 4–2. Herpangina: ovoid ulcerations with whitish-gray central area surrounded by an erythematous halo involving the tonsillar pillars.

Therapy

1. The disease is self-limiting, and acute symptoms generally persist for about 3 days.

2. Oral lesions heal in 7 to 10 days without scarring.

3. Treatment is palliative and includes bed rest, antipyretics, and analgesics. A palliative mouthrinse may be helpful.

4. Oral fluids should be encouraged to prevent dehydration. A soft diet is suggested for patient comfort.

5. Isolation of the infected individual is warranted to prevent spread of the disease.

HAND, FOOT, AND MOUTH DISEASE

Causative Agent: Coxsackie A Virus. The disease is usually caused by coxsackie A-16 virus and tends to occur in epidemics. Although it usually affects children between 1 and 10 years of age, it may occur in adults.

Evaluation. Recent exposure to an infected person should be determined.

Diagnosis

Subjective Findings. There is an incubation period of 2 to 6 days followed by a viral prodrome of low-grade fever and malaise.

Objective Findings. Painful, multiple, small vesicles develop that subsequently ulcerate, generally involving the hard palate, tongue, and buccal mucosa (Fig. 4–3). Multiple small, painful vesicles on the palms and soles and on the ventral surfaces of fingers and toes may be visible (Figs. 4–4 and 4–5). Lymphadenopathy may be present.

Therapy. The disease is self-limiting and re-

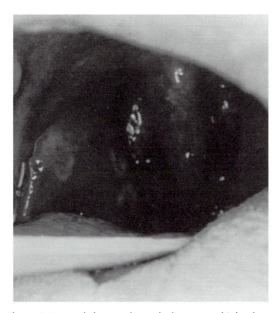

Figure 4–3. Hand, foot, and mouth disease: multiple ulcerations involving the soft palate and tonsillar pillars.

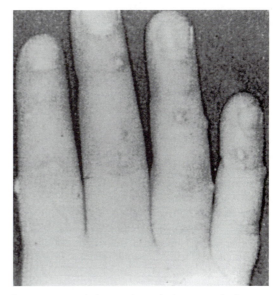

Figure 4–4. Hand, foot, and mouth disease: multiple vesicles involving the fingers.

solves spontaneously in 7 to 14 days. Treatment is palliative and may include antipyretics, analgesics, and mouthrinses. Lesions heal without scarring.

IMPETIGO

Causative Agents: Streptococci or Staphylococci. Impetigo is classified into two distinct types: bullous and nonbullous. The nonbullous type is characterized by crusted lesions that are caused primarily by streptococci and that may be secondarily infected by staphylococci. Bullous impetigo is characterized by bullae or by relatively clean eroded lesions caused by staphylococci. Glomerulonephritis may result from the nonbullous type.

Evaluation. A Gram stain is helpful in bullous impetigo but not in nonbullous impetigo because secondary infection of the latter is common. Throat and skin cultures may be indicated for family members and close contacts because nephritogenic strains are propagated by direct contact.

Diagnosis

Subjective Findings. There is often a history of mild trauma, insect bites, or exposure to other

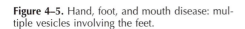

Figure 4–5. Hand, foot, and mouth disease: multiple vesicles involving the feet.

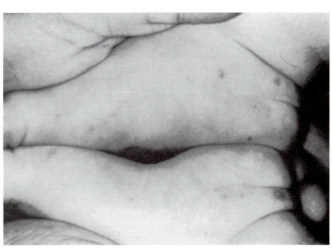

infected persons. The lesions are usually asymptomatic, but occasionally pruritus is a prominent feature.

Objective Findings. In the nonbullous type, multiple lesions develop, which often involve the face and extremities. They are characterized by a thick, adherent, yellowish-brown crust. These lesions may spread and coalesce into large, irregularly shaped lesions. Lymphadenopathy may be present.

In the bullous type of impetigo, flaccid, large bullae may occur anywhere on the body. After 2 to 3 days these bullae rupture, leaving discrete, round lesions. These lesions subsequently coalesce into polycyclic areas that tend to clear centrally. Gram staining of bulla contents reveals gram-positive cocci.

Therapy

Nonbullous Type. For minimal disease, cool water soaks are used to remove crusts, and the infected area is washed with an antiseptic cleaner. This is followed by application of a topical antibiotic two to three times a day. If lesions do not heal quickly with this therapy, systemic antibiotics are indicated.

For moderate or excessive disease, penicillin G or erythromycin is usually effective. Even if penicillin-resistant staphylococci are present, this therapy is usually effective.

Bullous Type. Because the causative organism is generally a penicillin-resistant strain of staphylococci, a semisynthetic penicillinase-resistant penicillin is indicated (i.e., dicloxacillin).

SCARLET FEVER

Causative Agents: Beta-Hemolytic Streptococci. Manifestations of the disease are due to a lack of immunity to erythrogenic toxins elaborated by the streptococci. Immunity to these toxins does not protect against streptococcal infection, however.

Evaluation. Recent exposure of the patient to a person with streptococcal infection should be determined.

Diagnosis

Subjective Findings. Prodromal features of sore throat, fever, and vomiting are regular subjective findings.

Objective Findings. A bright red papular skin rash beginning in skin folds and spreading to the remainder of the body is present. The rash appears 2 to 3 days after the initial symptoms become visible. The tongue is covered with a white coating, with the papillae being erythematous and prominent (strawberry tongue). This coating of the tongue is soon lost, leaving an erythematous, smooth, glistening surface. A grayish-white exudate may cover the tonsils and faucial pillars. Lymphadenopathy is usually present. The skin rash slowly fades and is followed by desquamation of the skin. Throat cultures reveal streptococcal infection.

Therapy

1. Penicillin is the drug of choice.
2. Palliative mouthrinses may be helpful.
3. Early diagnosis and treatment are important to prevent complications, which include local abscess formation, rheumatic fever, arthritis, and glomerulonephritis.

CANDIDIASIS

Causative Agent: *Candida albicans.* In approximately 50% of the population, this organism is part of the normal oral flora. Usually, the presence of this organism is of no clinical significance. In newborns, however, debilitated patients, asthmatic patients on steroid inhalers, or persons on long-term antibiotics whose normal oral flora has been altered, infection may occur.

Evaluation. It is important to identify the underlying etiology, which may include systemic diseases such as diabetes mellitus, leukemia, uremia, aplastic anemia, immunodeficiency syndromes, and immunosuppression.

Diagnosis

Subjective Findings. In cases with esophageal involvement, the patient may complain of sore throat. Otherwise, the patient may be asymptomatic or may complain of a burning or coating sensation in the mouth.

Objective Findings

1. The pseudomembranous form of the infection is characterized by raised, white, curdy plaques, which may appear to lump together in heaps (Fig. 4-6). The erythematous (atrophic) form is characterized by the presence of erythematous surface most commonly involving the palate or tongue. In severe cases there may be erosions and vesicles associated with these changes.
2. Scraping the lesions of the pseudomembranous form leaves a raw, bleeding surface.
3. Lesions may occur on any mucosal surface.
4. Potassium hydroxide (KOH) preparation of a smear reveals hyphae when observed microscopically.

Therapy

1. *Mild disease:* topical antifungal agent (i.e., nystatin)

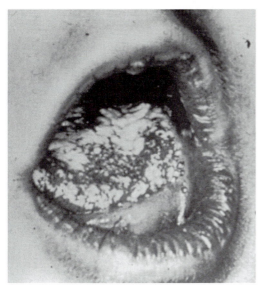

Figure 4–6. Candidiasis: white, curdy plaques coating the tongue.

2. *Moderate disease:* a systemic antifungal agent may be indicated (i.e., ketoconazole).

3. *Severe disease:* systemic antifungal agent (i.e., amphotericin B). This medication requires intravenous administration and is highly nephrotoxic.

Case Study

A 13-year-old male with a history of asthma presents for his recall appointment. An update of his medical history reveals a change in asthma medications to beclomethasone, an inhaled steroid preparation. Your examination reveals a patchy white area with an erythematous border on the palate (Fig. 4–7). When you ask the patient about the lesion, he states that he was unaware of it, although he has had a sore throat for the past several days. A smear of the lesion prepared with 10% KCH reveals the presence of hyphae when observed microscopically.

Diagnosis

The patient's medical history, clinical presentation, and microscopic findings are all consistent with a diagnosis of candidiasis. One of the more common side effects of inhaled steroid therapy is increased susceptibility to candidial infections.

Treatment

Because of the likely esophageal involvement, the patient was placed on fluconazole with total resolution of the infection.

DIABETES MELLITUS

Type I, or insulin-dependent, diabetes mellitus is the most common form in children. Approximately 2 in 1000 children between the ages of 5 and 18 years have the disease.

The development of Type I diabetes is the result of viral or toxic insults to the pancreatic islets in the child genetically predisposed to developing the disorder. The presence of islet cell antibodies in the patient in whom diagnosis has recently been confirmed suggests an autoimmune mechanism in the destruction of the insulin-producing beta cells. Although symptoms of diabetes may develop suddenly, the initial insult may take months to years to manifest clinically.

Evaluation. The suspicion of diabetes usually arises by one or more of the following:

1. *Family history:* Relatives of patients with diabetes are two and a half times more likely to develop the disease than the population at large.

2. *Symptoms:* Polydipsia, polyuria, weight loss with polyphagia, enuresis, recurrent infections, and candidiasis are common findings.

3. Glycosuria may be present.

4. Ketoacidosis and coma are possible.

Diagnosis. Subjective findings include a history of polydipsia, polyuria, polyphagia, and weight loss.

Objective findings include a fasting blood glucose level above 120 mg/dl. The oral glucose tolerance test result is abnormal, and glycosylated hemoglobin test values are elevated.

Periodontal disease is the most consistent oral finding in patients with poorly controlled diabetes mellitus. These patients exhibit increased alveolar bone resorption and inflammatory gingival changes, which may mimic the clinical manifestations of juvenile periodontosis. Xerostomia and

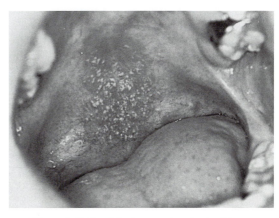

Figure 4–7. Candidiasis secondary to steroid use.

recurrent intraoral abscesses may be present. Enamel hypocalcification and hypoplasia along with reduced salivary flow can predispose these patients to an increased frequency of caries. An altered oral flora with an increase in *Candida albicans,* hemolytic streptococci, and staphylococci is also encountered. Both advanced eruption and delayed eruption of permanent dentition have been reported.

Therapy. The goal of treatment is to control blood glucose to as normal a level as possible, thereby reducing the potential complications of hyperglycemia and ketoacidosis. This generally involves the administration of an intermediate-acting insulin (NPH and Lente). An exciting new treatment modality currently under investigation is pancreatic transplantation.

Dental management of the well-controlled diabetic consists of the following:

1. Advise the patient to eat a normal meal before the appointment to avoid hypoglycemia.

2. If the dental procedure is anticipated to be stressful, consult the patient's physician regarding adjustment of the insulin dosage.

3. Consider using prophylactic antibiotics for surgery, endodontics, and periodontal therapy to minimize the risk of infection.

4. Have a glucose source available to treat the onset of hypoglycemia.

ACUTE LYMPHOBLASTIC LEUKEMIA

Causative Agent. The cause of acute lymphoblastic leukemia (ALL) is unknown, although several theories have been postulated involving viruses and immune surveillance. This disease is the most common childhood malignancy, occurring in approximately 4 in 100,000 children.

Evaluation. The manifestations of ALL are related to the functionally myelosuppressed state of the patient, which results from the overwhelming presence of malignant cells in the bone marrow. These patients demonstrate the pallor of anemia, purpura or bleeding secondary to thrombocytopenia, and prolonged or unusual infections owing to neutropenia.

Diagnosis. Subjective findings include fever, malaise, and occasionally bone pain.

Oral objective findings include the following:

1. Gingival oozing, petechiae, hematoma, or ecchymosis formation is common.

2. Cervical and submandibular lymphadenopathy are possible.

3. Oral ulceration, pharyngitis, and gingival

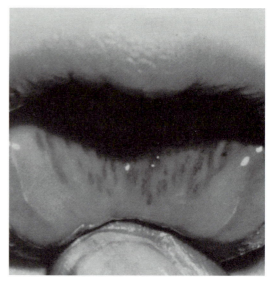

Figure 4–8. Acute lymphoblastic leukemia: large, painful ulceration secondary to chemotherapy.

infection unresponsive to conventional therapy are also important diagnostic determinations.

Systemic objective findings include the following:

1. A peripheral blood smear may show leukoerythroblastic changes.

2. Bone marrow aspiration and biopsy establish a definitive diagnosis.

Therapy. The goal of therapy is to destroy the leukemic cells and allow normal cells to repopulate the marrow. This is generally accomplished with chemotherapy, which may be supplemented with radiotherapy.

Oral complications of therapy include pain, ulceration, hemorrhage, and secondary infections. The prognosis for ALL is constantly improving, with 5-year survival rates of 60% to 80% (Fig. 4–8).

SICKLE CELL ANEMIA

Sickle cell anemia is a hereditary disorder whose clinical manifestations result from an abnormality of the beta chains of the hemoglobin S molecule. Hemoglobin S forms a linear polymer upon deoxygenation, which results in sickling of the red blood cells. Approximately 10% of black Americans carry the trait, and 0.2% have the homozygous form of the disease. Approximately 75,000 people in the United States have the disease.

Evaluation. The disease usually has no clinical

manifestation until a high proportion of the red blood cells contain hemoglobin S. This generally occurs around 6 months of age. An exception to this is the increased risk of infection in infants with the disorder.

Diagnosis

Subjective Findings. Often the earliest clinical presentation is painful swelling of the dorsum of the hand or foot owing to ischemic necrosis of the metacarpal or metatarsal bones. Other manifestations include hepatosplenomegaly, pallor, cardiomegaly, and icterus. Progressive episodes of infarction and scarring in the spleen cause it to decrease in size over time, eventually rendering the patient functionally asplenic.

Objective Findings. Laboratory findings include severe anemia (hemoglobin 5 to 9 g/100 ml) associated with sickled red blood cells, reticulocytosis, and variable hyperbilirubinemia.

Dental findings invariably relate to the extramedullary erythropoiesis, which is demonstrated by the following radiographic changes:

1. Decreased radiodensity with increased prominence of the lamina dura and a coarse trabecular pattern (stepladder appearance)
2. "Hair on end" effect of skull
3. Enamel hypomineralization
4. Increased prevalence of periodontal disease

Therapy. Infections, dehydration, acidosis, and hypoxia can all result in initiation of a painful crisis in patients afflicted with this disorder. Until recently transfusion therapy was the only effective way to manage these complications of the disease. Newly developed therapeutic stategies in treating this disease include pharmacologic approaches, bone marrow and cord blood transplantation, and improved supportive and preventive management. Dental management should ensure adequate hydration and the prevention of infection. Use of an aggressive prevention program, stress-reducing protocols including shorter appointments, and nitrous oxide sedation should be considered. Because diagnosis takes place at birth by neonatal screening, these patients are excellent candidates for an infant dental health program.

Prophylactic antibiotics are indicated for any oral surgical procedure to diminish the potential development of osteomyelitis or postoperative wound infections. (It should be noted that many children with this disorder are placed on daily prophylactic penicillin because of the risk of *Streptococcus pneumoniae* infection; thus, some modification in antibiotic coverage may be indicated for dental procedures.)

HISTIOCYTOSES (HISTIOCYTOSIS X)

The histiocytoses of childhood include a variety of disorders of mononuclear phagocytes and related cells that resemble histiocytes. The disorder probably results from immune dysregulation rather than from a neoplastic condition. The disease is frequently indolent and relapsing, and spontaneous remissions occur. Most patients with this disease are under 15 years of age, although the disease may afflict adults and the elderly. The spectrum of the disease ranges from local involvement of a single bone site to lesions affecting the skin, lymph nodes, lung, thymus, liver, spleen, bone marrow, gastrointestinal tract (including the oral cavity), and the central nervous system. Genetic studies reviewed by Hartman (1980) show that these various clinical manifestations reflect a varied spectrum of a single disease.

Evaluation. Patients with histiocytosis historically have been grouped into three general categories:

1. *Eosinophilic granuloma:* occurs in older children and adults and is characterized by localized lesions confined to bone. This category is currently called benign localized or polyostotic histiocytosis.
2. *Hand-Schüller-Christian disease:* occurs in younger children (aged 2–5 years) with a classic triad of manifestations of skull lesions, diabetes insipidus, and exophthalmos. Bone lesions are common, as is involvement of the gingiva and mandible, which may result in premature loss of teeth. This disease is currently called chronic progressive histiocytosis.
3. *Letterer-Siwe disease:* occurs in infants and is characterized by prominent skin and visceral lesions rather than bone lesions. The spleen, lymph nodes, liver, lungs, and bone marrow are commonly involved, and organ dysfunctions are frequent. This disease is currently called acute or subacute disseminated histiocytosis.

Diagnosis

Benign Localized or Polyostotic Histiocytosis

Subjective Findings. The syndrome is found predominantly in older children as well as adults. There is often an inability to bear weight and tender swelling owing to tissue infiltrates overlying bone lesions.

Objective Findings. The syndrome is characterized by solitary or multiple bone lesions. Radiographically, these lesions appear as destructive radiolucencies, usually with well-defined margins (punched-out lesions) (Fig. 4-9). Dental

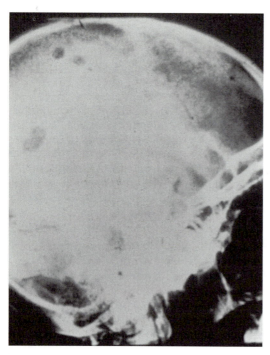

Figure 4–9. Histiocytosis X: punched-out lesions involving the cranium.

findings may include an intraoral mass or swelling, pain, gingivitis, and loose teeth. Oral lesions most often involve the posterior mandible. Histologic examination reveals proliferation of essentially normal, well-differentiated histiocytes. Multinucleated histiocytes are often present. Other inflammatory cells, such as granulocytes, eosinophils, lymphocytes, and plasma cells, are present in varying quantities. The Langerhans cell is prominent in the histologic examination of these lesions.

Chronic Progressive Histiocytosis

Subjective Findings. The disease is found predominantly in younger children aged 2 to 5 years. There are multiple sites of involvement with a chronic relapsing course. Exophthalmos as a result of orbital bone involvement and loss of teeth from gingival infiltration and mandibular involvement are not uncommon.

Objective Findings. Diabetes insipidus with polydipsia and polyuria may result from infiltration of the posterior pituitary. Chronic otitis media owing to involvement of the mastoid and petrous portion of the temporal bone and otitis externa are not uncommon.

Dental findings include histolytic involvement of the teeth and gingiva, often beginning in the periapical region of the teeth. Destruction of the lamina dura results in the radiographic appearance of "floating teeth." Gingival involvement

may also result in premature loss of teeth. The entire mandible may be involved, with bone loss leading to diminished mandibular rami height. Histologic findings are identical to those of benign localized histiocytosis.

Acute Disseminated Histiocytosis

Subjective Findings. Typically, an infant less than 2 years of age is presented with a scaly, seborrheic, eczematoid, sometimes purpuric rash involving the scalp, ear canals, abdomen, intertriginous areas, and face. The rash may be maculopapular or nodulopapular, and ulceration is present.

Objective Findings. Frequently, there are draining ears, lymphadenopathy, hepatosplenomegaly, and, in severe cases, hepatic dysfunction with hypoproteinemia and abnormal clotting factors. Pulmonary symptoms may include cough, tachypnea, and pneumothorax. Anemia and thrombocytopenia occur secondary to involvement of the hematopoietic system. Dental findings include intraosseous jaw lesions, most commonly in the posterior mandibular region. In addition, necrotic and ulcerative soft tissue lesions involving the gingiva are common. Histologic findings are identical to those of benign localized histiocytosis.

Therapy. The following therapies are used for the treatment of histiocytosis:

1. *Surgery:* This modality has a limited role, involving curettage of accessible lesions.
2. *Radiotherapy:* Localized therapy is used, with care to avoid irradiating potentially sensitive normal structures.
3. *Chemotherapy:* Various chemotherapeutic agents have been used to treat these disorders. Careful monitoring of blood counts and clinical status is vital prior to any dental procedures because chemotherapeutic toxicity can cause severe complications in these already immunocompromised patients.

Prognosis. The prognosis for patients with histiocytosis depends on three factors:

1. *Age at onset.* An age of 2 years portends a good prognosis, whereas patients less than 2 years of age tend to do poorly.
2. *Number of organs involved.* Localized disease, with less than four organ systems involved, is a good prognostic sign.
3. *Degree of organ dysfunction.* The specific involvement of three organ systems (hepatic, pulmonary, and hematopoietic), as manifested by organ dysfunction, has been found to be the most important prognostic indicator.

HEMOPHILIA (HEMOPHILIA A; FACTOR VIII DEFICIENCY)

Hemophilia is an X-linked recessive deficiency of factor VIII.

Evaluation. A positive family history is common in most mild to moderate cases. The personal history in these cases often is negative unless the patient has experienced some traumatic or surgical incident (i.e., a persistent oral bleeding episode). In many cases, a positive family history is lacking, but the personal history is significant for multiple bleeding episodes dating from about the age of 1 year or earlier.

Diagnosis

Subjective Findings. Mild to moderate cases may include a history of persistent bleeding, often involving the oral cavity. The sites most commonly involved are the maxillary lip, lingual frenum, and tongue. The onset of these bleeding episodes generally is not until the toddler stage. Subjective findings in severe cases may include chronic joint deformities and contractures secondary to bleeding into joints and muscles.

Objective Findings. Results of laboratory studies include normal bleeding time, normal platelet count and platelet aggregation, normal prothrombin time, and prolonged partial thromboplastin time. An assay is used to determine the severity of factor VIII deficiency. A concentration of factor VIII that is 5% to 30% of normal constitutes a mild deficiency, a level that is 2% to 5% of normal reflects a moderate deficiency, and a concentration that is less than 2% of normal constitutes a severe factor VIII deficiency.

Therapy. Factor VIII–containing materials raise plasma levels of factor by 2% for each unit of factor administered. Such materials include the following:

1. *Fresh frozen plasma.* The amount used is limited by volume considerations.
2. *Cryoprecipitate.* Factor concentration is approximately 20 times that of fresh frozen plasma.
3. *Lyophilized factor VIII preparations* have concentrations of factor that vary from 20 to 100 times that of fresh frozen plasma. Preparations of pooled plasma involve a greater risk of hepatitis and acquired immunodeficiency syndrome (AIDS) compared with cryoprecipitate, which is prepared from single units of plasma.

Nonfactor Products. Epsilon-aminocaproic acid (EACA) inhibits fibrinolysis by blocking the activation of plasminogen to plasmin. Consequently, a formed clot remains intact longer in the presence of EACA.

Recent reports and studies suggest that 1-deamino-8-D-arginine-vasopressin (DDAVP) may be a useful adjunct in the management of hemophilia. It has been shown that the administration of DDAVP results in a transient increase in plasma factor VIII levels and is particularly effective in mild and moderate hemophilia.

Complications of Therapy. Patients with hemophilia should avoid drugs that interfere with platelet function (i.e., aspirin, antihistamines).

Antibodies to factor VIII develop in approximately 8% to 16% of patients receiving factor VIII preparations. The presence of inhibitors is suggested when apparently adequate replacement therapy is ineffective. The presence of inhibitors can be documented via inhibitor assays.

Management of patients who develop inhibitors may involve the following:

1. Administration of products such as Proplex or Konyne, which have activated factors that bypass factor VIII and allow coagulation to occur
2. Massive doses of factor VIII in an attempt to overwhelm the inhibitors
3. Plasmapheresis to remove the inhibitor, in combination with high doses of factor VIII

Dental Considerations. The dentist must consider the severity of the hemophilia (mild, moderate, or severe) and the dental procedure to be performed. A consultation with a hematologist is mandatory prior to any treatment in these patients.

Low-risk procedures generally requiring no replacement therapy in all levels of hemophilia include the following:

1. Dental prophylaxis without deep scaling
2. Infiltration, pericemental, and intrapulpal administration of local anesthesia
3. Operative dentistry during which careful consideration is given to preventing soft tissue trauma
4. Pulpotomy and pulpectomy procedures
5. Placement of orthodontic appliances
6. Normal exfoliation of primary teeth
7. Preventive program (flossing and toothbrushing)
8. Oral radiographs

Moderate-risk dental procedures that may require replacement therapy include the following:

1. Dental prophylaxis with deep scaling
2. Removal of mobile, exfoliating primary teeth
3. Operative dentistry during which soft tissue trauma is anticipated (i.e., placement of stainless steel crowns, utilization of 8A or 14A rubber dam clamps)

High-risk procedures requiring replacement therapy include the following:

1. Block administration of local anesthesia
2. Simple extractions, curettage, and gingivoplasty
3. Multiple extractions, flap surgery or gingivectomy, extraction of bone-impacted teeth, and apicoectomy
4. Orthognathic surgery
5. Endotracheal or nasotracheal intubation

Precautions for hepatitis and AIDs are indicated for all hemophiliacs who have received blood products.

PEDIATRIC HUMAN IMMUNODEFICIENCY VIRUS INFECTION

Causative Agent. Human immunodeficiency virus (HIV) is the causative agent responsible for the disease called AIDS. The effects of this virus render the host immunocompromised and susceptible to opportunistic infections as a result of a loss of T4 lymphocytes. Current epidemiologic research implies that the virus may be spread most commonly through contaminated blood, semen, vaginal secretions, and breast milk. Although the virus has been cultured from other secretions, including tears, saliva, and urine, data suggest that exposure to these fluids rarely results in infection. Consequently, the virus is not easily transmitted by casual contact such as shaking hands; sharing food, eating utensils, drinking glasses, or towels; or hugging and kissing on the cheeks or lips.

Two major groups of pediatric patients may be afflicted with this disease. First, infants may acquire the virus perinatally. This maternal-infant transmission occurs in approximately 7000 pregnant women in the United States annually. A greater than 20% transmission rate of HIV from mother to child previously resulted in approximately 1500 children born with the infection annually. The prognosis for these children was extremely poor with the thought that most would succumb quickly to opportunistic infections. Recent advances have resulted in a marked improvement in these statistics. Zidovudine, an antiviral agent, when administered to HIV-infected pregnant women and their newborns, has been shown to reduce HIV transmission from over 20% to under 10%. Studies have found that children born with HIV infection have a 50%

chance of developing severe signs or symptoms by 5 years of age and a 75% chance of surviving beyond 5 years of age. The estimated time from birth to onset of severe symptoms is 6.6 years, and the mean survival time is 9.4 years. Table 4–1 displays the transmission categories for children less than 13 years of age. Second, adolescents and teenagers may acquire the virus through sexual contact (including sexual abuse) or intravenous drug abuse. Table 4–2 displays the transmission categories for adolescents and adults (HIV/AIDS Surveillance, 1991). Approximately 73,000 people over the age of 13 years were diagnosed with HIV or AIDS between January 1994 and June 1997. Seventeen percent of these people (7853) were between the ages of 13 and 24 years. The number of people diagnosed in this age group has remained relatively constant since 1995. Because of the relatively long incubation period of this virus, it is likely that many of these adults actually acquired the infection during their teenage years.

Evaluation. Like adults, children over 15 months of age may be diagnosed with HIV infection via an anti-HIV antibody assay (an enzyme-linked immunosorbent assay—ELISA) and the Western blot assay. Children under this age present a diagnostic dilemma, however, owing to the placental transfer of maternal anti-HIV anti-

TABLE 4–1. Pediatric AIDS Transmission Categories

Pediatric (<13 Years Old) Exposure Category: Transmission Group Cases	Percentage of Cumulative Total of Pediatric AIDS Cases
Hemophilia/coagulation disorder	5
Mother with/at risk for HIV infection	84
IV drug use	
Sex with IV drug user	
Sex with bisexual male	
Sex with person with hemophilia	
Born in Pattern II country*	
Sex with person born in Pattern II country	
Sex with transfusion recipient with HIV infection	
Sex with HIV-infected person, risk not specified	
Receipt of blood transfusion, blood components, or tissue	
Has HIV infection, risk not specified	
Receipt of blood transfusion, blood components, or tissue	9
Undetermined	2

HIV/AIDS Surveillance Report, 1997 (reprinted in Federal Register *9*(1):8, 1997).
*See explanation at Table 4–2.

TABLE 4–2. Adult and Adolescent AIDS Transmission Categories

Transmission Group	Percentage of Cumulative Total of AIDS Cases for Adults/Adolescents
Homosexual/bisexual men	59
Intravenous drug users (female and heterosexual male)	22
Homosexual/bisexual contact and IV drug users	7
Hemophilia/coagulation disorder	1
Heterosexual contact:	5
Sex with IV drug user	
Sex with person with hemophilia	
Sex with bisexual male	
Sex with transfusion recipient with HIV infection	
Sex with HIV-infected person, risk not specified	
Born in Pattern II country*	
Sex with person born in Pattern II country*	
Receipt of blood transfusion, blood components, or tissue†	2
Other/undetermined‡	4

*Pattern II transmission is observed in areas of central, eastern, and southern Africa and in some Caribbean countries. In these countries, most of the reported cases occur in heterosexuals, and the male-to-female ratio is approximately 1:1. Intravenous drug use and homosexual transmission either do not occur or occur at a low level.

†Includes 14 transfusion recipients who received blood screened for HIV antibody and 1 tissue recipient.

‡"Other" refers to three health care workers who underwent seroconversion to HIV and experienced AIDS after occupational exposure to HIV-infected blood. "Undetermined" refers to patients whose mode of exposure to HIV is unknown. This includes patients under investigation; patients who died, were lost to follow-up, or refused interview; and patients whose mode of exposure to HIV remained undetermined after investigation.

HIV/AIDS Surveillance, August 1991, p. 9. Reprinted in Federal Register 56(235):64015, 1991.

bodies. Consequently, research is currently being directed toward developing more specific assays to aid in the diagnosis of this disease in this age group.

Diagnosis

Subjective Findings. Most recent data suggest a bimodal pattern for the development of AIDS in congenitally acquired disease. Approximately one fifth of infected children present with an AIDS-defining illness in the first 9 months of life. After the first year there appears to be a steady but slower rate of progression to AIDS.

AIDS. Children with HIV infection display a wide variety of symptoms, signs, and pathologic conditions. Certain of these features are common and specific to the pediatric population, such as lymphocytic interstitial pneumonitis. Other common early findings include persistent fever, prolonged and unexplained diarrhea with subsequent weight loss, failure to thrive, generalized lymphadenopathy, hepatosplenomegaly, and recurrent infections. Among these infections, *Pneumocystis carinii* is the most commonly encountered. Oral findings include parotid swelling, frequent candidal infections, and gingivitis characterized by intense erythema of the marginal gingiva. Additionally, severe herpetic gingivostomatitis has been observed in several pediatric patients with AIDS. The emergence of acyclovir-resistant strains of herpes simplex has been reported in both children and adults.

Objective Findings. The presentation of a severe opportunistic infection such as *P. carinii* pneumonia along with a high CD4 (T helper cell) count during the first year of life is considered a distinguishing feature of pediatric HIV infection. Other significant findings include a depressed T-suppressor lymphocyte count, with a polyclonal elevation of immunoglobulins.

Therapy. Although no therapy is currently available for the underlying immunodeficiency, prevention and treatment of complications and antiviral therapy may improve survival.

Dental Considerations. As with any immunocompromised patient, a dental infection may be life-threatening to the child with AIDS. Therefore, an aggressive prevention program is imperative. Additionally, consultation with the patient's physician is strongly recommended to determine the individual's immune status, current medications, and need for prophylactic antibiotics. Specific oral conditions afflicting these patients and their therapy are outlined in Table 4–3. Oral candidiasis is the most common opportunistic infection in children with HIV. The clinical manifestation of this infection may take several forms, including pseudomembranous, erythematous, hyperplastic variants, and angular cheilosis. A significant percentage of these patients also experience esophageal involvement characterized by profound dysphagia. The severity of the infection dictates the treatment modality of topical or systemic antifungal agents (see earlier section on candidiasis).

Bacterial infections generally take the form of an atypical gingivitis characterized by a linear erythematous appearance of the facial and interproximal gingival margins. These lesions are generally unresponsive to conventional oral hygiene measures but may improve with twice-daily rinsing with 0.12% chlorhexidine.

Viral infections afflicting these patients generally belong to the herpes virus groups, namely herpes simplex, varicella-zoster, cytomegalovirus, and Epstein-Barr. Although all of these are un-

TABLE 4–3. Oral Conditions Afflicting AIDS Patients

Condition	Therapy	Child	Adolescent/Adult

Candidiasis	Antifungals—
	  Nystatin (topical)
	  Miconazole (topical)
	  Chlortrimazole (topical)
	  Ketoconazole (systemic)
	  Fluconazole (systemic)
	  Amphotericin B (systemic)
		Common	Common

HIV-associated gingivitis	Plaque removal/control, chlorhexidine rinses	Uncommon	Common
HIV-associated periodontitis	Plaque/removal, debridement, povidone-iodine, metronidazole, chlorhexidine	Uncommon	Common
Necrotizing stomatitis	Debridement, povidone-iodine, metronidazole, chlorhexidine	Rare	Uncommon
Herpes simplex	Oral acyclovir if not self-limiting, if prolonged, or if frequently recurrent	Uncommon	Uncommon
Herpes zoster	Oral and/or intravenous acyclovir	Rare	Uncommon
Aphthous ulceration	Steroid, usually topically, less commonly intralesionally, rarely systemically	Uncommon	Common
Hairy leukoplakia	Does not usually require treatment; oral acyclovir for severe case	Rare	Common
Xerostomia	Salivary stimulation (sialogogues)	Rare	Common
Kaposi's sarcoma	Palliative excision, chemotherapy, radiation therapy	Rare	Common
Oral warts	Excision	Rare	Uncommon
Parotid swelling	Does not usually require treatment; severe enlargement may respond to systemic steroids	Common	Rare

Modified from Greenspan JS, et al: Oral manifestations of HIV infection. Oral Surg 73:142–144, 1992.

common in children, herpes simplex (herpetic gingivostomatitis) is the most frequent of these infections encountered in the child with HIV infection. The clinical manifestations of this infection are described elsewhere in this chapter, and management in the HIV-infected patient includes administration of the antiviral drug acyclovir, which has been shown to be effective in treating viral infections in the immunocompromised host.

The clinician should appreciate that HIV-infected patients may present with atypical manifestations of common infections or infections with atypical causes. It is incumbent upon the practitioner to recognize these conditions to facilitate appropriate treatment or referral.

BIBLIOGRAPHY

Bernick SM, Cohen W, Baker L, Laster B: Dental disease in children with diabetes mellitus. J Periodontol 46:241, 1975.

Burns JC: Diagnostic methods for herpes simplex infection: A review. Oral Surg 50:346, 1980.

Conner EM, Sperling RS, Gelber R, et al: Reduction of maternal-infant transmission of human immunodeficiency virus type 1 with zidovudine treatment. N Engl J Med 331:1173, 1994.

Charache S, Terrin ML, Moore RD, et al: Effect of hydroxyurea on the frequency of painful crises in sickle cell anemia. N Engl J Med 332:1317, 1996.

Diagnosis and reporting of HIV and AIDS in states with integrated HIV and surveillance, United States, January 1994–June 1997. MMWR 47:309, 1998.

Epstein JB, Pearsall NN, Truelove EL: Oral candidiasis: Effects of antifungal therapy upon clinical signs and symptoms, salivary antibody and mucosal adherence of *Candida albicans.* Oral Surg 51:32, 1981.

Evans BE: Dental Care in Hemophilia. New York, National Hemophilia Foundation, 1977.

Fallon J, Eddy J, Wiener L, Pizzo PA: Human immunodeficiency virus infection in children. J Pediatr 114:1–30, 1989.

Friedman A: Superficial bacterial and fungal infections of the skin. Adv Pediatr Infect Dis 5:205–219, 1990.

Gershon A: Second episodes of varicella: Degree and duration of immunity. Pediatr Infect Dis J 9:306, 1990.

Gershon AA: Management of infections due to herpes simplex virus. Pediatr Infect Dis 3 (3 Suppl):S24, 1984.

Greenspan JS, et al: Oral manifestations of HIV infection. Oral Surg 73:142–144, 1992.

Hartman KS: Histiocytosis X: A review of 114 cases with oral involvement. Oral Surg 49:38, 1980.

HIV/AIDS Surveillance, August 1991, p 9 (reprinted in Federal Register 56[235]:64015, 1991).

Huebner RJ, et al: Herpangina, etiologic studies of a specific infectious disease. JAMA 145:628, 1951.

Keys DS: Hand, foot, and mouth disease. Aust Dent J 19:1, 1974.

King DL, Steinhauer W, Garcia-Godoy F, Elkins CJ: Herpetic gingivostomatitis and teething difficulty in infants. Pediatr Dent 14:82, 1992.

Kline MW: Oral manifestations of pediatric human immunodeficiency virus infection: A review of the literature. Pediatrics 97:380, 1996.

Kolmich JR: Oral candidiasis. Oral Surg 50:411, 1980.

Leggott PJ: Oral manifestations of HIV infection in children. Oral Surg 73:187–192, 1992.

Mannucci PM, Ruggeri ZM, Pareti FI, Capitanio A: 1-Deamino-8 D-arginine vasopressin: A new pharmacological approach to the management of hemophilia and von Willebrand's disease. Lancet 1:869, 1977.

Mintz GA, Rose SL: Diagnosis of oral herpes simplex virus infections. Oral Surg 58:486, 1984.

Nichols C, Laster LL, Bodak-Gyovai LZ: Diabetes mellitus and periodontal disease. J Periodontol 49:85, 1978.

Perna JJ, Eskinazi DP: Treatment of oro-facial herpes simplex infections with acyclovir: A review. Oral Surg Oral Med Oral Pathol 65:689, 1988.

Peters RB, Bahn AN, Barens G: *Candida albicans* in the oral cavities of diabetics. J Dent Res 45:771, 1976.

Petersen DE, Sonis ST: Oral Complications of Cancer Chemotherapy. Boston, Martinus Nijhoff, 1983.

Powell D: General dental management. *In* Boone DC (ed): Comprehensive Management of Hemophilia. Philadelphia, FA Davis, 1976.

Sanger RG, Bystrom EB: Radiographic bone changes in sickle cell anemia. J Oral Med 32:32, 1977.

Sanger RG, McTique DJ: Sickle cell anemia—pathology and management. J Dent Handicap 3:9, 1978.

Schwentker FF, et al: The epidemiology of scarlet fever. Am J Hyg 38:27, 1943.

Ship I, Miller MF, Ram C: A retrospective study of recurrent herpes labialis in a professional population, 1958–1971. Oral Surg 44:723, 1977.

Shklar G: Oral reflections of infectious diseases. Postgrad Med 49:87, 1971.

Sonis A, Musselman RJ: Oral bleeding in classic hemophilia. Oral Surg 53:363, 1982.

Spruance SL: Prophylactic chemotherapy with acyclovir for recurrent herpes labialis. J Med Virol Suppl 1:27–32, 1993.

Spruance SL, Rea TL, Thoming C, et al: Penciclovir cream for the treatment of herpes labialis. A randomized, multicenter, double-blind, placebo-controlled trial. JAMA 277:1374, 1997.

Stafford R, Sonis ST, Lockhart PB, et al: Oral pathoses as diagnostic indicators in leukemia. Oral Surg 50:134, 1980.

Vierrou AM, de la Fuente B, Poole AE, Hoyer LW: DDAVP (desmopressin) in the dental management of patients with mild or moderate hemophilia and von Willebrand's disease. Pediatr Dent 7:297, 1985.

Walters MC, Patience M, Leisenring W, et al: Bone marrow transplantation for sickle cell anemia. N. Engl J Med 335:369, 1996.

Wagner JE, Keman NA, Steinbuch M, et al: Allogeneic sibling umbilical-cord-blood transplantation in children with malignant and non-malignant disease. Lancet 346:214, 1995.

Wegner H: Increment of caries in young diabetics. Caries Res 9:91, 1975.

Willman CL, Busque L, Griffith BB, et al: Langerhans'-cell histiocytosis (histiocytosis X): A clonal proliferative disease. N Engl J Med 331:154, 1994.

Chapter 5

Topics in Pediatric Physiology

Dianne M. McBrien

Chapter Outline

The treatment of children presents particular challenges to the health care professional. The body of the pediatric patient is not simply a miniaturized version of his adult counterpart; child physiology and anatomy significantly differ from those of adults. Pediatric dentists must consider these differences when making therapeutic choices about young patients, especially when treatment includes drug therapy. Route and rate of drug administration, dosage, onset and duration of action, and possibility of toxicity are all influenced by the unique physiology of childhood.

This chapter reviews basic principles of pediatric physiology—including pharmacokinetic characteristics of the child—and anatomy. In the interests of simplicity, the material is presented by organ system. Because a comprehensive review of these subjects is beyond the scope of this chapter, the text stresses only those principles that differ significantly from those of the adult patient. Wherever possible, clinical applications to pediatric dentistry are discussed.

RESPIRATORY SYSTEM

Anatomy

Several anatomic features of the pediatric respiratory tract predispose the young patient to obstruction and collapse of both large and small airways.

A child's upper respiratory tract is prone to obstruction at several sites. The narrow nasal passages, tongue/oral cavity disproportion, and decreased airway diameter characteristic of infants and young children predispose this patient population to partial or complete upper airway obstruction. Additional risk may be generated by routine office procedures: A tightly clamped mask over the nares, a mouth pack depressing the oral cavity floor, or a retractor displacing the tongue posteriorly all may increase the likelihood of upper airway obstruction (Campbell et al., 1982). The secretions and edema associated with upper respiratory infections can also compromise the pediatric airway and should be kept in mind when an acutely ill child reports for an elective procedure. Postponement of the procedure is generally recommended until the child has been free of symptoms for 1 week.

Anatomic differences in the child's chest cage can also contribute to respiratory problems. The child's chest wall is more elastic than that of an adult, which means that lower ventilation pressures are needed to expand the lungs. The sternum is less rigid, which means that ribs and intercostal muscles have less support. In a resting position, the child's ribs are more horizontally placed than those of the adult; this positional difference makes intercostal muscle retraction inefficient. Thus, the diaphragm becomes the primary breathing muscle in the pediatric patient. Anything that limits diaphragmatic excursion should therefore be avoided, including the supine position that promotes gastric organ pressure on the diaphragm. Instead, a 20- to 30-degree head-up position is recommended by many authors to avoid such pressure and thereby minimize risk of regurgitation and aspiration (Campbell et al., 1982).

Lung infrastructure is different in the pediatric population as well. The majority of alveoli are formed after birth; indeed, the adult number of alveoli is generally present only at about the sixth year of life (Johnson et al., 1978). Although ratios of lung volume to body size are similar throughout the lifespan, children have a greater proportion of alveolar surface area to lung size.

Physiology

Because of this relative difference in alveolar surface area, children have a greater rate of *alveolar ventilation* (AV) per unit of area—proportionally greater exchange of gas across the alveoli.

The total volume of gas exchanged, however, is less than that of the adult, as is the *functional residual capacity* (FRC). FRC is defined as the volume of gas remaining in the lungs at the end of a normal expiration.

Drug Considerations

The ratio of AV to FRC helps to determine the rate at which changes in inspired gas concentration effect a clinical response. Although AV transports inhaled gas through the bloodstream and to the brain, FRC determines how much gas remains in the lungs during normal breathing. Thus, as the AV/FRC ratio increases, the body reacts more quickly to changes in inhaled gas concentration.

Given the child's high AV and low FRC, the pediatric AV/FRC ratio is almost five times that of an adult (Lerman, 1993). This ratio difference means that children react more rapidly to inhaled gases, such as nitrous oxide and halothane, and can be adequately anesthetized with lower gas concentrations than those required for adult patients. For this reason and because of some unique aspects of the pediatric heart discussed later in this chapter, children are at higher risk for overdose effects from inhalants, including hypotension, bradycardia, and hypoventilation. Careful monitoring of vital signs is therefore essential in children undergoing inhalant anesthesia for dental procedures.

CARDIOVASCULAR SYSTEM

Physiology

Immediately after birth, the infant cardiovascular system begins a series of complex changes that will continue for the next decade (Johnson et al., 1978). After umbilical cord clamping and the first extrauterine breaths, pulmonary vascular resistance falls and the heart itself undergoes several changes including closure of the ductus arteriosus and foramen ovale.

Other physiologic changes continue throughout infancy and childhood. The heart rate, which averages about 120 in the newborn, decreases throughout childhood: by 4 years of age, rates are less than 100. Adult heart rates are generally reached by 10 to 12 years of age (Table 5-1).

Cardiac output, defined as the product of heart rate and *stroke volume*—the amount of blood pumped by one contraction of the left ventricle—is influenced by several variables in the child. The infant heart is relatively inelastic and cannot make rapid changes in stroke volume. Thus, the heart rate is a much more important determinant of cardiac output in infants and

TABLE 5–1. Changes in Heart Rate During Development

Age	Mean Heart Rate
Newborn	115–170
6 months	100–150
1 year	90–135
3 years	80–125
5 years	80–120
10 years	75–110
15 years	70–110
Adult	70

young children than it is in adults; a significant drop in heart rate can result in decreased cardiac output and hypotension. At the same time, parasympathetic tone is more marked in the immature nervous system, which means that this age group is more prone to significant bradycardias with vagal stimulation. Examples of maneuvers producing vagal stimulation include defecation, bladder distension, pressure on the eyeballs, application of throat packs, and tracheal intubation. Because of the potential for vagally induced bradycardia with intubation, children undergoing manipulation of the airway are frequently premedicated with atropine or a similar parasympathetic blocking agent (Anderson, 1991; Campbell et al., 1982).

Blood pressure, in contrast, tends to rise throughout childhood. Mean systolic blood pressure in newborns ranges from 75 to 85 mm Hg; there is a 5 to 10 mm Hg increase over the first several weeks of life. Adult blood pressure values are generally reached by early adolescence. Table 5-2 displays average blood pressures for children.

Cardiac output also changes with age. Cardiac output per kilogram of body weight is highest in the newborn and gradually declines in the first several weeks of life. The relatively noncompliant infant myocardium adapts poorly to sudden changes in afterload; fluid overload and systemic hypertension produce cardiac failure more quickly in infants (Anderson, 1991).

Drug Considerations

Changes in cardiac output can dramatically affect the uptake of inhaled anesthetic agents. Sudden decreases in heart rate result in decreased cardiac output, which in turn increases the rate of inhaled anesthetic uptake. Because 40% of a child's cardiac output perfuses the brain, increases in inhaled anesthetic uptake associated with decreased cardiac output can significantly depress the central nervous system. These depressant effects can include central reduction in vasomotor tone and peripheral vasodilation, which can worsen the hypotension associated with significant bradycardia (Campbell et al., 1982).

Because of these potential adverse effects, inhaled anesthetics should be used carefully in the pediatric population. These agents act more rapidly in children than in adults, and children are adequately sedated by lower gas concentrations than those required for adults.

To minimize the hypotensive response associated with potential drops in heart rate, pediatric patients should be well-hydrated prior to procedures requiring inhaled or intravenous sedation. Recurrent vomiting, diarrhea, or poor oral intake in the days prior to the procedure are appropriate indications to reschedule.

GASTROINTESTINAL SYSTEM

The gastrointestinal tract undergoes continuous developmental change from birth to old age. Because many drugs are absorbed and metabolized by the gut, these changes must be considered when administering medications to children. There are several important physiologic differences in the child's gastrointestinal system:

Decreased Acidity. In infants and young children, immature gastric mucosa secretes low levels of acid; adult levels of gastric acidity are generally not reached until 3 years of age (Morselli, 1976). Before this time, the low acidity of the infant gut favors absorption of weakly acidic drugs, such as penicillins and cephalosporins, whereas the absorption of weakly basic drugs such as the benzodiazepines is delayed.

Altered Motility. Gastric emptying times are significantly longer during infancy. Average emptying times in the young infant can reach 8 hours and only reach adult values—2 to 3 hours—between 6 and 8 months of age (Morselli, 1976). Longer emptying times combined with the irregular peristalsis of infancy generally result in slower gastric drug absorption.

Altered Hepatic Metabolism. Many drugs are metabolized by the liver. Hepatic enzymes may act to detoxify a drug or to alter it into a more potent form. Because infants and young children are relatively deficient in these enzymes, they are at high risk for toxicity if not dosed correctly. Low levels of cytochrome P-450 en-

TABLE 5–2. Changes in Blood Pressure During Development

Age	Mean Systolic Blood Pressure (mm Hg)
Newborn	60–75
6 months	80–90
1 year	96
3 years	100
5 years	100
10 years	110
15 years	120
Adult	125

zymes are associated with sluggish oxidation of diazepam, phenytoin, and phenobarbital in the neonate; all of these drugs thus have prolonged clinical effects in this age group. Glucuronyl transferase, which acts to conjugate drugs into excretable form, is also deficient in the neonate but reaches adult levels after the first month of life. Morphine, acetaminophen, steroids, and sulfa antibiotics are all conjugated by glucuronyl transferase and thus are used with caution in the neonate (Morselli, 1976; Radde and Kalow, 1993).

The infant liver is also deficient in pseudocholinesterase: enzyme levels are at 60% of adult levels for the first several months of life. Even when calculated on an adjusted body weight scale, succinylcholine doses do not reach adult levels until after 2 years of age (Nightingale et al., 1966). Succinylcholine is therefore administered with caution to infant patients, who may respond with prolonged apnea.

RENAL SYSTEM

Although drugs can be excreted by a number of physiologic routes—examples include sweat, bile, and feces—the vast majority undergo renal excretion. Because of its immature capacity, the young kidney is less competent to excrete drug. Most renally excreted drugs are cleared by glomerular filtration, tubular transport, or a combination of both processes.

The *glomerular filtration rate* (GFR)—the volume of fluid filtered by the kidney per unit of time—doubles its newborn value by 2 months of age; adult levels are roughly five times the newborn level and are approached at about 12 months of age (Coulthard, 1985; Radde, 1993b). The GFR participates in the excretion of such commonly used pediatric drugs as the penicillins, short-acting barbiturates, and phenobarbital; recommended dosages of these agents for infants and toddlers are calculated to consider the low infant GFR.

Tubular transport describes a group of mechanisms that transfer drug and drug metabolites across renal tubular epithelium. Drugs in which tubular transport plays an excretory role include morphine, atropine, and sulfa antibiotics (Radde, 1993b). Many such drugs have decreased tubular transport rates in young infants and thus have narrower margins of toxicity in this patient population.

BLOOD AND BODY FLUIDS

Terminology

Drug metabolism and excretion are profoundly affected by the size of various body fluid compartments. Fluid distribution among these compartments is significantly different in infancy and childhood, which in turn alters the action of certain drugs in this age group.

A brief review of body fluid nomenclature may be helpful at this point. The *total body water* space consists of *intracellular* (ICF) and *extracellular* (ECF) fluid compartments. The *volume of distribution* (Vd) is that volume into which a drug is distributed in the body at equilibrium. Although Vd is usually measured in plasma—the volume of plasma at a given drug concentration that is required to account for all drug in the body—many drugs are distributed into body tissues as well. Thus, the Vd often may be estimated as greater than the total plasma volume.

Physiology

Alterations in Body Fluids. As the child grows, changes in body mass are accompanied by changes in body fluid compartments. Although total body water equals 80% of the infant's weight, it makes up only 50% to 60% of normal adult body weight (Table 5–3). Much of this volume loss comes from the ECF compartment. Because so much of infant weight is water, any water-soluble drug must be dosed at higher levels per unit of body weight to attain therapeutic concentration in this age group (Anderson, 1991).

Plasma Protein Differences. A number of plasma proteins function to bind drug in the bloodstream. Plasma proteins both transport drug and render it less physiologically active while bound. Several of these proteins, including serum albumin and plasma globulin, are deficient in the newborn and young infant. Certain drugs that are highly protein-bound, such as warfarin

TABLE 5–3. Differences in Distribution of Body Fluids Between Infants and Adults

	Infants	Adults
Total body water	80%	50% (males), 60% (females)
Extracellular fluid	35–40%	20%
Intracellular fluid	40–45%	40%

and digoxin, must be dosed at relatively low levels per unit of body weight in these patients (Radde, 1993a).

BODY HABITUS AND INTEGUMENT

Children are obviously smaller than adults. It makes intuitive sense that they need smaller drug doses to maintain therapeutic drug concentrations and that smaller doses are needed to produce toxicity. The "maximum safe dose" listed in standard drug reference manuals is frequently enough to overdose a pediatric patient; weight-based formulas are much safer in the pediatric population and are appropriate in all but the smallest neonates.

Not only is the pediatric patient smaller, but his or her proportions are also different from those of the adult. Because a child's height triples from birth to adulthood, but weight increases 20-fold during that same period, many professionals think that *body surface area* (BSA) is a more accurate parameter on which to base drug dosage (Crawford, 1950). Measured in square meters, BSA is estimated by plotting the child's height and weight on a nomogram. The ratio of BSA to body weight is highest in the neonate and falls to about one sixth of this level when adult proportions are reached just before puberty (Cole, 1993). Although BSA is rarely used in the clinical setting—it is inconvenient to calculate and unwieldy to use—it has been shown to be proportional to multiple physiologic variables, such as fluid requirements, oxygen consumption, metabolic rate, and cardiac output.

The tissue composition of infants and children differs as well, depending on developmental stage. Fat makes up 10% to 15% of full-term newborn weight, increases to 20% to 25% during the first several months of life, and then declines during the toddler and preschool years as the child becomes more active. Some commonly used dental sedatives—the benzodiazepines and barbiturates—are lipid-soluble and are extensively bound by fatty tissue, which decreases serum drug levels. It follows that children with lower percentages of body fat may be more sensitive to these agents (Morselli et al., 1973).

REFERENCES

Anderson JA: Physiologic principles in pediatric dentistry. *In* Pinkham JR (ed): Pediatric Dentistry, Principles in Pediatric Dentistry. Philadelphia, WB Saunders, 1991.

Campbell RL, Weiner M, Stewart LM: General anesthesia for the pediatric patient. J Oral Maxillofacial Surg *40:*497–506, 1982.

Cole CH (ed): The Harriet Lane Handbook, A Manual for Pediatric House Officers, 11th ed. Chicago, Year Book, 1993.

Coulthard MG: Maturation of glomerular filtration in preterm and mature babies. Early Hum Dev *11:*281–293, 1985.

Crawford JD, et al: Simplification of drug dosage calculation by applications of the surface area principle. Pediatrics *5:*783–789, 1950.

Johnson TR, Moore WM, Jeffries JE: Children are Different: Development Physiology. Columbus, OH, Ross Laboratories, 1978.

Lerman J: Anesthesia. *In* Radde I, Macleod S (eds): Pediatric Pharmacology and Therapeutics. St. Louis, CV Mosby, 1993, pp 476–479.

Morselli PL, Principi N, Tognoni G, et al: Diazepam elimination in premature and full term infants, and children. J Perinatol Med *1:*133–141, 1973.

Morselli P: Clinical pharmacokinetics in neonates. Clin Pharmacokinet *1:*81–98, 1976.

Nightingale DA, Glass A, Bachman L: Neuromuscular blockade by succinylcholine in children. Anesthesiology *27:*736, 1966.

Radde IC: Drugs and protein binding. *In* Radde I, Macleod S (eds): Pediatric Pharmacology and Therapeutics. St. Louis, CV Mosby, 1993a, pp 31–36.

Radde IC: Renal function and elimination of drugs during development. *In* Radde I, Macleod S (eds): Pediatric Pharmacology and Therapeutics. St. Louis, CV Mosby, 1993b, pp 87–103.

Radde IC, Kalow W: Drug biotransformation and its development. *In* Radde I, Macleod S (eds): Pediatric Pharmacology and Therapeutics. St Louis, CV Mosby, 1993, pp 60–65.

Chapter 6

Nonpharmacologic Issues in Pain Perception and Control

Stephen Wilson

Chapter Outline

The English word *pain* is derived from an ancient Greek word meaning penalty and a Latin word which meant punishment as well as penalty. When the term pain is used in clinical dentistry or medicine, it is synonymous with strong discomfort. It is important to realize that despite the distress experienced by the person in pain, pain has a uniquely purposeful and necessary function. Pain signals real or apparent tissue damage that thereby energizes the organism to take action in relieving or alleviating its presence. In this sense, it is a desirable experience for maintaining and guiding the activities in life.

It is important to understand that pain is more than just a sensation and a consequential response. It is a highly complex, multifaceted interaction of physical, chemical, humoral, affective (emotional), cognitive, psychological, behavioral, and social elements. Certainly, the determinants of how an individual interprets and reacts to pain are not clearly understood. The body of knowledge surrounding the understanding of pain, however, recently has begun to evolve and is accelerating rapidly into a scientific and useful discipline.

An interesting and clinically relevant paralleling experience to pain is the presence of anticipatory responses secondarily acquired from the pain experience. These are conceptualized and broadly referred to as "stress" and "fear." Children and adults can be profoundly influenced by the processes attending many events perceived as fearful, stressful, or both, including various dental procedures. For example, the 2-year-old child who presents with painful, abscessed maxillary anterior teeth due to nursing bottle caries and poorly endures the injection of local anesthesia and extractions while restrained in a papoose board will most likely develop strong disruptive and avoidance behaviors. Such behaviors may include crying with or without tears, placing hands over the mouth, refusing to open the mouth, kicking, screaming, shaking of the head, spitting, and biting. These may manifest during subsequent dental appointments.

Likewise, adult patients who have been hurt either as a child or as an adult by an inconsiderate, unempathetic dentist may have difficulty making and keeping appointments.

DEFINITION OF PAIN

Pain is a highly personalized state attending tissue damage that is either real (e.g., skin laceration) or apparent (e.g., excess bowel distention) as a result of an adequate stimulus. Under normal circumstances, the state of pain implies that there is a simultaneous activation of cognitive, emotional, and behavioral consequences that provides both motivation and a direction to action.

Pain can fluctuate in intensity and quality as a consequence of the passage of time. This may be as significant to the individual as the original insult. For instance, the intensely sharp, shooting pain in the lower back of a person who used an improper weight-lifting technique may change over time (and therapies) to an intermittent deadening, dull ache that may significantly interfere with a routine lifestyle.

Physiologically, pain involves neural signals that are transmitted over a multitude of pathways involving neurons that are specialized in space, biochemistry, size, and shape. These signals induce a host of secondary responses that may become organized in a hierarchy of systems involving portions of the central nervous system (CNS). At the physiologic level, some of these responses involve further transmission of neural signals and the release of neurochemicals and humorally active chemicals (e.g., gamma amino butyric acid [GABA, a neurotransmitter] and endogenous opioids [enkephalins]). Other systems within this response hierarchy include those which activate motor activities for purposeful escape; still others result in emotional and cognitive appreciation of the pain experience.

Research is discovering that the emotional and cognitive elements in the pain process play critical roles in the degree of pain awareness and, possibly more importantly, in the individual's ability to induce self-control while enduring the suffering or its consequences (Weisenberg, 1989). For instance, cognitive mechanisms (e.g., cognitive dissociation) that reduce the *perceived* quality and quantity of discomfort can be effectively taught to a patient prior to the experience of clinical or laboratory-induced pain. Children, through the process of suggestion, can be taught (to varying degrees) to ignore or to inhibit responsiveness to painful stimuli during cancer therapies (Weisenberg, 1977; Zeltzer and LeBaron, 1982).

THEORIES OF PAIN PERCEPTION: WHY AND HOW IT IS EXPERIENCED

Specificity

In the late 19th century, it was believed that the pain experience was merely a function of activating a particular set of neurons that resulted, metaphorically speaking, in a "ringing of the bell" at higher levels of the CNS signifying discomfort (Melzack and Wall, 1965; Sternbach, 1968). The neural receptors (i.e., free nerve endings) and their pathways were considered specifically specialized for the process of pain, just as other elements and pathways were rigidly designed as passages for other sensory information (i.e., pressure sensation).

Portions of this theory are in fact reasonably accurate descriptions and therefore remain prominent in our understanding of the pain mechanism, but the simplicity of the theory is inadequate in explaining the multifaceted nature of the pain experience (e.g., the phantom pain experienced by an amputee in the missing limb).

Pattern

A slightly more sophisticated model of pain mechanisms arose as a consequence of the technological ability to record stimulus-induced activity within neural pathways. Neural activity recorded and amplified on an oscilloscope allowed some appreciation of the changes in timing and grouping of nerve action potentials as a consequence of modification in stimulus parameters. A light stroking across a patch of skin may provoke one or two isolated action potentials in large-diameter neurons servicing the area, whereas a hot thermistor (warming element) may cause an initial burst followed by a steady discharge of action potentials in smaller neurons.

It was theorized that the recognition of painful stimuli by the individual was based primarily on the pattern of nervous activity that entered the CNS. Again, this theory was found inadequate in explaining the complexity of the pain experience, but it contributed significantly to the advancement of knowledge regarding pain mechanisms (Melzack and Wall, 1965; Sternbach, 1968).

Gate Control Theory

The gate control theory of pain was developed by Melzack and Wall in 1965 and has been the most influential, comprehensive, and adaptive conceptualization of pain and its consequences to date. The essence of the theory proposes that various "gates" controlling the level of noxious input via small-fiber neurons to the spinal cord can be modulated by other sensory, large-fiber neurons, higher CNS input, or both. Postulated mechanisms for the gates include presynaptic inhibitory effects on secondary transmission cells in the spinal cord. In essence, this implies that large fibers (e.g., those for touch) can cause partial depolarization of the nerve terminals of small fibers (for pain) that innervate transmission cells in the spinal cord. This results in the release of fewer "packets" of neurotransmitter molecules and a decreased likelihood that transmission cells will summate and fire.

A simplistic example would be the ameliorative inhibitory effect of the parent's rubbing a "bumped" area of the knee immediately following a toddler's fall. The light rubbing disproportionately activates greater numbers of large fibers that inhibit previously activated small fibers. In dentistry, a shaking of the lip during insertion of the needle and delivery of local anesthesia is commonly believed by many to distract or lessen the associated discomfort.

Transcutaneous electrical nerve stimulation (TENS), or the use of low-intensity electrical stimulation at peripheral sites, has been shown to provide pain relief (Woolf, 1989). Although the mechanism for TENS is not known, it has been suggested that its segmental effects may be due to activation of large-diameter, primary afferent fibers that in turn inhibit small-fiber transmission as predicted by the gate theory. A similar mechanism may account for the effects of acupuncture. TENS has been shown to produce partial analgesia to electrical tooth pulp stimulation in school age children (Abdulhameed et al., 1989).

Proportionately more emphasis has been placed on the role and influence of higher CNS modulation of pain perception and reactivity (LaVigne et al., 1986a, 1986b; Weisenberg, 1989). This reorientation is partially the result of more sophisticated studies suggesting the need for a more comprehensive explanation of cognitive, behavioral, and emotional influences in pain perception and control (Rasnake and Linscheid, 1989). Discoveries of endogenous opioids, widespread locations of opioid receptors throughout the CNS, and unnatural (i.e., electrical) stimulation of CNS sites resulting in pain-threshold elevations also have sparked renewed interest in pain research.

Additionally, animal studies have documented the presence and influence of descending supraspinal mechanisms on modulating painful input at the level of the spinal cord (Guilbaud et al., 1989). Interestingly, a phenomenon called stimulation-produced analgesia (SPA) has been demonstrated in both humans and animals. SPA results in specific inhibition of pain or avoidance behaviors during electrical stimulation of discrete brain sites (e.g., periaqueductal gray area of the medulla) and has few side effects. SPA of the periaqueductal gray area has been shown to inhibit jaw-opening reflexes due to tooth pulp stimulation in cats (Oliveras et al., 1974).

CNS EFFECTS ON PAIN PERCEPTION AND CONTROL

An endogenous opioid system that is both complex in function and widespread throughout the mammalian CNS has been partially characterized and described (Fields and Basbaum, 1989). Endogenous opioids are peptides that are naturally synthesized within the body and cause effects similar to opiates (e.g., morphine). β-Endorphin is one of the most potent peptides and has an N terminal identical to that of met-enkephalin, which was one of the first opioid peptides isolated.

The active opioid peptides are cleaved from larger precursors and act at various CNS opioid-receptor sites, including the spinal cord. The peptides are not equally potent, but all are inactivated by naloxone, a narcotic antagonist, and each may contribute in selective and specialized mechanisms underlying the pain perception process.

Correspondingly, there have been at least three opiate receptors characterized (μ, δ, and κ) throughout the CNS. The contribution of each in producing analgesia is not clear, however. Opioid ligands that bind to μ receptors produce potent analgesia when injected into the periaqueductal grey (PAG) area of the medulla. Other sites, extending from the hypothalamus to the rostral ventromedial medulla including the PAG, produce analgesia when properly stimulated electrically or by opiates. Curiously, the analgesic effects of nitrous oxide are believed either to be partially mediated by endogenous opioid ligands or capable of directly activating opiate receptors (Eger, 1985).

Theoretically, this system could mediate changes in the appreciation, motivation, and reactive processes of pain perception at higher levels of the CNS. Additionally, spinal cord influences in terms of either synaptic effectiveness or neuronal sensitivity are possible.

There is evidence to suggest that this system develops early in the CNS and thus should be functional in younger children. The extent of its influence and the conditions necessary for its activation are not understood. Future studies probably will underscore the means and usefulness of activating this system in addressing clinical pain states.

COGNITIVE ELEMENTS OF PAIN PERCEPTION

Cognition is a complex process resulting in an appreciation and often subsequent recognition of potential consequences as a function of "knowing." Knowing involves a multitude of processes including but not limited to perceiving, organizing, judging, meaning, reasoning, and responding.

Cognition implies an awareness of internal and external environmental influences on oneself. It also insinuates that steps can be taken to gain or command control over those influences and use the control to alter one's responsiveness (e.g., coping). For instance, one may be experiencing some discomfort but can possibly diminish the degree of discomfort by practicing mental processes (e.g., imagining pleasant events or counting holes in a ceiling tile).

A person can cope with a variety of conditions including stressful environments, depending on his or her perception of the situation. Factors such as consequences and repercussions of the situation, its timing, and individual resources apparently are important to the outcome of coping strategies. Coping, whether realized or not, is a statement of personal success that is most rewarding.

Coping strategies may include hypnosis and relaxation techniques, imagery, modeling, distraction, and reconceptualization. Typically, therapeutic coping strategies of pain management have a number of common elements including (1) an assessment of the problem, (2) reconceptualization of the patient's viewpoint, (3) development of appropriate skills (e.g., breathing and relaxation), (4) generalization and maintenance of those skills in preventing relapse, and (5) measurement of therapeutic success (Turk and Meichenbaum, 1989).

Evidence supports the notion that coping skills in the context of pain and anxiety can be taught even to children, and the effectiveness of cognitive training can be evaluated through self-report, physiologic, or behavioral measures. In one study, children who were undergoing restorative procedures were taught distraction and self-sup-

port techniques prior to undergoing dental procedures and subsequently compared to a group of children who were read stories. Self-report of anxiety for specific procedures (e.g., the injection) was less in those who received the cognitive training than in those who did not (Siegel and Peterson, 1980). This lends credence to the idea that school age children who have had opportunities to exercise self-control in anxiety-provoking circumstances may do better if they know that they are to receive an injection as part of their treatment rather than to proceed without any forewarning. This forewarning permits the child to invoke his or her own personalized coping skills in preparation for the "dreaded event."

Knowing ahead of time about impending discomfort, however, can have a detrimental effect under certain conditions. For instance, the less time between informing a young child who cognitively is incapable of significant coping strategies (i.e., 3 years or less) of a procedurally related painful stimulus (i.e., injection) and doing it allows correspondingly less time for interference behaviors to occur. It is even possible that the length of emotional outburst prior to and following the procedure may be reduced under these circumstances.

Some studies indicate that adults who are led to believe that they have some control over impending discomfort do exhibit more tolerance of painful stimuli (Weisenberg, 1989). A strong *belief* in their ability to gain self-control, however, is apparently an important factor in modulating the degree of discomfort. Those who lack this ability may place more trust in others (e.g., physician) and "suffer less" under their care.

Cognitive development and maturation are key to the success of cognitive strategies. There is evidence that anxiety reduction can be attained in the medical and dental environment as a function of age in school age cohorts. The extent to which these strategies can be successfully applied to preschoolers is yet to be determined. Younger children are capable of significant pain modulation through processes resembling cognitive strategies, however. In one study, play therapy with needles and dolls prior to venipuncture resulted in a significantly more rapid return of heart rate and less body movement within 5 minutes of blood drawing compared with controls. This finding was interpreted as evidence of reduced anxiety in the children (Young and Fu, 1988).

EMOTIONAL ELEMENTS OF PAIN PERCEPTION

Although pain and the anticipation of painful stimuli (i.e., anxiety) invoke a personalized emotional experience, most humans have a common understanding of the attendant emotions of such experiences. Certainly, we are adept at recognizing another's sufferings and possibly even better attuned to appreciating another person's anticipation of discomfort.

The expression of emotional content during or preceding painful experiences is most likely a complex combination of a partially inherited yet learning-tempered phenomenon that occurs early in life. An infant's expression of discomfort resulting from inoculations changes with aging from a more diffuse, crying, and reflexive response to one of anticipation, attentiveness toward the noxious object, and sometimes expression of anger (Craig et al., 1984; Izard et al., 1987).

An injured child may not be too terribly upset until she or he notices an adult's emotional outpouring over her or his condition. This is an important consideration when allowing parents to observe injections, extractions, and other treatment procedures. Careful assessment by the practitioner of the parents' concerns and likely response mode is most important. If one anticipates that the parent will not be stoic or supportive of the procedure, it may be advisable for the parent to leave the area or have the "more stoic" parent stay with the child.

The social response to pain can be a commanding and attention-gathering entity (Frodi and Lamb, 1978). For example, the toddler who skins his or her knee during a fall initially may not react as if in pain until the parent secondarily reacts to the injury. Depending on the parental response, the child may burst into tears if the parent looks upset or "toughen up" with the support of the parent's verbal encouragement.

Although one might conceive of the emotional elements of pain as being secondary to the pain itself, the emotional overtones may act in concert to modulate painful experiences. Indirect and anecdotal evidence suggests that certain pharmacologic agents (i.e., nitrous oxide and benzodiazepines) act on areas of the CNS responsible for emotional influence. A person feels the pain but is not particularly annoyed by it.

In contrast, emotional distress in anticipation of discomfort is known to lower pain thresholds and increase reactivity. Cognitive strategies designed to elicit positive emotional states can be effective in reducing anxiety and the degree of responsiveness to painful stimuli.

CHILDREN AND PAIN

Surprisingly, little is known about children and pain. Studies suggest that the developmental changes in response to painful stimuli occur early in infancy. In fact, anticipatory fears of sharp objects can be seen in children around one year of age (Barr, 1989). As a child matures, develops a broader vocabulary, and witnesses a variety of environments, his or her ability to communicate feelings becomes increasingly adept and surprisingly sophisticated. Paralleling and reflecting the child's cognitive development are signs manifesting the evolution of coping skills (Brown et al., 1986). In general, pain threshold tends to decline and the self-management of pain becomes more effective with increasing age (Katz et al., 1980). Similar self-management trends are noteworthy in the young dental patient (Zachary et al., 1985). This phenomenon undoubtedly results from the interactions of multiple factors, including the maturation of coping skills, appreciation of self-control, and social influences.

The pain associated with dental or other medically imposed procedures might be instrumental in invoking the opportunity for the development and testing of certain self-control and coping mechanisms (Cordh, 1973). Many children are efficient with their coping skills and tolerate mild discomfort with little overt expression. A few lack good coping skills and display hysterical behaviors (i.e., extreme panic, screaming, and struggling) in anticipation of or during minor discomforts. Consequently, any assessment of a child's behavioral and cognitive responses to the

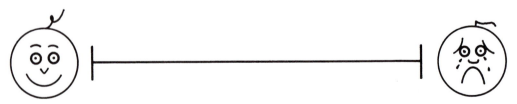

Figure 6–1. An example of a visual analog scale that can be used to measure the degree of discomfort in children. Note that the line is 100 mm long and is anchored at either end by happy-sad faces. The child is instructed to make a mark on the line that best describes how much pain he or she is having. The distance from the left end bar to the mark made by the child is the measure of discomfort for the child.

TABLE 6–1. Factors Exacerbating Children's Pain

Intrinsic Factors

Child's anxiety, depression, and fear
Previous experience with inadequately managed pain
Child's lack of control
Experience of other aversive symptoms (nausea, fatigue, and dyspnea)
Child's negative interpretation of situation

Extrinsic Factors

Anxiety and fears of parents and siblings
Poor prognosis
Invasiveness of treatment regimen
Parental reinforcement of extreme under-reaction (stoicism) or overreaction to pain
Inadequate pain management practices of health care staff
Boring or age-inappropriate environment

From McGrath PJ, Beyer J, Cleeland C, et al: Report of the Subcommittee on Assessment and Methodologic Issues in the Management of Pain in Childhood Cancer. Pediatrics 86:814–817, 1990.

dental environment should be considered in light of age-appropriate expressions, specific procedures, and the use of cognitive probes.

It may appear difficult to measure the degree of pain or discomfort in a young child, especially preschool children, because of their level of cognitive and language development. Several tools have been developed for this purpose, including nonverbal self-report techniques. Thus, the intensity of pain may be represented by the number of poker chips selected, the ranking of variable expressions on happy-sad faces, the rating along a "pain thermometer" scale, and color selections.

An accumulation of evidence indicates that the visual analog scale (VAS) is one of the most reliable and valid measurement tools for self-report of pain in children. Typically, a VAS is a line approximately 100 mm in length with each end being anchored by extreme descriptors (e.g., "no pain" vs. "worst pain imaginable") or happy-sad faces. The patient indicates the degree of perceived pain by making a mark on the line. The length of the line from the left-hand margin to the mark determines the magnitude of pain for that individual (Fig. 6-1). Certain physiologic measurements, especially heart rate, in conjunction with self-report of discomfort is thought to add another important dimension to the characterization of response specificity to painful stimuli (Winer, 1982).

Family and cultural elements are apparent in the mediation of pain-related expressions and their effects. An infant's cry may elicit protective and indulging types of behavior or, sadly, abusive behaviors in adult caretakers. Family members may respond differentially to a child's painful expressions with females being more supportive and soothing and males more coarse and distracting. Some societies are highly sensitive to infant distress while others are less.

In summary, many factors may contribute to a child's perception of pain. McGrath and colleagues (1990) have listed factors that tend to exacerbate the pain in children with cancer and suggest developmental considerations for quantification of pain (Tables 6-1 and 6-2).

BEHAVIOR MANAGEMENT TECHNIQUES

A variety of techniques can be used to manage the behavior of a child in the dental environment. The establishment of communication combined with a caring attitude is the key building block for developing sound rapport with any patient. Consequently, the great majority of children require minimal management efforts other than providing information on what is going to happen (e.g., tell, show, and do). *An important caveat is that every child responds to his or her environment with an individualized style. Practitioners must be perceptive and flexible with the use of their management techniques and optimize the likelihood of a successful encounter by matching their selection of techniques to that of the patient's style of interactive activities.*

TABLE 6–2. Age and Measures of Pain Intensity

Age	Self-Report Measures	Behavior Measures	Physiologic Measures
Birth to 3 years	Not available	Of primary importance	Of secondary importance
3 to 6 years	Specialized, developmentally appropriate scales available	Primary if self-report not available	Of secondary importance
>6 years	Of primary importance	Of secondary importance	Of secondary importance

From McGrath PJ, Beyer J, Cleeland C, et al: Report of the Subcommittee on Assessment and Methodologic Issues in the Management of Pain in Childhood Cancer. Pediatrics 86:814–817, 1990.

TABLE 6–3. American Academy of Pediatric Dentistry's Standards of Care for Behavior Management

Management Type	Description	Objectives	Indications	Contraindications
1. Communicative Management				
a) Tell-Show-Do	Explanations tailored to cognitive level; followed by demonstration; followed by actual procedure	a. Allay fears b. Shape patient's responses c. Give expectations of behavior	All patients who can communicate regardless of method of communication	None
b) Voice Control	Modulation in voice volume, tone, or pace to influence and direct patient's behavior	a. Gain patient's attention b. Avert negative or avoidance behaviors c. Establish authority	Uncooperative or inattentive, but communicative child	Children who are unable to understand due to age, disability, medication, or emotional immaturity
c) Positive Reinforcement	Process of shaping patient's behavior through appropriately timed feedback (e.g., praise, facial expression)	a. Reinforce desired behavior	Any patient	None
d) Distraction	Diverting patient's attention from perceived unpleasant procedure	a. Decrease likelihood of unpleasantness perception/threshold	Any patient	None
e) Nonverbal Communication	Conveying reinforcement and guiding behavior through contact, posture, and facial expressions	a. Enhance effectiveness of other Communicative Management techniques b. Gain and/or maintain patient's attention and compliance	Any patient	None
2. Conscious Sedation*	Pre- or intra-operative administration of sedative agents	a. Reduce or eliminate anxiety b. Reduce untoward movement/reaction c. Enhance communication d. Increase tolerance for longer periods e. Aid treatment of mentally, physically, or medically compromised patient	Any ASA Class I or II patients who cannot cooperate due to lack of psychological/emotional maturity; mental, physical or medical disability	a) Patient with minimal dental needs b) Medical contraindication to sedation
3. General Anesthesia*	Use of general anesthetics (intravenous, intramuscular, inhalation) for care intra-operative	a. Provide safe, efficient and effective dental care	Patients with certain physical, mental, or medically compromising conditions; local anesthesia is ineffective because of acute infection, allergy; extremely uncooperative, fearful, anxious or uncommunicative child or adolescent in which dental care cannot be deferred; extensive orofacial/dental trauma; protection of developing psyche	a) Healthy, cooperative patient with minimal dental needs b) Medical contraindication to general anesthesia

Technique	Description	Indications	Contraindications
4. Hand-Over-Mouth (HOM)*	Placement of hand over mouth while explaining behavioral expectations; removing hand when appropriate behavior is to be reinforced; reapplication if necessary	a. Gain child's attention for establishing communication b. Eliminate inappropriate avoidance responses c. Enhance child's self confidence in coping during treatment d. Ensure child's safety during delivery of care	A healthy child who is able to understand and cooperate, but elects to display defiant, obstreperous or hysterical avoidance behaviors	Children who are unable to understand due to age, disability, medications, or emotional immaturity
5. Nitrous Oxide-Oxygen Inhalation*	Inhalation of nitrous oxide/oxygen through nasal hood	a. Reduce or eliminate anxiety b. Reduce untoward movement/reaction c. Enhance communication d. Increase tolerance for longer periods e. Aid treatment of mentally, physically, or medically compromised patient f. Reduce gagging	Fearful, anxious, or obstreperous patients; certain mentally, physically, or medically compromised patients; gag reflex is hyperactive; profound local anesthesia cannot be obtained	Chronic obstructive pulmonary diseases; severe emotional disturbances; 1st trimester of pregnancy; drug or disease induced pulmonary fibrosis
6. Physical Restraint*	Partial or complete immobilization of patient's body or portions thereof	a. Reduce or eliminate untoward movement b. Protect patient/staff from injury c. Facilitate delivery of care	Cannot cooperate due to immaturity; mental or physical disability; failure of other management techniques; safety to patient/practitioner would be at risk	Cooperative patient; those who have medical or systemic conditions contraindicating restraint

*Requires informed consent.

The information within this table was taken with the permission and encouragement of the American Academy of Pediatric Dentistry: Guidelines for behavior management. Pediatr Dent, special issue: Reference manual 18:40-44, 1997.

The American Academy of Pediatric Dentistry (1997) has published guidelines on the management of children and special patients. That publication includes definitions, rationales, and descriptions of techniques that are commonly used to manage the behavior of these patients (Table 6–3). The list of techniques is not exhaustive but represents the major body of empirically and scientifically derived knowledge presently available on patient management. It is probable that newer techniques as well as refinements of those presently in existence will be developed with the goal of providing both a pleasant experience and positive learning. Some of these techniques are discussed further in Chapter 23, Patient Management.

Behavioral and physiologic findings suggest that the three most feared or anxiety-producing stimuli in the dental operatory are the injection of local anesthesia, application of the rubber dam, and initiation of tooth preparation with the high-speed handpiece (Badalaty et al., 1990; Currie et al., 1988; Doring, 1985; Houpt et al., 1985). Knowledge of these findings should prepare the dentist and staff to anticipate and manage disruptive behaviors that may accompany these procedures. For instance, the dental assistant should passively place his or her arms slightly above the torso and arms of the patient during the injection. In this fashion, assistants are prepared to intercept the child's hands if she or he attempts to grab the dentist's hands. Otherwise, the patient may inadvertently cause trauma to themselves or the dental staff. (See Chapter 28, Fig. 28–2, for an example of this procedure.)

Natural fears of bright lights, loud noises, sudden movements, and strange environments are easily aroused in and produce the most overt expressions of anxiety during the first 3 years of a child's life. These stimuli are found in every dental operatory! Consequently, the dentist and assistant should anticipate disruptive behaviors in the very young child. Taking time for development of rapport and trust, using instruments that are familiar to these patients (e.g., toothbrush), and allowing the child to use them initially is a fairly successful method of gaining the young child's confidence.

Nitrous oxide/oxygen (N_2O/O_2) can be effective for children who are mildly to moderately anxious, can respond to guidance, and have no medical contraindications to N_2O/O_2 administration. In sedative concentrations (30–45%), the patient can derive from N_2O/O_2 both a calming effect and some analgesia (although local anesthesia is usually required). Key elements to improve the effectiveness of N_2O/O_2 include proper patient selection, maximizing nasal breathing, minimizing oral shunting of air during crying episodes, snug fit of the nasal hood over the nose, soft flexible rubber hoods that adapt to the young child's face, adequate titration, and clinical monitoring.

Nitrous oxide is not without its perils. Results of laboratory studies as well as prolonged continuous clinical exposure or recreational abuse have been associated with significant sequelae, including bone marrow depression; teratogenic, mutagenic, and carcinogenic effects; spontaneous abortions; and neuropathies (Eger, 1985).

The immediate and long-term goals for the use of any behavioral management technique are to provide as pleasant an experience as possible for the patient, instill the understanding of the attainment and maintenance of a positive oral health attitude, and promote and foster lifelong care-seeking and preventive behaviors. Hence, the dentist's attitudes and demeanor toward his or her patients are most critical to the development of a positive dental attitude in those patients.

SHORT- AND LONG-TERM CONSEQUENCES OF BEHAVIOR MANAGEMENT

Unfortunately, few well-controlled studies have addressed the impact of behavioral management techniques used in childhood on behaviors later exhibited in the adult patient. Anecdotally, it has been noted that some aggressive techniques do not interfere with a patient's seeking of future care, especially if the child was relatively young when the technique was used. On the other hand, more aggressive techniques applied in childhood have been implicated as being prominent factors in the behavior of adult phobic dental patients. Frankly, there is not enough information available to satisfactorily define this issue, but considerations of lifestyle, personality development, and extenuating circumstances should be addressed before any significant conclusions are drawn.

In one study, the use of hand-over-mouth in preschool children judged successful on a short-term basis by the practitioner was not found to be a significant deterrent to the development of positive attitudes of the children toward dental care (Hartmann et al., 1985).

As for short-term effects, positive reinforcement has been shown to produce decreased disruptive behavior within a treatment session in children who have variable levels of baseline disruptive behaviors. Positive reinforcement may include patient praise, tokens or "stickers," and privileged socially related events (e.g., gaining the opportunity to watch a sibling or friend undergo dental treatment).

Time out (i.e., the separating of the child from the social environment or procedure that provokes disruptive behavior) appears to decrease patient disruptiveness in selected cases. The degree of success of time out varies, and factors such as the time-out period and the frequency of applied time out episodes are important considerations. Apparently, if time out is to be effective, it should be short and only used once or twice in attempts to gain the acceptable behavior. Longer periods and numerous uses on any given child doom the success of the technique.

Variables such as parenting style, personality, temperament, and sociability have not been studied systematically. Nonetheless, it is recognized that each child is unique in "how" they respond and has a distinguishable background; thus, future studies will no doubt prove the importance of these variables in the child's expression of behaviors (Schechter et al., 1991).

It should be emphasized that the great majority of pediatric dental patients can be managed by simple, nonaggressive techniques. However, even the use of tell-show-do, which is perceived as the most innocuous technique, is no guarantee that the patient will not become a dental phobic or that the parent won't react strongly to its use on their child if described as a "technique." It is the wise and competent practitioner who knows children's behaviors and parents' expectations.

Chapter 23 discusses behavior management in terms of verbal and nonverbal techniques, predictors of child misbehavior, and related themes.

REFERENCES

Abdulhameed SM, Feigal RJ, Rudney JD, Kajander KC: Effect of peripheral electrical stimulation on measures of tooth pain threshold and oral soft tissue comfort in children. Anesthesia Progress 36:52-57, 1989.

American Academy of Pediatric Dentistry: Guidelines for behavior management. Pediatric Dentistry, Special Issue: Reference Manual, 18:40-44, 1997.

Badalaty MM, Houpt MI, Koenigsberg SR, et al: A comparison of chloral hydrate and diazepam sedation in young children. Pediatric Dentistry 12:33-37, 1990.

Barr RG: Pain in children. In Wall PD and Melzack R (eds): Textbook of Pain. New York, Churchill Livingstone, 1989.

Brown JM, Okefe Saunders SH, Baker B: Developmental changes and children's cognition of stressful and painful situations. Pediatr Psychol 11:343-357, 1986.

Corah NL: Effect of perceived control on stress reduction and pedodontic patients. J Dental Res 52:1261-1264, 1973.

Craig KD, McMahon RJ, Morison JD, Zaskow C: Developmental changes in infant pain expressions during immunization injections. Soc Sci Med 19:1331-1337, 1984.

Currie WR, Biery KA, Campbell RL, Mourino AP: Narcotic sedation: An evaluation of cardiopulmonary parameters and behavior modification in pediatric dental patients. J Pedodont 12:230-249, 1988.

Doring KR: Evaluation of an alphaprodine-hydroxyzine combination as a sedative agent in the treatment of the pediatric dental patient. JADA 111:567-576, 1985.

Eger EI: Nitrous Oxide. New York, Elsevier Science, 1985.

Fields HL, Basbaum AI: Endogenous pain control mechanisms. In Wall PD, Melzack R (eds): Textbook of Pain. New York, Churchill Livingstone, 1989.

Frodi AM, Lamb ME: Sex differences and responsiveness to infants: A developmental study of psychophysiological and behavioral responses. Child Dev 49:1182-1188, 1978.

Guilbaud G, Peschanski M, Besson JM: Experimental data related to nociception and pain at the supraspinal level. In Wall PD, Melzack R (eds): Textbook of Pain. New York, Churchill Livingstone, 1989.

Hartmann C, Pruhs RJ, Taft TB Jr: Hand-over-mouth behavior management technique in a solo pedodontic practice: A study. J Dent Child 52:293-296, 1985.

Houpt MI, Koenigsberg SR, Weiss NJ, Desjardins PJ: Comparison of chloral hydrate with and without promethazine in the sedation of young children. Pediatr Dent 7:292-296, 1985.

Izard CE, Hembree EA, Heubner RR: Infants' emotion expressions to acute pain: Developmental change and stability to individual differences. Dev Psychol 23:105-113, 1987.

Katz ER, Kellerman J, Seagle SE: Behavioral distress in children with cancer undergoing medical procedures: Developmental considerations. J Consult Clin Psychol 48:356-365, 1980.

Lavigne JV, Schulein MJ, Hahn YS: Psychological aspects of painful medical conditions in children: I. Developmental aspects and assessment. Pain 27:133-146, 1986a.

Lavigne JV, Schulein MJ, Hahn YS: Psychological aspects of painful medical conditions in children: II. Personality factors, family characteristics and treatment. Pain 27:147-169, 1986b.

McGrath PJ, Beyer J, Cleeland C, et al: Report of the subcommittee on assessment and methodologic issues in the management of pain in childhood cancer. Pediatrics 86:814-817, 1990.

Melzack R, Wall PD: Pain mechanisms: A new theory. Science 150:971-979, 1965.

Oliveras JL, Woda A, Guilbaud G, Besson JM: Inhibition of the jaw-opening reflex by electrical stimulation of the periaqueductal gray matter in the awake, unrestrained cat. Brain Res 72:328-331, 1974.

Rasnake LK, Linscheid TR: Anxiety reduction in children receiving medical care: Developmental considerations. J Dev Behav Pediatr 10:169-175, 1989.

Schechter NL, Bernstein BA, Beck A, et al: Individual differences in children's response to pain: Role of temperament and parental characteristics. Pediatrics 87:171-177, 1991.

Siegel LJ, Peterson L: Stress reduction in young dental patients through coping skills and sensory information. J Consult Clin Psychol 48:785-787, 1980.

Sternbach RA: Pain: A psychophysiological analysis. New York-London, Academic Press, 1968.

Turk DC, Meichenbaum DH: A cognitive-behavioural approach to pain management. In Wall PD, Melzack R (eds): Textbook of Pain. New York, Churchill Livingstone, 1989.

Weisenberg M: Pain and pain control. Psychol Bull 84:1008-1041, 1977.

Weisenberg M: Cognitive aspects of pain. *In* Wall PD, Melzack R (eds): Textbook of Pain. New York, Churchill Livingstone, 1989.

Winer GA: A review and analysis of children's fearful behavior in dental settings. Child Dev *53*:1111–1133, 1982.

Woolf CF: Segmental afferent fibre-induced analgesia: Transcutaneous electrical nerve stimulation (TENS) and vibration. *In* Wall PD, Melzack R (eds): Textbook of Pain. New York, Churchill Livingstone, 1989.

Young MR, Fu VR: Influence of plan and temperament on the young child's response to pain. Child Health Care *18*:209–215, 1988.

Zachary RA, Friedlander S, Huang LN, et al: Affects of stress-relevant and -irrelevant filmed modeling on children's responses to dental treatment. J Pediatr Psychol *10*:383–401, 1985.

Zeltzer L, LeBaron S: Hypnosis and nonhypnotic techniques for reduction of pain and anxiety during painful procedures in children and adolescents with cancer. J Pediatr *101*:1032–1035, 1982.

Pain and Anxiety Control (Part I: Pain Perception Control)

*Stephen Wilson, Diane C. Dilley, William F. Vann, Jr.,
and Jay A. Anderson*

Chapter Outline

Pain is a complex, multidimensional phenomenon mediated by physicochemical processes in the peripheral and central nervous system. Its perception can be significantly modified by any of a host of mechanisms including, among others, drugs, environmental stimuli, cognitive and emotional processes, and social and cultural conditions. In terms of a conceptual context, pain may be thought of as a continuum whose boundaries are limited yet variable for each individual. On the lower end of the continuum is the pain perception threshold. The pain perception threshold can be defined as the least amount of stimulation applied to tissue that an individual can barely detect as being unpleasant. The pain tolerance threshold is a notable point of intensely noxious stimulation on the pain continuum above which the individual cannot reasonably endure and will seek definitive measures to relieve the pain. Determination of the pain perception threshold usually is associated with experimental conditions; however, more intense stimulation approaching or exceeding the pain tolerance threshold is more characteristic of clinical conditions.

The overwhelming majority of pharmacologic agents used in dentistry are used to control anxiety and pain. Generally, the elimination of pain sensation in the dental setting requires blocking of pain perception either peripherally using local anesthesia or centrally with general anesthesia. Anxiety is controlled, in part or completely, by using sedation that may involve pharmacologic or nonpharmacologic techniques or both. Anxiety and pain control in actual clinical practice overlap to a significant degree.

There is no single *best* technique for control of anxiety and pain. A practitioner may have a favorite technique, but one technique is not useful for all dental patients in all situations. The prudent and wise dentist has a working knowledge of several techniques and selects, on an individual basis, the one that appears to be the most appropriate for a particular patient. In some cases, this may necessitate referral.

GENERAL ANESTHESIA

General anesthesia renders the patient unconscious through depression of the central nervous system, thus eliminating patient cooperation as a factor.

There are categories of patients in whom the only reasonable anesthetic alternative for safe treatment is general anesthesia. Examples may include the very young, precooperative children, and severely mentally retarded children unable to cooperate for complicated or extensive dental procedures.

General anesthesia should be administered under the direction and supervision of an individual who has completed an American Medical Association (AMA) or American Dental Association (ADA) accredited training program, usually at the postdoctoral level, which provides comprehensive and appropriate training necessary to manage general anesthesia cases. Such persons must be licensed by state law to administer general anesthesia.

LOCAL ANESTHESIA

Mechanisms of Action

Pain perception may be altered at the peripheral level by blocking propagation of nerve impulses via local anesthesia. One dimension of the process of pain perception involves production of nerve impulses, or action potentials, by a noxious stimulus that activates specific receptors (nociceptors) at nerve endings. The nerve impulses travel along the nerve fibers via a physicochemical process involving ion transport across the neuronal membrane. The primary effect of local anesthetic agents is to penetrate the nerve cell membrane and block receptor sites that control the influx of sodium ions associated with membrane depolarization (Malamed, 1997). It is currently thought that the sequence of events involved in local anesthetic block consists of (1) binding of the local anesthetic to a receptor site that exists on the inside of the cell membrane, (2) blockade of the sodium channels through which the sodium ions would normally enter during depolarization, (3) decrease in sodium conductance, (4) depression of the rate of electrical depolarization, (5) failure to achieve threshold potential, and (6) lack of development of a propagated action potential and thus blockade of conduction of the nerve impulse (Covino, 1976). In general, small nerve fibers are more susceptible to the onset of action of local anes-

thetics than large fibers. Accordingly, the sensation of pain is one of the first modalities blocked, followed by cold, warmth, touch, and pressure.

Local anesthetic agents are weak chemical bases and are supplied generally as salts such as lidocaine hydrochloride. The salts may exist in one of two forms, either the uncharged free base or the charged cation. The free-base form, which is lipid-soluble, can penetrate the nerve cell membrane. Penetration of the tissue and cell membrane is necessary for the local anesthetic to have an effect because the receptor sites are located on the inside of the cell membrane. This explains in part why local anesthetic agents are not as effective in areas of an acute infection where the local tissues are acidic in pH. Once the free base has penetrated the cell, it re-equilibrates, and the cation is thought to be the form that then interacts with the receptors to prevent sodium conductance.

Local Anesthetic Agents

ESTERS

Discovered in 1860, cocaine was the first local anesthetic. Because of the number of adverse side effects associated with cocaine, attempts were made to develop alternatives that retained the local anesthetic properties of cocaine while eliminating the side effects. Several other benzoic acid ester derivatives were developed, including benzocaine, procaine (Novocain), tetracaine (Pontocaine), and chloroprocaine (Nesacaine). The major problem with the ester class of local anesthetics is their propensity for producing allergic reactions.

AMIDES

The amides, a relatively new class of local anesthetics, were introduced with the synthesis of lidocaine in 1943. These compounds are amide derivatives of diethylaminoacetic acid. They are relatively free from sensitizing reactions. Since lidocaine was synthesized, several other local anesthetics have been introduced. All are amides and include mepivacaine (Carbocaine), prilocaine (Citanest), bupivacaine (Marcaine), and etidocaine (Duranest).

Local Anesthetic Properties

Individual local anesthetic agents differ from each other in their pharmacologic profiles (see

Table 7-1). They vary in their potency, toxicity, onset time, and duration. All these characteristics may be clinically important and all vary as a function of the intrinsic properties of the anesthetic agent itself and the regional anesthetic procedure employed. Further, these characteristics may be modified by the addition of vasoconstrictors.

POTENCY

The intrinsic potency of a local anesthetic is the concentration required to achieve the desired effect of nerve blockade. Procaine has the lowest intrinsic potency; lidocaine, prilocaine, and mepivacaine have intermediate potency; tetracaine, bupivacaine, and etidocaine are of high potency. It is important to note that these types of local anesthetics do not necessarily come in the same percentage of concentration; hence, caution is needed to prevent exceeding toxic doses of local anesthesia, especially when used in combination with other agents affecting the cardiovascular and central nervous system (e.g., sedatives).

ONSET TIME

Onset time is the time required for the local anesthetic solution to penetrate the nerve fiber and cause complete conduction blockade. Clinically, it must be understood that conduction blockade requires time for onset; otherwise, needless pain may be produced by beginning a procedure too soon.

DURATION

Duration of anesthesia is one of the most important clinical properties considered when choosing an appropriate local anesthetic agent for a given procedure. A local anesthetic with increased protein-binding capacity and a vasoconstrictor has a longer duration than an agent with decreased protein binding and no vasoconstrictor. Generally, procaine and chloroprocaine, which are used primarily for spinal anesthesia, are considered of short duration. Lidocaine, mepivacaine, and prilocaine have an intermediate duration, and bupivacaine and etidocaine have a long duration.

REGIONAL TECHNIQUE

A major factor that determines drug characteristics is the type of regional (local) anesthetic procedure employed. Depending on whether topical, infiltration, or a major or minor nerve block

is employed, onset and duration of the various agents vary. Potency is not affected.

Onset. Local anesthesia of the soft tissues by the infiltration technique occurs almost immediately with all of the local anesthetics. As more tissue penetration becomes necessary, the intrinsic latency of onset previously discussed plays a greater role. Generally, in dentistry, for any given drug the onset time required is shortest with an infiltration block, longer with a peripheral (minor) nerve block, and longest for topical anesthesia.

Duration. Duration of anesthesia varies greatly with the regional technique performed. This profile may differ for different agents, depending on their intrinsic pharmacologic properties. For example, lidocaine (1%) with epinephrine (1:200,000) has a duration of 416 minutes with infiltration, 178 minutes with ulnar nerve block, 156 minutes with epidural anesthesia, and 94 minutes with spinal block (Covino, 1976).

OTHER FACTORS

Dose. The quality, onset time, and duration of a local anesthetic block may be improved by increasing the dose of the agent by using a higher concentration or greater volume. Increases in dose must be limited by anesthetic toxicity; however, for consistently effective local anesthetic block, an adequate concentration and volume must be administered as close to the target nerves as possible.

Vasoconstrictors. Onset time, duration, and quality of block are also affected by the addition of vasoconstrictor agents to the local anesthetic solution. Vasoconstrictor agents such as epinephrine decrease the rate of drug absorption by decreasing blood flow to the tissues, prolonging the duration of the anesthesia produced, and increasing the frequency with which adequate anesthesia is attained and maintained. Toxic effects of local anesthetics are reduced as a result of delay in absorption into the circulation. Onset time of anesthesia is sometimes shortened as well.

In pediatric dental patients, a vasoconstrictor is necessary because the higher cardiac output, tissue perfusion, and basal metabolic rate tend to remove the local anesthetic solution from the tissues and carry it into the systemic circulation faster, producing a shorter duration of action and a more rapid accumulation of toxic levels in the blood. Finally, vasoconstrictors produce local hemostasis following local anesthetic infiltration into the operating field. This assists in postoperative hemorrhage control, an advantage in the management of young children undergoing dental extractions.

Vasoconstrictors are all sympathomimetic agents that carry their own intrinsic toxic effects. These include tachycardia, hypertension, headache, anxiety, tremor, and arrhythmias. It has been shown that 2% lidocaine containing a concentration of 1:250,000 epinephrine is as effective in increasing the depth and duration of local anesthesia block as higher concentrations of epinephrine such as 1:100,000 or 1:50,000 (Keesling and Hinds, 1963). To avoid vasoconstriction toxicity in children, a concentration of 1:100,000 epinephrine should not be exceeded. The pharmacologic properties of the local anesthetics commonly used in dentistry are summarized in Table 7-1.

Toxicity

The use of local anesthetics is so common in dentistry that the potential for toxicity with these agents can be easily overlooked. Dentists who treat children should always be mindful of local anesthetic toxicity. Toxic reactions to local anesthetics may be due to overdose, accidental intravascular injection, idiosyncratic response, allergic reaction, or interactive effects with other agents (e.g., sedatives).

The dental practitioner should be familiar with the maximum recommended dose for all local anesthetic agents that are used on a dose per body weight basis (i.e., milligrams per kilogram). Simply knowing a total milligram amount for the average adult is not adequate and may lead to overdosage in pediatric patients. Maximum safe doses for local anesthetics are listed in Table 7-1.

CENTRAL NERVOUS SYSTEM REACTIONS

Local anesthetic agents cause a biphasic reaction in the central nervous system as blood levels increase. Although local anesthetics have depressant effects in general, they are thought to selectively depress inhibitory neurons initially, producing a net effect of central nervous system excitation. Subjective signs and symptoms of early anesthetic toxicity include circumoral numbness or tingling, dizziness, tinnitus (often described as a buzzing or humming sound), cycloplegia (difficulty in focusing), and disorientation. Depressant effects may be evident immediately. These include drowsiness or even transient loss of consciousness. Objective signs may include muscle twitching, tremors, slurred speech, and shivering followed by overt seizure activity.

Generalized central nervous system depression characterizes the second phase of local anesthetic toxicity, accompanied sometimes by respiratory depression.

CARDIOVASCULAR SYSTEM REACTIONS

The cardiovascular response to local anesthetic toxicity is also biphasic. During the period of central nervous system stimulation, the heart rate and blood pressure may increase. When plasma levels of the anesthetic increase, vasodilatation is followed by myocardial depression, with a subsequent fall in blood pressure. Bradycardia, cardiovascular collapse, and cardiac arrest may occur at higher levels of the agents. Most local anesthetics used in dentistry cause little cardiovascular alteration even at levels associated with seizure activity. The depressant effect on the myocardium is essentially proportional to the inherent potency of the local anesthetic, procaine being least toxic, lidocaine and mepivacaine being of intermediate toxicity, and bupivacaine and etidocaine being the most cardiotoxic.

The use of local anesthetic in pediatric dentistry has changed the quality and quantity of procedures possible as much as any other advance in the field. In children who are properly prepared psychologically, high-quality local anesthesia is usually all that is necessary to eliminate pain completely. One must be ever mindful of the pharmacokinetics of the agents used with children. Because of the higher cardiac output, higher basal metabolic rate, and higher degree of tissue perfusion in children, the agents tend to be absorbed more rapidly from the tissues. The less mature liver enzyme systems in young children may detoxify these chemicals at a slower rate than in adults. And the immature central nervous and cardiovascular systems probably are more susceptible to toxicity at lower drug levels than in adults. For these reasons, a precise local anesthetic technique should be used, aspiration techniques should be practiced, a vasoconstrictor is necessary, and a thorough knowledge of the intrinsic properties of local anesthetic agents is essential. *Above all, the recommended maximum safe dose of local anesthetic should be calculated precisely for each patient and must never be exceeded.*

ANALGESICS

Occasionally, pharmacologic relief of pain is necessary for the child dental patient. The agents used for pain relief are called analgesics. Ideally,

TABLE 7–1. Properties of Common Dental Local Anesthetics

Generic Name	Brand Name	Type	Concentration	Vasoconstrictor	Max. Rec. Dose (mg/kg)	Absolute Max. (mg)	Av. Duration Pulpal Tissue (min)	Av. Duration Soft Tissue (hr)
Propoxycaine with procaine	Ravocaine Novocain	Ester Ester	0.4% 2%	1:20,000 levonordefrin (Neo-Cobefrin)	6.6	400	30-60	2.3
Lidocaine	Xylocaine	Amide	2%	1:100,000 epinephrine	4.4	300	60	3-5
Mepivacaine	Carbocaine	Amide	3%		4.4	300	60-90	2-3
Mepivacaine	Carbocaine	Amide	2%	1:20,000 levonordefrin (Neo-Cobefrin)	4.4	300	60-90	3-5
Prilocaine	Citanest	Amide	4%		6.0	400	10 (infil) 60 (block)	1½-2 2-4
Prilocaine	Citanest Forte	Amide	4%	1:200,000 epinephrine	6.0	400	60-90	3-8
Bupivacaine	Marcaine	Amide	0.5%	1:200,000 epinephrine	1.3	90	90-180	4-12
Etidocaine	Duranest	Amide	1.5%	1:200,000 epinephrine	8.0	400	90-180	4-9
Articaine*	Ultracaine D-S	Amide	4%	1:200,000 epinephrine	7.0 (adult) 5.0 (child)	500	*Infil:* 220 (adult) 150 (child) *Block:* 270 (adult) 225 (child)	NA
Articaine*	Ultracaine D-S Forte	Amide	4%	1:100,000 epinephrine	7.0 (adult) 5.0 (child)	500	*Infil:* 180 (adult) 150 (child) *Block:* 285 (adult) 230 (child)	NA

*Available in Europe and Canada.
NA, Not available.

analgesic drugs should relieve pain without significantly altering consciousness. Analgesics act either in the peripheral tissues or centrally in the brain and spinal cord. Narcotic analgesics are thought to act primarily in the central nervous system. Non-narcotic analgesics, such as aspirin, are thought to act in the periphery at the nerve endings. The great majority of dental pain in pediatric patients can be managed using non-narcotic agents of relatively low potency. Children of all ages are capable of experiencing pain, however, and recently concern has been expressed that younger children and infants may be undermedicated after some clinical procedures.

Non-Narcotic Analgesics

Generally, the non-narcotic analgesics are useful for mild to moderate pain, which constitutes 90% of the pain of dental origin. The non-narcotic analgesics differ from the narcotics in their site of action, their lesser degree of toxicity and side effects, and their absence of drug dependence. These drugs exert their effects primarily at the peripheral nerve endings. The standard prototype drugs in this class are aspirin, acetaminophen, and nonsteroidal anti-inflammatory drugs (NSAIDs).

ASPIRIN

Since its introduction in 1899, aspirin, a salicylate (acetylsalicylic acid), has enjoyed widespread use for its analgesic, antipyretic, and anti-inflammatory properties. Despite the advent of many newer drugs, aspirin remains a standard drug of choice for treatment of mild pain.

The most significant side effects of aspirin include alterations of coagulation by inhibition of platelet aggregation, gastric distress and dyspepsia, occult blood loss, and, very rarely, sensitivity reactions such as urticaria, angioneurotic edema, asthma, or anaphylaxis. The anticoagulant properties of aspirin are rarely a problem in children; however, because a single dose of aspirin can increase bleeding time, aspirin should not be used prior to surgery. Aspirin should be avoided in patients with bleeding or platelet disorders and in those taking warfarin-type drugs (Coumadin).

The gastrointestinal effects of aspirin are the problems most commonly encountered and may be modulated by administering the drug with food or by using a buffered or enteric-coated preparation, although absorption may be affected. The more severe allergic-type reactions have been shown to occur more often in patients with pre-existing asthma, atopy, or nasal polyps, and aspirin should probably be avoided in patients with such a history. The possible association of aspirin with certain viral illnesses and the development of Reye's syndrome has resulted in many practitioners opting for aspirin substitutes.

Dosage. The recommended dosage for analgesia and antipyretic purposes in children is 10 to 15 mg/kg/dose given at 4-hour intervals up to a total of 60–80 mg/kg/day, with a maximum limit of 3.6 g/day.

ACETAMINOPHEN

Acetaminophen (e.g., Tylenol, Tempra, Datril) is the most common analgesic used in pediatrics in the United States today. It is an effective analgesic and antipyretic that is as potent as aspirin for treatment of mild pain. Unlike aspirin, acetaminophen does not inhibit platelet function (Shannon and Berde, 1989). It also promotes less gastric upset and has not been implicated in Reye's syndrome. The primary disadvantage of acetaminophen is that it has no clinically significant anti-inflammatory properties.

Toxicity as a result of overdosage may result in acute liver failure with serious or fatal hepatic necrosis. It is estimated that 15 g of acetaminophen is required in an adult to produce liver damage, or more than 3 g for a child under 2 years of age. Allergic reactions are rare. Acetaminophen is a good alternative analgesic in patients who do not require an anti-inflammatory effect.

Dosage. The recommended dosage for acetaminophen is as follows:

Adult: 300–650 mg every 4 hours
Children: 10–15 mg/kg/dose every 4–6 hours
Maximum dose: 1000 mg every 6 hours

NONSTEROIDAL ANTI-INFLAMMATORY DRUGS (NSAIDs)

A series of drugs called nonsteroidal anti-inflammatory agents (NSAIDs)—principally derivatives of phenylalkanoic acid—are available. They exert their analgesic effects peripherally by inhibiting prostaglandin synthetase. These agents possess analgesic and anti-inflammatory properties that are superior to those of aspirin, especially for arthritis, and are effective for the treatment of acute pain following minor surgery or trauma. The NSAIDs produce fewer bleeding problems than aspirin because their inhibition of platelet aggregation is reversible as soon as they have been excreted fully. Other side effects reported include gastrointestinal upset, rash, headache, dizziness, eye problems, hepatic dysfunction, and renal dysfunction. There are relatively few clinical drug trials evaluating NSAIDs in children, but common agents approved by the Food and Drug Administration (FDA) for children are ibuprofen (PediaProfen, Children's Advil) 4–10 mg/kg every 6 hours; naproxen (Naprosyn) 5–7 mg/kg two to three times per day; and tolmetin (Tolectin) 5–7 mg/kg three to four times per day. Both ibuprofen and naproxen are available in oral suspension form.

Narcotic Analgesics

The narcotics or opioids have been shown to interact with opioid receptors in the central nervous system, spinal cord, and in the periphery (Tyler, 1994). These interactions result in the pharmacologic effects characteristic of the narcotics, including analgesia, sedation, and cough suppression. Narcotics are significantly more effective against severe and acute pain than the non-narcotic analgesics. They carry the serious drawbacks, however, of a much greater incidence of adverse effects, such as sedation, respiratory depression, and dependence and abuse. There are many narcotic analgesics available, including morphine, meperidine (Demerol), fentanyl (Sublimaze), codeine, oxycodone (Percodan), and hydromorphone (Dilaudid). Most of these drugs must be administered parenterally. Meperidine, oxycodone, and codeine are available in an oral form. Only codeine is discussed in this section.

CODEINE

Codeine is the standard of comparison for oral narcotics and is the most commonly prescribed narcotic for moderate to severe pain. It is absorbed well when given orally and may be used for more severe pain that is not responsive to aspirin, acetaminophen, or the NSAIDs. Codeine is much less potent than its relative morphine. It has far less addictive potential because it does not alter mood significantly. Side effects include nausea, sedation, dizziness, constipation, and cramps. When given in low doses, its antitussive effect makes it an important drug for the treatment of cough. If given in high doses or over prolonged periods of time, codeine may produce the more serious side effects of respiratory depression and dependence seen with the other, more potent narcotics.

Codeine may be given alone or in combination with another analgesic. Because the narcotics act at a central site and the non-narcotic analgesics act at a separate peripheral site, it is prudent to combine the two types of analgesics for enhanced activity. An example is acetaminophen with codeine (Tylenol No. 3).

Dosage. It is recommended that codeine be given in combination with acetaminophen when it is given orally for pediatric analgesia. The recommended dosage is as follows:

Children: 0.5–1.0 mg/kg/dose given at 4- to 6-hour intervals as needed
Adults: 30–60 mg/dose given at 4- to 6-hour intervals as needed

It has been reported that 17% of children undergoing invasive restorative treatment and 22% of children needing tooth extraction require postoperative analgesia (Acs, 1992). It is rare that the recommended doses of acetaminophen or NSAIDs will not control dental pain. Should this situation occur, codeine in combination with acetaminophen usually provides the needed relief. In the very rare situation in which dental pain is refractory to these modalities, a more potent agent such as meperidine may be used. The duration of such drug use should always be very brief and embarked upon carefully. Definitive dental therapy must be provided expediently.

REFERENCES

Acs G, Drazner E: The incidence of postoperative pain and analgesic usage in children. ASDC J Dent Child 59:48-52, 1992.

Covino BG: Local Anesthetics: Mechanism of Action and Clinical Use. New York, Grune & Stratton, 1976.

Keesling GR, Hinds EC: Optimal concentration of epinephrine in lidocaine solutions. JADA 66:337, 1963.

Malamed SF: Handbook of Local Anesthesia, 4th ed. St Louis, CV Mosby, 1997.

Shannon M, Berde CB: Pharmacologic management of pain in children and adolescents. Pediatr Clin North Am 36(4):855-871, 1989.

Tyler DC: Pharmacology of pain management. Pediatr Clin North Am 41(1):59-71, 1994.

Chapter **8**

Pain and Anxiety Control (Part II: Pain Reaction Control— Conscious Sedation)

Stephen Wilson, William F. Vann, Jr., Diane C. Dilley, and Jay A. Anderson

Chapter Outline

The vast majority of pediatric dental patients can be managed in the conventional dental environment. By establishing good rapport with the patient and parent and by relying on sound behavior management techniques (see Chapter 23), the anxiety and pain of most pediatric dental patients can be managed effectively using only local anesthesia. In a few children, the anxiety and pain control needs to go beyond behavioral modification and physicochemical blockade of the anatomic pathways because these few are unable to tolerate dental procedures comfortably despite patient encouragement and adequate local anesthesia. For these patients, additional steps must be taken to control anxiety. Pharmacologic management is indicated for children who cannot be managed with traditional behavioral management techniques and local anesthesia.

The primary purpose of pharmacologic management of young patients is to minimize or eliminate anxiety. General anesthesia, to our knowledge, totally eliminates anxiety and the pain reaction threshold. Sedation, depending on its depth, produces a relative reduction in anxiety facilitating (1) the opportunity for inviting the patient to use learned coping skills and (2) the raising of the pain reaction threshold. Sedation and general anesthesia are not without significant risks against which the benefits of these techniques must be measured, however. The degree of sedation depends on a host of factors, the more prominent being dose, rate, and route of drug administered and patient metabolic rate, surface area, age, and general health. Thus and importantly, sedation represents a continuum whose effects vary from very mild anxiolysis to a deep sedation indistinguishable from general anesthesia. Traditionally, this continuum has been divided into the broad classes of conscious and deep sedation based on conventional wisdom. For the practitioner who uses sedation, education and training beyond most dental school curricula involving sedation techniques are necessary for deep sedation and some levels of conscious sedation.

In 1985, the American Academy of Pediatric Dentistry (AAPD) and the American Academy of Pediatrics jointly endorsed *Guidelines for the Elective Use of Conscious Sedation, Deep Sedation, and General Anesthesia in Pediatric Patients* (AAPD, 1985). These *Guidelines* set the current standard of care for those who practice these sedation techniques for pediatric patients. The AAPD has twice revised the *Guidelines,* with the latest revision being in 1997. The revised *Guidelines* are unique in the sense that they use descriptive levels of sedation, based on behavioral and clinical indices, to refine the traditional concepts and definitions of "conscious" and "deep" sedation (Table 8-1).

The *Guidelines* emphasize that the goals of sedation are to (1) facilitate the provision of quality care, (2) minimize the extremes of disruptive behavior, (3) promote a positive psychological response to treatment, (4) promote patient welfare and safety, and (5) return the patient to a physiologic state in which safe discharge, as determined by recognized criteria, is possible.

This chapter focuses on conscious sedation and its use as an adjunct in the management of anxiety and pain control in pediatric patients. Because of the potential overlap of conscious sedation with deep sedation and general anesthesia, the latter modalities must be discussed and clarified in the context of defining what conscious sedation is and, more important, what it is not.

Before discussing conscious sedation, we spell out several key definitions and delineate the fundamental differences among conscious sedation, deep sedation, and general anesthesia. These terms are defined clearly in the *Guidelines* as follows.

CONSCIOUS SEDATION

Conscious sedation is a minimally depressed level of consciousness in which the patient's ability to maintain a patent airway independently and continuously and to respond appropriately to physical stimulation or verbal command such as "Open your eyes." For the very young or handicapped person who is incapable of the usually expected verbal responses, a minimally depressed level of consciousness should be maintained. The caveat that loss of consciousness should be unlikely is a particularly important part of the definition of conscious sedation, and the drugs and techniques used should carry a margin of safety wide enough to render unintended loss of consciousness unlikely. Note that level 3 of conscious sedation suggests that a child may be in a state not unlike natural sleep and must be arousable to the degree that crying and withdrawal reflexes should follow a mild to moderate painful stimulus such as an injection of local anesthetic. If arousal, as described earlier, does not occur, especially after a repeated mild to moderate painful stimulus (e.g., trapezius muscle pinch), the child is in a state of deep sedation and must be monitored accordingly. The minimal monitoring requirement for most levels of conscious sedation is a pulse oximeter.

DEEP SEDATION

Deep sedation is a controlled state of depressed consciousness or unconsciousness from which the patient is not aroused easily. Deep sedation may be accompanied by a partial or complete loss of protective reflexes, including the ability to maintain a patent airway independently and respond purposefully to physical stimulation or verbal command. Young patients who are in deep sedation may respond with only a reflex withdrawal to an intensely painful stimulus, if at all. Monitoring requirements for deep sedation require a minimum of a pulse oximeter, capnograph, precordial stethoscope, and blood pressure cuff.

TABLE 8–1. Definitions and Characteristics for Levels of Sedation and General Anesthesia

	Conscious Sedation		Deep Sedation	
Functional level of sedation	Mild sedation (anxiolysis) (Level 1)	Interactive (Level 2)	Non-interactive/arousable with mild/moderate stimulus (Level 3)	Non-interactive/non-arousable except with intense stimulus (Level 4)
Goal	Decrease anxiety; facilitate coping skills	Decrease or eliminate anxiety; facilitate coping skills	Decrease or eliminate anxiety; facilitate coping skills; promote sleep	Eliminate anxiety; coping skills overridden
Responsiveness	Uninterrupted interactive ability; totally awake	Minimally depressed level of consciousness; eyes open or temporarily closed; responds appropriately to verbal commands	Moderately depressed level of consciousness; mimics physiologic sleep (vitals not different from those of sleep); eyes closed most of time; may or may not respond to verbal prompts alone; responds to mild/moderate stimuli (e.g., repeated trapezius pinching or needle insertion in oral tissues elicits reflex withdrawal and appropriate verbalization [complaint, moan, crying]); airway only occasionally may require readjustment via chin thrust.	Deeply depressed level of consciousness; sleep-like state, but vitals may be slightly depressed compared to physiologic sleep; eyes closed; does not respond to verbal prompts alone; reflex withdrawal with no verbalization when intense stimuli occur (e.g., repeated, prolonged, and intense pinching of the trapezius); airway expected to require constant monitoring and frequent management
Personnel	2	2	2	3
Monitoring equipment	Clinical observations	PO; precordial recommended*	PO, precordial, BP; capno desirable*	PO & capno, precordial, BP, ECG; defibrillator desirable
Monitoring info	None	HR, RR, O$_2$ Pre-; during (q15min); post, as needed	HR, RR, O$_2$, BP; [CO$_2$] if available Pre-; during (q10min); post till stable/discharge criteria	HR, RR, O$_2$, BP, [CO$_2$] Pre-; during (q5min); post till stable/discharge criteria

Monitors: PO (pulse oximetry); capno (capnography); BP (blood pressure cuff); ECG (electrocardiogram). HR = heart rate; RR = respiratory rate.
It should be noted that clinical observation should accompany any level of sedation and general anesthesia.
*"Recommended" and "desirable" should be interpreted as not a necessity, but as an adjunct in assessing patient status.
Guidelines for the Elective Use of Pharmacologic Conscious Sedation and Deep Sedation in Pediatric Dental Patients. Pediatric Dentistry, Reference Manual 1996–97: *1830-34, 1997.*

GENERAL ANESTHESIA

General anesthesia is a controlled state of unconsciousness accompanied by a loss of protective reflexes, including the ability to maintain an airway independently and respond purposefully to physical stimulation or verbal command.

CONSCIOUS VERSUS DEEP SEDATION: A CRITICAL QUESTION

The difference between conscious and deep sedation is a concept that must be comprehended thoroughly by those who sedate pediatric dental patients. Practitioners must realize that the goal of conscious sedation is a level of sedation that does not render the patient unconscious or unresponsive to repetitive mild or moderately painful stimuli. A reflex withdrawal alone to repeated mild or moderately painful stimuli is not appropriate for conscious sedation. The patient under conscious sedation can respond appropriately to verbal commands or mildly noxious stimuli and can maintain a patent airway at all times. If sedation techniques are practiced in this manner, the patient's cardiovascular and respiratory functions should always be well maintained.

Why is it a problem for the practitioner to move from the threshold of conscious sedation to deep sedation? The answer is simple: The patient has a much more serious risk of cardiovascular or respiratory misadventures. When the patient has a partial or complete loss of protective reflexes and cannot maintain an airway independently, apnea or hypoxemia may be a serious or life-threatening outcome (Anderson and Vann, 1988). Because the separation between conscious and deep sedation is sometimes difficult to discern, the wise practitioner obtains proper training in sedation and monitoring techniques before routinely using pharmacologic management of children.

For those practitioners who choose to practice deep sedation for pediatric patients, the *Guidelines* are specific about requirements for a higher level of personnel training as well as a higher level of vigilance in monitoring the sedated child. They spell out requirements for personnel, the operating facility, intravenous access, monitoring procedures, and recovery care that carry a higher level of expectation and training than is the case with the use of conscious sedation (AAPD, 1997). In short, for practitioners who choose to use deep sedation, the standard of care specified in the *Guidelines* is nothing less than stringent, and it is doubtful that many general practitioners or

pediatric dentists currently have the training or facilities to undertake deep sedation in an office-based setting.

RELIANCE ON THE *GUIDELINES* AS THE STANDARD OF CARE FOR CONSCIOUS SEDATION

The *Guidelines* have established a new standard of care for conscious sedation of pediatric patients. Because they were promulgated in the relatively recent past (1985), it is instructive to examine those areas that have been affected most dramatically. In considering presedation events, the *Guidelines* focus on parental instructions, dietary precautions, and a preoperative health evaluation. Essentially, the *Guidelines* intensify the presedation activities with a keen eye toward eliminating the possibility of sedation misadventures. They call also for documentation and recording of events during treatment (i.e., vital signs, medications given, and patient response).

The three standards in the *Guidelines* that have changed the manner in which pediatric conscious sedation is practiced most dramatically relate to (1) personnel, (2) patient monitoring, and (3) pre-procedural prescriptions. Relative to personnel, the *Guidelines* specify that an assistant other than the dental operator must participate in the conscious sedation procedure and that this assistant must be trained to monitor appropriate physiologic parameters and assist in any support or resuscitation measures required. Relative to intraoperative monitoring procedures during conscious sedation, the *Guidelines* specify continuous monitoring by a trained person. A precordial stethoscope and pulse oximeter are considered the minimum equipment needed for obtaining continuous information on heart rate and respiratory rate. According to fairly recent research in this area, the pulse oximeter is currently considered the standard of care for monitoring pediatric patients under conscious sedation (Anderson and Vann, 1988; Wilson, 1990).

Pre-procedural prescriptions refer to the practitioner writing a prescription for the parent to administer an agent outside of the treatment facility. The revised *Guidelines* indicate that only minor tranquilizers (e.g., diazepam) may be administered outside of the treatment facility. Chloral hydrate and meperidine are not considered minor tranquilizers and thus should not be administered to a child outside of the dental office.

In summary, the *Guidelines* have had a major impact on how the practitioner must approach the conscious sedation of children. There are no systematic evaluations of the impact of the *Guidelines* on safety in pediatric conscious sedation; however, it is our opinion that these Guidelines are dramatically improving the safety of sedation in the dental office environment. Unfortunately, significant morbidity and mortality have occurred; however, no deaths have occurred, to our knowledge, when the *Guidelines* have been faithfully followed by the practitioner.

ROUTES OF ADMINISTRATION

The primary routes of administration for conscious sedation are (1) inhalational, (2) enteral (e.g., oral or rectal), and (3) parenteral (e.g., intramuscular, subcutaneous, submucosal, intranasal, or intravenous). In our review of these techniques, only the primary advantages and disadvantages are discussed briefly.

Inhalational Route (Nitrous Oxide)

ADVANTAGES

The primary advantages of nitrous oxide for conscious sedation in pediatric dentistry are as follows.

Rapid Onset and Recovery Time. Because nitrous oxide has a very low plasma solubility, it reaches a therapeutic level in the blood rapidly, and, conversely, blood levels decrease rapidly when it is discontinued.

Ease of Dose Control (Titration). There are two ways to initially administer nitrous oxide to children. One is the standard titration technique used on adults, and the other is the rapid induction technique. For the standard titration technique, nitrous oxide should be started at 10% concentration, then administered in increments of concentration ranging from 5% to 10% until the patient becomes comfortable and some clinical signs of optimal sedation are noted. The signs of optimal sedation include slight relaxation of the limb and jaw muscles; ptosis of the eyelids; a blank stare as if looking up at a star-filled evening sky; palms open, warm, and slightly moist; slight change in the pitch of the patient's voice; and patient reports of being comfortable and relaxed. Each time the clinician increases the concentration, he or she should wait approximately 30 seconds while talking with the child and watching for classic signs of optimal sedation before deciding to increase the concentration again. The end point in terms of maximal con-

centration of nitrous oxide usually should not exceed 50% for children. Most children seem comfortable and demonstrate optimal signs of sedation in the concentration range of 35% to 50% of nitrous oxide. The standard titration technique is primarily used for mildly anxious but cooperative children.

A second option to the standard titration techniques of nitrous oxide administration is the rapid induction technique. This technique is usually indicated for the mild to moderately anxious, potentially cooperative child who needs to be controlled quickly by the clinician. The technique involves administering 50% nitrous oxide immediately to the patient without any titration steps.

In either technique, nitrous oxide should be discontinued if the child becomes disruptive and no longer breathes through the nitrous oxide hood or if the child becomes nauseated, vomits, or both. Also, good nitrous oxide hygiene is always indicated and includes a scavenging system, large operatories, rapid room-air exchanges, supplemental movement of air (i.e., fans), and a nasal hood that adapts closely to the nose area of the face.

Lack of Serious Adverse Effects. Nitrous oxide is considered to be inert and nontoxic when it is administered with adequate oxygen. The most commonly encountered side effect is nausea, which should be rare unless high concentrations of nitrous oxide are used. Poor technique with high concentrations may also result in an excitement phase, in which the patient may become uncomfortable, uncooperative, and delirious.

DISADVANTAGES

The use of nitrous oxide in pediatric dentistry also has several disadvantages.

Weak Agent. Attempts to push the concentration of nitrous oxide up in order to control moderately or severely anxious patients will be fraught with failure and will not be pleasant for the operator or the patient.

Lack of Patient Acceptance. There are some patients (adults and children) who do not find the effects of nitrous oxide pleasant. These patients may become overtly noncompliant, removing the nasal mask or becoming otherwise uncooperative.

Inconvenience. In some areas, such as the maxillary anterior teeth, the use of the nitrous oxide nasal mask may hinder exposure of the area. This may be a problem, especially in small children.

Potential Chronic Toxicity. Retrospective survey studies of dental office personnel who were exposed to trace levels of nitrous oxide suggest a possible association with an increased incidence of spontaneous abortions, congenital malformations, certain cancers, liver disease, kidney disease, and neurologic disease. These results underscore the necessity of scavenging (removing) waste gases adequately from the dental operatory. It should be noted that it can be difficult to scavenge nitrous oxide adequately in the uncooperative child because gases that are exhaled through the mouth cannot be scavenged effectively.

Potentiation. Although nitrous oxide is a weak and safe agent when used with oxygen, deep sedation or general anesthesia may be easily produced if nitrous oxide is added to the effects of other sedative drugs given by another route. The combination of nitrous oxide with any other conscious sedation technique must be undertaken with extreme care by a person who has the proper training and experience.

Equipment. Equipment must be purchased, installed, and maintained. The level of nitrous oxide may be adjusted in small increments to produce the desired effect.

Practical Use of Inhalation Sedation Techniques

Nitrous oxide analgesia is relatively safe and effective for the treatment of children in the dental office. It is useful for decreasing mild levels of anxiety and is indicated for patients who have the capacity to be compliant and follow instructions during nitrous oxide administration. Children who have nasal obstructions or are uncooperative when directed to breathe through the nose are poor candidates for nitrous oxide administration. The analgesic properties of nitrous oxide help to raise the pain threshold and may be used to lessen the discomfort during a local anesthetic injection. Nitrous oxide does *not* eliminate the need for local anesthetic pain control in most children, however, except for very minor dental procedures (i.e., small Class V preparations).

Nitrous oxide changes the patient's perception of the environment and the passage of time and is therefore helpful in managing children with short attention spans. This mild dissociation may be perceived by some children as unpleasant, in which case the level of nitrous oxide should be decreased or discontinued.

A total liter flow rate per minute of gases should be established first with 100% oxygen. An adult will require 5–7 liters/minute, whereas a 3- to 4-year-old will require 3–5 liters/minute. While adjusting the controls, the dentist should use the "tell-show-do" technique with terminology appropriate for the age level of the child. The nosepiece should be introduced with instructions to breathe nasally (i.e., "smell the happy air"). Light finger pressure under the lower lip to produce an oral seal and gentle tapping of the nosepiece can be helpful to encourage nasal breathing in the young child.

After stabilization of the nosepiece and delivery of 100% oxygen for 3 to 5 minutes, the nitrous oxide level should be increased to 30% to 35% and administered for 3 to 5 minutes for the induction period. While administering the nitrous oxide, the dentist should talk gently to the child to promote relaxation and reinforce cooperative behavior. Although asking older children and adults if they feel tingling sensations in the fingers and toes is appropriate for verification of early signs of central nervous system (CNS) effects from the nitrous oxide, these suggestive questions to the young child may lead to undesirable body movements. An indication of such CNS effects would be slight movements of the fingers and toes in the young child.

Most dentists prefer to increase the level of nitrous oxide to 50% for 3 to 5 minutes to provide maximum analgesia for the local anesthetic injection; however, concentrations of nitrous oxide in excess of 50% are contraindicated for dental office sedation. When the dental injection is completed, the nitrous oxide level should be reduced to 30% to 35% for a maintenance dose during the dental treatment; alternatively, 100% oxygen may be administered when the nitrous oxide is only needed for behavior management related to the dental injection.

Upon termination of nitrous oxide administration, inhalation of 100% oxygen for not less than 3 to 5 minutes is recommended. This allows diffusion of nitrous oxide from the venous blood into the alveoli through the respiratory tract. Adequate oxygenation, especially following long procedures, enables the patient to return without incident to pretreatment activities. Inadequate oxygenation may produce such postoperative side effects as nausea, light-headedness, or dizziness, all of which can be reversed with continued oxygen administration.

It is important for the dentist to recognize that nitrous oxide analgesia should not be used as a substitute for the traditional nonpharmacologic approach to child management problems in the dental office. Nitrous oxide should be considered an adjunct to aid in management of mild anxiety in the child who is capable of cooperating in the dental chair.

Oral Route

A route of administration used commonly for conscious sedation in pediatric dentistry is oral premedication.

ADVANTAGES

Convenience. Usually oral drug administration is easy and convenient, especially if the medication tastes good and can be delivered in low volume. The drug may be given at home or in the office depending on the classification of drug used. Giving it in the office has the advantages of supervision (to be certain that the proper dose is given at the appropriate time) and medicolegal safety. Usually it is best to administer oral premedications in a separate quiet, dimly lit room with a soft chair or rocking chair, where induction of sedation can be facilitated by the parent in a conducive environment.

Economy. To administer oral premedications, no special office equipment needs to be purchased or maintained. Special equipment is needed to monitor patients under conscious sedation as specified in the *Guidelines,* however.

Lack of Toxicity. If appropriate doses are calculated for each patient (keeping the previous discussion on pharmacokinetics in mind) and single drugs are used in single doses, the oral route of sedation is extremely safe. If, however, drug combinations are used or if two routes are combined (e.g., oral premedication followed by intravenous or inhalational medications), the chances of adverse side effects increase dramatically.

DISADVANTAGES

Variability of Effect. The biggest disadvantage of oral premedication is the fact that a standard dose must be used for all patients on a weight or body surface area (BSA) basis. Individuals of the same weight (or BSA), however, may respond differently to the same dose of drug, depending on many variables. Absorption of the drug from the gastrointestinal tract can be altered by several factors, such as the presence of food, autonomic tone, fear, emotional make-up, fatigue, medications, and gastric emptying time. The patient may not cooperate in ingesting the medication or may vomit, making estimation of

the dose actually received impossible. If an inadequate dose has been given, a paradoxical response may occur, which may be due to a direct effect or loss of emotional inhibitions. The patient may become agitated and more uncooperative rather than sedated and cooperative. These factors make the oral route of administration least dependable as far as certainty of effect is concerned. A second dose of oral medication to offset a presumably inadequate dose should never be given. Titration is not possible or safe with oral medication. If absorption of the initial dose has been delayed for any reason and a second dose is subsequently given on the assumption that the first dose was ineffective, both doses will eventually be absorbed, possibly resulting in a high serum level of the CNS-depressant drug and leading to possible serious consequences, such as respiratory arrest, cardiovascular collapse, and death.

Onset Time. Oral drug administration has the longest time of onset of any route of drug used for conscious sedation. The lag time, which is from the time of administration until treatment is attempted, varies from 15 to 90 minutes depending on the type of drug used.

Oral premedication is useful in pediatric dentistry, but its limitations must be clearly understood. An adequate dose must be given and enough time must be allowed to elapse for absorption to take place before the desired effect can be expected.

Intramuscular Route

The intramuscular route of drug administration involves injection of the sedative agent into a skeletal muscle mass. It also involves certain advantages and disadvantages when used in pediatric dentistry.

ADVANTAGES

Absorption. Absorption from an injection deep into a large muscle is much faster and more dependable than absorption from the oral route.

Technical Advantages. Technically, the intramuscular route of administration might be considered the easiest of all routes. It requires no special equipment except a syringe and needle. Patient cooperation is required for the oral route of administration, sometimes making it difficult to give a full dose of a bitter-tasting medication to an uncooperative child. When intramuscular medications are administered, little or no patient cooperation is required, and the full calculated dose is given with a high degree of certainty. Even when a child requires restraint, intramuscular injections are easier to accomplish technically than placement of an intravenous cannula.

DISADVANTAGES

Onset. Absorption of the injected drug can be decreased or delayed by several factors. A patient who is cold or very anxious may experience peripheral vasoconstriction in the area of the injection, significantly decreasing the rate of absorption. Perhaps the biggest variable in onset is related to where the drug is actually deposited. If the drug is deposited deep into a large muscle mass, the high degree of vascularity there will allow rapid uptake. If, however, some or all of the drug is deposited between muscle layers, in the surface of the muscle, or not in the muscle at all (all distinct possibilities in small, struggling children), absorption may be unpredictable.

Effect. As with the oral route, a standardized dose is used, calculated on the patient's weight or BSA. Drug effect cannot be titrated safely by administering additional doses for much the same reason as that described for the oral route—that is, the possibility of cumulative overdose. A standard dose may have little or no effect in some children, whereas it may sedate others heavily.

Trauma. Injection sites that are devoid of large nerves and vessels are used for intramuscular injections, such as the mid-deltoid region, the vastus lateralis muscle of the thigh, and the gluteus medius muscle. Proper selection of the injection site and proper technique should minimize the possibility of tissue trauma.

Intravenous Access. The potential for side effects and toxicity is higher with the intramuscular route than with the inhalational or oral route. Compared with the intravenous route, a major disadvantage of the intramuscular route is the lack of a means of access (an intravenous catheter) in the event of a medical emergency.

Liability Costs. Malpractice insurance carriers charge a higher premium for dentists who administer parenteral sedatives in the dental office. In addition, many state dental practice acts have established requirements for permits for dentists who administer parenteral medications.

Subcutaneous Route

Occasionally, the subcutaneous route of administration is used in pediatric dentistry for con-

scious sedation. In this situation, the drug is injected into the subcutaneous or submucosal space, not into the muscle. Generally, similar advantages and disadvantages apply to this route as to the intramuscular route with the following exceptions.

ADVANTAGES

Site. For dental procedures, some drugs may be injected submucosally within the oral cavity, usually into the buccal vestibule. This may be less objectionable to some patients and parents than multiple injection sites, and it may be more comfortable and convenient for the dentist to perform.

DISADVANTAGES

Technical Disadvantages. The rate of absorption is slower with the subcutaneous route than with the other parenteral routes. Blood supply to the subcutaneous tissue often is sparse compared with muscle. Within the oral cavity, however, vascularity is abundant and absorption is seldom a problem.

Tissue Slough. Because the drug is deposited close to the surface of the skin or mucosa, tissue sloughing is possible. For this reason, only nonirritating substances should be given subcutaneously, and large volumes of solution should not be injected.

Liability Costs. Administration of parenteral medications increases the costs of malpractice coverage and may be subject to state dental laws that require permits for the use of parenteral sedation.

Conscious Sedation via the Intravenous Route

The intravenous route is the optimal and ideal route for administration of conscious sedation.

ADVANTAGES

Titration. Among the parenteral routes, only the intravenous route allows exact titration to a desired drug effect. Because the drug is injected directly into the blood stream, absorption is not a factor. Within a few circulation times, the intravenous drug exerts its maximal effect. Small, incremental doses may be given over a relatively short period of time until the desired level of sedation is achieved, thus avoiding under- or over-dosing with a standardized single bolus dose, as is necessary with oral, intramuscular, or subcutaneous injections.

Test Dose. With the intravenous route, a very small initial test dose can be administered, and a short period of time is allowed to pass to observe for an allergic reaction or extreme patient sensitivity to the agent.

Intravenous Access. In the event of a medical emergency, administration of emergency drugs is almost always best accomplished through the intravenous route. Establishing intravenous access after an emergency can be difficult and can consume precious time.

DISADVANTAGES

The intravenous route would be used for all patients requiring conscious sedation if it did not involve serious disadvantages.

Technical Disadvantages. Establishment of intravenous access (venipuncture) is technically the most difficult skill that must be mastered in the practice of conscious sedation. Placing and maintaining an intravenous catheter in children can be difficult even for a seasoned pediatrician. The procedure requires both training and extensive practice.

Potential Complications. Because potent drugs are injected directly into the blood stream, the intravenous route carries an increased potential for complications. Extravasation of drug into the tissues, hematoma formation, and inadvertent intra-arterial injections are possible complications of a misplaced intravenous catheter. If the medication is injected too rapidly, exaggerated effects may be produced. An immediate anaphylactic allergic reaction becomes life-threatening more rapidly if it is due to an intravenous bolus of a drug than if it is due to an oral or intramuscular dose. These complications should be all avoidable by using a test dose and a proper, careful technique. Thrombophlebitis is a rare complication that is attributable directly to the intravenous cannula.

Patient Monitoring. Because of the previously discussed increased potential of rapidly developing complications, the patient receiving intravenous sedation requires the highest level of monitoring.

Liability Costs. Again, because the intravenous route is a parenteral route, the liability costs are considerably higher than those for oral administration. With the additional monitoring and the armamentarium required, intravenous sedation is considered by many to be cost-prohibitive for the routine practice of general dentistry.

PHARMACOLOGIC AGENTS FOR CONSCIOUS SEDATION

A large number of drugs are available for use in sedation and anesthesia. In this chapter individual drugs or techniques are put into perspective rather than discussed in detail. Three primary groups of drugs are used for conscious sedation in pediatric dentistry: the sedative-hypnotics, the antianxiety agents, and the narcotic analgesics (Table 8–2). Each group acts primarily in a different area of the brain and should be expected to produce a distinctive primary effect. The wise practitioner of conscious sedation understands which specific effect to expect from a given drug and uses the drug principally to achieve that effect.

Sedative-Hypnotics

The sedative-hypnotics are drugs whose principal effect is sedation or sleepiness. As the dose of a sedative-hypnotic drug is increased, the patient becomes increasingly drowsy until sleep (hypnosis) is produced. Further increasing the dose can produce general anesthesia, coma, and even death. It is important to note that the primary effect of these drugs is not to decrease anxiety or to raise the pain threshold (analgesia). In fact, a sedative-hypnotic used alone may lower the pain reaction threshold in some cases by removing inhibitions, and in inadequate dosages it may simply produce a patient who is more responsive to pain stimulation. The principal action of the sedative-hypnotics results from the initial primary effect of these drugs on the reticular activating system, an area of the brain involved in maintaining consciousness. Further increases in dose affect other brain areas, especially the cortex.

The sedative-hypnotic drugs fall into two categories: the *barbiturates,* such as pentobarbital, secobarbital, and methohexital; and the *nonbarbiturate hypnotics,* which include drugs such as chloral hydrate and paraldehyde.

TABLE 8–2. Conscious Sedation: Pharmacologic Agents

Group	Site of Primary Effect	Effect
Sedative hypnotics	Reticular activating system	Sedation/sleep
Antianxiety agents	Limbic system	Decrease in anxiety
Narcotics	Opioid receptors	Analgesia

Oral chloral hydrate, alone or in combination with other drugs, is the most common sedative agent used in pediatric dentistry. When used in low doses (25–40 mg/kg), chloral hydrate can produce mild sedation, or it can have the opposite effect, producing a resistive and agitated patient, as occurs also with barbiturate sedation in children. Higher doses (50–60 mg/kg), especially in combination with other premedications such as hydroxyzine (Atarax or Vistaril) or meperidine (Demerol), can produce good sedation, but patients must be monitored closely, according to the *Guidelines,* because of the increased risk of respiratory depression and loss of consciousness (Nathan and West, 1987). Another characteristic of chloral hydrate is that it causes relaxation of the tongue muscles. Thus, the airway must be examined for hypertrophied tonsils because a relaxed tongue can easily drop back against enlarged tonsils, blocking the airway in a supine, sedated patient (Fishbaugh et al., 1997). In fact, the airway and size of the tonsils should be examined in every child who is being considered for sedation. Children with tonsils greater than 50% of the potential airway should not be sedated and other means of pharmacologic management should be considered (i.e., general anesthesia). Chloral hydrate is bitter-tasting, which can produce management problems during administration. A final disadvantage is that chloral hydrate can induce nausea and vomiting secondary to gastric irritability.

Antianxiety Agents

Previously the antianxiety agents were called minor tranquilizers (the major tranquilizers are the antipsychotic drugs). These drugs have the primary effect of removing or decreasing anxiety. The primary site of action of these agents is the limbic system, which is the "seat of the emotions." Theoretically, a dose exists for each antianxiety agent at which anxiety is decreased without producing significant sedation. As doses are increased, however, the reticular activating system and then the cortex are affected, producing sedation and sleep as well. Because anxiety is often the primary problem in people with dental phobias, a primary effect against anxiety appears to be desirable, especially in reasonably cooperative adults. Antianxiety drugs possess a flatter dose-response curve pharmacologically than many of the sedative-hypnotics (especially barbiturates), allowing for a safer therapeutic index. This means that for most antianxiety drugs (e.g., diazepam), a larger difference exists between the

dose that produces loss of consciousness than is the case with a rapid-acting sedative-hypnotic (e.g., methohexital), which has a steep dose-response curve—that is, the difference between a mildly sedating dose and general anesthesia is small. Drugs such as methohexital (Brevitol) should not be used for conscious sedation for this reason. The antianxiety agents produce no analgesia.

The antianxiety agents consist primarily of the benzodiazepines, and the two most commonly used benzodiazepines are diazepam (Valium) and midazolam (Versed). This group of agents is principally used for conscious sedation in adults. Unfortunately, there is a lack of extensive clinical experience and research on these agents in children, but clinical evidence is increasing for the potential of these drugs in pediatric patients (Moore, 1985). Both can be administered orally; however, midazolam is more potent, has a more rapid onset (usually notable signs can be seen within 10 minutes), and shorter duration of action than diazepam. Profound respiratory depression has been associated with midazolam use, especially when administered in combination with narcotics. Also noteworthy is an "angry" response that occurs in many children after the administration of midazolam. Characteristically, these children become irritable, uncontrollable, and angry with others in their presence approximately 45 minutes after administration.

Some of the antihistamines, such as hydroxyzine (Atarax, Vistaril) and diphenhydramine (Benadryl), possess both antianxiety and sedative-hypnotic properties. They are often classified with the antianxiety agents. These drugs are not very useful for conscious sedation when used alone but are useful in combination with other drugs such as the sedative-hypnotics and potentiating agents. They may also be used as co-medicaments because of their antiemetic properties.

Narcotics

The narcotics were discussed previously in the section on analgesics. These drugs are used also as part of conscious sedation techniques for their primary action of analgesia. The site of action of the narcotics is the opioid receptors of the central nervous system. These drugs modify the interpretation of the pain stimulus in the CNS and therefore raise the pain threshold. As the dose of the narcotic is raised, other effects such as sedation occur. It should be recognized that sedation per se is not the principal end point sought from a narcotic. If narcotic dosage is pushed to achieve sedation, serious side effects are encountered, the most frequent of which are respiratory depression and apnea, which can lead to hypoxia. If sedation is desired, it should be accomplished with a drug that produces sedation as its primary effect.

Narcotics may produce nausea and vomiting, especially when used alone. In high doses, narcotics may also produce cardiovascular depression. Narcotics are powerful potentiators of other CNS depressant drugs. The principal use of narcotics in conscious sedation should, therefore, be to augment the effects of the sedative-hypnotic or antianxiety agents and to contribute some degree of analgesia that other agents do not provide. It should be noted, however, that the analgesia obtained with narcotics cannot be used as a substitute for adequate local anesthesia.

Narcotics used in conscious sedation techniques include morphine, meperidine (Demerol), and fentanyl (Sublimaze). Alphaprodine (Nisentil) was formerly a popular synthetic narcotic for pediatric sedation but was withdrawn from the U.S. market in 1986 owing to multiple adverse reactions resulting in death or severe morbidity. When considering the use of narcotics in pediatric dentistry, it is wise to remember the definition of conscious sedation as spelled out in the *Guidelines*. To reiterate, the caveat that loss of consciousness should be unlikely is a particularly important part of the definition of conscious sedation. The drugs and techniques used should carry a margin of safety wide enough to render unintentional loss of consciousness unlikely (AAPD, 1997). Narcotics have steep dose-response curves. They must be used with extreme caution for conscious sedation because they carry a high risk of producing respiratory depression and loss of consciousness, especially if they are combined with other agents such as nitrous oxide.

Ketamine

The dissociative agent ketamine has had periods of popularity in pediatric dental practice. It produces a cataleptic state with profound analgesia and amnesia. Because ketamine acts primarily on the thalamus and cortex, not on the reticular activating system, the patient does not appear to be asleep but rather dissociated from the environment. Respirations usually are not depressed with proper dosages. Profound stimulatory cardiovascular changes usually are produced, so tachycardia and increased blood pressure can be expected.

Ketamine is mentioned primarily to point out that it is classified as a general anesthetic because the patient under its influence is incapable of making appropriate responses to verbal commands or stimulation. It may cause respiratory depression and arrest in some patients as well as delirium and hallucinations. Ketamine should be used only by practitioners qualified to administer general anesthesia.

MONITORS

A host of monitors are used during sedation and general anesthesia (Wilson, 1995). The most common are pulse oximeters, capnographs, blood pressure cuffs, precordial stethoscopes, electrocardiographs, temperature probes, and defibrillators. The mix of monitors required for any sedation depends on the final depth of sedation. The most common monitors for conscious sedation are pulse oximeters, precordial stethoscopes, and blood pressure cuffs. These are briefly outlined.

Pulse Oximeter

A pulse oximeter is a self-contained instrument that noninvasively monitors the degree of oxygen saturation of hemoglobin molecules in the patient's blood and the patient's heart rate. Oxygen sensors placed across perfused tissue beds in which a pulse can be detected (e.g., the fingertip) determine oxygen saturation by measuring differences in the absorption of red and infrared light that is emitted by the sensors. Normally, the hemoglobin in arteries of healthy children and adults is approximately 97% saturated. Several factors, however, can cause "false alarms" or indications of desaturation when, in fact, the hemoglobin molecule is completely saturated with oxygen. Such factors may include patient movement artifacts, cold tissue beds, poor perfusion of tissue beds, and crying.

Precordial Stethoscope

Precordial stethoscopes are essentially stethoscopes whose bell is temporarily attached to the chest wall. By listening through the stethoscope, the clinician can determine the quality and relative quantity of air movement during breathing as well as the heart sounds. The closer the bell of the stethoscope is placed to the precordial notch (i.e., in the soft tissue area immediately above the manubrium of the chest), the louder are the breathing sounds compared with heart sounds. Partially occluded airways or restrictive airways have different qualities of sounds, including wheezing, stridor, or crowing. The precordial stethoscope is especially sensitive to competing operatory sounds (e.g., the pitch of the high-speed handpiece), and the operator must rely frequently on other clinical signs or physiologic monitors (e.g., capnographs) to determine the stability and condition of the patient.

THE FUTURE

The level of training required for a dentist to administer sedation or anesthesia safely is currently under debate and is changing throughout the United States. In many states special permits are required to practice certain anesthetic techniques. The suggested minimum educational requirement for training necessary to administer conscious sedation is 60 hours of instruction and clinical experience in an accredited program (AAPD, 1985), and some states are considering the adoption of educational and clock-hour requirements for practitioners who use office-based conscious sedation.

Deep sedation and general anesthesia are grouped together for training requirements, medicolegal reasons, and purposes of malpractice insurance. *Remember:* A sedation technique from which a patient is not easily aroused and may not respond purposefully to verbal commands at all times is, by definition, deep sedation. The suggested educational requirements for administration of deep sedation or general anesthesia is a minimum of 1 year of advanced study or its equivalent as described in Part II of the American Dental Association's *Guidelines for Teaching the Comprehensive Control of Pain and Anxiety in Dentistry* (NIH, 1985). Many states have adopted requirements for deep sedation and general anesthesia.

In summary, a pharmacologic approach to managing the behavior of uncooperative children in the dental office with conscious sedation is complex and requires additional training beyond the scope of this textbook. An undersedated child may continue to be a management problem, whereas an oversedated child may quickly become a life-threatening emergency in the dental office.

REFERENCES

AAPD: Guidelines for the elective use of conscious sedation, deep sedation, and general anesthesia in pediatric patients. Pediatr Dent 7:334-337, 1985.

AAPD: Guidelines for the Elective Use of Pharmacologic Conscious Sedation and Deep Sedation in Pediatric Dental Patients. Pediatric Dentistry, Reference Manual 1996-97: 18:30-34, 1997.

Anderson JA, Vann WF: Respiratory monitoring during pediatric sedation: Pulse oximetry and capnography. Pediatr Dent 10:94-101, 1988.

Fishbaugh DF, Wilson S, Preisch JW, Weaver JM II: Effect of tonsil presence and size on an airway blockage maneuver in children during sedation. Pediatr Dent 19:277-281, 1997.

Moore PA: Monitoring and management: Adult vs. pediatric patients (scientific abstract). Anesth Prog 32:168-169, 1985.

Nathan JE, West MS: Comparison of chloral hydrate-hydroxyzine with and without meperidine for management of the difficult pediatric patient. J Dent Child 54:437-444, 1987.

NIH Consensus Development Conference Statement on Anesthesia and Sedation in the Dental Office. JADA 111:90-93, 1985.

Wilson S: Conscious sedation and pulse oximetry: False alarms? Pediatr Dent 12:228-232, 1990.

Wilson S: Review of monitors and monitoring during sedation with emphasis on clinical applications. Pediatr Dent 17:9-14, 1995.

Chapter 9

Antimicrobials in Pediatric Dentistry

Michael W. Roberts and Wilma A. Lim

Chapter Outline

The second most commonly prescribed group of drugs for use in dentistry after the local anesthetics are the antibiotics. Various infections involving the teeth and oral cavity can become severe and even life-threatening if not properly treated. Treatment of infections usually involves a definitive dental or surgical procedure and often requires the use of antibiotics. Antimicrobials are substances that kill or suppress the growth or multiplication of microorganisms, whether bacteria, viruses, or fungi. Antibiotics are substances produced by microorganisms or by synthetic chemical methods that can produce an antimicrobial action. Antibiotics are indicated for diseases in which a specific microbial agent has been identified, for a clinical situation that points clearly to a probable microbial cause, and for use as a lifesaving measure in a gravely ill patient. Prophylactic use of antibiotics is also indicated in some specific instances, such as prophylaxis

against bacterial endocarditis for patients with congenital heart disease. Antibiotic therapy is maximally successful if the causative pathogen is known or has been positively identified (by culture or serology) and the therapeutic agent most active against that pathogen (confirmed by sensitivity testing) is used in appropriate doses.

ANTIMICROBIAL CLASSIFICATION

A vast array of antimicrobials are available for use in pediatric dentistry. They may be classified in several different ways.

Microbial Target Category

Antimicrobial agents are often categorized according to microbial target group. The principal emphasis of this chapter is on antibacterial agents (i.e., antibiotics). Antibiotics are considered to be either of narrow or wide spectrum. Narrow-spectrum antibiotics are effective primarily against either gram-positive or gram-negative organisms. Broad-spectrum drugs are effective against a wider range of organisms (Table 9–1). The overlap in effectiveness can be considerable with the broad-spectrum drugs. Efficacy against a particular microorganism is ideally determined by testing the sensitivity of the actual causative pathogen (obtained by culture) to specific antibiotics. Unfortunately, culturing may take 24 hours to several days and would delay initiation of antimicrobial therapy. This requires that a best guess be made for specific clinical situations as to which pathogen is most likely the causative agent and which antibiotic is usually most effective against that organism. This antibiotic, or combi-

nation of antibiotics, is used until culture and sensitivity results are available. Dental and periodontal infections are most commonly caused by bacteria that normally colonize the mouth, throat, and upper alimentary canal (e.g., aerobic and anaerobic streptococci, *Micrococcus* species, anaerobic gram-negative bacteria [*Bacteroides, Fusobacteria,* and *Veillonella* species], and occasionally staphylococci or spirochetes). These organisms are typically sensitive to penicillin. Hence, penicillins remain the single most useful class of antibiotics for dental and periodontal infections. Occasionally, dental infections are caused by aerobic gram-negative bacteria, *Actinomycetes,* or fungi. In these cases, other antimicrobials are needed for optimal therapy.

Convenient tables listing antimicrobial treatment recommended for various medical and dental clinical syndromes and sites of infection are

TABLE 9–1. Antimicrobial Spectrum and Preferred Therapeutic Agents

Microbial Spectrum	Class of Preferred Antimicrobial	Examples
Gram-positive aerobic bacteria	Natural penicillins	Penicillin G, Penicillin V K
	Penicillinase-resistant penicillins	Oxacillin, nafcillin, methicillin
	Aminopenicillins	Ampicillin, amoxicillin
	Macrolides	Erythromycin, clarithromycin, azithromycin
	Glycopeptides	Vancomycin, teicoplanin
	Cephalosporins	Cefazolin, cephalothin, cephalexin, cefaclor
	Lincosamides	Clindamycin
	Topicals	Bacitracin, mupirocin
Gram-negative aerobic bacteria	Aminoglycosides	Gentamicin, tobramycin, amikacin
	Extended-spectrum penicillins	Azlocillin, mezlocillin, piperacillin
	Antipseudomonal penicillins	Carbenicillin, ticarcillin
	Monobactams	Aztreonam
	Carbapenems	Imipenem, meropenem
	Cephalosporins	Ceftazidime
	Sulfonamides	Trimethroprim-sulfamethoxazole
Broad-spectrum antibacterial	Third-generation cephalosporins	Cefotaxime, ceftizoxime, ceftriaxone, cefoperazone
	β-lactam + β-lactamase Inhibitor combinations	Ampicillin + sulbactam Amoxicillin + clavulanate Ticarcillin + clavulanate Piperacillin + tazobactam
	Quinolones	Ciprofloxacin, ofloxacin, sparfloxacin, norfloxacin
	Carbapenems	Imipenem + cilastin
	Tetracyclines	Tetracycline, chlortetracycline
	Chloramphenicol	Doxycycline, minocycline
Anaerobic Bacteria	Penicillins	Penicillin G
	Cephalosporins	Cefotetan, cefoxitin
	Carbapenems	Imipenem + cilastin
	Lincosamides	Clindamycin
	Chloramphenicol	Chloramphenicol
	Metronidazole	Metronidazole
Fungal Infections	Polyenes	Amphotericin B
	Azoles	Fluconazole, ketoconazole, itraconazole
	Topical antifungal agents	Nystatin, clotrimazole, miconazole, tolnaftate
Viral Infections	Anti-herpesvirus agents	Acyclovir, ganciclovir, foscarnet, famciclovir
	Topical anti-herpes agents	Trifluridine, idoxuridine

published and updated periodically. An example is the *Pocketbook of Pediatric Antimicrobial Therapy* by J.D. Nelson.

Mode of Action

Antimicrobials may also be categorized according to their mode or site of action. There are seven different modes of action described for antimicrobial agents (Table 9–2): (1) inhibiting synthesis of the bacterial cell wall, which is required for bacterial survival, (2) inhibiting protein synthesis at one of several possible steps, (3) acting as an antimetabolite by interfering with the metabolism of folic acid and thus interfering with bacterial growth, (4) interfering with cell membrane permeability, (5) inhibiting nucleic acid synthesis, (6) inhibiting bacteria topoisomerase enzymes, and (7) inhibiting cytochrome P-450 sterol. By these mechanisms of action, the antibiotics produce toxic effects that selectively interfere with the life cycle of the bacteria while not causing significant alterations in the human host (Reed et al., 1995).

TABLE 9–2. Antimicrobials: Mode of Action

Inhibition of Cell Wall Synthesis
  Penicillins
  Cephalosporins
  Monobactams
  Carbapenems
  Glycopeptides
  Azole antifungals

Inhibition of Protein Synthesis
  Bind 50s ribosome
    Macrolides
    Chloramphenicol
    Lincosamides
  Bind 30s ribosome
    Aminoglycosides
    Tetracyclines

Antimetabolites
  Sulfonamides

Alteration of Cell Membrane Permeability
  Polymixins
  Clotrimazole (antifungal)
  Polyene antifungals

Inhibition of Nucleic Acid Synthesis
  Rifampin
  Griseofulvin
  Nucleoside antivirals

Topoisomerase Inhibitors
  Nalidixic acid
  Quinolones

Inhibition of Cytochrome Sterol
  Azoles (antifungal)

TABLE 9–3. Bactericidal and Bacteriostatic Antibiotics

Bactericidal	Bacteriostatic
Penicillins	Macrolides
Cephalosporins	Tetracyclines
Glycopeptides	Chloramphenicol
Carbapenems	Sulfonamides
Monobactams	Lincosamides
Aminoglycosides	Rifampin
Quinolones	

Bactericidal Versus Bacteriostatic Antibiotics

Antibiotics may also be classified as bactericidal or bacteriostatic. Bactericidal antibiotics actually kill the microorganisms, whereas bacteriostatic antimicrobials inhibit bacterial growth or multiplication and depend on the normal host defense mechanisms (immune system) to eliminate the microorganism. Bactericidal agents are preferable in most situations. Bacteriostatic agents should not be used in immunocompromised patients because their diminished host resistance may be unable to kill the offending microorganisms. Table 9–3 lists the agents in these categories.

Resistance

Bacterial resistance to antibiotics has been a continuing and evolving problem. It has been exacerbated by widespread indiscriminate use of antibiotics in veterinary, medical, and dental applications. Some of the most common current mechanisms of bacterial resistance to antibiotics are summarized in Table 9–4.

Current issues in bacterial resistance include increasing resistance of staphylococci to penicillinase-resistant penicillins (e.g., methicillin, oxacillin), resistance of pneumococci to penicillins by alteration of bacterial penicillin-binding proteins, resistance of enterococci to glycopeptide antibiotics (i.e., vancomycin), and multidrug resistance among gram-negative bacteria due to bacterial modifying enzymes and extended-spectrum beta-lactamases. Fortunately, the oral flora causing most dental and periodontal infections have rarely manifested these types of antibiotic resistance to date.

The development of resistant bacterial strains may be minimized by consistent use of an appropriate antibiotic dosage for an adequate period of time. For gram-negative infections, especially *Pseudomonas* infections, or infections with en-

TABLE 9–4. Mechanisms of Bacterial Resistance

Antibiotic Class	Common Mechanisms of Resistance
Penicillins	Hydrolysis by bacterial beta-lactamases, altered bacterial binding proteins
Cephalosporins	Hydrolysis by extended-spectrum beta-lactamases cephalosporinases
Macrolides	Methylation of bacterial ribosomes with altered binding of macrolides
Aminoglycosides	Modification by bacterial hydroxylases, methylases, acetylases
Glycopeptides	Modification of bacterial cell wall precursors, with decreased binding
Trimethoprim-sulfamethoxazole	Resistant bacterial enzymes in folate pathway

terococci, treatment with combinations of antibiotics (e.g., a beta-lactam and aminoglycoside) may help to avoid the emergence of resistant strains. Antibiotic combinations may also be necessary for infections with mixed types of bacteria. When planning combination drug therapy, it is important to select antibacterial agents that have synergistic or additive activity. Drugs that are antagonistic in combination may result in suboptimal clinical outcomes and an increased likelihood of the emergence of resistant strains (Gold and Moellering, 1996).

In most university-related clinical settings, the use of antibiotics is increasingly scrutinized by formulary committees and antibiotic review panels. One hopes that such efforts will promote an increased rational and appropriate use of antibiotics to minimize the spread of bacterial resistance.

ANTIBIOTIC AGENTS

The antibiotic agents that are used most commonly in pediatric dentistry include the penicillins, the macrolides, and the cephalosporins.

Penicillins

In 1928, Sir Alexander Fleming discovered that penicillin mold lysed gram-positive microorganisms. This observation did not gain clinical usefulness until the 1940s, when the antibiotic era began. The penicillins are a group of antibiotics that differ in their pharmacologic properties. They are primarily active against gram-positive aerobic and anaerobic bacteria, but their spectrums of coverage can vary. As a group, they are the most allergenic antibiotics, and all exhibit cross-allergenicity.

Penicillin G. Penicillin G was the prototype of this group of antibiotic agents and continues to be the drug of choice for many infections. Its coverage is limited primarily to gram-positive organisms and selective gram-negative cocci.

Penicillin G has two primary unfortunate properties. First, it is poorly absorbed orally, owing to its destruction by gastric acid, so it is best given by the intramuscular route. Second, it is readily destroyed by penicillinase-producing microorganisms. Semisynthetic penicillins have been developed in order to expand coverage and to overcome some of these disadvantages.

Penicillin V. The primary advantage of penicillin V is that it is stable at gastric pH, allowing for much improved absorption when it is administered orally. Its spectrum of coverage is the same as for penicillin G except for slightly less efficacy against *Neisseria gonorrhoeae* and some anaerobes. It is also inactivated by penicillinase, however. Penicillin V is the primary oral antibiotic used to treat dental infections.

Ampicillin and Amoxicillin. Ampicillin has a broader spectrum of coverage than penicillin G or V, covering more gram-negative organisms, including *Escherichia coli, Haemophilus influenza,* and *Salmonella.* It is, however, less effective against some gram-positive organisms. Ampicillin is used commonly in pediatrics, owing to the frequency of *H. influenza* infections. Although ampicillin is absorbed better orally than penicillin G, significant degradation occurs in the gut, and diarrhea or gastrointestinal upset is common. Nine percent of children develop a maculopapular rash after receiving ampicillin. Amoxicillin has the same spectrum of coverage as ampicillin but is absorbed better orally and causes less diarrhea. Despite the usefulness of these drugs in pediatrics, they are not indicated over penicillin G or penicillin V for use against dental infection. Development of resistance to these agents, especially by *H. influenza,* is becoming increasingly problematic.

Penicillinase-Resistant Penicillins. Some strains of staphylococci produce an enzyme, penicillinase, which destroys penicillins, resulting in drug resistance. Several penicillins have been developed that are resistant to destruction by penicillinase, including oxacillin, methicillin, nafcillin, cloxacillin, and dicloxacillin. Methicillin is not well absorbed orally. These drugs should be reserved for infections involving penicillinase-producing staphylococci and are not indicated for common dental infections.

Erythromycin

Erythromycin is a macrolide antibiotic that was introduced in 1952. Its spectrum of coverage is similar to penicillin's with the addition of some penicillinase-producing staphylococci, chlamydiae, *Legionella*, mycoplasma, and others. It is well absorbed orally. The free base form is unstable at gastric pH, however, so it is administered with an enteric coating or in a salt form (stearate or estolate). Gastrointestinal upset in the form of diarrhea is common. The major disadvantage of erythromycin is that it is bacteriostatic rather than bactericidal. Despite this disadvantage, erythromycin is an effective drug for dental infections and is considered by many dentists to be the drug of choice.

Cephalosporins

The cephalosporins are a newer group of bactericidal antibiotics that are chemically related to penicillin. They are broad-spectrum in coverage and are divided into three "generations" by coverage. They are basically equivalent to penicillins in their activity against gram-positive organisms (except *Streptococcus faecalis*) and are resistant to penicillinase. First-generation cephalosporins have limited activity against gram-negative enterobacteria. The second-generation drugs extend their spectrum to include more of these organisms, and the third generation cephalosporins have enhanced activity against many gram-negative bacilli. The cephalosporins exhibit some cross-sensitivity in patients allergic to penicillin.

The oral cephalosporins include cephalexin, cefaclor, cefadroxil, cefixime, and several newer agents. They have fewer side effects than penicillins and taste less bitter when given orally. The cephalosporins are effective against oral pathogens but generally have less anaerobic activity than penicillins and at best similar activity against aerobic oral flora. Therefore, cephalosporins generally offer no advantage over penicillins for most dental infections and are usually more expensive. Cephalosporins should be reserved for severe infections involving gram-negative organisms or mixed infections.

Summary

Most dental and periodontal bacterial infections are caused by gram-positive aerobes, facultative streptococci, and occasionally staphylococci. Other occasional pathogens include anaerobic gram-negative organisms such as *Bacteroides, Veillonella, Fusobacterium,* gram-negative aerobes, and diphtheroids (Cieslak, 1995). The initial drugs of choice continue to be penicillin and erythromycin. Streptococci, most staphylococci, and most anaerobic pathogens continue to remain sensitive to both penicillin and erythromycin. Owing to their bactericidal action, penicillin V (oral) or penicillin G (intramuscular) is usually recommended as the primary drug of choice for dental and periodontal infections. Erythromycin or clindamycin is usually the alternative drug of choice in patients allergic to penicillin (Drug Information Handbook for Dentistry, 1997).

BACTERIAL ENDOCARDITIS PROPHYLAXIS

Bacterial endocarditis is a microbial infection of the endocardium (inner layer of the cardiac muscle). Certain patients with congenital cardiac lesions or acquired cardiac defects are believed to be at high risk for this condition if a procedure or manipulation causes transient bacteremia. The blood-borne bacteria may lodge on the abnormal endocardium or heart valves and result in serious endocardial infection. Recommended prophylactic antibiotic regimens are based on in vitro studies, clinical experience, animal models, and assessment of the bacteria common to a particular site and those most commonly identified with endocarditis (American Academy of Pediatrics, 1994). In 1997, an ad hoc writing group appointed by the American Heart Association for their expertise in endocarditis and treatment published updated recommendations regarding antibiotic prophylaxis of bacterial endocarditis. The cardiac conditions for which antibiotic prophylaxis is and is not recommended to prevent bacterial endocarditis are listed in Table 9–5. Antibiotic prophylaxis is recommended for *all* dental procedures likely to cause significant bleeding from soft and hard tissues, including professional oral prophylaxis and initial placement of orthodontic bands (but not bracket placement), in at-risk patients. Simple orthodontic adjustments that are unlikely to cause bleeding and spontaneous shedding of deciduous teeth are thought not to present a significant risk of endocarditis;

TABLE 9–5. Cardiac Conditions Associated with Endocarditis

Endocarditis Prophylaxis Recommended

High-risk category
Prosthetic cardiac valves, including bioprosthetic and homograft valves
Previous bacterial endocarditis
Complex cyanotic congenital heart disease (e.g., single ventricle states, transposition of the great arteries, tetralogy of Fallot)
Surgically constructed systemic pulmonary shunts or conduits
Moderate-risk category
Most other congenital cardiac malformations (other than above and below)
Acquired valvar dysfunction (e.g., rheumatic heart disease)
Hypertrophic cardiomyopathy
Mitral valve prolapse with valvar regurgitation and/or thickened leaflets

Endocarditis Prophylaxis Not Recommended

Negligible-risk category (no greater risk than the general population)
Isolated secundum atrial septal defect
Surgical repair of atrial septal defect, ventricular septal defect, or patent ductus arteriosus (without residua beyond 6 mo)
Previous coronary artery bypass graft surgery
Mitral valve prolapse without valvar regurgitation
Physiologic, functional, or innocent heart murmurs
Previous Kawasaki disease without valvar dysfunction
Previous rheumatic fever without valvar dysfunction
Cardiac pacemakers (intravascular and epicardial) and implanted defibrillators

From Dajani AS, et al: Prevention of bacterial endocarditis. JAMA 277:1794-1801, 1997. Copyright 1997, American Medical Association.

therefore, prophylaxis is not recommended in these situations.

Bacterial endocarditis after dental manipulations is most commonly caused by alpha-hemolytic streptococci. Therefore, prophylaxis is specifically directed against these organisms. Gingivitis, periodontitis, and periapical infections can be the source of a bacteremia. Excellent oral hygiene and maintenance of dental health are important to reduce the potential for bacterial seeding in the bloodstream of at-risk patients.

The dental and other procedures for which antibiotic prophylaxis is and is not recommended are given in Tables 9-6 and 9-7. The antibiotic prophylaxis regimens for dental, oral, respiratory treatment or esophageal procedures are described in Table 9-8.

There are significant changes from previous recommendations. Additional guidelines have also been provided, including the following:

1. In the case of delayed healing or of a procedure that involves infected tissue, additional doses of antibiotics may be necessary, even though bacteremia rarely persists longer than 15 minutes after the procedure is completed.

2. Amoxicillin is the preferred oral antibiotic because it is better absorbed from the gastrointestinal tract and provides higher and more sustained serum levels.

3. If a patient is taking amoxicillin chronically for some reason (e.g., rheumatic fever prevention), oral clindamycin, azithromycin, clarithromycin, or one of the other parenteral regimens should be used.

4. If a high-risk patient (e.g., a patient with a prosthetic valve) has maintained a "high level" of oral health, oral antibiotic prophylaxis may be used for simple dental procedures, rather than the parenteral regimen. Some physicians, however, may still prefer parenteral antibiotic administration for these high-risk patients. The patient's physician should be consulted when planning

TABLE 9–6. Dental Procedures and Endocarditis Prophylaxis

Endocarditis Prophylaxis Recommended*

Dental extractions
Periodontal procedures including surgery, scaling and root planing, probing, and recall maintenance
Dental implant placement and reimplantation of avulsed teeth
Endodontic (root canal) instrumentation or surgery only beyond the apex
Subgingival placement of antibiotic fibers or strips
Initial placement of orthodontic bands but not brackets
Intraligamentary local anesthetic injections
Prophylactic cleaning of teeth or implants where bleeding is anticipated

Endocarditis Prophylaxis Not Recommended

Restorative dentistry† (operative and prosthodontic) with or without retraction cord‡
Local anesthetic injections (nonintraligamentary)
Intracanal endodontic treatment; post placement and buildup
Placement of rubber dams
Postoperative suture removal
Placement of removable prosthodontic or orthodontic appliances
Taking of oral impressions
Fluoride treatments
Taking of oral radiographs
Orthodontic appliance adjustment
Shedding of primary teeth

*Prophylaxis is recommended for patients with high- and moderate-risk cardiac conditions.
†This includes restoration of decayed teeth (filling cavities) and replacement of missing teeth.
‡Clinical judgment may indicate antibiotic use in selected circumstances that may create significant bleeding.
From Dajani AS, et al: Prevention of bacterial endocarditis, JAMA 277:1794-1801, 1997. Copyright 1997, American Medical Association.

TABLE 9–7. Other Procedures and Endocarditis
....

Endocarditis Prophylaxis Recommended

Respiratory tract
  Tonsillectomy and/or adenoidectomy
  Surgical operations that involve respiratory mucosa
  Bronchoscopy with a rigid bronchoscope
Gastrointestinal tract*
  Sclerotherapy for esophageal varices
  Esophageal stricture dilation
  Endoscopic retrograde cholangiography with biliary
    obstruction
  Biliary tract surgery
  Surgical operations that involve intestinal mucosa
Genitourinary tract
  Prostatic surgery
  Cystoscopy
  Urethral dilation

Endocarditis Prophylaxis Not Recommended

Respiratory tract
  Endotracheal intubation
  Bronchoscopy with a flexible bronchoscope, with or
    without biopsy†
  Tympanostomy tube insertion
Gastrointestinal tract
  Transesophageal echocardiography†
  Endoscopy with or without gastrointestinal biopsy†
Genitourinary tract
  Vaginal hysterectomy†
  Vaginal delivery†
  Cesarean section
  In uninfected tissue:
    Urethral catheterization
    Uterine dilatation and curettage
    Therapeutic abortion
    Sterilization procedures
    Insertion or removal of intrauterine devices
Other
  Cardiac catheterization, including balloon angioplasty
  Implanted cardiac pacemakers, implanted defibrillators,
    and coronary stents
  Incision or biopsy of surgically scrubbed skin
  Circumcision

---

*Prophylaxis is recommended for high-risk patients; optional for medium-risk patients.
†Prophylaxis is optional for high-risk patients.
From Dajani AS, et al: Prevention of bacterial endocarditis, JAMA *277*:1794–1801, 1997. Copyright 1997, American Medical Association.

dental care for high-risk persons. Clindamycin phosphate is recommended for parenteral administration in patients known to be allergic to amoxicillin or ampicillin.

ANTIFUNGAL AGENTS

Candida species, especially *Candida albicans,* can often be found on the healthy mucous membranes of the body. Multiplication of the *Candida* species and invasion of the tissues rarely occur unless the immunity of the host is compro-

mised, however. Candidiasis is common in children receiving oncology treatment, particularly during periods of severe immunosuppression and neutropenia. The extensive use of broad-spectrum antibiotics, steroids, chemotherapy-associated immunosuppression, and inadequate oral hygiene and nutrition alter the balance of the oral microflora and place children at risk for candidiasis.

The clinical management of oral candidiasis in children is similar to that in adults and consists principally of antifungal agents. Suspected *Candida* infections should be confirmed by culture, potassium hydroxide smear, or both prior to the initiation of prompt and aggressive therapy in immunosuppressed patients. The medicament and route of administration is determined by the severity of the infection. Oral and esophageal candidiasis is usually treated with topical suspensions or troches of antifungal agents (e.g., nystatin or clotrimazole).

All antifungal agents formulated for oral topical use contain sweeteners that can promote caries if used for an extended period of time. Daily use of topical fluorides is recommended to reduce the caries potential.

Nystatin. Nystatin is available as an oral suspension (100,000 units/ml), tablet (500,000 units), and pastille/troche (200,000 units). A dose of 1–3 million units/day in three to five divided doses for 10 to 14 days is recommended.

Clotrimazole. Clotrimazole is a fungicidal agent that is available only as a 10-mg troche for intraoral application. An oral suspension can be compounded from the vaginal tablets, however. The recommended dose is 1 troche dissolved slowly in the mouth five times a day for 14 days to achieve maximum effectiveness. The child must be of age and maturity to comprehend and follow instructions to use the troche vehicle. Liver toxicity has been reported in patients using clotrimazole, and clinical studies have not been conducted to establish the safety of the drug for children below 3 years of age.

Ketoconazole. Ketoconazole is reserved for treating more severe infections. A single daily tablet (200 mg) of 3.3–6.6 mg/kg taken with food for 10 to 14 days is recommended. Significant hepatotoxicity has been associated with ketoconazole. The drug should be limited to children 2 years of age or older unless the potential benefit outweighs the risks because safety has not been established for younger children. Ketoconazole is not indicated for patients that are also taking antacids or phenytoin.

Amphotericin B and Fluconazole. Disseminated candidiasis can be life-threatening and can

TABLE 9–8. Prophylaxis Regimens for Dental, Oral, Respiratory Tract, or Esophageal Procedures

Situation	Agent	Regimen*
Standard general prophylaxis	Amoxicillin	Adults: 2.0 g; children: 50 mg/kg orally 1 h before procedure
Unable to take oral medications	Ampicillin	Adults: 2.0 g intramuscularly (IM) or intravenously (IV); children: 50 mg/kg IM or IV within 30 min before procedure
Allergic to penicillin	Clindamycin *or*	Adults: 600 mg; children: 20 mg/kg orally 1 h before procedure
	Cephalexin† or cefadroxil† *or*	Adults: 2.0 g; children; 50 mg/kg orally 1 h before procedure
	Azithromycin or clarithromycin	Adults: 500 mg; children: 15 mg/kg orally 1 h before procedure
Allergic to penicillin and unable to take oral medications	Clindamycin *or*	Adults: 600 mg; children: 20 mg/kg IV within 30 min before procedure
	Cefazolin†	Adults: 1.0 g; children: 25 mg/kg IM or IV within 30 min before procedure

*Total children's dose should not exceed adult dose.

†Cephalosporins should not be used in persons with immediate-type hypersensitivity reaction (urticaria, angioedema, or anaphylaxis) to penicillins.

From Dajani AS, et al: Prevention of bacterial endocarditis, JAMA 277:1794–1801, 1997. Copyright 1997, American Medical Association.

require aggressive treatment with intravenous amphotericin B. Serious side effects develop frequently with this drug, including azotemia and nephrotoxicity. Unlike other antifungal agents, fluconazole can be administered orally (100 mg/tablet) or intravenously and has fewer reported side effects, the most common being gastrointestinal distress.

Most practitioners have moved toward the preferential use of fluconazole instead of ketoconazole for mild to moderate deep-seated candidiasis. The use of other azole agents as monotherapy for serious visceral candidiasis remains incompletely established. It is still believed to be preferable to use systemic amphotericin B for life-threatening visceral candidiasis. Fluconazole should not be used in combination with phenytoin. The efficacy and safety of fluconazole compared with amphotericin B in children younger than 3 years has not been established.

ANTIVIRAL AGENTS

Primary herpetic gingivostomatitis is the most commonly recognized manifestation of the herpes simplex virus (HSV) type I. It is an acute illness often with concomitant fever, malaise, irritability, and cervical lymphadenopathy together with the characteristic oral and perioral ulcerative lesions involving the gingiva and mucous membranes of the mouth. HSV gingivostomatitis

in healthy children resolves spontaneously within 10 to 14 days and requires only supportive therapy. Primary or reactivation of latent HSV infections in immunosuppressed patients require more aggressive therapy, however. Ulcerated herpetic lesions may be a portal for bacteria and fungi, resulting in serious disseminated infection.

Acyclovir. Treatment of HSV infection in immunosuppressed patients consists of oral or intravenous acyclovir. Prophylactic acyclovir should be considered in patients seropositive for HSV and at high risk for reactivation. The recommended oral dose in adults is 200 mg three to five times daily for the duration of immunosuppression. In children with severe HSV, acyclovir should be used at 10 mg/kg given three times per day (30 mg/kg/day). Acyclovir is not indicated for patients at low risk for reactivation. Although the likelihood of acyclovir resistance is low, potential side effects of intravenous administration include encephalopathy secondary to renal insufficiency and nephrotoxicity. Adverse effects encountered with oral administration include headaches and nausea.

REFERENCES

Cieslak TJ: Intraoral and dental infections. *In* Jenson HB, Baltimore RS (eds): Pediatric Infectious Diseases: Principles and Practices. Norfolk, CT, Appleton and Lange, 1995.

Dajani AS, et al: Prevention of bacterial endocarditis. JAMA 277:1794–1801, 1997.

Drug Information Handbook for Dentistry, 2nd ed. Wynn RL, Meiller TF, Crossley HL (eds). Hudson, (Cleveland), Lexi-Comp Incorporated, 1997.

Gold HS, Moellering RC Jr: Antimicrobial-drug resistance. N Engl J Med *335*:1445–1453, 1996.

Nelson JD: Pocketbook of Pediatric Antimicrobial Therapy, 12th ed. Baltimore, Williams and Wilkins, 1996.

Reed MD, Goldfarb J, Blumer JL: Anti-infective therapy. *In* Jenson HB, Baltimore RS (eds): Pediatric Infectious Diseases: Principles and Practices. Norfolk, CT, Appleton and Lange, 1995.

Report of the Committee on Infectious Diseases, 23rd ed. Elk Grove, IL, American Academy of Pediatrics, 1994.

Chapter **10**

Medical Emergencies

Kaaren G. Vargas and Jay A. Anderson

Chapter Outline

Dentistry is an invasive surgical specialty that is often associated with high levels of patient anxiety. These factors combine to produce a situation that may be conducive to medical emergencies, especially those that are induced or aggravated by stress. Also, pharmacologic agents are used routinely in the dental office. All drugs, whether local anesthetics, antibiotics, sedatives, or analgesics, carry the potential of producing toxicity or allergy.

The specter of medical emergencies is often frightening and bewildering to dental students because of the implication that they will be called upon to diagnose and treat medical conditions that they are not trained or equipped to handle. It may be comforting to realize that the dentist is not expected to diagnose the underlying cause of all emergencies accurately and immediately render curative treatment. The accurate diagnosis of a medical condition often, in fact, requires hours to days to determine in the hospital setting. The primary responsibilities of the dentist in the area of medical emergencies fall into the area of prevention, preparation, basic life support, and procurement of help and transport.

PREVENTION OF MEDICAL EMERGENCIES

Perhaps the most important aspect of dealing with medical emergencies is preventing their occurrence. Prevention of medical emergencies can generally be accomplished, as much as possible, by an adequate history and physical examination, medical consultation (when indicated), and vigilant patient monitoring.

History and Physical Examination

A thorough knowledge of all existing medical conditions, physical or psychological, that may predispose the patient to development of a problem will prevent the vast majority of emergency situations. This knowledge is gained through the medical history and physical examination. The easiest way to obtain a medical history is to have the patient complete a simple medical history questionnaire, such as the short form available through the American Dental Association (ADA). Included are questions pertaining to any present or past medical conditions, allergies, hospitalizations, medications, and so forth. The dentist reviews this form, notes positive findings, and conducts a brief interview with the patient to clarify any questions and expand upon the questionnaire.

The physical examination should include baseline vital signs (heart rate, respiratory rate and character, and blood pressure in older children), a thorough head and neck examination, and observation of general appearance (e.g., gait, mental status, skin tone, and color). Further physical evaluation should be dictated by the dentist's training and expertise. If a practitioner uses sedation techniques that may depress the patient's cardiovascular or respiratory function, it is recommended that the practitioner possess skills in the physical diagnosis of the cardiovascular and pulmonary systems (e.g., chest and heart auscultation).

A thorough history and physical examination should make the dentist aware of any preexisting conditions that may lead to a medical emergency. This knowledge should allow the development of a treatment protocol for the patient that will make such an event highly unlikely. This may involve the use of conscious sedation for stress-induced conditions such as asthmatic attacks or epileptic seizures, proper timing of appointments, bacterial endocarditis prophylaxis, or even performing the needed procedures in the hospital operating room if deemed necessary.

Medical Consultation

If any questions arise regarding the management of a medically compromised child, it is highly desirable to contact the patient's physician by telephone for guidance.

PATIENT MONITORING

The level of monitoring that is necessary to treat a pediatric dental patient safely varies, depending on the patient's condition and the patient management technique being used. Patient monitoring involves the observation of physiologic parameters over time in order to detect any change and deal with it before a potentially dangerous situation develops. The dentist should always monitor (observe) the general appearance of the patient, including the level of consciousness, level of comfort, muscle tone, color of the skin and mucosa, and respiratory pattern. For the majority of healthy patients being treated with local anesthesia alone, this is all the monitoring that is necessary.

When conscious sedation is used, especially in children in whom a much narrower margin of safety often exists because of smaller degrees of respiratory and cardiovascular reserve, additional monitoring should be routinely employed. The primary systems to be monitored during dental treatment with conscious sedation or deep sedation are the central nervous system (CNS), respiratory system, and the cardiovascular system. Presedation vital signs, including heart rate, respiratory rate, blood pressure, and temperature, must always be obtained. The heart sounds and breath sounds should be continuously monitored via a precordial stethoscope in all patients undergoing conscious sedation (Fig. 10–1). This allows continuous auscultation by the dentist of the patient's heart rate and rhythm and respiratory pattern without having to look consciously at a monitor screen for data.

In addition to these essential monitors, several other devices are available that further enhance one's ability to monitor the patient's vital functions. For cardiovascular monitoring, blood pressure and heart rate may be conveniently monitored via noninvasive blood pressure devices that can measure systolic, diastolic, and mean blood pressure and heart rate at predetermined inter-

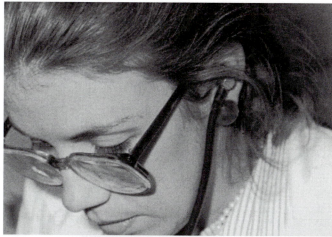

Figure 10–1. Use of a precordial stethoscope.

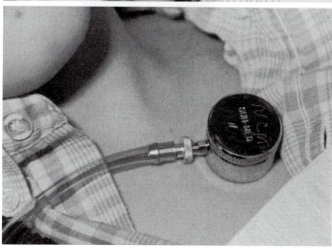

vals and display the data digitally. Several devices have been advocated for respiratory monitoring, including the capnograph, pulse oximeter, ear oximeter, impedance plethysmograph, and the transcutaneous oxygen and carbon dioxide monitors. Of these devices, the pulse oximeter is the most useful and accurate for detecting developing hypoxia and the capnograph is the most sensitive and accurate system to determine whether the patient is breathing. The pulse oximeter measures oxyhemoglobin saturation instantaneously and provides immediate feedback on the status of the patient's oxygenation. The capnograph continuously analyzes the carbon dioxide content of respired gases, providing a breath-to-breath representation of the presence or absence of air flow.

Whenever deep sedation or general anesthesia is used, more sophisticated monitoring is essential. In addition to the essential observations and precordial stethoscope, monitoring during deep sedation should include recording of vital signs at a minimum of 5-minute intervals (including blood pressure), continuous temperature monitoring, and an electrocardiogram (ECG). Placement of an intravenous catheter is also highly recommended. The use of restraining devices in small children makes monitoring especially difficult. When these devices are used, the dentist should observe at least one extremity and the face for color, check head position frequently to ensure a patent airway, and monitor heart and breath sounds continuously with a precordial stethoscope. The use of a pulse oximeter and capnograph should be standard.

PREPARATION FOR EMERGENCIES

Despite preventive measures, medical emergencies do occasionally occur. The dental practitioner must be adequately prepared for such events. Preparation involves personal, staff, and office preparation.

Personal Preparation

As previously stated, it cannot be expected that the practicing dentist will be able to diagnose and treat every possible medical emergency. It is, however, possible to anticipate with some certainty which emergency situations are most likely to arise in the dental office and be well prepared to deal with them. Examples include syncope, hyperventilation, seizures, hypoglycemia, postural hypotension, asthma, allergic reactions, and airway obstruction. Certainly, any emergency situation that might logically occur as a direct result of medications or techniques being used must be anticipated, well understood, and prepared for. Examples include local anesthetic reactions and respiratory depression secondary to sedation. Personal preparation for the dentist should include, as a minimum, a good working knowledge of the signs, symptoms, course, and therapy for these common treatable conditions. Training in basic life support (cardiopulmonary resuscitation, CPR) should be considered essential for any practicing health professional. If conscious sedation techniques are to be used, advanced cardiac life support training is desirable.

Staff Preparation

Office personnel should be trained in the recognition and treatment of common medical emergencies. It is desirable to require that all office staff members be certified in basic CPR. A team approach to medical emergencies will provide for organized management of emergency situations. Each staff member should have a preassigned role in case of an emergency so that emergency equipment will be brought (and maintained) by an assigned person, emergency drugs will be prepared by another, and all tasks will be performed in an organized fashion. Because medical emergencies, fortunately, occur relatively rarely in the dental office, it is desirable to run mock medical emergency drills regularly in order to keep the team protocol running smoothly and to reduce panic in an actual emergency.

Office Preparation

Every dental office contains a great deal of equipment and supplies. A minimal amount of additional equipment is essential for every office to be properly prepared for medical emergencies.

These essentials can be divided into emergency equipment and emergency drugs.

EMERGENCY EQUIPMENT

Keeping in mind the dentist's primary responsibilities of basic life support and transport in most situations, it should be apparent that very little equipment is necessary to deal with medical emergencies. First of all, oxygen must be readily available. An oxygen source capable of delivering greater than 90% oxygen at flows in excess of 5 liters/minute for a minimum of 1 hour must be available. This means that an "E" cylinder is the minimum size required. The initial primary goal of basic life support is establishment and maintenance of proper respiratory function. Hypoxemia (low oxygen content in the arterial blood) is the final common pathway leading to morbidity and mortality in the majority of severe medical emergency situations. Adequate oxygenation must be ensured by the administration of supplemental oxygen. If the patient is breathing adequately spontaneously, oxygen may be delivered by way of a face mask, nasal mask, or nasal prongs. The patient may cease breathing during an emergency situation, however, making artificial ventilation necessary. A positive pressure oxygen delivery system (bag-valve-mask) is, therefore, also considered essential equipment in order to deliver oxygen to the apneic patient.

A high-volume suction device is the third piece of equipment that is considered essential to treat medical emergencies. Emergency situations, especially those involving an obtunded patient, often induce vomiting. The aspiration of vomitus can be disastrous. This can usually be prevented by proper positioning and suctioning. Most dental offices, of course, contain high-volume suction equipment for restorative purposes.

Other emergency equipment items that are desirable and recommended include syringes and needles, the armamentarium for establishing an intravenous line; cricothyrotomy equipment; oral and nasal airways; a laryngoscope; and endotracheal tubes.

EMERGENCY DRUGS

Most medical emergencies in the dental office do not require the use of drugs. The practitioner's thought process should be primarily directed toward basic life support measures and should turn to drug therapy only when clearly indicated. The contents of an appropriate emergency drug kit may be quite different for individual dentists, depending upon the drugs used in the office, their individual level of training, and the level of medical support immediately available. It is expected that pharmacologic agents be available to definitively treat any medical emergency that may be expected to arise as a direct result of any drug that is used to treat patients. This includes the use of local anesthetics, which may produce toxic or allergic reactions.

The dentist should be well familiarized with each drug in the emergency kit. Commercially available emergency kits are not only very expensive, they are also almost never optimal as far as which drugs are included for any individual practitioner's purposes. One of the biggest dangers of owning a commercially available emergency kit is gaining a false sense of security simply by purchasing it. If the practitioner does not know the uses, doses, and probable side effects of each drug in the kit and keep this information up to date, the kit may in actuality be more dangerous than potentially beneficial. A good drug kit should contain as few drugs as possible and should be simple, neat, and readily available. The dentist should be familiar with every drug, including its dose, indications, and side effects.

The following list is my recommendation for drugs that might be included in a basic emergency drug kit for the dentist who treats children. The list contains only superficial information and must be expanded upon as recommended previously.

Drugs to Treat Allergy

EPINEPHRINE

Use. Epinephrine is the most important drug in any emergency kit. It is the treatment of choice for life-threatening anaphylactic reactions and for severe asthmatic reactions, and it is a basic cardiac life support drug. If a dentist is administering any drugs to patients, including local anesthetics, epinephrine must be available in case of allergy.

Action. Epinephrine is a sympathomimetic that stimulates both alpha and beta receptors. Epinephrine increases heart rate and blood pressure, relaxes bronchial smooth muscle, and has an antihistaminic action.

How Supplied. 1:1000 ampule (1 mg/ml) or 1:10,000 preloaded syringe (0.1 mg/ml).

Dose. 0.01 mg/kg (0.1 ml/kg of 1:10,000 IV) (0.01 ml/kg of 1:1000 IM); may need to repeat

after 5 to 10 minutes as needed. Single pediatric doses should not exceed 0.3 mg. Administration of the agent is either subcutaneous or intramuscular/intralingual.

Side Effects. Side effects of epinephrine include hypertension, cardiac arrhythmias, anxiety, and headache.

DIPHENHYDRAMINE (BENADRYL)

Use. Diphenhydramine is used for allergic reactions of slower onset or less severity than anaphylaxis and as an adjunct to epinephrine in severe allergic reactions.

Action. H_1 antagonist that blocks the response of the H_1 receptor to histamine.

How Supplied. 50 mg in 1-ml ampule or 10 mg/ml vial.

Dose. 1–2 mg/kg, IV or IM.

Side Effects. Sedation, anticholinergic.

Benzodiazepine Antagonist

FLUMAZENIL (ANEXATE, ROMAZICON)

Use. Flumazenil is used to reverse the respiratory depression or other undesirable effects of several benzodiazepines, including methylclonazepam, diazepam, flunitrazepam, and midazolam.

Action. Benzodiazepine receptor antagonist.

How Supplied. Flumazenil injection is supplied in multiple-dose vials of 5 ml and 10 ml.

Dose. The recommended initial dose is 0.2 mg IV over 15 seconds. If the desired level of consciousness is not obtained within 60 seconds, a further dose of 0.1 mg can be injected and repeated at 60-second intervals, up to a maximum total dose of 1 mg. The usual dose is between 0.3 and 0.6 mg.

Side Effects. Very rarely, the following side effects occur: agitation, anxiety, dizziness, hypertension, tachycardia, nausea, and vomiting.

Anticonvulsant

DIAZEPAM (VALIUM)

Use. Diazepam is used for treatment of status epilepticus (recurrent seizures).

Action. Anticonvulsant.

How Supplied. 5 mg/ml vial or preloaded syringe.

Dose. <5 yr: 0.3 mg/kg, with initial dose not exceeding 0.25 mg/kg to a maximum of 0.75 mg/kg total dose for episode, slow IV (or deep

IM):* maximum total dose, 5 mg. > 5 yr: 1 mg/
dose, slow IV;* maximum total dose, 10 mg.
Adults: 5–10 mg/dose, slow IV;* maximum total dose, 30 mg.
Side Effects. Sedation, respiratory depression.

Narcotic Antagonist

NALOXONE (NARCAN)

Use. Naloxone is used to reverse respiratory
depression or other undesirable effects of narcotic analgesics. This drug is essential if any narcotics are administered.
Action. Narcotic antagonist.
How Supplied. 0.4 mg/ml ampule.
Dose. 0.01 mg/kg, IV or IM; may repeat with
a subsequent dose of 0.1 mg/kg if needed.
Side Effects. Very rarely, cardiac arrest has
been reported with the use of naloxone.

Steroid

HYDROCORTISONE SODIUM SUCCINATE
(SOLU-CORTEF)

Use. The inclusion of a corticosteroid is recommended in order to treat acute adrenal insufficiency if it should occur in a steroid-dependent
patient, or as an adjunctive treatment for a severe
anaphylactic reaction or asthmatic attack.
Action. An adrenal corticosteroid: anti-inflammatory and membrane stabilization.
How Supplied. 50 mg/ml in 2-ml Mix-O-Vial.
Dose. 0.2–1 mg/kg. Higher doses may be
needed for severe acutely life-threatening situations.

Antihypoglycemics

50 PERCENT DEXTROSE

Use. If loss of consciousness or obtundation
occurs as a result of hypoglycemia, the treatment
of choice is to obtain intravenous access and
administer 50% dextrose to raise serum glucose
levels.
Action. Directly raises serum glucose levels
(immediately).
How Supplied. Dextrose 50% in sterile
water—50-ml bottle (1 ml = 0.5 g).
Dose. 0.5–1 gm/kg (1–2 ml/kg), IV, until patient regains consciousness.

GLUCAGON

Use. If intravenous access cannot be established, the hormone glucagon may be used. It
must be kept in mind that restoration of consciousness may require a delay of 10 to 20
minutes.
Action. Raises serum glucose levels by encouraging glycogenolysis.
How Supplied. 1 mg/ml solution.
Dose. 0.5–1 mg, IM (0.025–0.1 mg/kg); may
repeat dose after 20 minutes if needed. Maximum single dose is 1 mg.

Vasopressors

Especially if intravenous sedation techniques are
being used, a drug to raise blood pressure in
case of severe hypotension is advisable. If hypotension should occur, the situation must be assessed before any drug is given. If hypotension
is due to a cardiac arrhythmia, the arrhythmia
must first be treated with appropriate therapy. If
hypotension is due to a drug effect (vasodilatation), appropriate fluid therapy with or without a
vasopressor is indicated. Two possible alternative
vasopressors are given.

EPHEDRINE

Use. Ephedrine is used to raise blood pressure
and heart rate from shock levels.
Action. Indirect alpha and beta sympathomimetic actions by release of endogenous catechol-
amines.
How Supplied. 25 or 50 mg/ml ampule.
Dose. 0.5 mg/kg, IV or IM.
Side Effects. Hypertension, tachycardia, arrhythmias, headache.

METHOXAMINE (VASOXYL)

Use. Methoxamine is used to raise blood pressure from shock levels.
Action. Methoxamine has a direct alpha sympathomimetic effect only. The drug produces an
increase in blood pressure by peripheral vasoconstriction, without direct cardiac effects. Reflex bradycardia can be produced by methoxamine.
How Supplied. 10 mg/ml vial or 20 mg/ml
ampule.
Dose. 0.25 mg/kg, IM, or 0.08 mg/kg, slow IV.
Side Effects. Bradycardia, hypertension, headache.

---

*May repeat dose every 15 minutes as needed, to maxi-
mum dose.

Analgesics

For acute emergencies in which the presence of pain and anxiety may significantly worsen the clinical situation, a narcotic analgesic may be indicated. This situation is primarily the case with acute myocardial infarction, which is obviously principally a problem of elderly patients. Morphine, meperidine (Demerol), or many other narcotics may be used.

Advanced Cardiac Life Support (ACLS) Drugs

If the dentist has training in advanced cardiac life support (ACLS), or if he or she performs deep sedation or general anesthesia, basic ACLS drugs may be included in the emergency kit. An ECG monitor and a defibrillator should be available when these drugs are used.

ATROPINE

Use. Atropine is used in the treatment of bradycardia.

Action. Atropine is a parasympathetic (vagal) blocking agent; therefore, it increases the patient's heart rate.

How Supplied. 0.4 mg/ml ampule or vial.

Dose. 0.01 mg/kg, IV or IM. For advanced cardiac life support, 0.02 mg/kg, IV or IM.

Side Effects. Tachycardia, arrhythmia, dry mouth.

SODIUM BICARBONATE

Use. Acidosis, cardiac arrest.

Action. Raises blood pH directly.

How Supplied. 1 mEq/ml.

Dose. 1 mEq/kg, slow IV at 10-minute intervals, as needed during resuscitation.

Side Effects. Alkalosis, hypernatremia.

CALCIUM CHLORIDE

Use. Asystole, hypotension, electromechanical dissociation (EMD).

Action. Increased cardiac contractility.

How Supplied. 10% solution (100 mg/ml).

Dose. 0.2 ml/kg of 10% calcium chloride, IV, will provide 20 mg/kg, every 10 minutes as needed.

Side Effect. Phlebitis.

LIDOCAINE (XYLOCAINE)

Use. Lidocaine is used to treat ventricular arrhythmias (ventricular extrasystoles and ventricular tachycardia).

Note: Only "cardiac lidocaine" may be used for this purpose. Dental lidocaine should not be injected intravenously.

Action. Lidocaine depresses automaticity and suppresses ectopic ventricular pacemakers.

How Supplied. 1% (10 mg/ml) or 2% (20 mg/ml) vial or prefilled syringe.

Dose. 1 mg/kg, IV.

Side Effects. Sedation, local anesthetic toxicity in high doses (seizures).

Other Drugs

Other agents that are not injectable drugs but that might be included as part of the emergency drug kit include (1) a respiratory stimulant, such as aromatic ammonia inhalants, (2) sugar (to treat hypoglycemia in an awake patient), (3) a vasodilator such as nitroglycerin, and (4) a "medihaler" of metaproterenol (Metaprel), albuterol (Ventolin, Proventil), or isoetharine (Bronkosol) to treat an asthmatic attack.

BACKUP MEDICAL ASSISTANCE

The final essential component of office preparation for medical emergencies involves securing back-up medical assistance in advance. This involves having the current telephone numbers of the nearest rescue squad and emergency room facility conveniently displayed where they will be immediately available if needed. When feasible, arrangements should be made with a physician whose office is nearby for immediate assistance should an emergency arise. Such a relationship must be prearranged, not assumed.

MANAGEMENT OF MEDICAL EMERGENCIES

The management of basically all medical emergencies, especially those involving a change in the state of consciousness, should be approached in a similar fashion, keeping certain priorities in mind (Table 10–1). Not only will this approach make patient management more efficient and effective, it will also make it less anxiety-provoking and confusing for the dentist.

TABLE 10–1. Management of Medical Emergencies
....

Position	*Circulation*
Airway	*Definitive therapy*
Breathing	

Position

For emergencies involving obtundation of consciousness or hypotension, the best position for managing the situation is to place the patient lying flat on his or her back with the feet raised slightly above the level of the heart. This will minimize the work of the heart, increase return of pooled blood from the extremities, and increase vital blood flow to the brain. Fortunately, this position is easily accomplished in the dental chair. For medical emergencies in the conscious patient involving respiratory distress (e.g., asthmatic attack) or chest pain (angina), the semisitting position is generally preferred by the patient.

Airway ("A")

The first priority in the management of all medical emergencies is the establishment of a patent, functioning airway. If the supply of oxygen to the lungs is cut off for even a short period, especially in a child, rapid neurologic and cardiovascular deterioration will ensue, leading to cardiac arrest, brain cell damage, and death. The airway may be obstructed by progressive swelling, trauma, a foreign body, or other causes.

By far the most common cause of airway obstruction, however, involves the tongue. When a patient becomes obtunded or unconscious, the musculature supporting the mandible and tongue becomes lax, allowing the base of the tongue to fall back against the posterior pharynx, thus blocking the airway between the oral and nasal cavities and the trachea. Extending the head on the neck and thrusting the jaw forward while opening the patient's mouth (head tilt-chin lift or jaw thrust maneuver) is usually adequate to open the airway that is obstructed by the tongue. An oral or nasal airway device may be useful in keeping the tongue forward in the unconscious or deeply obtunded patient. These devices, however, should not be used in conscious patients owing to their propensity to produce laryngospasm, gagging, and vomiting.

If the airway is obstructed by a foreign body, such as a cotton roll or dental restoration, management depends on the patient's condition. In the conscious patient, the initial step should be to deliver four sharp blows with the heel of the hand to the patient's back, between the scapulae, over the spine. Sharp back blows will rapidly raise intrathoracic pressure, causing a burst of air to be expelled through the larynx, hopefully dislodging the obstruction. The four back blows should be delivered in rapid succession and should immediately be stopped if the patient begins to cough up the foreign body. If the back blows are not successful, the abdominal thrust (Heimlich maneuver) should be attempted. In the sitting or standing position, the operator positions himself behind the patient, places one fist below the xiphoid process over the mid-upper abdomen, clenches it with the other hand, and pulls up and back forcefully. This maneuver pushes the diaphragm up and produces a more sustained and forceful increase in intrathoracic pressure, expelling air through the larynx and hopefully dislodging the obstruction. Four abdominal thrusts are performed in rapid succession. The abdominal thrust may be modified for the patient who is lying down (as in the dental chair) in that the rescuer delivers the thrust with the heel of the hand from the side or front of the patient.

The abdominal thrust should not be performed with small children because of their relatively large abdominal organs (especially the liver), which could be damaged. In these cases, a chest thrust maneuver should be delivered instead, with the heel of the hand positioned over the child's midsternum, as would be the position for chest compressions during CPR. Chest thrusts are also used with pregnant females and the obese. The sequence of four back blows followed by four abdominal thrusts is repeated until success in dislodging the obstruction is attained or the patient loses consciousness.

In the unconscious patient with an obstructed airway, the patient is positioned supine (face up), the airway is positioned by tilting the head back and elevating the chin, and an attempt is made to ventilate the patient manually via either mouth-to-mouth resuscitation or a bag-valve-mask system. Although back blows and abdominal thrusts may have been unsuccessful in dislodging an obstruction up to this point, the mechanism of positive pressure breathing is different because the air flow is in the opposite direction and may dislodge the obstruction. If the attempt to ventilate manually is unsuccessful, the sequence of four back blows (accomplished by rolling the patient toward the rescuer temporarily) and four abdominal or chest thrusts (from the side or front) is delivered. With an unconscious patient, these maneuvers are followed by sweeping a finger from the side of the patient's mouth deep into the oropharynx in order to remove any foreign body that may have been dislodged. An attempt at positive pressure ventilation is again made. This sequence is repeated until it is successful in establishing a patent airway or until an invasive technique is deemed necessary.

INVASIVE TECHNIQUES

In children, total airway obstruction leads to cardiac arrest and brain dysfunction quite rapidly. In most small children, total airway obstruction will not be tolerated longer than 1 minute. If the sequences described earlier are not successful in opening the airway rapidly and the patient is displaying signs and symptoms of hypoxia (cyanosis, arrhythmias), an invasive technique for opening the airway must be used.

The initial invasive tool in the dentist's armamentarium for dealing with airway obstruction should be direct laryngoscopy via the laryngoscope. Use of the laryngoscope requires a certain amount of training and skill. With the laryngoscope, the larynx may be exposed so that any foreign body may be removed under direct vision. The trachea may then be intubated with an appropriate endotracheal tube for manual ventilation as needed.

Opening of the airway via cricothyrotomy is the last resort method of airway control. The cricothyroid membrane between the thyroid cartilage and the cricoid bone is either incised with a scalpel or punctured with a large-bore needle in order to ventilate the trachea with a flow of oxygen or allow respiration to be assisted. This technique, along with the critical anatomic landmarks, should be understood thoroughly by every dentist.

Breathing ("B")

The second priority in dealing with medical emergencies, once a patent airway is established, is to ensure that adequate breathing is present. The chest should be observed for expansion and the nose and mouth observed for air flow during respiration by feeling and listening. If the patient is not breathing, rescue breathing should be initiated immediately. Initially, four rapid breaths are given in order to expand the lungs, followed by one breath every 3 seconds for children or one breath every 5 seconds for adults, until spontaneous respirations resume.

Rescue breathing may be accomplished by the mouth-to-mouth or the bag-valve-mask tech-

nique. Mouth-to-mouth ventilation is sometimes necessary in the emergency situation, but its efficacy is severely limited by the fact that exhaled air, containing a maximum of 15% to 18% oxygen, is delivered to the hypoxic patient's lungs.

Use of a positive pressure breathing system (bag-valve-mask), which can deliver close to 100% oxygen, is highly preferable. A mask is used, which fits tightly over the patient's mouth and nose. The mask is attached to a one-way valve, which allows oxygen to enter the patient when the reservoir bag is squeezed forceably. The empty bag then refills with oxygen only. The technique entails securing a tight mask fit on the patient's face and opening the airway with one hand and compressing the bag with the other, forcing oxygen by positive pressure into the patient's lungs. Exhalation is passive. This technique of rescue breathing is much more efficient than mouth-to-mouth resuscitation and should be mastered by all dentists. A bag-valve-mask system, such as an Ambu bag, is considered essential emergency equipment for every dental office.

Circulation ("C")

Once the airway and breathing have been established, the condition of the patient's circulatory system should be established. The most rapid, convenient, and accurate method of assessing circulation is to palpate the carotid pulse. The carotid artery should be felt just under the sternocleidomastoid muscle in the neck. One should never palpate both carotid arteries simultaneously because pressure on the baroreceptors of the carotid sinuses may precipitate reflex bradycardia. The quality, rate, and rhythm of the pulses should be noted. If the pulse is absent, CPR should be initiated immediately. If the pulse is present, a more accurate assessment of cardiovascular status should be obtained by measuring blood pressure and heart rate.

Definitive Therapy ("D")

Only after the "A," "B," and "C" of emergency management have been satisfied should one consider definitive drug therapy. Whether or not definitive drug therapy should be embarked upon by the dentist depends on several factors, including his or her training and expertise, the availability of medical assistance, and the situation that the dentist is presented with. If the emergency is very acute and life-threatening, especially if the cause is clear or was precipitated by treatment or a drug that was administered, definitive therapy may be indicated and essential. Some common medical emergencies for which definitive therapy is indicated will be briefly discussed.

SYNCOPE

Vasodepressor syncope, or the simple faint, is probably the most common cause of loss of consciousness in the dental office. It is, however, much less common in children than in young adults. Syncope is a maladaptive stress reaction that is usually triggered by anxiety. As the patient becomes anxious, the fight-or-flight response of the sympathetic nervous system is triggered, and endogenous epinephrine and norepinephrine are released into the circulation. This response involves a large increase in blood flow to the muscles of the body. If the muscles are contracting, as would be the case if a person is running, blood flow is maintained. In the dental chair, however, little or no muscle contraction occurs and the blood is, therefore, pooled in the muscles, especially in the lower extremities, effectively decreasing the relative blood volume available to the central circulation and, therefore, the brain. The heart rate reflexively increases in an attempt to maintain the blood pressure, and the blood vessels in the periphery constrict, producing the typical cold, pale, and sweaty skin. As blood flow to the brain decreases in the upright position, the patient feels dizzy or faint. This phase of the condition is called presyncope. It may begin rapidly and last a few minutes.

If it is recognized in a susceptible patient and dealt with quickly, loss of consciousness may be avoided. Management of presyncope consists of positioning the patient flat on the back, lowering the head, and raising the feet to augment blood flow to the brain by gravity. Encouraging the patient to contract muscles, especially in the legs, also augments return of pooled venous blood from the musculature. Administration of oxygen is appropriate in any emergency involving a decrease in brain perfusion. The use of an ammonia inhalant to stimulate the patient may be of some benefit.

If the process of syncope continues, the sympathetic nervous system fatigues and the parasympathetic nervous system suddenly becomes dominant. This vagal response results in a sudden, severe decrease in heart rate and blood pressure, often to startlingly low levels. Blood flow to the brain is decreased, and consciousness is lost. Breathing becomes irregular, the pupils dilate, and convulsive movements are often noted. The muscles relax, and the airway may become obstructed. Loss of consciousness from syncope is usually rapidly responsive to positioning as previously mentioned. Oxygen should be administered; airway, breathing, and circulation maintained; tight and constrictive clothing loosened; and vital signs monitored.

Consciousness is usually regained fairly quickly, but heart rate and blood pressure may be slow in recovering. If recovery of consciousness is delayed beyond 5 minutes or is incomplete after 15 to 20 minutes, medical assistance should be sought. Drug therapy is usually not indicated with syncope unless the heart rate or blood pressure remains dangerously depressed after positioning. In such a case, atropine to increase heart rate or a vasopressor to increase blood pressure may be necessary.

ALLERGIC REACTION

Allergic reactions involve hypersensitivity responses by the immune system to antigens that are recognized as foreign, with subsequent antibody formation. There are several different types of allergic responses, ranging from mild, delayed rashes to severe, sudden, life-threatening anaphylaxis. The primary agents employed in pediatric dentistry that might provoke an allergic reaction are the penicillins, intravenous sedative agents, or the ester-type local anesthetics.

The anaphylactic reaction is mediated primarily by the release of histamine from sensitized mast cells. Histamine is a potent toxic agent that produces inflammation and vascular effects. The body systems primarily involved in a clinical allergic reaction are the skin, respiratory system, and cardiovascular system. Skin involvement is the most common reaction and may range from a mild erythematous rash to urticaria (hives) to angioedema (severe swelling).

In general, the more rapid the onset and the more intense the symptoms, the more severe the generalized reaction can be expected to become. Angioedema that involves the face and neck may be rapidly progressive, leading to airway obstruction and death. The respiratory system is usually involved after the skin reaction starts in generalized anaphylaxis. The primary problem is constriction of bronchial smooth muscle, producing respiratory distress owing to airway obstruction, primarily expiratory in nature. The principal recognizable sign is wheezing, a distinctive breathing sound associated with bronchoconstriction. As the obstruction worsens, the patient has increasing difficulty in exchanging adequate volumes of air; usually becomes panicked, which worsens the situation; and may become severely hypoxic. Other smooth muscles also contract and may produce symptoms of abdominal cramps, nausea and vomiting, or incontinence. As anaphylaxis progresses, the cardiovascular system is affected. Hypotension is produced by the vasodilating effect of histamine and other mediators of the response. Reflex tachycardia, arrhythmias, and eventually cardiac arrest may follow.

Management of allergic reactions depends on the time course and severity of the symptoms. If symptoms are immediate or severe, epinephrine at 0.01 mg/kg should be administered, preferably intravenously in the 1:10,000 dilution or intramuscularly in the 1:1000 dilution. Epinephrine counteracts most of the effects of histamine. It produces bronchodilatation (countering bronchoconstriction) and raises blood pressure and heart rate by its alpha and beta effects. It also counters skin rash, urticaria, and angioedema by an unknown mechanism.

Diphenhydramine (Benadryl), a histamine receptor blocker, should also be administered. This antihistamine will not reverse to any great extent histaminic effects that have already occurred, but it may prevent further progression or recurrence of symptoms. If the reaction is delayed or mild, diphenhydramine may be all that is necessary to prevent progression of the allergic reaction. Diphenhydramine should also be administered orally at 6-hour intervals for 24 to 48 hours after any allergic reaction. Oxygen should always be administered if any respiratory symptoms are present. Use of an aerosolized sympathomimetic agent such as epinephrine, isoproterenol, or metaproterenol (Metaprel) to treat bronchospasm may also be of benefit. If the reaction is severe, the patient should be transported to the hospital, and supplemental use of a corticosteroid, such as hydrocortisone sodium succinate, should be considered. Ideally, the steroid preparation should be given early in the course of the reaction.

SEIZURES

Of the multiple types of seizures, the tonic-clonic (grand mal) type is the most frightening and the one that most often requires treatment. Only this type is considered here. Grand mal seizures are manifested in four phases: the prodromal phase, the aura, the convulsive (ictal) phase, and the postictal phase.

The prodromal phase consists of subtle changes that may occur over minutes to hours. It is usually not clinically evident to the practitioner or the patient. The aura is a neurologic

experience that the patient goes through immediately prior to the seizure. It is specifically related to the trigger areas of the brain in which the seizure activity begins. It may consist of a taste, a smell, a hallucination, motor activity, or other symptoms. A given patient's aura is often the same for all seizures. As the CNS discharge becomes generalized, the ictal phase begins. The patient loses consciousness, falls to the floor, and tonic, rigid skeletal muscle contraction ensues. As the chest wall musculature contracts, air is expelled through the larynx, producing vocalization called the epileptic cry. Clonic movements then begin, producing rapid jerking of the extremities and trunk. Breathing may be labored during this period, and patients may injure themselves. This clonic phase usually lasts 1 to 3 minutes. As the clonic phase ends, the muscles relax and movement stops. A significant degree of CNS depression is usually present during this postictal phase, and it may result in respiratory depression. The patient has amnesia from the prodromal phase throughout the entire seizure.

Management of a seizure consists of gentle restraint and positioning of the patient in order to prevent self-injury, ensuring adequate ventilation, and supportive care, as indicated, in the postictal phase, especially airway management. Single seizures do not require drug therapy because they are self-limiting. Should the ictal phase last longer than 5 minutes or if seizures continue to develop with little time between them, a condition called status epilepticus has developed. This may be a life-threatening medical emergency because the uncontrolled muscle activity can result in hyperthermia, increased oxygen consumption, tachycardia, hypertension, impaired ventilation, and cardiac arrhythmias. This condition is best treated with intravenous diazepam, and transport should be arranged to take the patient to the hospital.

HYPERVENTILATION

Hyperventilation syndrome, like syncope, is a maladaptive anxiety reaction that primarily occurs in apprehensive young females who attempt to hide their anxiety. It is much less common in males and is rare in young children. The syndrome is often triggered by an anxiety-provoking event such as the local anesthetic injection. The patient is usually unaware of the fact that she is beginning to hyperventilate. The respiratory rate may increase to 25 to 30 breaths per minute, with an increase in tidal volume as well. The patient may complain of difficulty in getting her breath. The increased ventilation causes carbon dioxide to be eliminated from the blood. The decrease in the Pa_{CO_2} in the blood (hypocarbia) causes a physiologic vasoconstriction of the arteries supplying the brain with a consequent decrease in blood flow to the brain. The patient begins to feel dizzy and light-headed, which further enhances the anxiety, worsening the condition in a vicious cycle. Other symptoms include numbness and tingling of the extremities and perioral area, muscle twitching and cramping, seizures, and loss of consciousness.

Management of hyperventilation involves early recognition of the patient's anxiety and discussing it openly with the patient. Reassurance, patient rapport, and calmly coaching the patient to breathe slowly may stop the process. Oxygen should not be administered. If the cycle cannot be broken, steps should be taken to increase the Pa_{CO_2}. This can be accomplished simply by having the patient breathe into a paper bag, which causes rebreathing of exhaled CO_2-containing air, thus raising the Pa_{CO_2} and reversing the process. This should not be done for an extended period of time, of course, owing to the possibility of producing hypoxia. Occasionally, use of an antianxiety agent, such as intravenous diazepam, is helpful.

ASTHMA

The primary type of asthma in children is allergic or extrinsic asthma, which is IgE antibody mediated. This type of asthma is usually outgrown by the late teens or early twenties. The asthma attack in this case is usually triggered by specific allergens, such as pollens, dust, and molds. The tracheobronchial tree is quite hyperreactive in asthma and contains increased amounts of tenacious secretions. During an acute asthmatic attack, constriction of the smooth muscle in the bronchial walls causes bronchospasm and the characteristic wheezing. Thick secretions are produced, which can plug the small airways, and bronchial wall edema may develop rapidly, further compromising the airway. This process may produce various signs and symptoms varying from mild wheezing and coughing to severe dyspnea, cyanosis, and death.

In adults, the primary type of asthma is called extrinsic asthma. With extrinsic asthma, attacks may be precipitated by infections, irritants, exercise, and, importantly, stress. Some overlap in these asthma types certainly occurs. With any asthmatic patient, a thorough history should be taken, including how often attacks occur, how severe they have become (if hospitalization has been required), what triggers attacks, and what medications are being taken. All attempts should be made to avoid precipitating factors. If the patient is taking medications, he or she should be instructed to continue taking them prior to the dental appointment. If patients use a Medihaler to self-administer aerosolized medications (Isuprel, Metaprel), they should bring it to their appointment.

If patients with asthma begin to wheeze and develop any respiratory distress in the dental chair, they should be given oxygen and allowed to sit up (if they are more comfortable sitting). If they have a Medihaler, they should use it, which will usually abort the attack. If aerosolized adrenergic agents fail to reverse the bronchospasm, 0.01 mg/kg (maximum dose, 0.5 mg) of epinephrine (1:1000) should be injected subcutaneously. This should reverse the attack in most cases. If no relief has been afforded after two doses of epinephrine, emergency transport to the hospital should be arranged. If the attack becomes very severe, intravenous aminophylline may be initiated in an attempt to relieve bronchospasm. A loading dose of 5.6 mg/kg is infused over 10 minutes, followed by a continuous intravenous infusion of 1 mg/kg/hour. Any patient requiring parenteral drug administration to control an asthma attack should be transported to the hospital. Early administration of a corticosteroid (hydrocortisone or dexamethasone) may also be helpful in severe attacks.

DIABETES MELLITUS

Diabetes mellitus is a disorder involving poor insulin production and consequently disorders of carbohydrate, fat, and protein metabolism. It is characterized by hyperglycemia if it is untreated. Diabetes mellitus occurring in children is called juvenile onset diabetes mellitus and usually carries the worst prognosis. These patients have little or no pancreatic beta cell function and therefore require parenteral insulin daily. Blood glucose levels may be difficult to control. The principal emergencies that develop are due to either hypoglycemia or hyperglycemia. If plasma insulin levels remain low or absent for a prolonged period of time, blood glucose levels become extremely elevated. The glucose, however, is unable to enter the cells as a result of the lack of insulin, and the cells metabolize fat and proteins to produce more glucose as well as ketones and other metabolic acids. A condition known as diabetic ketoacidosis occurs, which may lead to coma and death if it is left untreated. The important fact to realize concerning ketoacidosis is that it requires several days to develop, during which time the patient is ill. It does not occur suddenly in a previously alert and well patient.

If a diabetic patient who is doing well experiences a sudden deterioration in the dental office, the condition is far more likely to be due to acute hypoglycemia, or insulin shock. The usual scenario involves a patient who has taken his or her morning insulin and has forgotten to eat a meal or has ingested inadequate carbohydrate. Exercise and stress may also increase carbohydrate utilization and lower blood glucose concentrations. Glucose and oxygen are the primary metabolites for brain cells. As the serum glucose level begins to decrease, neurologic symptoms may begin to appear. Most diabetic patients are well attuned to this phenomenon and carry a carbohydrate source to be ingested in this event. If carbohydrate is not ingested and the blood glucose concentration continues to decrease, evidence of deteriorating cerebral function ensues. The patient may become lethargic, have a change in mood, act strangely, or become nauseated. The sympathetic nervous system becomes hyperactive in an attempt to raise the blood glucose level, producing symptoms of tachycardia, hypertension, anxiety, and sweating. The patient develops slurred speech, ataxia, mental obtundation, and eventually loss of consciousness. Seizures may occur.

Management of hypoglycemia involves the administration of glucose. The oral route is used only if the patient is fully conscious and is experiencing early symptoms. Sugar dissolved in juice or a sugar-containing soft drink may be used. If the patient has become mentally obtunded, an intravenous catheter should be established and 50% dextrose administered until consciousness is regained. Alternatively, glucagon may be administered intramuscularly if establishment of intravenous access is not possible. It must be remembered that consciousness will be regained more slowly when glucagon is used. The dentist should never attempt to administer glucose orally to a mentally obtunded or unconscious patient.

> It is recommended that the dental practitioner further expand upon this material, becoming familiar with other medical emergency situations that may occur in the dental office, especially those drug-related emergencies that may result from pharmacologic agents being used in daily practice.

REFERENCES

Goodson JM, Moore RA: Life-threatening reactions after pediatric sedation: An assessment of narcotic, local anesthetic, and anti-anxiety drug interaction. JADA *107*:239–245, 1983.

Malamed SF: Handbook of Medical Emergencies in the Dental Office, 2nd ed. St. Louis, CV Mosby, 1982.

Malamed SF: Sedation: A Guide to Patient Management, 3rd ed. St. Louis, CV Mosby, 1995.

11

Dental Public Health Issues in Pediatric Dentistry

M. J. Kanellis

Chapter Outline

DEFINITION OF DENTAL PUBLIC HEALTH

ROLE OF THE INDIVIDUAL PRACTITIONER

ACCESS TO CARE

CHILDREN AND DENTAL PUBLIC HEALTH

Barriers to Care for Infants and Toddlers from Low-Income Families

Project Head Start

School-Based Dental Care

The Challenge of Adolescence

SUMMARY

Increasingly, one of the primary challenges facing the dental profession is ensuring that all children and adults enjoy the benefits of good oral health. Although the majority of dental needs of children can be successfully addressed one-on-one within a dental office, certain needs may be more efficiently addressed on a community-wide basis. This chapter provides an overview of dental public health and outlines ways in which the oral health of children is enhanced by various public health activities.

DEFINITION OF DENTAL PUBLIC HEALTH

Dental public health is defined as "the science and art of preventing and controlling dental diseases and promoting dental health through organized community efforts" (American Board of Dental Public Health, 1992). A common misconception about dental public health is that its primary objective is the delivery of dental care to low-income persons. Although this is im-

portant, the actual delivery of dental care is only one aspect of dental public health.

The three major core functions of public health, as identified by the 1988 Institute of Medicine study, are assessment, policy development, and assurance (National Academy of Sciences, 1988). The major activities of dental public health can be divided into these same categories. Examples of core dental public health activities that affect the oral health of children are given in Table 11-1.

ROLE OF THE INDIVIDUAL PRACTITIONER

It is important for the individual practitioner to understand that the oral health status and needs of children receiving care in a private practice setting may not represent *all* children in the community. The challenge for all dentists, therefore, is to look beyond the individual dental office and make a broad assessment of their community's needs while assessing their own role in

TABLE 11–1. Examples of Dental Public Health Activities Affecting Children

Assessment

1. Documenting the oral health status of children
2. Assessing the supply and availability of dentists to meet the needs of children
3. Assessing the status of water fluoridation in communities
4. Assessing the need for dental care for children with special health care needs
5. Identifying barriers to dental access
6. Screening children before entering school

Policy Development

1. Developing policies and advocating for legislative action to ensure access to oral health services for low-income, underserved, hard-to-reach, and vulnerable children
2. Developing programs that focus on primary and secondary prevention
3. Developing programs to provide dental care to children with special health needs or without access to adequate dental care
4. Adopting state rules mandating oral health screening for children entering school for the first time

Assurance

1. Encouraging and coordinating efforts to provide oral health education and promotion in schools, clinics, community settings, and other settings
2. Expanding or establishing new dental clinical sites or developing promotional activities by the State Health Agency to meet the oral health needs of a specific target group or community
3. Targeting topical and systemic fluoride programs to areas with nonfluoridated water supplies and high-risk populations
4. Including an oral health component in all school health initiatives
5. Establishing school-based prevention programs and school-based or school-linked dental clinics as components of comprehensive school health
6. Establishing programs to train medical professionals and other health related workers to recognize oral health problems, including early childhood caries (ECC)
7. Integrating oral health services into appropriate health, education, and social service programs (e.g., Maternal and Child Health, nutrition, WIC, health promotion, PATCH program, school health)

Adapted from Association of State and Territorial Dental Directors' Guidelines for State & Territorial Dental/Oral Health Programs: Essential Public Health Services to Promote Oral Health in the United States. January 3, 1997.

enhancing the oral health of the entire community. Dental public health activities in which practitioners are frequently involved include advocating fluoridation of community water supplies, participating in school and community health promotion activities, advising policymakers regarding dental care programs (including Medicaid), and participating in oral health screening and community assessment activities. Support and guidance for the individual practitioner becoming involved in dental public health activities can be sought from a variety of sources, including the oral health components of state public health agencies, county boards of health, and various community boards and organizations.

One important issue practitioners often find themselves involved with is enhancing access to dental care for members of their communities. This topic is discussed in the following paragraphs.

ACCESS TO CARE

Although regular dental care contributes substantially to healthy mouths for millions of children,

a significant number of children and adults have serious problems receiving the care they need. These children are most often from low-income or minority families and unfortunately these groups tend to experience more oral disease than other children (Call, 1989; Rizk et al., 1994; Kaste et al., 1996). Some of the factors that can limit access to dental care for these children are (1) lack of finances (including lack of third-party coverage), (2) lack of transportation, (3) language and cultural barriers, and (4) lack of perceived need for care.

Historically, financial limitations have been among the most formidable barriers for low-income children in receiving health care. In 1965, the federal government attempted to reduce these financial barriers by creating the Medicaid program (Title XIX), which pays for medical and dental care for eligible low-income people. Adult dental coverage under Medicaid is optional, and covered services vary widely from state to state. Coverage for child dental services is mandatory, however, because of a 1968 amendment to the Medicaid program creating the Early and Periodic Screening, Diagnostic and Treatment (EPSDT) program (U.S. Congress, 1968). The purpose of the EPSDT program is to identify the health problems of children as early as possible and to provide comprehensive preventive and remedial care.

Dental care is a mandatory part of the EPSDT program and covers diagnostic, preventive, and restorative services for all Medicaid-enrolled children up to 21 years of age. The EPSDT program requires that children receive oral health evaluations from their primary care provider beginning at birth, with a referral to the dentist at age 3. States have the option of requiring earlier referrals, with some states requiring referral to a dentist at 1 year of age.

CHILDREN AND DENTAL PUBLIC HEALTH

This textbook is organized by children's developmental stages. It works well to discuss dental public health issues within this same developmental context. The remainder of this chapter is devoted to introducing some dental public health issues as they relate to children of different age groups.

Barriers to Care for Infants and Toddlers from Low-Income Families

Dental care for infants and toddlers from low-income families presents a dilemma for several reasons. These children often (1) lack financial access to care, (2) have care givers who fail to recognize the importance of early dental visits, (3) have difficulty finding a dentist who will accept Medicaid, and (4) have difficulty finding a dentist who will see children under the age of 3 years.

As stated elsewhere in this text, dental care for children should begin in infancy. This is especially true for low-income children who are at higher risk for disease. Although it is true that many children never experience decay in their primary dentition, others experience severe decay. For young children, particularly those under age 3, such treatment often requires hospitalization and general anesthesia. Thus, for low-income children with severe decay, the costs of treatment can be very high and present a major barrier to patients, parents, and practitioners.

Despite EPSDT program requirements that eligible children visit a dentist by age 3 (or younger in some states), the use of dental services by low-income children ages 0 to 3 remains extremely low (Damiano et al., 1996). Continuing

efforts are needed to convey the importance of early dental visits for this group of children. In addition, oral health screening and counseling should be a part of existing public health programs where young children appear for other services. Successful integration of oral health activities, including prevention, education, and screening, has already occurred in many public health programs, including Maternal Child Health Clinics and Women, Infants, and Children (WIC) Clinics.

Although dental components are often an integral part of public health programs, rarely are public health clinics established solely to meet the needs of low-income infants. At least one international model exists for a clinic designed specifically for the oral health care of infants, however. In Brazil, a state-sponsored infant oral health clinic has been in existence since 1986.

Project Head Start

Prior to beginning kindergarten or first grade, large numbers of children in the United States participate in formal preschool programs. Preschools provide a unique opportunity to study the oral health status of children in the 3- to 6-year-old age group (Edelstein and Douglass, 1995) and for increasing access to services for low-income children. The largest preschool program in the country is Project Head Start, which primarily serves children from low-income families and children with disabilities. Head Start, established in 1965, is administered by the Department of Health and Human Services (DHHS), and in fiscal year 1995, over $3 billion were allocated for Head Start programs serving over 750,000 children.

Project Head Start has historically maintained a strong commitment to the health of children enrolled in its programs and has a mandatory dental component that requires that all enrolled children receive a dental examination complete with prophylaxis as well as follow-up care for necessary restorative treatment. Head Start programs establish and maintain dental records for children enrolled in their program, but the necessary dental treatment is usually provided by dentists in the community. Head Start pays for necessary dental treatment for children enrolled in their program who are not eligible for funding from Medicaid or other sources. This unique public-private partnership has been instrumental in helping ensure access to care for low-income preschool children nationwide. One of the stated goals of Head Start is to attempt to link families

A Dental Clinic for Babies: A Success Story

Karin Weber

In 1983, a group of professors in the Department of Pediatric Dentistry at the State University of Londrina, Paraná, Brazil initiated a project addressing dental care during the first years of life. There had been a significant increase in the numbers of families with very young children (birth to 5 years) contacting the Pediatric Dentistry Department. Most of these children were referred by dentists and physicians who were able to identify the need for treatment but clinically unprepared to serve this particular age group. The project obtained formal approval in 1986, and the Baby Clinic (*Bebê-Clínica*) was officially inaugurated. Since then, major changes in the area of dental health education have come about in Brazil. These changes have been instrumental in raising the population's consciousness of the importance of early dental care and have resulted in the currently accepted concept of "early attention to and maintenance of oral health." The Baby Clinic was readily accepted by the surrounding community as well as the area's pediatric dentists. In 1989, the Baby Clinic started to serve not only as a clinical opportunity for educating dental professionals but as a regional reference center for dental care of a population from birth to 5 years of age. All fundamental developmental research was finished in 1991. Since achievement of the primary objectives—research, teaching, and community care—the Baby Clinic has worked toward the application of its results, transmitting knowledge and experience to other universities, public health services, and dental professionals in Brazil and other countries. In 1993, the research group *CNPO/ UEL/BABY CLINIC (Conselho Nacional de Desenvolvimento Científico e Technológico/ Universidade Estadual de Londrina/Bebê-Clínica)* was created, and during the Second National Conference on Oral Health held in Brasília-DF (*Distrito Federal*) in September of 1993, dentistry for small children was recognized as a right for every Brazilian citizen.

The group of professors at the Baby Clinic also are responsible for the invention of the "Macri," a piece of equipment used to facilitate clinical examination of infants and toddlers (Fig. 11-1). This sling/chair-like device does not require the cooperation of the child but provides a comfortable position with minimal restraint as well as excellent visualization of the oral cavity. Parents are always welcome to remain near the child to provide encouragement and support. In addition to the Macri used for clinical examination, a Macri was also developed particularly for radiographic purposes. This apparatus spins 360 degrees around its own axis to facilitate the child's positioning for radiographic procedures.

Box continued on following page

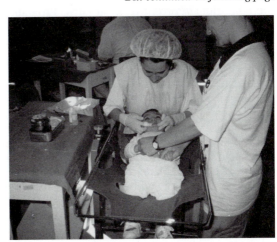

Figure 11–1. A young child being examined in a Macri.

A Dental Clinic for Babies: A Success Story *continued*

Early prevention of dental caries is based on education as well as treatment. Health professionals, especially pediatricians and pediatric dentists, carry a responsibility to provide educational programs to parents on oral care during the first year of life, with subsequent and additional programs directed toward the child as the child grows and matures.

The Baby Clinic uses a three-step process. This process starts with the *Educational Program,* a presentation directed at parents. At this first stage, parents receive an overview of all the factors involved in oral health: tooth eruption patterns, oral cleaning, breast feeding, nutritive and non-nutritive sucking, the caries process, types of fluorides, diet, and feeding practices. Parents are also informed of the types of treatments available for their children at the Baby Clinic. Emphasis is placed in the role and responsibility of the parents in preventing dental disease. The second step of the process is the *Preventive Program.* Both an oral and general assessment are performed to evaluate the child's oral and physical health. This is the optimal time to assess the child's risk of dental disease through an analysis of current diet, oral hygiene practices, and family and social environment. According to the individual child's perceived degree of risk, parents are given more specific recommendations pertaining to methods and timing of providing oral care. Time of recall is also determined by degree of risk and can vary from 1 week to 6 months. The third step in the process is the *Restorative Program* and consists of any necessary dental treatment, including treatment under sedation and general anesthesia.

Children with special needs (up to age 21) are also treated at the Baby Clinic. Emergency dental care is also available to children ages birth to 5 years on a 24-hour basis.

It is extremely important to note that *all* children receive all these types of services free of charge. The Baby Clinic is affiliated with the State University of Londrina, which in turn is financially supported by the Paraná state government.

The success of the Baby Clinic has proven the value of an interdisciplinary, multifaceted project involving multiple health care providers. The Baby Clinic has demonstrated a team approach to early dental care, integrating the actions of health care providers such as pediatric dentists, speech pathologists, nutritionists, pediatricians, and psychologists. Currently, the Baby Clinic is the only research group in Brazil in the field of dentistry for babies and serves as a national center of reference for the discipline.

The concept of dentistry for children in Brazil, previously based solely on an early restorative treatment, has evolved to take a preventive and educational approach to the maintenance of early oral health. This fact has been well observed at the Baby Clinic through the years. In 1985, 78% of parents bringing their children to the Baby Clinic sought restorative treatment, and only 22% sought information on oral health maintenance (Walter and Nakama, 1992). At present, 88% of parents seek information, and only 12% do so purely for restorative treatment. It has been shown that maximum effectiveness of the Educational/Preventive/Restorative Program and best oral health results occur when care is initiated at 6 months of age (with an upper safety limit of around 12 months of age). Reduction in caries prevalence is 85% in children for whom care was initiated in the first year of life and who were subsequently followed for a period of 4 years (Walter, 1995). In addition, Walter and Nakama (1993) have shown that, of the children who previously participated in the three-step program at the Baby Clinic, 65% seen between the ages of 5 and 6 years are caries-free. This regional finding surpasses the national goal, proposed by the World Health Organization for the year 2000, that 50% of Brazilian children be free of dental caries.

The Baby Clinic at the State University of Londrina-Paraná was the first research group in Brazil in the field of dentistry for babies and still serves as a national center of reference for the discipline. Currently, an ambitious project is progressing in conjunction with the State Department of Public Health and the State University of Londrina. At the end of 1997, 200 general dentists working in county public health dental clinics throughout the state were trained at the Baby Clinic to deliver early dental care to infants and younger children. These dentists are also being trained to organize and institute infant oral health programs in 210 public health dental clinics in addition to the 39 public health dental clinics currently offering infant oral health care in Paraná state.

As a result of the pioneering work in Londrina, other Baby Clinics have been established in Brazil. Twenty-seven universities throughout the country have programs providing infant oral health care. The Brazilian Armed Forces has also joined the movement and established infant oral health care programs at five Brazilian military bases.

Seven other countries in South America have also recognized the importance of early dental intervention and Baby Clinics are being maintained or starting up in Peru, Venezuela, Colombia, Ecuador, Paraguay, Uruguay, and Bolivia.

The guiding philosophy of the Baby Clinic is that maintaining the oral health of children is a necessary antecedent to the prevention of dental disease. Proper oral health maintenance offers a practical, simple, effective, and low-cost approach.

REFERENCES

Nakama R, Walter LRF: Prevention of dental caries in the first year of life [Abstract]. J Dent Res 73(4):773, 1993.

Walter LRF: Modern paediatric dentistry. *In* World Congress of the International Association of Dental Students and Young Dentists Worldwide, São Paulo, Brazil. Official Program, 42, 1995, p 9.

Walter LRF, Nakama L: Pacientes de Alto Índices de Cárie × Pacientes de Alto Risco: Qual a conduta? *In* Bottino MA, Feller C (eds): Atualizacão na Clínica Odontológica: O Dia a Dia do Clínico Geral. São Paulo, Artes Médicas, 1992, pp 251–258.

to an ongoing health care system to ensure that the child continues to receive comprehensive health care even after leaving the Head Start program (U.S. Government Printing Office, 1995).

School-Based Dental Care

The reaching of school age presents another unique opportunity for enhancing the oral health of children. Schools are a logical site for promoting oral health through educational and prevention programs and delivering dental services to school age children because they provide a high concentration of children at the same location (Marx et al., 1998). The United States has enjoyed a long tradition of successfully implementing oral health activities into school settings. Examples of services that can be provided in a school-based setting include oral health education, fluoride mouth-rinsing, sealant placement, oral health screenings and referrals, and comprehensive restorative care.

Health education, including oral health education, has long been considered an important part of school curricula in the United States. Dentists and other dental health professionals often have the opportunity to contribute to these activities by visiting classrooms and participating in health fairs or other special events. Oral health informa-

tion presented in these forums can generate interest and stimulate changes in knowledge and attitudes. It is important for the oral health professional to understand that these changes are commonly short-lived, however, and that desired behavioral changes require regular, long-term follow-up (Striffler et al., 1983).

School-based fluoride mouth-rinsing programs in the United States have been a common public health prevention strategy for nearly 30 years. In 1988, an estimated 3.25 million children were participating in school-based fluoride mouth-rinsing programs in 11,683 schools (Burt and Eklund, 1992). Historically, school-based fluoride mouth-rinsing programs have been most commonly targeted at schools where the majority of children do not have access to fluoridated drinking water, regardless of the socioeconomic level of the students. The general decline in the caries rate among children has caused researchers to question the cost-effectiveness of these programs (Bohannan et al., 1985). These programs are most likely to be cost-effective when targeted at schools with additional risk factors besides a lack of water fluoridation (e.g., low-income status, high caries rate, lack of access to primary care). Typically, children participating in school-based fluoride mouth-rinsing programs rinse once a week with 10 ml of a 0.2% neutral sodium fluoride solution. Alternatively, children may rinse daily with 0.05% NaF. Mouth-rinsing activities are generally supervised by a classroom teacher, a school nurse, or other persons with appropriate training.

School-based sealant programs have become increasingly popular as a means of increasing the prevalence of sealants among low-income children (Bohannan et al., 1984; Cohen and Horowitz, 1993; Klein et al., 1985). Although pit and fissure sealants have been known to be effective in preventing dental decay for over 25 years (Simonsen, 1991), only 11% of American school children had dental sealants on their teeth in 1989 (U.S. Public Health Service, 1989) with sealant use even lower for children from low-income families (4.3% for children from families with incomes of less than $10,000—U.S. Public Health Service, 1989). In 1995, 109 school-based/school-linked dental sealant programs were identified in 27 states (Amini et al., 1995). These programs usually target schools with a high percentage of low-income children (based on eligibility for free and reduced meal programs). Certain grades are usually chosen to participate, based on the eruption patterns of the permanent molars. Because of the timing of eruption for first permanent molars, second grade is a common age to initiate sealant programs. The majority of sealant programs use a four-handed approach, with each sealant team generally providing sealants to 10 to 15 children a day (Fig. 11–2).

Oral health screenings are carried out in schools under a number of different circumstances. Often, oral health screenings are provided as part of health fairs, or in combination with other educational/promotional activities. The purpose of these screenings is generally to identify gross problems and to refer children for dental care. A minimum of equipment is needed for this level of screening, with a pen light and

tongue blade often sufficing. When screenings are performed in conjunction with school-based sealant programs or as part of surveys gathering data on the oral health status of children, the mirror and explorer examination is often more complete.

Following school-based oral health screenings, referrals for follow-up care are generally made to area dentists, public health agencies, or school-based clinics. Only rarely are school-based screenings or examinations intended to take the place of complete dental examinations by dentists outside the school. This information should be communicated to parents and guardians of children who are screened in school-based settings in order that they understand the intent of the school-based screening and the limitations of the procedures provided (e.g., no radiographs).

Comprehensive school-based dental care is not common in the United States, although some school-based programs providing a wide range of services have been in existence for more than 75 years. In Virginia, comprehensive school-based dental programs were first introduced in 1921, with ongoing programs in existence ever since (Day and Doherty, 1996). Although examples of school-based programs offering comprehensive care can be found in the United States, perhaps the best known model for comprehensive school-based dentistry is the School Dental Service of New Zealand, which has been in existence for over 60 years (Jones, 1984).

School-based dental care can provide a means for increasing both access and use of dental services for children who do not or cannot receive care in the private sector. School-based dental programs, regardless of scope, should involve careful planning in order to optimize chances for success. The most fundamental aspect of planning involves a careful assessment of the need for school-based dental services and ongoing evaluation of such programs. School-based programs should not attempt to replace services provided in the private sector, nor should they compete for patients that are adequately served by existing resources.

The Challenge of Adolescence

Providing oral health care to adolescents can be a rewarding experience for the practitioner. This is generally a very "teachable" age, with most adolescents acutely interested in their appearance and their health. For some adolescents, however, daily life challenges may make dental care a very low priority. Adolescence is a period

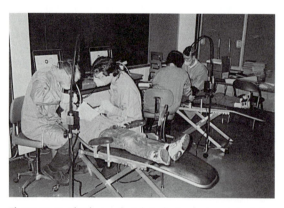

Figure 11–2. Third-year dental students placing sealants in a school-based sealant program.

School-Based Sealants: The Cincinnati Experience

Mark Siegal

One example of a successful school-based sealant program can be found in the city of Cincinnati, Ohio (Siegal, 1995). The Cincinnati program targets children in second and sixth grades in schools with at least 50% of children eligible for the free/reduced cost lunch program. All children in those grades are eligible for the program, with parental consent.

Individual arrangements are made with each school for two dental teams to set up a portable dental office in the schools. The equipment and supplies are delivered in a van and take about 45 minutes to set up. The portable dental office includes all of the infection control considerations necessary to meet state and Occupational Safety and Health Administration (OSHA) requirements. Depending on the enrollment and participation, the sealant program's stay ranges from a day to over a week.

After a dentist has evaluated each child's need for sealants and determined which teeth are to be sealed, the sealants are placed by a dental hygienist–dental assistant team. In Ohio, as in most states with sealant programs, a dentist need not be present while the sealants are placed. Some state dental practice acts, however, require the dentist's presence. On a typical school day, each team places sealants on 15 children in the Cincinnati program. The Cincinnati program has been a model for other Ohio programs.

---

of life typically associated with increased risks in the areas of health and education (Hechinger, 1992) and, in some estimations, adolescents today face greater risks to their current and future health than ever before (Gans and Blyth, 1990). Consider a few of the following statistics from 1995 concerning life for American teenagers (Cohen, 1996):

1. Every 22 seconds, an American teenager becomes pregnant
2. Every 47 seconds, an American child is abused or neglected, and about half are teens
3. Every 67 seconds, an American teenager has a baby
4. On any given day, 40,000 American teens are in jails or detention facilities
5. Every day, 6 teenagers commit suicide

Needless to say, the oral health needs of adolescents are often overshadowed by other pressing concerns.

The term "at risk" has become a general term used to describe people in trouble (Tidwell and Garrett, 1994) and is often used to categorize adolescents who are not likely to succeed in school or in life because of one or more factors (Capuzzi and Gross, 1989). Factors that can place an adolescent at risk may include but are not limited to chemical dependency, teenage pregnancy, poverty, disaffection with school and society, emotional and physical abuse, physical and emotional disabilities, and learning disabilities (U.S. Public Health Service, 1993).

Many of these same factors can affect an adolescent's oral health and ability or willingness to seek dental care. Low-income adolescents experience more decay than other adolescents (National Institute of Dental Research, 1989), and adolescents with risk factors of poverty, teenage pregnancy, low grades, or disaffection with school are less likely to use or receive dental care than other adolescents (Harvey, 1996).

As with other age groups, lack of finances is a significant barrier to oral health care for at-risk adolescents. It is estimated that one in five American teenagers lives in poverty (Cohen, 1996) and that one third of American teenagers living in poverty are not covered by Medicaid (Cohen,

Bright Futures—an Approach to Oral Health Supervision

Paul Casamassimo

In 1994, the Maternal and Child Health Bureau, in partnership with the Medicaid Bureau of the Health Care Financing Administration, both of the U.S. Department of Health and Human Services, published *Bright Futures: Guidelines for Health Supervision of Infants, Children, and Adolescents.* This set of guidelines was developed by a national panel of health professionals with expertise in the care of children, with support and consultation from a large number of child health and advocacy groups. These guidelines are meant to form the basis for preventive health supervision of children through the end of the millennium and beyond. They were envisioned to represent the best practice of care for children and to unify health professionals in approaching child health supervision comprehensively and across disciplines.

Dentistry's participation is noteworthy because of the key role of dentists in the development of this document directed to the general health of the pediatric patient. In many health arenas, oral health is an afterthought. Studies have demonstrated that the medical community dealing with children has only a marginal understanding of oral health issues and a poor performance record in provision of oral health education, fluoride prescription, and identification and referral of early dental disease. The promise of *Bright Futures* is that oral health considerations are now a part of child health supervision, beginning even in the prenatal period. Their placement and description in the overall paradigm for health supervision has been directed by dental professionals to ensure that interventions are age-appropriate and scientifically sound.

The first practical offshoot of *Bright Futures* is a sister document entitled *Bright Futures in Practice—Oral Health.* This is the first of several specific sets of guidelines that deal with various aspects of pediatric health such as oral health and nutrition. In *Bright Futures in Practice—Oral Health,* concepts such as risk assessment, measuring health outcomes, and interdisciplinary health supervision are explored. Risk assessment, for example, is a growing part of dental care science, with significant research and interest being devoted to identifying historical and clinical factors that can be used by providers in the care setting to rate patients' susceptibility to dental diseases such as caries or periodontal disease. *Bright Futures* proposes a set of risk factors that can be used by a variety of health professionals to apply preventive strategies more individually. These are grouped by age so that the changing habits and lifestyles of children and teens can be monitored.

Another innovation of *Bright Futures in Practice—Oral Health* is the concept of anticipatory guidance applied to oral health supervision. A box in this text (see Chapter 13) describes the application of this concept to pediatric dentistry in more detail.

A final innovation of this sister document is outcomes. In an age of accountability, what has been missing from oral health is a set of measurable health characteristics to indicate when patients are not only free of disease but on a path of preventive behaviors that most likely will keep them there. *Bright Futures* proposes a simple set of knowledge, behavior, and clinical outcomes that are understandable to both dental professional and parent and that can be common ground for demonstration, discussion, and assessment within a child's health supervision.

Bright Futures is a comprehensive approach to oral health supervision that has value for dental and other health professionals. We include it because the concept of developmental stages, so important in this book, is the basis for both general and oral health supervision in *Bright Futures.*

REFERENCES

Casamassimo PS (ed): Bright Futures in Practice—Oral Health. Arlington, VA, National Center for Education in Maternal and Child Health, 1996.

Green M (ed): Bright Futures: Guidelines for Health Supervision of Infants, Children, and Adolescents. Arlington, VA, National Center for Education in Maternal and Child Health, 1994.

1996). Nonfinancial barriers to care also exist and may include (1) low priority given to oral health, (2) no perceived need for dental care, (3) a "dislike" for going to the dentist, (4) lack of office hours that do not interfere with school and other activities, and (5) lack of transportation.

Addressing the oral health needs of at-risk teens is a relatively newly recognized problem, and strategies for dealing with this problem have not been as well developed as for other age groups. Possible strategies that may offer solutions include integrating oral health services into comprehensive school-based health centers, offering screening and referral programs in community settings frequented by teens, and maximizing the participation of adolescents in the EPSDT program (English, 1993).

REFERENCES

American Board of Dental Public Health: Informational brochure. Gainesville, FL, ABDPH, 1992.

Amini H, Bouchard J, Farquehar C, et al: Assessment of school-based/linked sealant programs in the U.S. J Dent Res 74 (AADR Abstract #267):45, 1995.

Association of State and Territorial Dental Directors' Guidelines for State & Territorial Dental/Oral Health Programs: Essential Public Health Services to Promote Oral Health in the United States. January 3, 1997.

Bohannan HM, Disney JA, Graves RC, et al: Indications for sealant use in a community-based preventive dentistry program. J Dent Educ 48(2):45-55, 1984.

Bohannan HM, Stamm JW, Graves RC, et al: Fluoride mouthrinse programs in fluoridated communities. JADA 111:783-789, 1985.

Burt BA, Eklund SA: Dentistry, Dental Practice, and the Community, 4th ed. Philadelphia, WB Saunders, 1992, p 182.

Call RL: Effects of poverty on children's dental health. Pediatrician 16:200-206, 1989.

Capuzzi D, Gross D: Youth at Risk. Alexandria, VA, American Association for Counseling and Development, 1989.

Cohen LA, Horowitz AM: Community-based sealant programs in the United States: Results of a survey. J Public Health Dent 53(4):241-245, 1993.

Cohen MI: Great transitions, preparing adolescents for a new century: A commentary on the health component of the concluding report of the Carnegie Council on Adolescent Development 19:2-5, 1996.

Damiano PC, Kanellis MJ, Willard JC, Momany ET: A report on the Iowa Title XIX dental program: Final report to the Iowa Department of Human Services. Iowa City, IA. The University of Iowa Public Policy Center and College of Dentistry, 1996.

Day KC, Doherty J: Celebrating 75 years of dental public health in Virginia. Virginia Dental J 73(3), 1996.

Edelstein BL, Douglass CW: Dispelling the myth that 50 percent of U.S. schoolchildren have never had a cavity. Public Health Rep 110:522-530, 1995.

English A: Early and periodic screening, diagnosis, and treatment program (EPSDT): a model for improving adolescents' access to healthcare. J Adolesc Health 14:524-526, 1993.

Gans JE, Blyth DA: America's Adolescents: How Healthy Are They? AMA Profiles of Adolescent Health Series. Chicago, American Medical Association, 1990.

Harvey HL: Factors affecting the utilization of dental services by adolescents. Thesis, The University of Iowa, 1996.

Hechinger FM: Fateful Choices: Healthy Youth for the 21st Century. Washington, DC, Carnegie Council on Adolescent Development, 1992.

Jones R: The school-based dental care systems of New Zealand and South Australia—a decade of change. J Pub Health Dent 44(3), 1984.

Kaste LM, Selwitz RH, Oldakowski RJ, et al: Coronal caries in the primary and permanent dentition of children and adolescents 1-17 years of age: United States, 1988-1991. J Dent Res 75(Spec Iss):631-641, 1996.

Klein SP, Bohannan HM, Bell RM, et al: The cost and effectiveness of school-based preventive dental care. Am J Public Health 75:382-390, 1985.

Marx E, Wooley SF: Health is Academic: A Guide to Coordinated School Health Programs. New York: Teachers College Press, 1998.

National Academy of Sciences, Institute of Medicine: The future of public health. Washington, DC, National Academy Press, 1988.

National Institute of Dental Research, U.S. Department of Health and Human Services: Oral Health of United States Children; The National Survey of Dental Caries in U.S. School Children: 1986-87, National and Regional Findings. NIH Pub. No. 89-2247. Bethesda, MD, National Institute of Dental Research, 1989.

Rizk SP, Christen AG: Falling between the cracks: Oral health survey of school children ages five to thirteen having limited access to dental services. ASDC J Dent Child 61(5-6):356-360, 1994.

Siegal M: School-based dental sealant programs expanding: Ohio among the leaders. ASTHO School Health Report 2(4):1-2, 1995.

Simonsen RJ: Retention and effectiveness of dental sealant after 15 years. JADA 122:34-42, 1991.

Striffler DF, Young WO, Burt BA: Dentistry, Dental Practice, and the Community, 3rd ed. Philadelphia, WB Saunders, 1983, p 491.

Tidwell R, Garrett SC: Youth at risk: In search of a definition. J Counsel Dev 72:444-446, 1994.

U.S. Congress, House: January 2, 1968. An act to amend the Social Security Act. Public Law 90-248, HR 12080.

U.S. Government Printing Office: Head Start program performance standards for operation of Head Start programs by grantees and delegate agencies. Chapter XIII—Office of Human Development Services, Department of Health and Human Services, 1995, p 231.

U.S. Public Health Service, National Center for Health Statistics: Dental services and oral health: United States, 1989. PHS Publ No 93-1511, Series 10 No 183. Washington, DC, Government Printing Office, 1992.

U.S. Public Health Service: Toward improving the oral health of Americans: An overview of oral health status, resources and care delivery. Public Health Reports, Nov./Dec., 1993.

Summary

One of the joys of practicing dentistry is observing children in a dental practice mature and grow into healthy adults. Dentists contribute to the oral health of these patients individually but can also contribute to good oral health for the entire community. When dentists turn their eyes to the community, they see numerous opportunities to enhance the oral health of the entire community through involvement with dental public health efforts affecting children of all ages.

I

Conception to Age Three

Without question, the development of a child from conception to age 3 years is the most dramatic with regards to growth and development. In an approximately 3 year, 9 month period of time, a single cell, the fertilized egg, develops into a human being, complete with feelings, emotional needs, ability to communicate, gross motor skills such as walking, and fine motor skills such as piling up blocks. Dentally, the edentulous neonate will, at age 3, have a complete primary dentition consisting of 20 teeth.

From a medical standpoint, these years are very important. The obstetrician monitors the development of the fetus and the welfare of the pregnant mother and is responsible for the neonate during birthing. The pediatrician or family physician will attend to the neonate (1-4 weeks postpartum), the infant (first year of life), the toddler (1-3 years), the child (3-12 years), and the adolescent (12-19 years). To some degree, the quality of life of any culture can be measured by the health and survival rate of children under age 3. Environmental, nutritional, or disease circumstances that compromise the mother and the developing fetus and neonate can have woeful consequences. Good medical care of the pregnant mother and the neonate is essential to produce the emergence of a healthy child and adolescent.

The importance of these years dentally cannot be overemphasized. Dental conditions such as cleft palate, disturbances in calcification, unusual numbers of teeth, oral habits, caries, and the development of malocclusions start during these years. The profession of dentistry has long recognized the importance of these years. Indeed, for years dental students have memorized the onset of calcification dates for all the primary and permanent teeth. More recently, guidelines addressing fluoride supplementation for children under age 3, nursing caries, and home care techniques for the young child have been developed. However, infant oral health and care of the child patient younger than age 3 have largely been approached didactically and not clinically.

If so much could be done to enhance dental health with effective preventive stategies implemented in the first year of life, then why hasn't dentistry been doing so? The answer to this question is simple and will be addressed here and in another chapter of this book. First, for most of the twentieth century, dentistry was not as prevention oriented as it was treatment oriented. The dentist who was not implementing prevention programs for patients had no reason to see patients until they had time to aggregate some disease. Because of the youth of these patients and the modest amount of time that the teeth had been in the oral cavity, it was often a poor chance that dentists could do much in children before 30-36 months of age. Second, if children did have teeth that needed restoration, because of their youth and inability to communicate and suppress their fears regarding a new and unknown situation, the dentist who was restoratively bound found himself with the dilemma of how to perform delicate restorative techniques on a child practicing avoidance behaviors such as crying, kicking, and wiggling.

Fortunately, contemporary dentistry is prevention oriented, and most dentists today understand their disease prevention obligations to their patients and seek prevention strategies that ensure maintenance of oral health for all their patients. With this in mind, then, it is obvious that *the child in the first year of life is a most desirable preventive patient in that whatever is done preventively for this patient will have a lifetime of effect.* Also, because the dentist is seeing the child primarily to help formulate a strategy toward the prevention of dental diseases, the behavior of the child is as incidental to the dentist as it is to the physician.

Today's family-oriented dentist is active in prenatal classes and the examination of babies. This dentist has established communications with family physicians and pediatricians within the community and stands poised and ready to dispense information that will help the physicians in the community understand what is entailed in infant oral health. In addition, children are recruited into the practice enthusiastically before the first birthday. If there are questions about oral hygiene, dietary fluoride supplementation, nutrition, and nursing, this dentist is ready to see the parents and their infant at any time. Lastly, this dentist understands the techniques of patient management and stabilization of the children in this age group so that he or she can, when needed, treat the dental disease or injuries that this age group can experience.

12

The Dynamics of Change

Chapter Outline

Physical Changes

Body

J. R. Pinkham

The gestation of a human being lasts approximately 9 months and begins at the moment the mother's ovum is fertilized by the father's sperm cell. At this moment of penetration of the ovum's wall, the sperm releases 23 chromosomes into the ovum, which also releases from a dissolving nucleus 23 chromosomes of its own. The human infant begins life with these 46 chromosomes. The fertilized cell begins to expand by the process of mitosis. The first division of the fertilized ovum into two cells usually takes place in 24 to 36 hours.

The time from conception to birth is often described in three phases. The first phase, the period of the ovum, is measured from fertilization until implantation. This period lasts until the dividing ovum, or blastocyst, becomes attached to the wall of the uterus. This period lasts for approximately 10 to 14 days. The next period lasts 2 to 8 weeks and is called the period of the embryo. This period is most important because of the cell differentiation that occurs during this time. It is during this period that all the major organs appear. The third and last period, which

TABLE 12–1. Cognition, Play, and Language

Piagetian Stage	Age	Object Permanence	Causality	Play	Receptive Language	Expressive Language
I	Birth to 1 month	Shifting images	Generalization of reflexes		Turns to voice	Range of cries (hunger, pain)
II	1–4 months	Stares at spot where object disappeared (looks at hand after yarn drops)	Primary circular reactions (thumb sucking)		Searches for speaker with eyes	Cooing Vocal contagion
III	4–8 months	Visually follows dropped object through vertical trajectory (tracks dropped yarn to floor)	Secondary circular reactions (recreates accidentally discovered environmental effects, e.g., kicks mattress to shake mobile)	Same behavioral repertoire for all objects (bangs, shakes, puts in mouth, drops)	Responds to own name and to tones of voice	Babbling Four distinct syllables
IV	9–12 months	Finds an object after watching it hidden	Coordination of secondary circular reactions	Visual motor inspection of objects Peek-a-boo	Listens selectively to familiar words Responds to "no" and other verbal requests	First real word Jargoning Symbolic gestures (shakes head no)
V	12–18 months	Recovers hidden object after multiple visible changes of position	Tertiary circular reactions (deliberately varies behavior to create novel effects)	Awareness of social function of objects Symbolic play centered on own body (drinks from toy cup)	Can bring familiar object from another room Points to parts of body	Many single words—uses words to express needs Acquires 10 words by 18 months
VI	18 months–2 years	Recovers hidden object after invisible changes in position	Spontaneously uses nondirect causal mechanisms (uses key to move wind-up toy)	Symbolic play directed toward doll (gives doll a drink)	Follows series of two or three commands Points to pictures when named	Telegraphic two-word sentences

From Zuckerman BS, Frank DA: *In* Levine MD, et al: Developmental-Behavioral Pediatrics. Philadelphia, WB Saunders, 1983, p 91.

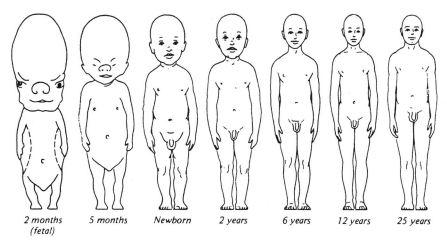

| 2 months (fetal) | 5 months | Newborn | 2 years | 6 years | 12 years | 25 years |

Figure 12–1. The changing proportions of the human body from 2 months in utero to adulthood. (From Jackson CM: Some aspects of form and growth. *In* Robbins WJ, Brody S, Hogan AF, et al [eds]: Growth. New Haven, Yale University Press, 1929, p 118.)

starts at 8 weeks and lasts until delivery at approximately 40 weeks, is called the period of the fetus. This period is characterized by maturation of the newly formed organs.

Figure 12-1 shows the difference in the proportions of the fetus at 2 and 5 months, the newborn's body, and the changes that are made during maturation. No year is more dramatic in growth than the first year of life, during which most children undergo a 50% increase in length and almost a 200% increase in weight. Toward the end of the first year of life, the growth rate slows. After the first birthday, the growth rate stays very stable and the height and weight increments of the child remain relatively predictable all the way until adolescence.

There are no good predictors of the child's final height before age 3. At age 3 however, correlations between the child's height and weight at maturity are fairly strong. The process of a newborn changing into an adult is one of elongation. The legs, at first shorter than the trunk, become longer. Also, the length of the child's trunk, compared with his or her breadth, becomes considerably greater.

As the body changes and matures, the infant is afforded increasingly sophisticated postural and locomotive actions. Table 12-1 shows some of the physical and cognitive developmental hallmarks of a child during his or her first 18 months of life. (Piagetian psychology as well as object permanency and causality is discussed in this chapter's section on cognitive development.)

By age 2, a child has the gross motor skills to run, climb, walk up and down steps, and kick a ball. His fine motor skills allow him to stack blocks (up to six), make parallel crayon strokes, and turn the pages of a book one page at a time. Table 12-2 shows a variety of motor skills and the mean age at which they are acquired.

The nervous system of the child grows dramatically from birth until age 3. In fact, by the end of his second year the child's brain has attained 75% of its adult weight (Hurlock, 1950).

TABLE 12–2. Median Age and Range in Acquisition of Motor Skills

Motor Skill	Age in Months		Motor Skill	Age in Months	
	Median	*Range**		*Median*	*Range**
Transfers objects hand to hand	5.5	4–8	Holds crayon adaptively	11.2	8–15
Sits alone 30 seconds or more	6.0	5–8	Walks alone	11.7	9–17
Rolls from back to stomach	6.4	4–10	Walks up stairs with help	16.1	12–23
Has neat pincer grasp	8.9	7–12	Walks up stairs both feet on each step	25.8	19–30
Stands alone	11.0	9–16			

*5th to 95th percentile.
Adapted from Bayley N: Manual for the Bayley Scales of Infant Development. New York, Psychological Corporation (1969). From Zuckerman BS, Frank DA: Infancy. *In* Levine MD, et al (eds): Developmental-Behavioral Pediatrics. Philadelphia, WB Saunders, 1983, p 89.

REFERENCE

Hurlock EB: Child Development. New York, McGraw-Hill, 1950.

Craniofacial Changes

Jerry Walker

INTRAUTERINE GROWTH AND DEVELOPMENT

The organization and complexity of growth and development are nowhere more evident than in the changes that take place in the head and face (Table 12–3). The human face begins its first observable growth during the fourth week of intrauterine life with the development of the branchial apparatus. The branchial apparatus is first seen as a series of ridges on the lateral aspect of the cephalic end of the embryo at approximately the third week of intrauterine life. A 1-month-old embryo has no real face, but the key primordia have already begun to gather. These slight swellings, depressions, and thickenings then rapidly undergo a series of mergers, rearrangements, and enlargements that transform them from a cluster of separate masses into a face (Stewart et al., 1982) (Fig. 12–2).

Sperber described the presomite stage of development (21 to 31 days), during which the 3-mm embryo develops at its cranial end five mesenchymal elevations or processes. The five mesenchymal elevations constitute the initial features of the face. These include the frontonasal process, two maxillary processes, and two mandibular arches. These processes grow differentially, and by obliterating the ectodermal grooves between them, they eventually contour the features of the face.

The oral cavity of the embryo is bounded by

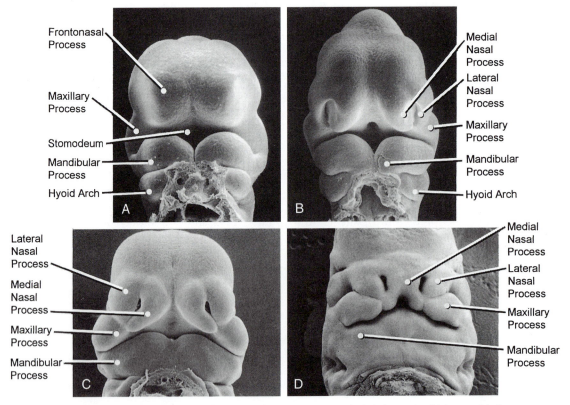

Figure 12–2. Scanning electron micrographs of mouse embryos (except *D*, which is human), which resemble human embryos at comparable stages of development. *A,* This stage is approximately 24 days post-conception in the human and shows the division of the first brachial arch into the maxilla and mandible and the hyoid arch. *B,* At approximately 31 days in the human, the medial and lateral nasal processes are recognizable alongside the nasal pit. *C,* Fusion of the median nasal, lateral nasal, and the maxillary processes form the upper lip. Fusion of the maxillary and mandibular processes establish the width of the mouth (approximately 36 days in the human). *D,* At 42 days gestation in humans, more definitive fusion has taken place, and the mouth and nose are readily evident. Still, this stage portrays a map of the potential cleft sites most commonly observed in facial development. (Courtesy Dr. K. Sulik. *A* and *B* reproduced with permission from Proffit WR: Contemporary Orthodontics. St. Louis, Mosby–Year Book, 1986.)

TABLE 12–3. Developing Structures of the Head and Face

Developing Structures	Initiation (Weeks in Utero)
Neural plate	2
Buccopharyngeal membrane	2
Mandibular arch initiation	3
Hypoglossal muscles (tongue)	5
Medial and lateral nasal processes	5
Lens of the eye	5
Retina	5
External carotid artery	6
Eustachian tube	6
Larynx	6
Maxillary process	6
External auditory meatus	7
Nasal septum	8
Two palatal shelves fuse together	8
Palatal shelves fuse with nasal septum	10
Ossification of craniofacial skeleton	10
Eyelids completely formed and closed	10
Eyelids open	28

the frontonasal process and by the maxillary and mandibular processes of the first branchial arch (Fig. 12–3). Each maxillary process moves toward the midline and joins with the lateral nasal

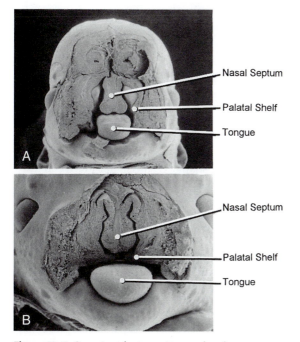

Figure 12–3. Scanning electron micrographs of mouse embryos sectioned in the frontal plane. *A,* Before elevation of the palatal shelves showing their margins extending to the level of the lateral borders of the tongue. *B,* Following elevation of the palatal shelves. (Courtesy Dr. K. Sulik. Reproduced with permission from Proffit WR: Contemporary Orthodontics. St. Louis, Mosby–Year Book, 1986.)

fold of the frontonasal process. As this is happening, a shelf-like process (the palatal process) develops on the medial side of each maxillary process. These two palatal processes move toward the midline, where they fuse. This palatal fusion is normally completed by the eighth intrauterine week. The mandibular processes fuse at the midline somewhat before the maxillary and nasal processes (Fig. 12–4). The palate grows more rapidly in width than in length during the fetal period as a result of midpalatal sutural growth and appositional growth of the lateral alveolar margins. A failure in the fusion of the processes gives rise to oral or facial clefts or both. In the mandible, the cartilaginous skeleton of the first branchial arch, known as Meckel's cartilage, provides a form for the development of the mandible.

The muscles of mastication, that is, the temporalis, the masseter, and the medial and lateral pterygoids, and the trigeminal nerve also are derived from the first branchial arch. At approximately 60 days of gestation, the embryo has acquired all of its basic morphologic characteristics and enters the fetal period, which is marked by osseous development.

Rapid orofacial development is characteristic of the advanced development of the cranial portion of the embryo compared with its caudal portion. The different rates of growth result in a pear-shaped embryonic disc, with the head region forming the expanded portion of the pear. Because of this early development of the cranial end of the embryo, the head constitutes nearly "one half" of the total body size during the postsomite embryonic period (fourth to eighth week).

The dominance of head growth and development in the embryonic period is not maintained in the fetal period. Accordingly, the proportions of the head are reduced from about one-half of the entire body length at the end of the embryonic period to about one-third at the fifth month.

During the fetal period, the eyeballs, following the neural pattern of growth, initially grow rapidly. This contributes to the widening of the face. Interestingly, the nasal cavity and the nasal septum are believed to have a considerable influence in determining facial form, by acting either as a matrix for development or as a biomechanical template.

The growth of the nasoseptal region contributes to frontomaxillary, frontonasal, frontozygomatic, and zygomaticomaxillary sutured changes. The expansion of the eyeballs, the brain, and the spheno-occipital synchondrosal cartilage also acts in separating the facial sutures. The overall

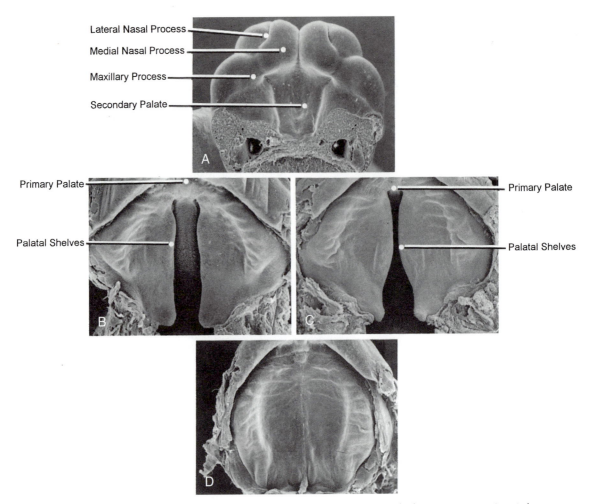

Lateral Nasal Process

Medial Nasal Process

Maxillary Process

Secondary Palate

Primary Palate

Palatal Shelves

Primary Palate

Palatal Shelves

Figure 12–4. These scanning electron micrographs of human specimens (except *A*, which is a mouse specimen) show several stages of palate closure from 53 to 59 days postconception. *A*, At the completion of primary palate closure; *B*, Palatal shelves during elevation; *C*, Just prior to fusion of the shelves; *D*, The secondary palate following fusion. (Courtesy Dr. K. Sulik. *A* reproduced with permission from Proffit WR: Contemporary Orthodontics. St. Louis, Mosby–Year Book, 1986.)

effect of these diverse forces of expansion is osseous buildup on the posterior surface of the facial bones (Sperber, 1978).

Unlike the embryonic period, during the fetal period the size of the maxilla relative to the mandible varies widely. Throughout the embryonic stage, the mandible is considerably larger than the maxilla. It is not until the fetal stage that the maxilla is more developed than the mandible. Subsequent to this, the mandible grows at a greater pace and equals the size of the maxilla by 11 weeks in utero. Between the thirteenth and the twentieth week in utero, mandibular growth again lags relative to the maxilla. At birth, the mandible tends to be retrognathic to the maxilla (Ranly, 1980). During the remainder of its intrauterine existence, the fetus undergoes a process of growth and maturation and a reorgani-

zation of the spatial relationships between various structures (Enlow, 1982).

Rapid and extensive growth characterizes the ensuing 7 months of fetal life. An expansion of the cranium occurs during this fetal period as the result of a combination of growth processes, including interstitial, endochondral, and sutural or translational growth. The cartilage remnants of the chondral cranium that persist between the bones are known as synchondroses.

In addition, the cranial base undergoes selective appositional remodeling by resorption and apposition. This process is mediated by activity on the part of the bone-forming cells, the osteoblasts, as well as by bone-destroying cells, the osteoclasts.

The major remodelling of the early facial skeleton that occurs throughout the remainder of the

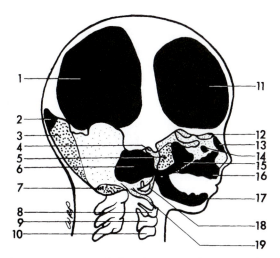

Figure 12–5. Human skull at about 3 months. Intramembranous bones are shown in black. Cartilage is represented by light stippling, and bones developing by endochondral ossification are indicated by darker stippling. Approximate time of appearance for each bone is indicated in parentheses. 1, Parietal bone (10 weeks). 2, Interparietal bone (8 weeks). 3, Supraoccipital (8 weeks). 4, Dorsum sellae (still cartilaginous). 5, Temporal wing of sphenoid (2 to 3 months; the basisphenoid appears at 12 to 13 weeks, orbitosphenoid at 12 weeks, and presphenoid at 5 months). 6, Squamous part of temporal bone (2 to 3 months). 7, Basioccipital (2 to 3 months). 8, Hyoid (still cartilaginous). 9, Thyroid (still cartilaginous). 10, Cricoid (still cartilaginous). 11, Frontal bone (7½ weeks). 12, Crista galli (still cartilaginous; inferiorly, the middle concha begins ossification at 16 weeks, the superior and inferior conchae at 18 weeks; the perpendicular plate of ethmoid begins ossification during the first postnatal year, the cribriform plate during the second postnatal year, the vomer at 8 fetal weeks). 13, Nasal bone (8 weeks). 14, Lacrimal bone (8½ weeks). 15, Malar (8 weeks). 16, Maxilla (end of sixth week; premaxilla, 7 weeks). 17, Mandible (6 to 8 weeks). 18, Tympanic ring (begins at 9 weeks, with complete ring at 12 weeks; petrous bone, 5 to 6 months). 19, Styloid process, still cartilaginous. (From Enlow DH: Handbook of Facial Growth. Philadelphia, WB Saunders Co, 1982. Modified from Patten BM: Human Embryology, 3rd ed. New York, McGraw-Hill, 1968.)

fetal period begins in the fetus at about 14 weeks. Before this time, the bones enlarge in all directions from their respective ossification centers. Remodelling, a process that accompanies growth, starts when the definitive form of each of the individual bones of the face and cranium is attained (Enlow, 1982) (Fig. 12-5).

GROWTH AND DEVELOPMENT AFTER BIRTH

At birth, the bony face and skull show little differentiation from child to child. Newborns have tiny mouths and virtually no chins. Their faces are small, although their eyes, in comparison with the small face, are exceedingly large. The forehead and top of the head are big. It is difficult to imagine the diversity of individual looks that will develop over the course of childhood and adolescence from such similar little infant faces (Fig. 12-6).

At birth, the maxilla is very low frontally and relatively small. By 9 months, the jaw has become considerably wider and higher. There is also a remarkable increase in the maxillary sinus. At birth, the bones that compose the cranium are not fused and are separated by six membrane-filled gaps called fontanelles (Fig. 12-7). Each of these areas is completely closed by ossification within 2 years after birth.

The face appears broad and flat at birth. The lower jaw seems underdeveloped and receded. The overall broadness of the face results from the lack of vertical growth, which is still to come. The horizontal dimensions are more nearly adult-like. The upper and total face heights are not even half completed at birth. According to Ranly (1980), they are 43% and 40%, respectively, which means that the most striking and complex growth of the head is associated with the face. After an initial spurt during the first 3 years, the rate of increase of these dimensions slows. It remains steady until the adult size is reached. The cranium, as represented by cranial width and length, is nearer to adult size than any other part of the head. This can be explained by the development of the brain, which by the eighth month of intrauterine life has all of the nerve

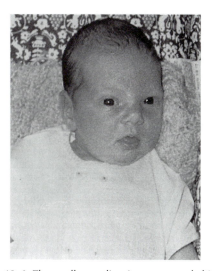

Figure 12–6. The small nose, lips, jaws, ears, and chin of this 3-week-old female baby are shared with other young babies. Babies have a uniformity of appearance. With growth, of course, the subtle differences between young babies' faces will become explicit and easily recognized.

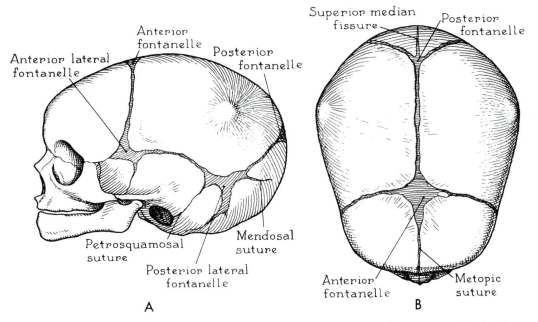

Figure 12–7. The cranium at birth. Note the fontanelles, one at each corner of the parietal bones. (Reproduced with permission from Silverman FN, et al [eds]: Caffey's Pediatric X-ray Diagnosis, 8th ed. Copyright 1985 by Year Book Medical Publishers, Inc, Chicago.)

cells it will ever have. The growth of the cranial vault is complete before that of the maxilla, and maxillary growth is complete before mandibular growth. This is an example of the cephalocaudal growth gradient, which indicates that the cranial structures are nearer their adult size during infancy and childhood than other body parts (Fields, 1991). Symphyseal growth increases the width of the mandible. By the second year, the symphysis is closed and growth becomes localized in the mandible as well as in the nasomaxillary complex. An enormous metamorphosis has taken place, but many more changes need to occur before the child's adult appearance is realized.

REFERENCES

Caffey J: Pediatric X-Ray Diagnosis. Chicago, Year Book, 1950.

Enlow DH: Handbook of Facial Growth. Philadelphia, WB Saunders, 1982.

Fields HW: Craniofacial growth from infancy through adulthood. Pediatr Clin North Am *38*:1053–1088, 1991.

Proffit WR: Contemporary Orthodontics. St. Louis, Mosby–Year Book, 1986.

Ranly DM: A Synopsis of Craniofacial Growth. New York, Appleton-Century-Crofts, 1980.

Sperber GH: Craniofacial Embryology. Bristol, John Wright and Sons, 1978.

Stewart RE, Barber TK, Troutman KC, et al: Pediatric Dentistry: Scientific Foundations and Clinical Practice. St. Louis, CV Mosby, 1982.

Dental Changes

C. A. Full

The purpose of this section is to address the growth, development, and eruption of each tooth unit from its initiation to complete eruption. By definition, *growth* signifies an increase, expansion, or extension of any given tissue. For example, a tooth grows as more enamel is deposited by ameloblasts. *Development* addresses the progressive evolution of a tissue. A tooth develops as the ameloblasts develop from less specific ectodermal tissue and as the dentinoblasts develop from unspecialized mesoderm.

Teeth are formed by tissues originating from both ectoderm and mesoderm. At approximately 6 weeks of age, the basal layer of the oral epithelium of the fetus shows areas of increased activity and enlargement in the areas of the future dental arches. This increase and expansion give rise to the dental lamina of the future tooth germ. As the tooth bud continues to develop, it reaches a point at which it is recognized as the cap stage. At this time, it will begin to incorporate mesoderm into its structure. Therefore, the tooth-forming organ is initially formed from ectoderm but shortly thereafter includes mesoderm.

The expansion of tissue on the epithelial borders represents the beginning of the life cycle of

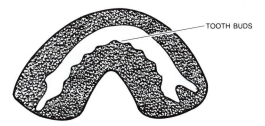

Figure 12–8. Diagrammatic representation of the tooth buds—approximately 8-week-old fetus.

the tooth. The ectoderm will become responsible for the future enamel, and the mesoderm will become primarily responsible for pulp and dentin. The tooth germ is accountable for the development of the following three formative tissues:

1. Dental organ (epithelial)
2. Dental papilla
3. Dental sac

The 6-week-old fetus demonstrates ten sites of epithelial activity on the occlusal (soft tissue) border of both the developing maxilla and the mandible (Brauer et al., 1959). These sites are lined next to each other and ultimately predict the position of the future 10 primary teeth in both the maxilla and the mandible (Fig. 12-8).

In addition to developing 20 primary teeth, each unit also develops a dental lamina that is responsible for the development of the future permanent tooth (Orban, 1957). Therefore, the primary centrals, laterals, and cuspids produce a dental lamina for the future permanent centrals, laterals, and cuspids. The first and second primary molars produce a dental lamina for the future first and second permanent premolars.

The unaccounted-for permanent molars develop from and on three successive locations on one dental lamina extending distally from each of the second primary molars (Fig. 12-9) (Orban, 1957).

An analysis of the successive periods of growth of the tooth germ can be organized by the following stages of the life cycle of the tooth (Orban, 1957):

Growth
  Initiation
  Proliferation
  Histodifferentiation
  Morphodifferentiation
  Apposition
Calcification
Eruption
Attrition

GROWTH

Initiation (Fig. 12-10)

The initiation stage is first noticed in the 6-week-old fetus. As the word initiation suggests, this stage is recognized by the initial formation of an expansion of the basal layer of the oral cavity immediately above the basement membrane. The basal layer is a row of organized cells lined up on the basement membrane, which is a tissue division line between the ectoderm (epithelium) and the mesoderm (Fig. 12-11). The cells of the basal layer are the innermost cells of the oral epithelium (ectoderm) adjacent to the basement membrane.

At 10 specific intermittent locations along the basement membrane, the cells of the basal layer

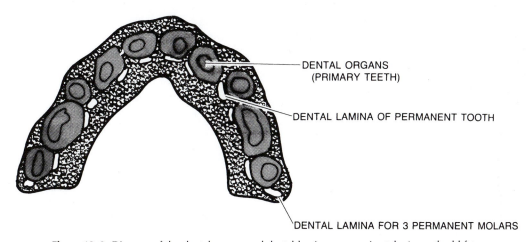

DENTAL ORGANS
(PRIMARY TEETH)

DENTAL LAMINA OF PERMANENT TOOTH

DENTAL LAMINA FOR 3 PERMANENT MOLARS

Figure 12–9. Diagram of the dental organs and dental lamina—approximately 4-month-old fetus.

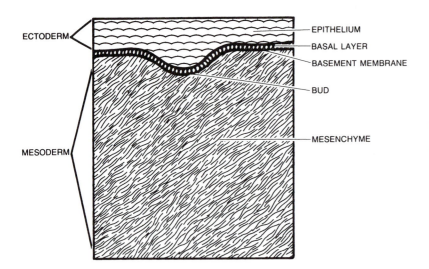

Figure 12–10. Diagram of the initiation stage of the life cycle of the tooth—approximately 5- to 6-week-old fetus.

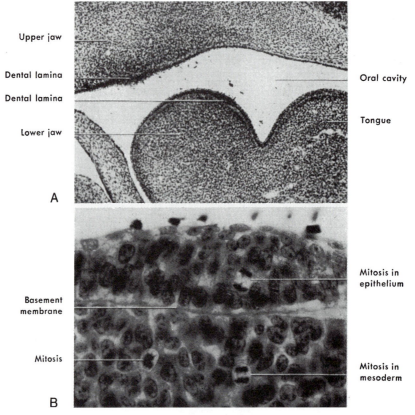

Figure 12–11. Initiation of tooth development. Human embryo 13.5 mm long, fifth week. *A,* Sagittal section through upper and lower jaws. *B,* High magnification of thickened oral epithelium. (From Orban B: Dental Histology and Embryology, 2nd ed. New York, McGraw-Hill, 1929.)

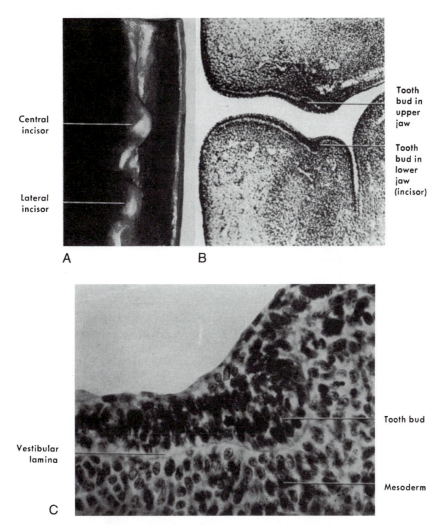

Central incisor

Lateral incisor

Tooth bud in upper jaw

Tooth bud in lower jaw (incisor)

A   B

Vestibular lamina

Tooth bud

Mesoderm

C

Figure 12–12. Bud stage of tooth development (proliferation stage). Human embryo 16 mm long, sixth week. *A,* Wax reconstruction of the germs of the central and lateral lower incisors. *B,* Sagittal section through upper and lower jaws. *C,* High-magnification view of the tooth germ of the lower incisor in bud stage. (From Orban B: Dental Histology and Embryology, 2nd ed. New York, McGraw-Hill, 1929.)

multiply at a much faster rate than the surrounding cells (Schour and Massler, 1940). This development occurs at that point on the oral epithelium that is the tooth bud and is responsible for the initial growth of that tooth (Fig. 12-12).

It can be noted that the times of initiation of the various teeth differ (Brauer et al., 1959). This period of tooth development is also recognized as the bud stage. Such a description assists in visually understanding the developmental process of the immature tooth.

Proliferation (Fig. 12-13)

Proliferation is really only a further multiplication of the cells of the initiation stage and an expansion of the tooth bud, resulting in the formation of the tooth germ. The tooth germ is a result of the prolific epithelial cells forming a cap-like appearance with the subsequent incorporation of the mesoderm. This incorporation of mesodermal tissue below and within the cap gives rise to the dental papilla.

The mesenchyme (mesoderm) surrounding the dental organ and dental papilla is the tissue that will form the dental sac. The dental sac ultimately gives rise to the supporting structures of the tooth. These structures are the cementum and periodontal ligament.

As the tooth germ continues to proliferate in an irregular fashion, it produces a cap-like appearance. This stage is called the cap stage because the structure takes on the form of a cap

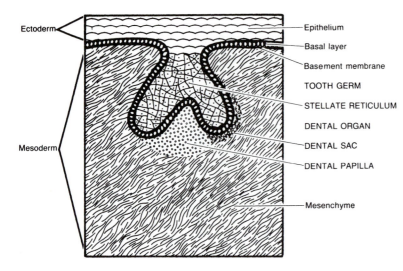

Figure 12–13. Diagram of the proliferation stage of the life cycle of the tooth—approximately 9- to 11-week-old fetus.

(Fig. 12–14). Like the bud stage, it is so referenced for visual identification. As the cap begins to form, the mesenchyme changes within the cap to initiate the development of the dental papilla.

The dental papilla evolves from the mesenchyme invaginating the inner dental epithelium and specializes to form the pulp and dentin.

The dental sac also comes into being by a

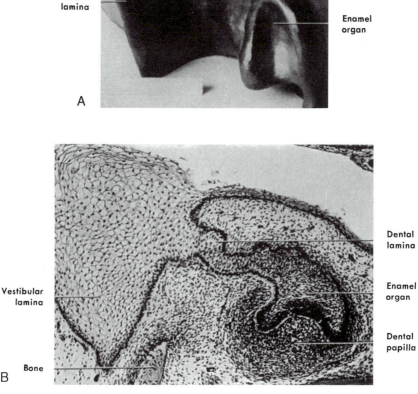

Figure 12–14. Cap stage of tooth development. Human embryo 60 mm long, eleventh week. *A,* Wax reconstruction of the dental organ of the lower lateral incisor. *B,* Labiolingual section through the same tooth. (From Orban B: Dental Histology and Embryology, 2nd ed. New York, McGraw-Hill, 1929.)

marginal condensation in the mesenchyme surrounding the dental organ and dental papilla.

The stellate (star-like) reticulum (network) is an organization of cells within the descending portion of the dental organ that is enamel-forming tissue and is called the enamel pulp.

Therefore, the tooth germ during this stage has all the necessary formative tissues to embrace the development of a tooth and its periodontal ligament (Orban, 1957).

In summary, the tooth germ consists of all the necessary elements for the development of the complete tooth. The germ is composed of the following three distinct parts: (1) dental organ, (2) dental papilla, and (3) dental sac. The dental organ produces the enamel. The dental papilla generates the dentin and pulp. The dental sac gives rise to the cementum and periodontal ligament (Orban, 1957).

Histodifferentiation (Fig. 12-15)

The histodifferentiation stage is marked by the histologic difference in the appearance of the cells of the tooth germ because they are now beginning to specialize. The cap continues to grow and takes more of the appearance of a bell. The image of a bell is registered because the extensions of the cap grow deeper into the mesoderm. This part of development is appropriately called the bell stage. The tissue within the bell is the tissue that gives rise to the dental papilla.

The dental organ is now completely surrounded by the basement membrane and is divided into an inner and outer dental epithelium. The dental organ ultimately becomes enamel.

The condensation of the tissue (mesoderm) adjacent to the outside of the bell is responsible for the dental sac. The dental sac ultimately gives rise to the cementum, which is the covering of the tooth's root, and to the periodontal ligament, which attaches the tooth to the bone around the tooth roots.

The dental lamina continues to shrink to look more like a cord. The dental lamina for the permanent successor becomes obvious as an extension of the dental lamina of the primary tooth. The basal layer continues its existence and is now divided into an inner and an outer dental epithelium. The stellate reticulum expands and organizes to incorporate more intercellular fluid in preparation for the formation of enamel (Figs. 12-16, 12-17 and 12-18).

Morphodifferentiation (Fig. 12-19)

The morphodifferentiation stage, as the name implies, is the stage at which the cells find an arrangement that ultimately dictates the final size and shape of the tooth (Brauer et al., 1959). This stage is called the advanced bell stage (see Fig. 12-19). The cells of the inner dental epithelium become the ameloblasts, which produce the enamel matrix. As the ameloblasts begin their formation, the tissue of the dental papilla immediately adjacent to the basement membrane begins to differentiate into odontoblasts (Figs. 12-20 and 12-21). The odontoblasts and the ameloblasts are responsible for the formation of dentin and enamel, respectively.

Although the development of dentin is not clearly understood, structures have been identified that show progressive changes. The change in dentin formation first seen is a thickening of the basement membrane of the inner dental epithelium and the pulp developed by the dental

Text continued on page 158

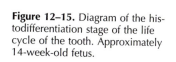

Figure 12–15. Diagram of the histodifferentiation stage of the life cycle of the tooth. Approximately 14-week-old fetus.

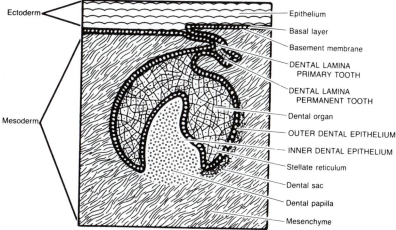

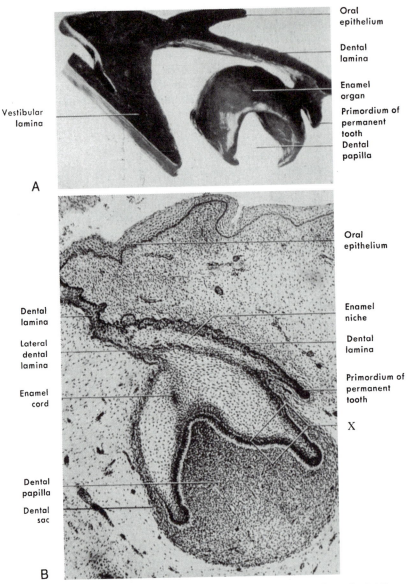

Oral
epithelium

Dental
lamina

Enamel
organ

Primordium of
permanent
tooth
Dental
papilla

Vestibular
lamina

A

Oral
epithelium

Dental
lamina

Lateral
dental
lamina

Enamel
cord

Enamel
niche

Dental
lamina

Primordium of
permanent
tooth

X

Dental
papilla

Dental
sac

B

Figure 12–16. Bell stage of tooth development. Human embryo 105 mm long, fourteenth week. *A,* Wax reconstruction of lower central incisor. *B,* Labiolingual section of the same tooth. "X" designates inset (see Fig. 12–17). (From Orban B: Dental Histology and Embryology, 2nd ed. New York, McGraw-Hill, 1929.)

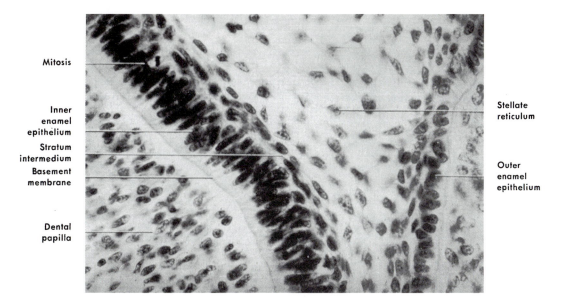

Figure 12–17. The four layers of the epithelial dental organ in high magnification (area "X" of Fig. 12–16). (From Orban B: Dental Histology and Embryology, 2nd ed. New York, McGraw-Hill, 1929.)

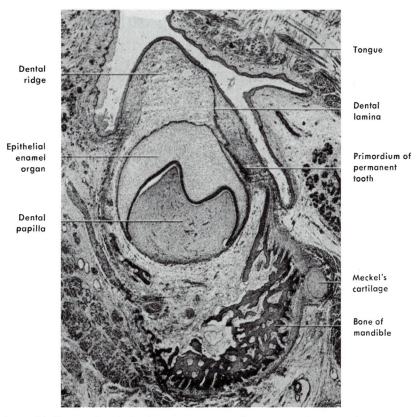

Figure 12–18. Advanced bell stage of tooth development. Human embryo 200 mm long, age about 18 weeks. Labiolingual section through the first primary lower molar. (From Bhaskar S: Synopsis of Oral Histology. St. Louis, CV Mosby, 1962, p 44.)

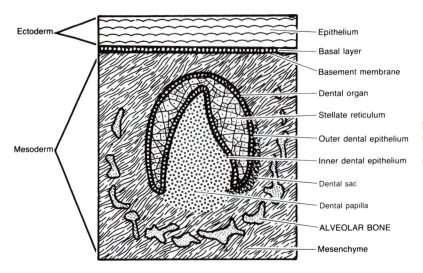

Ectoderm ——

Epithelium

Basal layer

Basement membrane

Dental organ

Stellate reticulum

Outer dental epithelium

Inner dental epithelium

Dental sac

Mesoderm

Dental papilla

ALVEOLAR BONE

Mesenchyme

Figure 12–19. Diagram of the morphodifferentiation stage of the life cycle of the tooth. Approximately 18-week-old fetus.

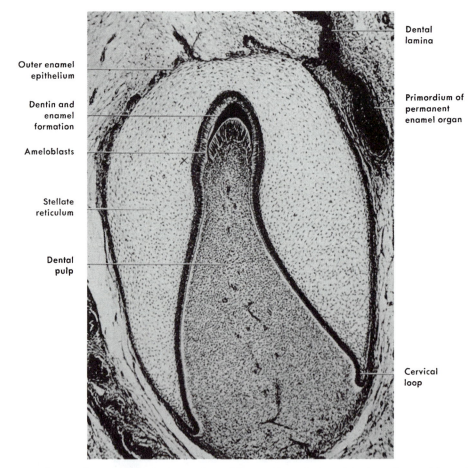

Outer enamel epithelium

Dentin and enamel formation

Ameloblasts

Stellate reticulum

Dental pulp

Dental lamina

Primordium of permanent enamel organ

Cervical loop

Figure 12–20. Tooth germ (lower incisor) of a human fetus (fifth month). Beginning of dentin and enamel formation. The stellate reticulum at the tip of the crown reduced in thickness. "X" designates inset (see Fig. 12–21). (From Diamond M, Applebaum E: J Dent Res *21*:403, 1942.)

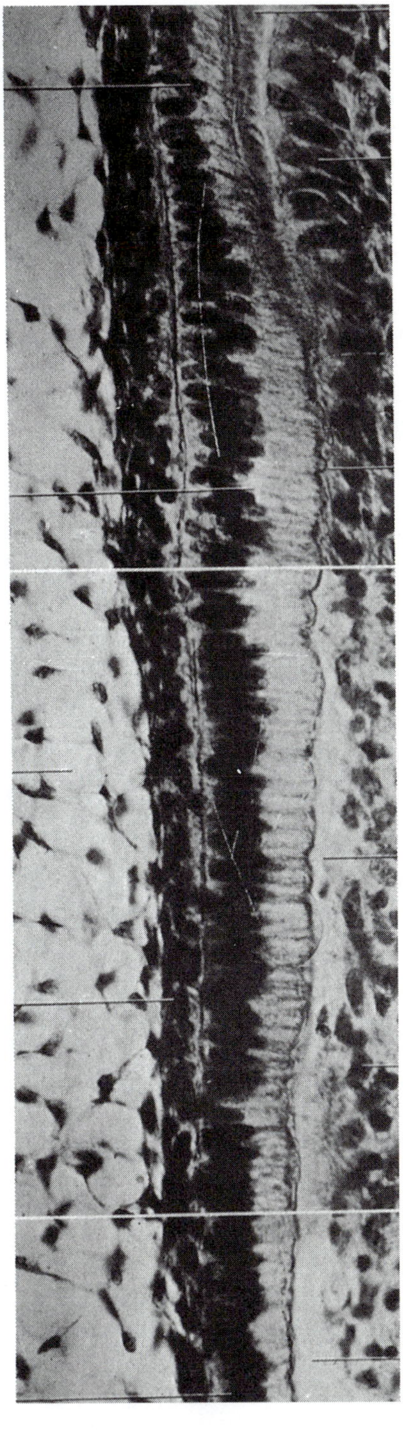

Ameloblasts

Cells of inner
enamel epithelium

Stellate reticulum

Stratum intermedium

Cells of inner
enamel epithelium

Dentin

Odontoblasts

Pulp cells and
inner enamel
epithelium
in contact

Cell-free
zone

Pulp

Cell-free
zone

Figure 12–21. High-magnification view of the inner dental epithelium from inset "X" in Figure 12–20. In the cervical region the cells are short, and the outermost layer of the pulp is cell-free. Occlusally, the cells are long and the cell-free zone of the pulp has disappeared. The ameloblasts are again shorter where dentin formation has set in and enamel formation is imminent. (From Diamond M, Applebaum E: J Dent Res *21*:403, 1942.)

papilla. The membrane from the mesenchyme of the pulp consists of fine reticular fibrils. A continuation of growth is noted by a formation of irregular spiraling fibers from deep in the pulp that entangle with the reticular fibrils from the mesenchyme of the pulp. These long spiraling fibers are known as Korff's fibers and assist in the structural support of the developing dentin (Fig. 12-22) (Orban, 1957).

The specialized cells of the previous stage now arrange themselves in a manner that gives each tooth its prescribed size and shape. There is a disappearance of the dental lamina except for the dental lamina proper immediately adjacent to the developing primary tooth.

The dental lamina proper continues to proliferate to the lingual of the primary tooth to begin the development of the permanent tooth. The primary tooth germ now becomes a free internal organ (Orban, 1957). The specialized cells found during the histodifferentiation stage and the organization of these specialized cells during the morphodifferentiation stage prepare the tooth for the development of various tissues of enamel, dentin, pulp, cementum, and periodontal ligament.

Apposition (Fig. 12-23)

Whereas the morphodifferentiation stage dictates the size and shape of the tooth, the appositional stage occurs when the network or tissue matrix of the tooth is formed. Cells that have the potential for the deposition of extracellular matrix fulfill the plan of the tooth germ established by previous stages. The growth is appositional, additive, and regular. This accounts for the layered or layered appearance of enamel and dentin (Orban,

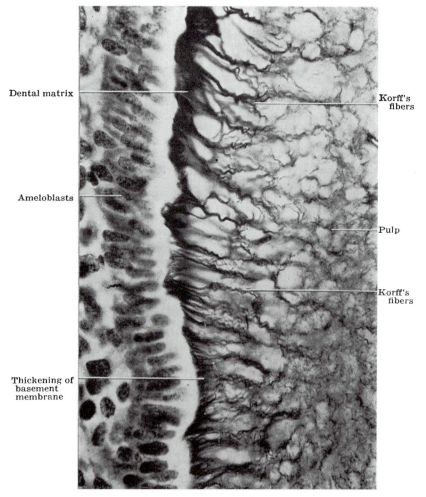

Figure 12–22. Thickening of the basement membrane between pulp and inner dental epithelium—development of Korff's fibers. (Reproduced by permission from Bevelander G: *In* Sicher H, Bhaskar SN (eds): Orban's Oral Histology and Embryology, 7th ed. St. Louis, CV Mosby, 1972.)

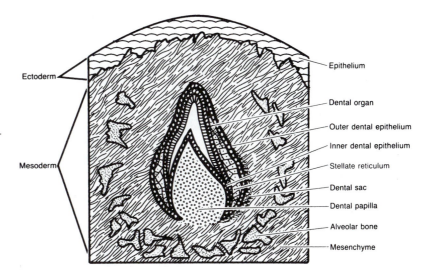

Figure 12–23. Diagram of the apposition stage of the life cycle of the tooth.

Ectoderm

Mesoderm

Epithelium

Dental organ

Outer dental epithelium

Inner dental epithelium

Stellate reticulum

Dental sac

Dental papilla

Alveolar bone

Mesenchyme

1957). The organized special tissues now deposit incremental layers of enamel and dentin matrix. The matrices layered by ameloblasts and odontoblasts begin from a growth center along the dentino-enamel and dentino-cemental junction (Figs. 12-24 and 12-25).

CALCIFICATION (Fig. 12-26)

Calcification occurs with an influx of mineral salts within the previously developed tissue matrix. The chemical structure of enamel consists of approximately 96% inorganic material and approximately 4% organic material and water. The inorganic portion is composed primarily of calcium and phosphorus, with a small portion of many other compounds and elements, such as carbon dioxide, magnesium, and sodium, to mention a few (Table 12-4).

Calcification begins with the precipitation of enamel in the cusp tips and incisal edges of the teeth and continues with the production of more

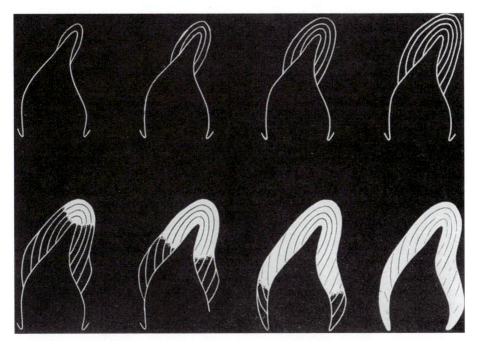

Figure 12–24. Diagram of enamel matrix formation and maturation. Formation follows an incremental pattern; maturation begins at the tip of the crown and proceeds cervically in cross-relation to the incremental pattern. (Modified from Diamond and Weinmann. Reproduced by permission from Orban B: Oral Histology and Embryology, 4th ed. St. Louis, CV Mosby, 1957.)

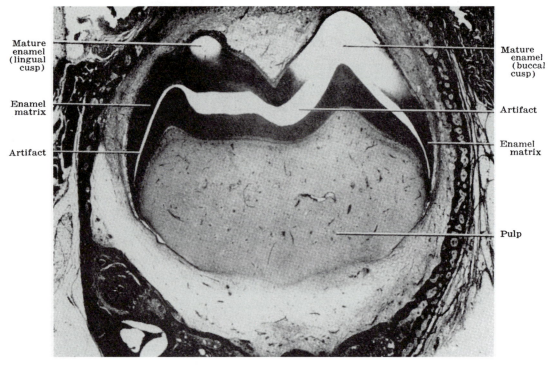

Figure 12–25. Buccolingual section through a deciduous molar. Maturation of the enamel has started in the lingual cusp; it has fairly well progressed in the buccal cusp. Note the gradual transition between the enamel matrix and the fully matured enamel. (Modified from Diamond and Weinmann. Reproduced by permission from Orban B: Oral Histology and Embryology, 4th ed. St. Louis, CV Mosby, 1957.)

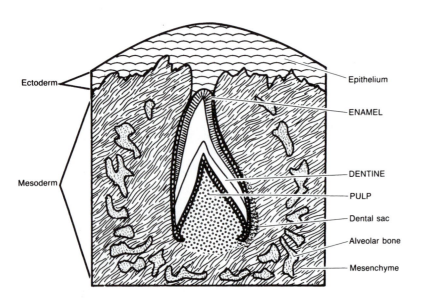

Figure 12–26. Diagram of the calcification stage of the life cycle of the tooth.

TABLE 12–4. Chemical Contents of Enamel, Dentin, Cementum, and Bone

	Enamel	Dentin	Cementum, Compact Bone
Water	2.3%	13.2%	32%
Organic matter	1.7	17.5	22
Ash	96.0	69.3	46
In 100 g of ash:			
Calcium	36.1 g	35.3 g	35.5 g
Phosphorus	17.3	17.1	17.1
Carbon dioxide	3.0	4.0	4.4
Magnesium	0.5	1.2	0.9
Sodium	0.2	0.2	1.1
Potassium	0.3	0.07	0.1
Chloride	0.3	0.03	0.1
Fluorine	0.016	0.017	0.015
Sulfur	0.1	0.2	0.6
Copper	0.01		
Silicon	0.003		0.04
Iron	0.0025		0.09
Zinc	0.016	0.018	

	Whole Teeth	Bone
Lead	0.0071 to 0.037	0.002 to 0.02

Small amounts of: Ce, La, Pr, Ne, Ag, Sr, Ba, Cr, Sn, Mn, Ti, Ni, V, Al, B, Cu, Li, Se

Reproduced by permission from Sicher H: Orban's Oral Histology and Embryology, 5th ed. St. Louis, CV Mosby, 1962. Compiled by Dr. Harold C. Hodge.

layers on these small points of origin. Therefore, the older or more mature enamel is found at the cusp tips or incisal edges and the new enamel is at the cervical region (see Figs. 12-24 and 12-25).

The calcification of enamel and dentin is a very sensitive process that takes place over a long period of time. Therefore, calcification irregularities noted in any fully developed tooth can often be equated with a specific systemic disturbance (Brauer et al., 1959). In the cross-section of the clinical crown of a tooth that has been prepared for histologic view, there are apparent lines or bands, which are called the incremental lines of Retzius (Fig. 12-27). Depending on how the section is prepared (either longitudinally or horizontally), the incremental lines of Retzius may appear as lines or circles (Fig. 12-28). These lines or circles represent the developmental pattern of the developing tooth.

The degree of variation of any line usually reflects a reaction to a change in the physiologic processes of growth and development of the tooth. For instance, in the primary teeth there is an incremental line of Retzius called the neonatal line or neonatal ring (Fig. 12-29). This neonatal line is due to the abrupt change in certain body processes of the fetus when it is born. At that time, there is enough of a change or insult to the newborn's systems to cause a growth change

that is reflected dentally as a neonatal ring (Orban, 1957). This ring is actually due to disturbances in the growth and calcification of the tooth.

In summary, the aspect of enamel maturation called calcification involves the hardening of the already previously formed matrix by the precipitation of mineral salts (inorganic calcium salts). This calcification is a slow, gradual process beginning at the cusp tip or incisal edge of the tooth (see Fig. 12-25).

ERUPTION (Fig. 12-30)

It is necessary to discuss briefly root development before addressing eruption. The developmental process of the crown of the tooth involves many overlying processes at one time. The same is true for the root. Root development has correlations with eruption. When the clinical crown of the tooth has completed its formation, the inner and outer epithelia appear to fold over at the cementoenamel junction and continue their growth without any tissue between them. Previously, stellate reticulum was there. The inner and outer dental epithelia without the stellate reticulum is now called Hertwig's epithelial root sheath, which is responsible for the size and shape of the root and eruption of the tooth (Fig. 12-31) (Orban, 1957).

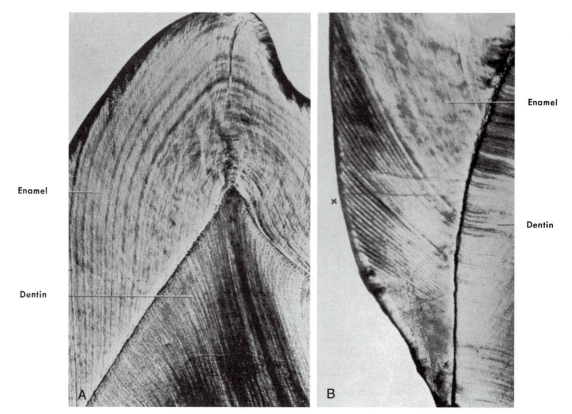

Figure 12–27. Incremental lines of Retzius in longitudinal ground sections. *A,* Cuspal region. *B,* Cervical region (x). (Reproduced by permission from Bhaskar SN [ed]: Orban's Oral Histology and Embryology, 10th ed. St. Louis, CV Mosby, 1986.)

Eruption can be categorized into three different phases: (1) preeruptive phase, (2) eruptive phase (prefunctional), and (3) eruptive phase (functional). The preeruptive phase is that period during which the tooth root begins its formation and begins to move toward the surface of the oral cavity from its bony vault. The prefunctional eruptive phase consists of that period of development of the tooth root through gingival emergence. Most eruption tables report the time that the tooth can be first seen in the mouth (Figs. 12–32 and 12–33). The tooth root is usually approximately one half to two thirds of its final length at the time of gingival emergence.

After the tooth has erupted into the oral cavity and meets its antagonist (opposing tooth in the opposite arch), it is considered to be in the functional eruptive phase. Teeth remain a dynamic unit in that some type of movement, no matter how slight, is always taking place. Teeth continue to move and erupt as necessary as the body continues to change throughout life (Orban, 1957).

There has been considerable speculation about the causes of tooth eruption. Some examples of causes of tooth eruption often cited are (1) root formation, (2) proliferation of Hertwig's epithelial root sheath, (3) proliferation of the connective tissue of the dental papilla, (4) simultaneous growth of the jaw, (5) pressures from muscular action, and (6) apposition and resorption of bone. Because of this myriad of processes happening at the time of eruption, it is difficult to single out any one process as the primary cause of tooth eruption.

The process of elimination of primary teeth is caused by the eruptive pressure of the permanent successor at the apex of the primary tooth and its surroundings. The eruptive pressure stimulates the development of osteoclasts. A progressive resorption of the tooth root, dentin, and cementum as well as adjacent bone is completed by the action of the osteoclasts.

ATTRITION (Fig. 12-34)

Attrition is the wearing of the teeth during function. It is the normal wearing of the teeth during contact with opposing teeth in occlusion. It is easy to understand why certain types of food and associated habits may cause more or less

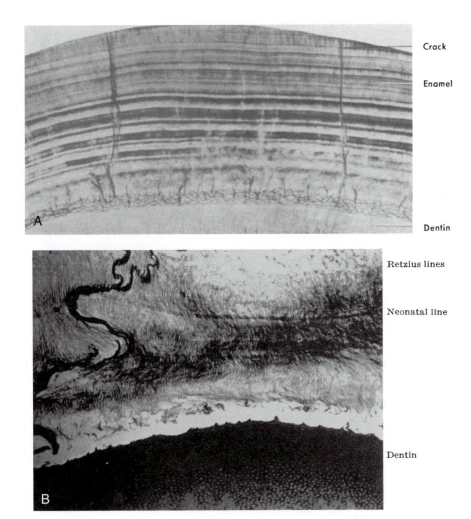

Crack

Enamel

Dentin

Retzius lines

Neonatal line

Dentin

Figure 12–28. *A,* Incremental lines of Retzius in transverse ground section, arranged concentrically. *B,* Decalcified paraffin section of exfoliated primary molar (× 20). Heavy dark lamella runs from darkly stained dentin to surface in an irregular course independent of developmental pattern. Roughly parallel to dentin surface a number of incremental lines are visible, one of which, the neonatal line, is accentuated. (Reproduced by permission from Bhaskar SN [ed]: Orban's Oral Histology and Embryology, 10th ed. St. Louis, CV Mosby, 1986.)

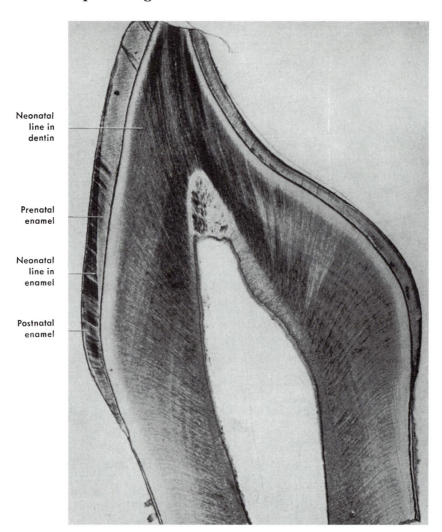

Neonatal
line in
dentin

Prenatal
enamel

Neonatal
line in
enamel

Postnatal
enamel

Figure 12–29. Neonatal line in the enamel. Longitudinal ground section of a primary cuspid. (From Schour I: J Am Dent Assoc *23*:1947–1950, 1936. Copyright by the American Dental Association. Reprinted by permission.)

wear, depending on the individual (Brauer et al., 1959). The effects of attrition on occlusion are adjusted for by further functional eruption.

Figure 12-35 is a diagram summarizing the life cycle of the tooth from initiation through attrition.

THE PRIMARY DENTITION TO AGE THREE

Table 12-5 demonstrates the various stages of development of the teeth from conception to adolescence (Finn, 1973). The primary teeth begin to form at 7 weeks in utero, and the enamel of all of the primary teeth is usually completed by the first year of age. All of the primary teeth generally have erupted by 24 to 36 months of

age. The root structure of these primary teeth is usually complete by age 3 (Finn, 1973).

At birth, histologic analysis of the teeth of the maxilla and mandible in most cases shows the appearance of some degree of calcification of 24 tooth units. The 24 tooth units are the 20 primary teeth and the four first permanent molars (Figs. 12-36 and 12-37).

The first primary tooth to erupt is the mandibular primary incisor. This tooth usually erupts in a vertical upright position (Brauer et al., 1959). As other primary teeth erupt, they may be spaced apart from each other, particularly in the incisor area. Spaces frequently recognized in the primary dentition are the primate spaces (Fig. 12-38). Primate spaces are the spaces between the mandibular primary cuspid and the first primary molar, and between the maxillary primary

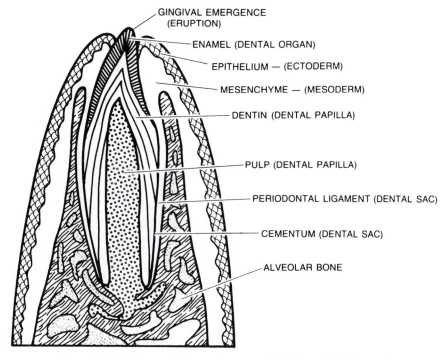

GINGIVAL EMERGENCE
(ERUPTION)

ENAMEL (DENTAL ORGAN)

EPITHELIUM — (ECTODERM)

MESENCHYME — (MESODERM)

DENTIN (DENTAL PAPILLA)

PULP (DENTAL PAPILLA)

PERIODONTAL LIGAMENT (DENTAL SAC)

CEMENTUM (DENTAL SAC)

ALVEOLAR BONE

Figure 12–30. Diagram of the eruption stage of the life cycle of the tooth.

Figure 12–31. Three stages in root development (diagrams). *A,* Section through a tooth germ showing the epithelial diaphragm and proliferation zone of the pulp. *B,* Higher-magnification view of the cervical region of *A. C,* Imaginary stage showing the elongation of Hertwig's epithelial sheath between diaphragm and future cemento-enamel junction. Differentiation of odontoblasts in the elongated pulp. *D,* In the cervical part of the root, dentin has been formed. The root sheath is broken up into epithelial rests and is separated from the dentinal surface by connective tissue. Differentiation of cementoblasts. (Reproduced by permission from Bhaskar SN [ed]: Orban's Oral Histology and Embryology, 10th ed. St. Louis, CV Mosby, 1986.)

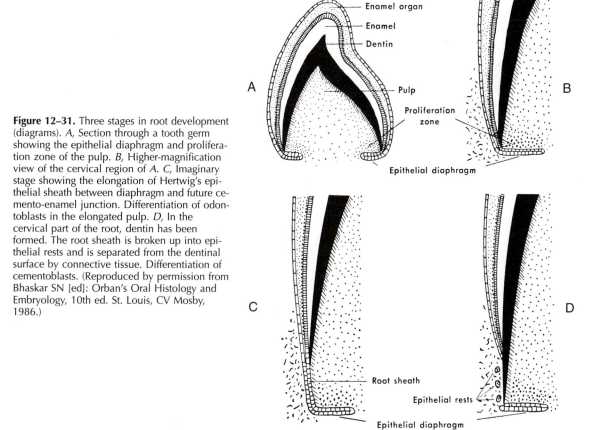

Enamel organ

Enamel

Dentin

Pulp

Proliferation zone

Epithelial diaphragm

Root sheath

Epithelial rests

Epithelial diaphragm

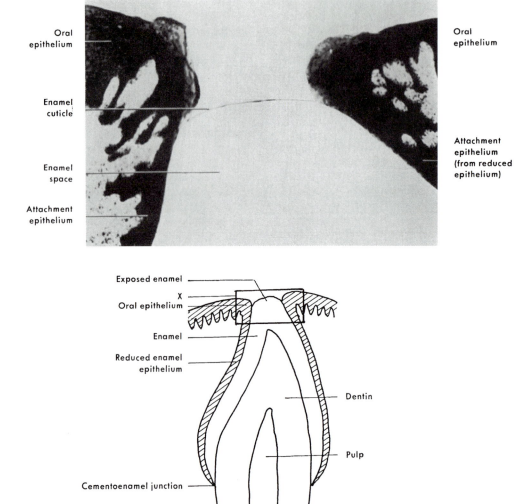

Figure 12–32. Tooth emerges through a perforation in the fused epithelia. "X" in diagram indicates area from which the photomicrograph was taken. (Reproduced by permission from Bhaskar SN [ed]: Orban's Oral Histology and Embryology, 10th ed. St. Louis, CV Mosby, 1986.)

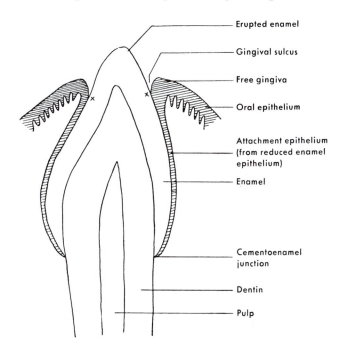

Figure 12–33. Diagram of the attached epithelial cuff and gingival sulcus at an early stage of tooth eruption. Bottom of sulcus is at "X." (Reproduced by permission from Bhaskar SN [ed]: Orban's Oral Histology and Embryology, 10th ed. St. Louis, CV Mosby, 1986.)

lateral incisor and the primary cuspid. The primary dentition remains relatively stable until it is influenced by the focus of the erupting permanent dentitions.

THE PERMANENT DENTITION TO AGE THREE

The first permanent molar is the first tooth to show germ formation at age 3½ to 4 months in utero. It is followed by the central and lateral incisors, which demonstrate formation at 5 to 5½ months in utero. The cuspid is the only other permanent tooth that begins its formation before birth at 5½ to 6 months in utero. The first and second bicuspids and the second and third molars demonstrate germ formation after birth.

At birth, the only teeth that show a trace of hard tissue formation are the first permanent molars (Brauer et al., 1959). With the exception of the third molars, all permanent teeth demonstrate hard tissue formation by 3 years of age (Finn, 1973) (see Table 12-5).

GLOSSARY

Ameloblast: One of a group of cells originating from the ectoderm from which the dental enamel is developed; an enamel cell. The ameloblasts cover the papilla of the enamel organ.

Apposition: Appositional growth is that stage of

the life cycle of the developing tooth during which a layer-like deposition of a nonvital extracellular secretion is laid down in the form of tissue matrix.

Attrition: A rubbing or friction. In dentistry, the term refers to the natural wearing away of the substance of a tooth under the stress of mastication.

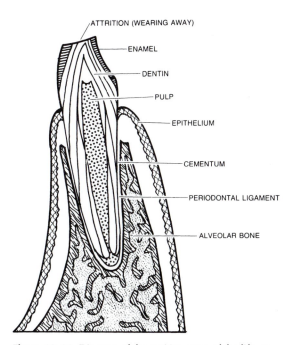

Figure 12–34. Diagram of the attrition stage of the life cycle of the tooth.

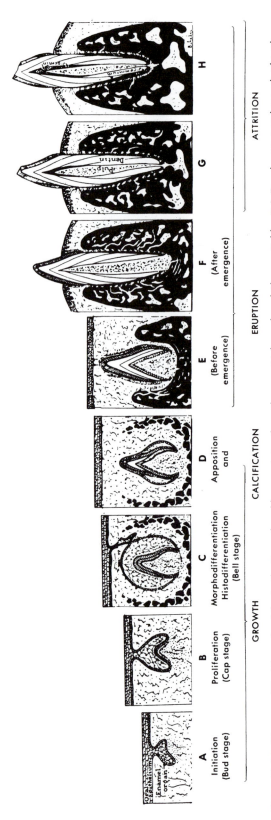

Figure 12–35. Diagram of the life cycle of the tooth. (Reproduced by permission from Sharawy, Mohamed, and Bhussry, Baldev Raj: Development and growth of teeth. *In* Bhaskar SN [ed]: Orban's Oral Histology and Embryology, 10th ed. St. Louis, CV Mosby, 1986. Modified from Schour I, Massler M: J Am Dent Assoc 27:1785, 1940. Copyright by the American Dental Association. Reprinted by permission.)

TABLE 12–5. Chronology of the Human Dentition

Tooth	Hard Tissue Formation Begins	Amount of Enamel Formed at Birth	Enamel Completed	Eruption	Root Completed
Primary Dentition					
Maxillary					
Central incisor	4 mo in utero	Five sixths	1½ mo	7½ mo	1½ yr
Lateral incisor	4½ mo in utero	Two thirds	2½ mo	9 mo	2 yr
Cuspid	5 mo in utero	One third	9 mo	18 mo	3¼ yr
First molar	5 mo in utero	Cusps united	6 mo	14 mo	2½ yr
Second molar	6 mo in utero	Cusp tips still isolated	11 mo	24 mo	3 yr
Mandibular					
Central incisor	4½ mo in utero	Three fifths	2½ mo	6 mo	1½ yr
Lateral incisor	4½ mo in utero	Three fifths	3 mo	7 mo	1½ yr
Cuspid	5 mo in utero	One third	9 mo	16 mo	3¼ yr
First molar	5 mo in utero	Cusps united	5½ mo	12 mo	2¼ yr
Second molar	6 mo in utero	Cusp tips still isolated	10 mo	20 mo	3 yr
Permanent Dentition					
Maxillary					
Central incisor	3–4 mo	. . . . . .	4–5 yr	7–8 yr	10 yr
Lateral incisor	10–12 mo	. . . . . .	4–5 yr	8–9 yr	11 yr
Cuspid	4–5 mo	. . . . . .	6–7 yr	11–12 yr	13–15 yr
First bicuspid	1½–1¾ yr	. . . . . .	5–6 yr	10–11 yr	12–13 yr
Second bicuspid	2–2¼ yr	. . . . . .	6–7 yr	10–12 yr	12–14 yr
First molar	at birth	Sometimes a trace	2½–3 yr	6–7 yr	9–10 yr
Second molar	2½–3 yr	. . . . . .	7–8 yr	12–13 yr	14–16 yr
Mandibular					
Central incisor	3–4 mo	. . . . . .	4–5 yr	6–7 yr	9 yr
Lateral incisor	3–4 mo	. . . . . .	4–5 yr	7–8 yr	10 yr
Cuspid	4–5 mo	. . . . . .	6–7 yr	9–10 yr	12–14 yr
First bicuspid	1¾–2 yr	. . . . . .	5–6 yr	10–12 yr	12–13 yr
Second bicuspid	2¼–2½ yr	. . . . . .	6–7 yr	11–12 yr	13–14 yr
First molar	at birth	Sometimes a trace	2½–3 yr	6–7 yr	9–10 yr
Second molar	2½–3 yr	. . . . . .	7–8 yr	11–13 yr	14–15 yr

After Logan and Kronfeld: JADA *20*, 1933 (slightly modified by McCall and Schour). Copyright by the American Dental Association. Reprinted by permission.

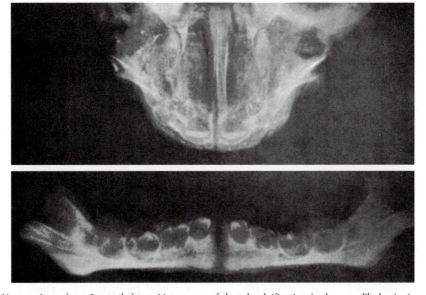

Figure 12–36. Wet specimen from 8-month fetus. Note areas of dental calcification in the mandibular incisors, cuspids, and first primary molars as well as in the maxillary central and lateral incisors and first primary molars. There is only slight calcification in the maxillary cuspids and cusp tips of the second primary molars. (From McCall JO, Wald SS: Clinical Dental Roentgenology, 4th ed. Philadelphia, WB Saunders, 1957, p 153.)

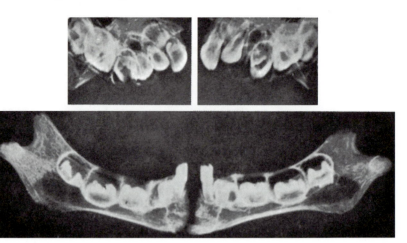

Figure 12–37. Wet specimen from infant at birth. Note areas of dental calcification similar to those shown in Figure 12–36. Maxillary calcification is slightly less advanced. (From McCall JO, Wald SS: Clinical Dental Roentgenology, 4th ed. Philadelphia, WB Saunders, 1957, p 154.)

Basal layer: Basal is an adjective meaning pertaining to or situated near a base. In the developing tooth, the basal layer is that tissue at the junction of the ectoderm and mesoderm.

Basement membrane: The delicate, transparent, membranous layer of cells underlying the epithelium of mucous membranes and secreting glands at the junction of the ectoderm and mesoderm.

Bud stage: The initial expansion of cells of the ectoderm in the developmental life cycle of the tooth.

Calcification: The process by which organic tissue becomes hardened by a deposit of calcium salts within its substance.

Cap stage: The step of tooth development after the bud stage and before the bell stage, which is caused by unequal growth of the cells of the basal layer descending into the mesoderm to form the appearance of a cap.

Cementoblast: One of the cells arising from the mesoderm from which the cementum of the tooth is developed.

Cementum: The layer of bony tissue covering

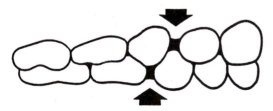

Figure 12–38. Primate spaces between the maxillary primary lateral incisor and primary canine and between mandibular primary canine and mandibular first molar. (From Finn SB: Clinical Periodontics, 4th ed. Philadelphia, WB Saunders, 1973; after Baume LJ: J Dent Res *29*:442, 1950.)

the root of a tooth. It differs in structure from ordinary bone by containing a greater number of Sharpey's fibers (see *Sharpey's fibers*).

Dental lamina: *Dental*—pertaining to a tooth or teeth; *lamina*—a thin leaf or plate of something, such as bone; *dental lamina*—dental ridge; a band of thickening of the epithelium along the margin of the gum, in the embryo, from which the enamel organ is ultimately developed.

Dental organ (enamel organ): A process of epithelium forming a cap over the dental papilla from which the enamel is developed.

Dental papilla: A process of condensed mesenchyme within the dental organ and cap from which the dentin and dental pulp are formed.

Dental sac: A process of condensed mesenchyme surrounding the dental organ and dental papilla from which the cementum and periodontal ligament are formed.

Dentinoblast: A cell found on the pulpal side of the dentinoenamel junction differentiated from an odontoblast to form dentin.

Ectoderm: The outer layer of the primitive (two-layered) embryo from which the epidermis and the neural tube are developed.

Enamel pulp: The soft material from which the dental enamel is developed.

Eruption: The act of breaking out, appearing, or becoming visible. For a tooth, it is the process of moving through alveolar bone into the oral cavity.

Hertwig's epithelial root sheath: An investment of epithelial cells around the unerupted tooth and inside of the dental follicle, which are derived from the enamel organ.

Histodifferentiation: A stage of the life cycle

of the tooth identified by the cells of the embryonic tissue becoming specialized. The proliferating cells of ectoderm and mesoderm take on a definite change in this stage in order to be able to produce enamel, dentin, and cementum.

Initiation: A stage of the life cycle of the tooth identified as the very first point of its development.

Mesenchyme: The embryonic connective tissue; that part of the mesoderm whence are formed the connective tissues of the body as well as the blood vessels and lymphatic vessels.

Mesoderm: The middle of three layers of the primitive embryo.

Morphodifferentiation: A stage of the life cycle of the tooth identified as that period producing form or shape.

Odontoblast: One of the cylindrical connective tissue cells that form the outer surface of the dental pulp adjacent to the dentin. They are connected with each other by protoplasmic processes. Each odontoblast has a long, thread-like process, the dental fibril (or fiber of Tomes), which extends through the dentinal tubule to the dentoenamel junction.

Odontoclast: One of the cells that help to absorb the roots of the primary teeth. They occur between the primary teeth and the erupting permanent teeth.

Periodontal ligament: *Periodontal*—situated or occurring around a tooth; pertaining to the periodontal membrane that attaches the tooth to alveolar bone.

Periodontal membrane: The connective tissue occupying the space between the root of a tooth and the alveolar bone and furnishing a firm connection between the root of the tooth and the bone.

Proliferation: The reproduction or multiplication of similar forms; a stage in the life cycle of the tooth bud just after the initiation stage.

Sharpey's fibers: Cementum is the covering of the tooth root surface. There is also a cementoid tissue covering the cementum, and it is lined with cementoblasts to maintain a dynamic state. There are connective tissue fibers passing through these cementoblasts from the periodontal ligament into the cementum. The embedded portion of the fiber in the cementum is the Sharpey fiber.

Stellate reticulum: *Stellate*—shaped like a star or stars; *reticulum*—a network, especially a protoplasmic network in cells; *stellate reticulum*—the reticular connective tissue-like epithelium forming the enamel pulp of the developing tooth.

Tooth bud: The very initial identification of the developing tooth by the expansion of certain cells in the basal layer of the oral epithelium (ectoderm only).

Tooth germ: The rudiment of a tooth, consisting of a dental sac and including the dental papilla and dental organ (enamel organ).

REFERENCES

Brauer JC, Demeritt WW, Higley LB, et al: Dentistry for Children. New York, McGraw-Hill, 1959.

Finn SB: Clinical Pedodontics. Philadelphia, WB Saunders, 1973.

Orban BJ: Oral Histology and Embryology. St. Louis, CV Mosby, 1957.

Schour I, Massler M: Studies in tooth development: The growth pattern of human teeth—Part II. J Am Dent Assoc *27:*1918-1931, 1940.

Cognitive Changes

J. R. Pinkham

Even relatively recently, the human infant has been regarded because of his or her helplessness as a cognitively incompetent creature. Many psychologists now recognize that there is cognitive ability in the newborn. In fact, there now is evidence that newborns can experience sensations of pain, touch, and changes in bodily position. Also, it is now known that infants can from the first day of life smell, see, and hear. Cognitive competence explains how and why an infant explores a nursing mother's fingers and studies her face.

In 1984, Mussen and coworkers noted that there are four major areas of cognitive development during the first year of a child's life. The first is the area of perception. Even very young infants have the ability to perceive movement, facial relationships, and color (see Table 12-1).

The second prominent cognitive area is the recognition of information. It is now known that infants can recognize certain stimuli such as a face when viewed from various and different observational angles. In such a case, it is contended that children have developed mental schemes or representations of things encountered in their consciousness and that these schemes contain some but not all of the crucial elements of the object or event. This allows them to recognize the similarity of new objects compared with old ones because of their ability to generalize on these crucial elements.

The third important cognitive focus is the ability to categorize. Children can group things together by way of their shape, color, and use even by the age of 1 year.

Enhancement of memory is the fourth cognitive development of the first year of life. Even very young infants can be shown to have some memory. At age 6 months and older, the ability to recall past experience appears obvious. At this age, most children have the ability to recall past events and to use the information gained from that event to help them form a reaction to things presently going on. Two theories are of interest in the study of cognition in infants. The first is learning theory. The term conditioning is the most important concept derived from that body of thought. There are two types of conditioning, classic and operant. *Classic conditioning* occurs when two stimuli are paired together. For instance, sucking the nipple, if paired often enough with hearing a lullaby, eventually leads the infant to initiate sucking when he hears the lullaby. *Instrumental* or *operant conditioning* occurs when a child's actions are reinforced or rewarded. This kind of learning is possible when the parents coo as a response to a child's chortles. It is also possible if the mother gives her crying daughter a cookie to quiet her down. It is contended that rewarded behavior is behavior that is likely to occur again.

The cognitive development theory of Jean Piaget is the other theory of interest in the attempt to understand infant cognition. According to Piaget, much of the intellectual attainments of the child from birth to the age of 2 years results from the actions of the child with objects in the environment. Although Piagetian theory is not without some controversy regarding its accuracy, it is extremely useful to researchers, clinicians, parents, and other observers of infants because Piaget based his conclusions on observations of his own children's behavior. The behaviors he saw are common to all children.

In 1954, Piaget described the first 2 years of life as a period of sensorimotor development, which he divided into six discrete stages. Piaget contended that during this time the child must develop knowledge in the following three areas:

1. Object permanence: Objects continue to exist even when they are not perceivable by the child.
2. Causality: Objects have uses, and events have causes. Piaget used the term circular reaction (primary, secondary, and tertiary) to describe the changes that occur in this area. A primary circular reaction describes recreating an already known satisfying action, such as thumb sucking. A secondary circular reaction is the recreating of an accidentally discovered cause and effect. Tertiary circular reactions involve experimentation, and, as one might guess, such behaviors often exasperate the child's parents.
3. Symbolic play: One object can represent another.

The language development of the infant is, at first, very slow. The mean expressive vocabulary of an 18-month-old is 10 words. At this time, the receptive vocabulary of the child is considerably higher than the expressive vocabulary. Toward the end of the second year, the expressive vocabulary of children develops extraordinarily quickly. In 1983, Levine and colleagues noted that at 3 years of age the mean vocabulary of a child is 1000 words.

Table 12-1 of the previous physical change section coordinates the six stages of the sensorimotor stage of development with cognition, play, and language development.

REFERENCES

Levine MD, Carey WB, Crocker AC, et al: Developmental Behavioral Pediatrics. Philadelphia, WB Saunders, 1983.
Mussen PH, Conger JJ, Kagan J, et al: Child Development and Personality, 6th ed. New York, Harper & Row, 1984.
Piaget J: The Construction of Reality in the Child. New York, Basic Books, 1954.

Emotional Changes

J. R. Pinkham

There are many human emotions, such as shame, guilt, anger, joy, fear, and sadness. Many more could be named. Emotions can be discerned by observing behavioral reactions (crying), measuring physiologic responses (faster heart rate), or ascertaining a person's thoughts and reactions ("I'm depressed").

In assessing the emotional state of young children, the latter two methods of discernment are of little or no value. As a general rule, in the first year of a child's life adults assign whatever emotion they feel that the child should feel in a particular situation. Thus, a wide range of interpretation exists. When an 18-month-old child spills his or her milk, one parent may interpret the child's crying as frustration over his or her awkwardness, another as guilt for the mistake, and another as fear of having nothing else to drink.

It is also evident that in older children and adults, the true description of an emotion is very much influenced by how a person reacts to, analyzes, and studies his or her own inner feelings. Thus, for the same stimulus one person may laugh and another may cry. In very young children, ascertaining such subtleties as these is not possible. The excited babbling of a 3-month-old, which parents label as joy, may more appropriately be called simply excitement.

There appears to be an awakening of emotional states within the child between 4 months and 10 months of age. In 1984, Mussen and colleagues noted that infants were capable of displaying fearful behavior as well as anger or frustration. As a child approaches his or her first birthday, sadness on separation from a parent, joy on reunion, and jealousy with peers or siblings become reliable findings.

Infant and childhood fears are interesting to clinicians who treat children and must be taken into account when formulating a strategy for dealing with the child. Uncertainty and certainty are a pair of elements that emerge early in infancy and can lead to fear or lack of fear. For instance, if the first time the jack in a jack-in-the-box jumps up, it startles the child, the child may avoid the toy until later, when he recognizes at what part of the tune the jack will jump out. Avoiding startling situations is important in helping children react in new environmental situations.

Fear of strangers is almost a universal finding after 7 to 12 months of age, although its intensity varies from child to child. Another very common fear in this age group is fear of separation from the parents. This fear starts around 6 months of age, peaks between 13 and 18 months of life, and then declines. The basis for the onset of this fear is probably the result of developing a remembrance of the parent even when the parent is not present, i.e., object permanence. Because of this mental process, separation becomes distressful. In 1974, Goin-DeCarie suggested that infants with a dysfunctional relationship with their mothers develop permanency much later than those whose mothers have been consistent and affectionate.

The onsets and peaks of separation anxiety appear to be the same in children from a variety of cultures, although the rate of diminishment of the fear varies greatly (Kagan et al., 1978). It should be noted that the problem of separation anxiety is fairly well controlled by most children by 36 to 40 months of age and by many children by 32 to 36 months of age. In 1967, Ainsworth concluded that children who have strong relationships with their primary caregivers can utilize that relationship as a place from which to venture into wider social circles by exploration. Conversely, children with poorly developed relationships with their caregivers are not able to undertake such exploration because they lack security.

REFERENCES

Ainsworth MDS: Infancy in Uganda: Infant Care and the Growth of Attachment. Baltimore, Johns Hopkins Press, 1967.

Goin-DeCarie T: The Infant's Reaction to Strangers. New York, International Universities Press, 1974.

Kagan J, Kearsley R, Zelaso P: Infancy: Its Place in Human Development. Cambridge, Harvard University Press, 1978.

Mussen PH, Conger JJ, Kagan J, et al: Child Development and Personality, 6th ed. New York, Harper & Row, 1984.

Social Changes

J. R. Pinkham

THE FIRST YEAR

In the first year of life, the child is utterly and completely dependent on the parents. Mothering is extremely important to the child at this time. In the first several months, the child does not show a clear differentiation among people. The baby may coo or smile at parents as well as strangers.

Nonreflexive smiling occurs at 2 to 3 months, and this represents the first major social behavior of the infant other than crying. With this smile, the child begins to understand what a behavior other than crying can do to expand his or her influence within the home.

The most important happenings socially during the first year of life are the development of strong and secure attachments to nurturing and caring adults. It should be noted that, according to available research, children who are started early in life in high-quality day care environments do not suffer developmental social consequences compared with children raised solely by their mothers at home.

THE SECOND YEAR

The 1-year-old child is capable of great social progress during his second year of development. The advent of language skills allows the child to learn and to relate to the family. Socially, children seek to exert their will. A need to test independence starts to surface. Effective and consistent parenting strategies become very important.

Role model observation becomes important at this age and remains so for years to come. Role models who display a consistent behavior are the most effective. Children who observe nonaggressive ways of handling frustration are likely to acquire that approach. Unfortunately, children who see violent, aggressive behaviors consistently are just as likely to adopt those approaches.

The maintenance of affection between parent and child and increasing verbal approval and disapproval are important at this age. Discipline should be educational, not punitive. Parents need to be reminded that 1- and 2-year-old children have not acquired internal controls and that often temper tantrums are normal and are best left unnoticed. Physical punishment, beyond an attention-getting technique by a parent (e.g., one painless thump on the buttocks), is usually contraindicated and can actually make a misbehaving child behave worse.

THE THIRD YEAR

Depending on the individual child, late in the second year or early in the third year the child starts to eat independently of the parents. The third year is when potty training generally starts. This should not be started too soon and should never become a conflict between the child and the parent. Parents should wait until the child is ready.

The third year is a demanding one for parents. The period for children between the second and third birthdays have been labeled "the terrible twos." The child in his third year may use the word "no!" anytime he or she cares to resist. The child is often an embarrassment to his or her parents because he does not hesitate to state his observations in front of everyone ("Aunt Jane is fat!"). Genital manipulation is not an uncommon practice at this age, and this may be trying for parents also.

By the end of the third year, the child is asking "how" and "why" questions. The child's unique identity is beginning to surface, and he or she can integrate the standards of others into his or her own life. Because of this and because of increased communication skills, the child by the third birthday is capable of a variety of social interchanges with other people. Because of this ability to communicate, for years the third birthday marked the entry date for many children into a program of dental care. Of course, one of the premises of this textbook is that from a prevention standpoint, age 3 is much too late for the first dental appointment.

Epidemiology and Mechanisms of Dental Disease

Steven M. Adair

Much progress has been made in the last half of the twentieth century in understanding the complex interactions of the dental caries process. Because of its multifactorial nature, however, there is still much to be learned regarding the initiation, progression, and prevention of dental decay. The relationships to caries among diet, microflora, saliva, host response, fluoride and other trace elements, the demineralization-remineralization phenomenon, and other factors all require further elucidation. We understand the process sufficiently, however, to enable most children with access to dental care to grow up free of caries, a disease that was once endemic in the population.

Current knowledge has led to a wealth of preventive regimens that can be applied on an individual or a public health basis. This has led to a dramatic reduction in the prevalence of dental caries among children in the United States (Brunelle and Carlos, 1982, 1990). A caries-free teenager is no longer a rarity but a realistic goal for the dental practitioner to hold for most child patients in the practice. This is particularly true for children whose prevention programs are initiated early in life.

This part of the chapter reviews the microbiology and histopathology of caries and discusses early caries during the establishment of the primary dentition.

CURRENT CONCEPTS OF THE CARIES PROCESS

Dental caries is a complex, multifactorial disease whose study has involved a multitude of basic science and clinical disciplines. A detailed discussion of current knowledge is beyond the scope of this chapter, but the following brief review should acquaint the reader with a basic understanding of the process.

Dental caries is a disease of the dental hard tissues, characterized initially by the decalcification of the inorganic portions of the tooth. Loss

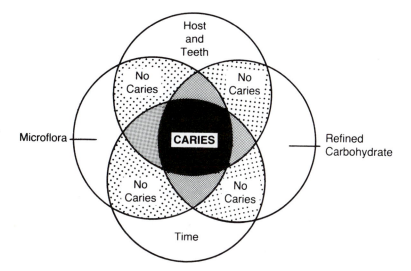

Figure 12–39. Venn diagram illustrating the relationship of the major factors involved in the caries process.

of the mineral content is then followed by breakdown of the organic matrix. This destructive process results from the metabolism of carbohydrates by oral microorganisms. In its simplest terms, the process can be visualized by a Venn diagram illustrating the following requirements: (1) a susceptible tooth, (2) presence of bacteria, (3) access to refined, fermentable carbohydrate, and (4) time. These requirements were first proposed in 1890 by Miller. Figure 12–39 illustrates the basis of the acidogenic, or chemicoparasitic, theory of dental caries. In this most widely accepted model, bacteria utilize dietary carbohydrates, principally sucrose, as a substrate for acid production. The resultant acids begin the process of demineralization.

MICROBIOLOGY OF DENTAL CARIES

In order to participate in the caries process, bacteria must not only be able to withstand an acidic environment (aciduric) but they may also contribute to that environment by producing organic acids (acidogenic). Of the many organisms present in the oral cavity, the genus most frequently implicated as a cause of caries is *Streptococcus.*

Several species of streptococci are know to be cariogenic in laboratory animals. These include *Streptococcus mutans, sanguis, salivarius,* and *milleri* (Drucker and Green, 1978; Fitzgerald, 1968). *Lactobacillus acidophilus* and *casei* have also been associated with the decay process. Some strains of *Actinomyces* are also capable, to a lesser extent, of producing coronal caries in some animal models as well as root surface caries in humans (Syed et al., 1975).

In humans, *S. mutans* has been correlated with caries in numerous cross-sectional epidemiologic studies and is currently presumed to play the major role in the initiation of the lesion, even though it is not the first to colonize on the tooth's surface (Loesche et al., 1975). Lactobacilli also have been correlated with dental caries. These species are minimally involved in lesion initiation but are believed to play a role in the caries progression. Increasing attention in recent cariology research is being given to the relative cariogenic potential of various combinations of plaque bacteria.

TRANSMISSION OF *STREPTOCOCCUS MUTANS*

Because its ecological niche is on the tooth surface, *S. mutans* does not appear in the mouth of infants until the later stages of primary tooth eruption (Berkowitz et al., 1980). Studies have demonstrated that a minimum infective dose of *S. mutans* is required to implant human strains into rats (van Houte et al., 1976). Subsequently it has been shown that mouth-to-mouth transmission of *S. mutans* takes place between mothers and their children (Berkowitz et al., 1981). Successful implantation into the infant is also related in part to the size of the inoculum. Infants appear to acquire a genotype of *S. mutans* that is identical to the mother's, although mothers harbor a more heterogeneous population of *S. mutans* than do their infants at the time of acquisition (Caufield and Walker, 1989). This "vertical transmission" appears to involve primarily the mother because the strains obtained from fathers are

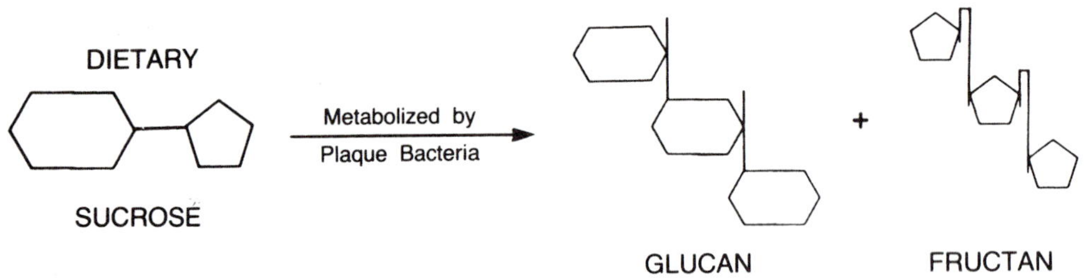

DIETARY

SUCROSE

Metabolized by
Plaque Bacteria

GLUCAN   FRUCTAN

Figure 12–40. The breakdown of dietary sucrose into glucan and fructan.

clearly distinct from those of the mother or the infant. The transmission can be delayed, perhaps even prevented, by instituting intensive preventive programs in prima gravida mothers who harbor more than 10^2 colony-forming units per milliliter of saliva (Kohler et al., 1983). Alaluusua and Renkonen (1983) have shown that early detection of *S. mutans* in an infant's mouth is related to a higher level of caries by age 4 years.

FORMATION OF PLAQUE

The initial colonization of teeth probably begins with organisms other than *S. mutans* (van Houte et al., 1971), which does not have great ability to adhere to teeth by itself. The mechanisms of initial colonization include (1) adherence of bacteria to pellicle or the enamel surface, (2) adhesion between bacteria of the same or different species, and (3) subsequent growth of bacteria from small enamel defects and from cells initially attached to tooth structure (Gibbons and van Houte, 1973). Plaque development continues with the formation of extracellular polymer chains via the breakdown of sucrose into its two main components, glucose and fructose (Fig. 12-40). The polymers are synthesized from each of these components. Chains of glucose and fructose are called glucans and fructans, respectively. These polysaccharides, particularly glucans, are sticky, gelatinous substances that further enhance the bacteria's ability to adhere to the tooth and to each other. Glucans and fructans also affect the rate at which saliva can enter the plaque to buffer the acid and reverse the demineralization process.

Intracellular metabolism of carbohydrates leads to the production of acids, chiefly lactic, that can depress plaque pH from a resting level of about 6 to a value of 4 within minutes of contact with a fermentable carbohydrate. Fructans, which are more soluble than glucans, may also serve as a reservoir of easily catabolized polysaccharide for the bacteria to utilize when other substrates are not available.

HISTOPATHOLOGY OF SMOOTH SURFACE LESIONS

The earliest clinical sign of the caries process on smooth enamel surfaces is the white spot lesion (Fig. 12-41), an area of white, chalky, opaque enamel typically seen under a layer of plaque at the gingival margin of tooth surfaces. It can also be seen on the proximal tooth surfaces that become exposed after exfoliation of an adjacent primary tooth. The white spot lesion is an indication that the underlying enamel has decalcified. In cross-section the lesion is conical, with its apex toward the dentin. During the early stages of development, the lesion may not be visible on a bitewing radiograph.

The enamel lesion has been divided by Silverstone and coworkers (Silverstone et al., 1981) into histologic zones that correspond to the

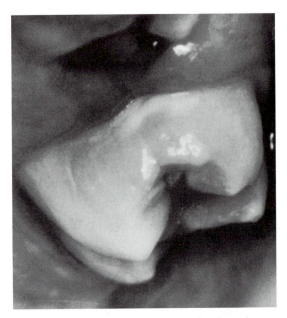

Figure 12–41. White spot lesion on mesial surface of permanent first molar, below the contact area. Created by long-standing plaque, it is now visible after exfoliation of primary second molar.

changes produced in the enamel (Fig. 12–42). The surface zone is the relatively unaffected superficial enamel that acts as a diffusion gradient, allowing minerals (fluoride, calcium, phosphate, and other ions) to pass in and out of the enamel. Only 5% to 10% of the mineral content is lost from the surface layer. Below this zone is the body of the lesion, the principal area of demineralization, representing about 60% mineral loss. In developed lesions, this area roughly corresponds to the radiographic image as seen on bitewing films. The third zone, called the dark zone because of its appearance under polarized light microscopy, represents an area of mineral loss intermediate to the two preceding zones. The advancing front of the lesion, the translucent zone, has sustained a mineral loss similar to the surface zone (5–10%). Unless steps are taken to arrest and reverse this process, the lesion continues to advance toward the dentin. As it approaches the dentinoenamel junction, the lesion spreads laterally and the previously intact surface layer breaks down, creating clinically detectable cavitation.

The histopathology of pit and fissure caries is somewhat different from that of smooth surface lesions; consequently, approaches to the prevention of the two types of caries are different. The use of fluoride in its various forms, improved oral hygiene, and dietary control are primarily effective in combating smooth surface lesions. Pit and fissure sealants and preventive resin restoration techniques are used to control pit and fissure lesions. The histopathology and prevention of pit and fissure lesions are discussed in Chapter 32.

DEMINERALIZATION AND REMINERALIZATION

One of the most important concepts that has evolved in cariology since the 1970s is the process of demineralization and remineralization of enamel. The caries process is no longer thought of as linear, beginning with acid demineralization of enamel and ending in a clinically detectable lesion. Rather, the process appears to be a dynamic one, involving both the loss of enamel mineral content and its replacement, with surface enamel functioning as a diffusion matrix. Enamel is composed of mineralized crystals surrounded by a water-protein-lipid matrix that occupies 10% to 15% of the total volume (Guggenheim, 1984). This matrix provides relatively large channels through which acids, minerals, fluoride, and other ions may pass in both directions.

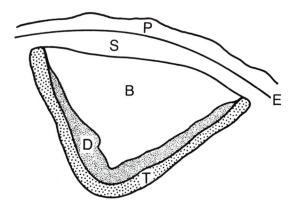

Figure 12–42. Diagram of an early enamel (white spot) lesion, illustrating: plaque (P), enamel surface and pellicle (E), intact surface layer (S), body of the lesion (B), dark zone (D), and translucent zone (T).

Under normal oral conditions, an equilibrium is established between mineral loss and mineral gain. The balance can be disturbed, however, by environmental factors in the oral cavity, such as plaque fluid pH and the presence or absence of fluoride. Acid production by plaque creates an environment with a lowered pH at the enamel surface, leading to dissolution of subsurface enamel crystals. Calcium, phosphorus, and other minerals diffuse out through the enamel surface in the process known as demineralization.

The presence of fluoride in the oral environment, even in very low concentration, can affect the equilibrium of this process in the opposite manner, leading to remineralization. This fluoride may come from the saliva, the plaque fluid, or from the demineralized enamel itself. During remineralization, fluoride facilitates the diffusion of calcium and phosphorus back into the lesion where partially dissolved hydroxyapatite crystals are rebuilt into fluoridated hydroxyapatite. This latter structure is now more resistant to acid dissolution than were the original crystals (Feagin et al., 1971). A true "repair" of the original early lesion takes place.

Thus, dental caries must be viewed as a dynamic process taking place on all plaque-covered surfaces. The initial demineralization is followed by remineralization, a process that is enhanced by fluoride ions in the saliva, plaque, and enamel. The resultant repaired crystals are less soluble than the original crystals. As long as the surface layer remains intact, remineralization of the lesions is possible and a restoration may be avoided. The clinician must recognize the importance of the surface layer of the white spot lesion and avoid the temptation to penetrate it with the explorer. Doing so creates an irreversible lesion

Text continued on page 183

Early Caries: The Importance of Recognition for Prevention and Treatment

David Johnsen

The introduction of water fluoridation and other fluoride modalities more than a generation ago has led to an overall reduction of dental caries, but specific kinds of caries patterns have persisted. This phenomenon holds implications for planning prevention and treatment programs suited to individual children. This section presents the timing and appearance of common kinds of dental caries experiences and the resulting considerations for prevention and treatment.

Figure 12-43 presents a schematic illustration of the earliest appearance of specific caries experiences. The first to appear is nursing caries, which appear before 20 months of age. This is almost invariably baby bottle tooth decay. Although it is impossible to state that no other type of caries could occur at this age, no other kind of caries pattern has been reported. The significance of this point is reflected in the commonly asked question, "When should a child's first visit to the dentist take place?" The traditional answer, age 3, has been based on the age at which most children can cooperate for a dental examination rather than the age at which the child may be developing extensive dental problems.

Bottle caries is rampant decay that springs from sleeptime bottle feeding combined with infection with *Streptococcus mutans*. It first affects the maxillary incisors. This disease pattern is important because extensive treatment is required before the child is old enough to cooperate for restorative dental care, necessitating physical restraint, sedation, or general anesthesia. The significance of the prevention of bottle decay is that

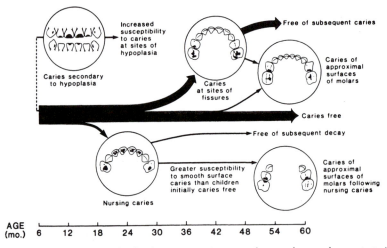

Figure 12–43. Schematic for different kinds of caries experiences and ages when each can start. A significant percentage of children remain caries free. Nursing caries (usually baby bottle tooth decay [BBTD]) begins between 1 and 2 years of age; children with BBTD are at significantly greater risk for future caries than are caries-free children. Pit and fissure caries usually begins after about age 3, with caries of approximating tooth surfaces beginning shortly after. (From Johnsen D. *In* Wei SH: Pediatric Dentistry: Total Patient Care. Philadelphia, Lea & Febiger, 1988.)

all other early caries patterns appear in children who are old enough for potential cooperation. Thus, dental health to age 2½ or so is a function of early counseling and establishment of proper feeding practices, in particular discontinuation of the sleeptime bottle. It is also significant for prevention planning to note that the child with bottle caries is more likely to develop subsequent smooth surface decay than the child without bottle caries.

Caries of the grooves and fissures of the posterior teeth is associated with an inability to clean defects that extend into the tooth. A large percentage of children now experience only caries of the grooves and fissures of the posterior teeth. In fluoridated areas and in areas where children have access to supplemental fluoride, this pattern of dental disease is more common than any other. Identification of children at risk for this type of dental caries is accomplished by visual and careful tactile inspection of the teeth for susceptible grooves and fissures. Prevention of this pattern is accomplished by the use of pit and fissure sealants.

Caries of the proximal surfaces of posterior teeth can begin after the molars move into adjacent contact. Children with this pattern of caries in the primary dentition have an uncontrolled infection of *S. mutans*. Susceptibility to smooth surface caries is significant for the dentist, who can then plan additional prevention measures, such as supplemental fluoride. An aggressive approach to restorative treatment may be necessary, requiring the placement of restorations at the earliest detection of lesions in the primary dentition.

In summary, early detection of caries and, more specifically, early identification of specific types or patterns of decay focuses the decision of the dentist on prevention and restorative procedures to the advantage of the patient and the satisfaction of the dentist.

The Persisting Problem

Norman Tinanoff

The seriousness and societal costs of early childhood caries (ECC) continue to be a significant health issue, especially for children from racial/ethnic minorities and from developing countries. Caries prevalence rates of 50% are commonly reported for 3- to 5-year-old children attending Head Start programs in the United States. There is considerable evidence these children with caries at an early age are not only at greater risk for new lesions in their primary and permanent teeth but may have other health problems. For instance, affected children have been shown to weigh less than their counterparts without caries. Perhaps the pain or infections associated with ECC may cause eating difficulties, or poor nutritional practices may be responsible for both the reduced body weight and caries. The consequences of this disease are not only a significant problem for the health and comfort of the affected child but are a considerable financial issue for the caretakers or the federal or state agencies paying for the dental care.

Box continued on following page

The Persisting Problem *continued*

Recently there have been challenges to the conventional wisdom that the bottle is the sole etiologic factor of this condition. Such concerns have given impetus to replacing terms for this condition, such as nursing caries and baby bottle tooth decay, with the words that reflect a less certain understanding of the etiology. It is still accepted that the group of cariogenic microorganisms, mutans streptococci, and frequent carbohydrate intake combines to produce abundant acid that demineralizes the child's teeth; and prolonged or night-time bottle-feeding practices in infants and toddlers may provide the carbohydrate source. Yet evidence suggests that bottle use per se may be an oversimplification of the cause of the rampant caries. Data from some developing countries, with high caries rates in infants and toddlers but few or no baby bottles, suggest that ECC cannot be attributed to inappropriate bottle use in these settings. Perhaps other factors, such as frequent carbohydrate exposure from nonbottle foods, relative caries risk of certain carbohydrates, and enamel hypoplasia due to malnutrition or premature birth, need further exploration.

Another controversial yet poorly documented caries risk is the potential cariogenicity of "at will" breast feeding. There are case reports associating prolonged or night-time breast feeding and ECC. One cannot dismiss a possible association between reported rampant caries in these cases and dietary practices other than breast feeding, however.

The prevention of ECC has focused on educational programs to alter children's feeding practices and methods to reduce levels of mutans streptococci infection in infants. There has been surprisingly little scientific effort to test these methods, however. The few studies that have evaluated educational programs to have parents decrease bottle use or to increase oral preventive behaviors have shown little long-term success. Perhaps other methods to foster preventive behaviors in parents whose children are at high risk for ECC need to be explored. Psychological approaches, such as self-efficacy enhancement and performance feedback techniques, may increase parents' confidence in their ability to perform oral health preventive behaviors for their children. Although these techniques have not been applied to behavioral changes required to prevent ECC, there is considerable literature showing their effects in other health areas.

Besides behavioral techniques to change adverse health behaviors, intensive preventive interventions that do not rely on patient compliance also should be examined as methods of reducing ECC. In some groups, lack of preventive behaviors and deeply entrenched feeding practices may be so difficult to change that it would not be practical to alter these behaviors. Studies of the efficacy of frequent professional tooth brushing or professional administration of an antimicrobial agent, or fluoride, are currently being evaluated. The focus of such programs is to place the responsibility for caries prevention on the dental health professional rather than on the parent.

Better knowledge of the cause of ECC and effective strategies to reduce its risk should produce enormous reductions in initial and long-term dental treatment costs, as well as the pain and suffering among affected children.

Medical Management of Infant and Toddler Dental Caries

Burton Edelstein

Dental therapies traditionally aim at two ends of the decay spectrum: prevention and repair. Increasing attention is now being given to the large middle ground—clinical management of underlying disease activity. This entails medical rather than surgical reparative therapies. Infant and toddler years are important in determining a child's likelihood of developing caries over time. It is early in life that cariogenic flora, dietary patterns, health behaviors, and even attitudes about personal health are initiated. Thoughtful medical management at this age holds tremendous promise for reducing oral disease throughout life. Appropriate medical interventions include diagnostic, pharmacologic, and behavioral interventions.

A careful look at the natural history of dental caries reveals a number of points along its progression where it can be prevented, mitigated, or reversed through medical interventions. Medical management can do the following:

- Delay initial acquisition of cariogenic flora during the first few years of life
- Reduce the intensity of caries activity once the disease process is established
- Reverse initial lesions by remineralizing decalcified enamel
- Arrest caries progression once cavitation occurs
- Minimize the extent of necessary restorations by creating sharper distinctions between carious and sound dentin and enamel
- Enhance the ease of restoring teeth in young children by significantly reducing tooth sensitivity, often negating the need for local anesthesia

The following table describes the various stages of disease progression and associated medical interventions:

Natural History of Caries	Medical Management with Examples of Evolving Therapies
Pre-dentate	Identify high-risk parents by history and culture; reduce salivary cariogenic flora reservoir (e.g., chlorhexidine mouth rinses for mother + parental information on limiting transmission)
Dentate, not yet infected with cariogenic flora	Identify high-risk children (family history), inhibit receptivity to cariogenic flora (e.g., topical application of bactericidal varnishes)
Dentate, infected with cariogenic flora	Identify presence of cariogenic flora (culture) and implement behavioral/lifestyle program to limit disease progression
Caries active	Identify children with high levels of cariogenic organisms, reduce levels (e.g., low-dose, high-frequency topical fluorides combined with eating/bottle behavior/lifestyle management)
Decalcifications present	Identify decalcifications as early lesions; implement recalcification regimens (e.g., apply recalcifying topical and adhesive agents (amorphous calcium phosphate in methacrylic base)
Cavitations present	Enhance topical agent effectiveness by sequential superficial excavation of necrotic tooth structure and application of topical fluorides or fluoride-releasing cements
Acute pain or infection	Utilize pharmacotherapies to manage pain, infection, and behavior in conjunction with traditional surgical approaches

Box continued on following page

Medical Management of Infant and Toddler Dental Caries *continued*

Because all therapies have some downside risks and impositions of time and expense, it is essential to intervene appropriately and tailor care to each child's level of disease and parental willingness to perform home treatments and make parenting changes. Medical interventions for behaviorally determined diseases demand meaningful education, motivation, reinforcement and health behavioral counseling. The more that is accomplished through medical management, the less needs to be accomplished through dental repair and the better the long-term outcome can be. Although dentists are unaccustomed to seeing predentate children, this is an ideal time to initiate medical management of dental caries by assessing parental dental history, salivary cariogenic flora, and attitudes about caries prevention. Counseling to prevent or delay initial transmission of cariogenic flora reduces the child's risk of cavities substantially.

Once a dentate child presents for evaluation, the child's decay status needs to be evaluated for both *"caries"*—the *disease process*—and *"cavities"*—the *lesions* that result from the caries process (Fig. 12-44). After this distinction is clear to the toddler's parent, it is possible to discuss separate treatments for these two components of decay, particularly for high-risk children. Upon determining both "caries" and "cavity" status, a child can be triaged as either caries-active, with or without cavities, or caries-inactive, with or without cavities. Many very young children with significant caries activity have simply not lived long enough for their disease to be expressed as cavities. Others who developed cavities early may have their caries process completely arrested yet retain evidence of earlier decay activity. Those children with neither activity nor lesions require the fewest interventions to maintain health.

The dental armamentarium for medical management of caries in infants and toddlers is limited by demands that suitable agents be topical; have high substantivity and low toxicity; be easy to administer by parents; and be effective and reasonably priced. There are no ideal medications or formulations for medical interventions in the caries process, but much can be accomplished with existing agents. New varnishes, recalcifying bondable materials, and fluoride-releasing cements hold increasing promise. Like many other lifestyle pathologies, however, the greatest success in subduing this chronic disease may

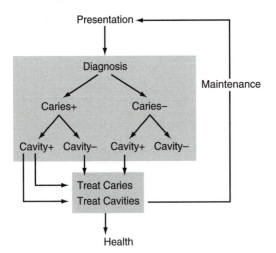

Figure 12–44. Chart for determining a dentate child's decay status.

take the form of behavioral interventions supplemented with medications rather than medications alone. Success depends on the following:

- Developing a "medical" mindset
- Focusing on the natural history of dental caries
- Using careful histories, acute clinical observation, and salivary cultures to identify risk
- Formulating tailored interventions to control the caries process
- Communicating clearly to parents
- Creating a therapeutic alliance with parents on behalf of their children
- Assessing the success of medical interventions
- Providing the least possible treatment consistent with desired outcomes
- Following up to reinforce success and limit failure.

Treating caries at the level of the disease process to prevent its expression, progression, and ultimate dental destruction is the highest calling and deepest challenge facing dentists who treat young children. Success in delaying caries initiation and suppressing its expression holds the greatest promise for children's long-term oral health.

that must be restored. The lesion in its early stages may not be detectable on a radiograph. Many small lesions radiographically limited to enamel can be treated noninvasively with fluoride, however. This is predominantly true in permanent teeth, which have a much thicker enamel layer than primary teeth. The clinician must also bear in mind that carious lesions are larger clinically than they appear on radiographs. Clinically cavitated lesions may also undergo remineralization, as is the case with some chronic carious lesions, but restorations obviously cannot be avoided in these situations.

REFERENCES

Alaluusua S, Renkonen O-L: *Streptococcus mutans* establishment and dental caries experience in children from 2 to 4 years old. Scand J Dent Res *14*:453-457, 1983.

Berkowitz RJ, Turner J, Green P: Primary oral infection of infants with *Streptococcus mutans*. Arch Oral Biol *25*:221-224, 1980.

Berkowitz RJ, Turner J, Green P: Maternal levels of *Streptococcus mutans* and primary oral infection of infants. Arch Oral Biol *26*:147-149, 1981.

Brunelle JA, Carlos JP: Changes in the prevalence of dental caries in U.S. school children, 1961-1980. J Dent Res *61*(Sp Issue):1346-1351, 1982.

Brunelle JA, Carlos JP: Recent trends in dental caries in U.S. children and the effect of water fluoridation. J Dent Res *69*(Sp Issue):723-727, 1990.

Caufield PW, Walker TM: Genetic diversity within *Streptococcus mutans* evident from chromosomal DNA restriction fragment polymorphisms. J Clin Microb *27*:274-278, 1989.

Drucker DB, Green RM: The relative cariogenicities of *Streptococcus milleri* and other viridans group streptococci in gnotobiotic hooded rats. Arch Oral Biol *23*:183-187, 1978.

Feagin F, Patel PR, Koulourides T, Pigman W: Study of the effect of calcium, phosphate, fluoride and hydrogen ion concentrations on the remineralization of partially demineralized human and bovine enamel surfaces. Arch Oral Biol *16*:535-548, 1971.

Fitzgerald RJ: Dental caries research in gnotobiotic animals. Caries Res *2*:139-146, 1968.

Gibbons RJ, van Houte J: On the formation of dental plaques. J Periodontol *44*:347-360, 1973.

Guggenheim B: Cariology Today. Basel, S Karger, 1984.

Kohler B, Bratthall D, Krasse B: Preventive measures in mothers influence the establishment of the bacterium *Streptococcus mutans* in their infants. Arch Oral Biol *28*:225-231, 1983.

Loesche WJ, Rowan J, Straffon LH, Loos PJ: Association of *Streptococcus mutans* with human dental decay. Infect Immun *11*:1252-1260, 1975.

Miller WD: The Microorganisms of the Mouth. Philadelphia, SS White Dental Manufacturing Co, 1890. Republished, K Knoig (ed), Basel, S Karger, 1973.

Silverstone LM, Hohnson NW, Hardie JM, et al: Dental Caries: Aetiology, Pathology, and Prevention. London, Macmillan Press Ltd, 1981.

Syed SA, Loesche WJ, Pape HL Jr, Grenier E: Predominant cultivable flora isolated from human root surface caries plaque. Infect Immun *11*:727-731, 1975.

van Houte J, Gibbons RJ, Pulkinen AJ: Adherence as an ecological determinant for streptococci in the human mouth. Arch Oral Biol *16*:1131-1141, 1971.

van Houte J, Burgess RC, Onose H: Oral implantation of human strains of *Streptococcus mutans* in rats fed sucrose or glucose diets. Arch Oral Biol *21*:561-564, 1976.

Chapter 13

Examination of the Infant and Toddler

Stephen Goepferd

Chapter Outline

Tradition in dentistry has recommended that a child's first dental visit occur after 3 years of age. This recommendation was based on the child's ability to cooperate in the dentist's office and the assumption that most children under 3 years of age didn't have any cavities. Although the prevalence of dental disease in school age children is decreasing (NIDR, 1989), there is substantial evidence that infants and toddlers experience dental disease (Kaste et al., 1996). One particularly destructive process in infants and toddlers is nursing caries. Dental decay found in 3- and 4-year-old children is initiated well before age 3.

Current knowledge in cariology, use of fluorides, and understanding the cariogenic potential of the diet, coupled with the fact that basic habits (i.e., preventive behaviors and dietary habits) are established very early in life (Anderson et al., 1977), justify efforts to prevent dental disease

during infancy. Furthermore, dental professionals, by virtue of early critical decision-making based on their knowledge of oral disease prevention, have been successful in assisting parents to keep their children caries-free. It is incumbent upon the dental profession to educate parents and other health care providers so that appropriate early decisions can be made in an effort to prevent oral disease in infants and toddlers.

A child's first visit to the dentist should occur no later than 12 months of age so that the dentist can evaluate the infant's oral health, determine the child's risk for developing dental disease, intercept potential problems, and educate parents in the prevention of dental disease in their child (AAPD, 1997; Nowak, 1997). An ever-increasing demand by parents for early dental evaluation of their infants and toddlers and for the acquisition of preventive knowledge requires the dental practitioner to be comfortable in examination of the infant and toddler (Goepferd, 1986b).

OBJECTIVES OF THE INFANT AND TODDLER EXAMINATION

The examination of the infant and toddler centers around three major objectives:

1. Introduction to dentistry
2. Risk assessment and oral examination
3. Prevention

Introduction to Dentistry. The initial examination of infants and toddlers should provide a foundation for the development of a positive attitude toward dentistry. The method of examining infants as well as the recommended environment can provide a pleasant, nonthreatening introduction to dentistry for the child and the parents.

Risk Assessment and Oral Examination. Medical history, analysis of current feeding and oral health practices, clinical findings, and the child's social and physical environment provide the basis for an estimate of the child's risk for developing dental disease. Examination of the infant begins with an evaluation of the head and neck region and an inspection of the oral cavity to detect any pathologic process or the early evidence of dental disease, leading to an assessment of the child's oral development.

Prevention. A major emphasis during the infant's initial visit should center around the counseling of parents regarding their role in preventing dental disease in the child. Preventive counseling should include dietary counseling with respect to feeding practices and snacking patterns, tooth cleaning procedures (positioning and timing), and fluoride assessment, all resulting in the development of an appropriate prevention program.

STEPS OF THE INFANT EXAMINATION

The examination of an infant should follow a logical sequence of events that results in a thorough yet expeditious procedure.

Preappointment Assessment

To provide the most complete and pertinent yet concise discussion during the visit, it is necessary to obtain and preview the following historical information. This information can be obtained from the parents through the use of a questionnaire, which is mailed to the parents and returned to the office prior to the appointment or in the office upon arrival.

Biographic Data and Family and Social History. This information lends insight into the family structure and provides an understanding of parent-child relationships, which is vital to the development of recommendations for dietary modifications and tooth cleaning procedures.

Prenatal, Natal, and Neonatal History. Information in these categories is helpful in explaining dental abnormalities that occur in the primary dentition and provides a means of documenting potential causative events while they are still relatively fresh in the parents' minds. Examples of such events are high-risk pregnancies, medication ingestion during pregnancy, preterm or low-birth-weight infants, and significant febrile episodes during early childhood.

Development History. Knowledge of the child's progress in attaining the various developmental milestones, including the eruption of the first tooth, assists the dentist in discovering significant growth alterations and provides a basis for answering the many questions that parents have regarding their child's dental development.

Medical History. An accurate medical history is as important for infants and toddlers as it is for older children and adults. Furthermore, a history of frequent episodes of otitis media and the accompanying frequent ingestion of antibiotic suspensions that contain high concentrations of sucrose, for example, influence recommendations for dietary management, tooth cleaning procedures, and possible topical fluoride applications.

Dental History. Knowledge of episodes of previous dental trauma, teething difficulties, nonnutritive sucking habits, and current patterns of home oral health care of the infant provides a basis for answering parents' questions and for developing recommendations for future management.

Feeding History. An overview of the infant's feeding history is important in assisting the practitioner in developing a relevant discussion of the dietary influences on dental caries and providing appropriate recommendations for altering potentially damaging feeding practices. Important information includes bottle and breast feeding, frequency and duration of feedings, use of a nighttime bottle or use of the bottle as a pacifier, the contents of the bottle, weaning from bottle or breast, and the transition to covered feeding cups.

The preappointment information aids the practitioner in tailoring the interview and counseling portion of the visit to meet the individual needs of the child and his or her parents.

Interview and Counseling

The interview and counseling portion of the visit is best accomplished prior to the examination of the infant or toddler.

- Specific concerns of the parents are identified so that they can be addressed during the examination, if appropriate.
- If the infant fusses during the examination (normal behavior), the parents predictably will direct their attention toward the child during the discussion that follows the examination and not toward the dentist.
- The child can be occupied with toys in a nonthreatening environment prior to the examination, and the parents can direct their attention toward the discussion.

Once the preappointment information has been reviewed, the dentist greets the child and the parents and discusses the parental concerns, the reason for seeking care, and any information from the preappointment information that requires further clarification. Based on the information, appropriate recommendations can be made regarding each aspect of an overall dental disease prevention program for the child.

The Examination Procedure

The clinical examination of the infant and toddler is made with the parent's assistance in a nonthreatening environment. Most often, it is neither necessary nor recommended that the dental chair be used for the infant examination. In fact, a pleasant location away from the busy dental operatory is appropriate. The parent and the dentist sit facing each other in a knee-to-knee position, supporting the child with the head cradled on the dentist's lap (Fig. 13–1). This position allows the parent to restrain the child gently if necessary and provides the parent as well as the dentist with good visualization of the child's oral cavity. This position is comfortable for the infant, and the parental contact provides a calming reassurance for the child. The psychological development of the child under 30 to 36 months of age is frequently insufficient to facilitate cooperation

in a dental setting, and some infants and toddlers cry or fuss during the examination, requiring minimal restraint by the parent. The dentist should reassure the parents that the child's behavior is normal and should not be considered inappropriate. The parents are fully aware that their child is likely to cry in other similar situations such as during a visit to the pediatrician's office or the barber shop. The crying or fussing should not interfere with the examination. Initially, the practitioner may be surprised at the number of infants and toddlers who remain calm during the entire examination. This is especially true with infants 12 months of age or younger.

Once the child is positioned properly, the dentist can perform a complete head and neck and intraoral examination. The dentist should begin with a general appraisal of the child, using a warm, gentle touch in a nonthreatening manner. The head and neck region should be evaluated for the presence of abnormalities in size, shape, and symmetry of the head; lymph nodes; facial symmetry; eyes, ears, and nose; and lips and mouth. The practitioner must always be aware of the possibility of child abuse when the infant or toddler shows evidence of head, neck, and facial bruising.

The examination of the mouth, with an artificial light source if needed, should begin with palpation and inspection of the lips, gingivae, and mucosa by placement of a forefinger along the cheek and positioning it on the gum pad distal to the most posterior maxillary tooth. The intraoral examination should include an evaluation of the soft tissues for the presence of any pathologic processes, such as inclusion cysts, congenital epulides, submucous clefts, traumatic ulcerations, frenum lacerations, and gingivitis. The examination of the dentition should include an evaluation of the jaw relationships, appropriate parameters of occlusion (overjet, overbite, molar relationships, midline deviations, and crossbites), presence or absence of spacing, presence of dental developmental abnormalities, hypoplastic or hypocalcified enamel, and dental caries.

Following the intraoral examination, the practitioner or a member of his or her staff should demonstrate positioning and technique for tooth cleaning in the infant. The child should then be positioned with the head on the parent's lap so that the parent can practice tooth cleaning under supervision and appropriate suggestions can be offered.

The findings of the clinical examinations are collated with the previous information gathered, the child's degree of risk for development of

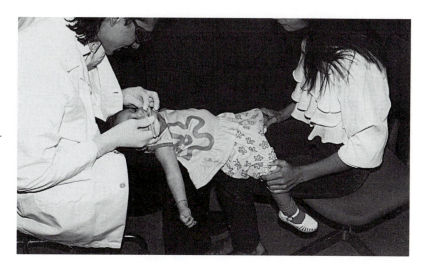

Figure 13–1. Examination of an infant in the knee-to-knee position.

dental disease is determined, and final recommendations about the parents' role in an optimal preventive program for the child and treatment recommendations, if any, are offered; finally, an appropriate recall schedule is determined.

Determining a Recall Schedule

The recall schedule is based on clinical findings and the results of the risk assessment. The appointment should be individualized and not determined by a traditional 6-month interval. Examples of suggested criteria for determining recall intervals are listed in Table 13–1. The presence of any one of the factors may be sufficient to justify placing the patient on a more frequent schedule.

At the recall visit, in addition to the clinical examination, the practitioner assesses the parents' tooth-cleaning efforts, evaluates feeding practices and snacking patterns, and investigates the degree to which the parents are following

the recommended prevention program that was previously outlined.

THE EMERGENCY EXAMINATION

Dental emergencies for infants and toddlers present a challenge for the dental office. In addition to treating the particular emergency, the office is faced with managing both the parents and the child. Most dental emergencies occurring in children 12 to 30 months of age are the result of trauma. Occasionally, the emergency is related to dental caries or to some systemic condition such as primary herpetic gingivostomatitis. In the case of a traumatic injury, before performing the examination the dentist must obtain certain vital information, including (1) a thorough medical history, (2) immunization status (especially against tetanus), and (3) a complete description of the traumatic incident. If the injuries are not adequately accounted for by a description of the accident, if they are inconsistent with the re-

TABLE 13–1. Criteria for Recall Schedule Determination

	Clinical Findings	Feeding or Diet Patterns	Dental Development
3 Months	Enamel decalcification Considerable plaque build-up Amelogenesis imperfecta Dentinogenesis imperfecta	Bottle used at bedtime or naptime Bottle used as a pacifier Bottle used past 12 months of age Frequent cariogenic snacking pattern	Stage of dental development has minimal influence on the 3-month interval recall category
6 Months	Posterior proximal contacts No previous tooth cleaning Primary dentition crowding Moderate plaque build-up	Relatively cariogenic diet or snacks	Second primary molar eruption is expected within 6 months
12 Months	Generalized spacing present Good oral hygiene exhibited Shallow occlusal anatomy	Good dietary habits exhibiting a low cariogenic potential	Second primary molar eruption is expected in 6–12 months

ported incident, or if evidence of multiple injuries in different stages of healing is noted, there may be probable cause to suspect child abuse. The historical information aids in the examination of the child and provides clues to the discovery of injuries that might otherwise go undetected. The emergency examination of the infant and toddler is performed in the knee-to-knee position, as previously described.

Nontrauma-related dental emergencies in infants and toddlers usually concern mouth pain and are often related to dental caries, especially nursing caries at this age. Thorough history-taking is important and often provides insight into the nature of a problem that may not be related to dental caries. It is important to remember that from the parents' perspective, most oral pain reported by children is interpreted as a toothache. If the nature of the emergency (trauma, deep caries) warrants radiographs, the child is positioned on a parent's lap with the parent stabilizing the child and film (Fig. 13–2) and appropriate radiation protection. Alternatively, the child may be stabilized by another means, such as any of the commercially available immobilization devices, but only after parental consent.

MANAGEMENT OF ELECTRICAL BURNS OF THE MOUTH

Electrical burns involving children's oral and perioral tissues require both immediate and long-term management by a multidisciplinary health team, wherein the dentist plays a key role. Most oral electrical burns are caused when a child bites on the live end of an electrical extension cord. Saliva acts as a conducting medium, producing an arc between the cord and the child's mouth. The heat generated can reach 2500–3000°C and causes extensive tissue damage. The commissure of the lip is the most common site of oral electrical burns, which occur most often in children under 4 years of age, the highest frequency of occurrence being between 18 and 24 months of age. Studies have shown, however, that older children (older than would generally be thought of as chewing on electrical cords) also are capable of inflicting this injury upon themselves (Canady et al., 1996). Education of preschoolers and kindergarten age children must include warnings of the dangers of electrical cords.

Nature of the Injury

Initially, the burn appears as charred, gray-white tissue with a centrally depressed area surrounded by elevated, erythematous margins. Swelling of

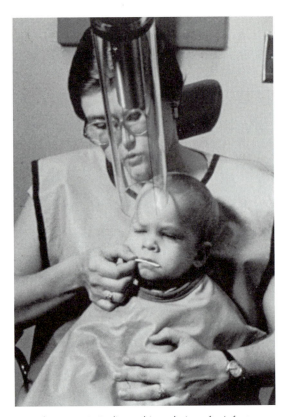

Figure 13–2. Radiographic technique for infants.

the tissues begins within hours and persists for 12 to 14 days. The burns are characterized by liquefaction of fat, coagulation of protein, and vaporization of fluids. Vascular damage causes further tissue damage at the borders of the wound by virtue of ischemia. Pain associated with the wound is usually minor owing to the destruction of neural tissue. The initial wound exhibits little or no bleeding because of electrical cauterization of the surrounding blood vessels. It is commonly reported that future bleeding from the labial artery can occur when sloughing of the necrotic tissue occurs any time from 4 to 21 days after the injury. A review of cases treated at the University of Iowa showed that this probably does not occur as often as would be expected, but parents should still be given first-aid instructions (direct pressure) to deal with this until help can be obtained in the nearest emergency room (Canady et al., 1997). Sloughing of the damaged tissue is completed within 2 to 3 weeks, and complete re-epithelialization occurs. Scarring of the wound results in contracture of the oral and perioral tissue and may lead to microstomia.

Treatment of Electrical Burns

An electrical burn to a child's mouth can be a severely disfiguring injury that can impede function and may result in a limited oral opening. Treatment objectives center around minimizing disfigurement and contraction. The following four main treatment approaches have been advocated: (1) immediate surgical excision of the wound, (2) delayed reconstructive surgery after 1 year of natural healing, (3) delayed primary reconstructive surgery after 2 weeks of healing, and (4) immediate postburn splinting of the oral commissure. The first three methods traditionally involve multiple surgical procedures over a period of years to achieve an esthetic result. Recent evidence indicates that immediate splinting of the commissure provides the best cosmetic result, minimizes contracture, and minimizes or eliminates the need for surgical reconstruction.

Initial Medical Management

The physician's immediate concerns are focused on the risk of bleeding, adequate nutritional and fluid intake, risk of bacterial infection, and risk of tetanus. Although the need for systemic antibiotics is controversial, there is apparent agreement that antibiotic therapy is appropriate for the most severe burns. Daily wound debridement followed by topical application of an antibiotic ointment is recommended. Diet management is aimed at minimizing trauma to the wound and depends on the severity of the injury and the child's ability to cooperate. Occasionally, the child may require hospitalization to accomplish these objectives if they cannot be attained on an outpatient basis.

Initial Dental Management

Dental management consists of fabricating a commissural splint early during the first 10 days after the injury. A number of appliance designs are available, and the selection depends on factors such as child behavior and cooperation, dental development, stability needed, and parental compliance. The appliance may be removable, fixed, or extraoral according to the needs and demands of the given situation (Czerepak, 1984; Holt et al., 1982; Josell et al., 1984; Silvergrade et al., 1982; Swain and Pinkham, 1983). The functional aspect common to all appliances is the presence of commissural wings. Wing placement depends on two critical measurements (Fig. 13–3). Measurement "a" is the distance from the midline to the unaffected commissure, and measurement "b" is the distance from the incisal edge to an imaginary intercommissural line,

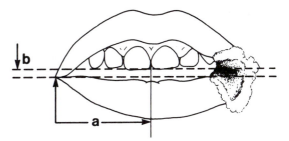

Figure 13–3. Measurements for a commissural splint.

thereby producing one horizontal and one vertical measurement to establish the position of the commissural wings. The appliance should exert slight tension on the lips at rest (Fig. 13–4). The appliance must be worn 24 hours a day (except for cleaning and eating with a removable appliance) for a period of 6 to 8 months and then for 12 hours a day (at night) for an additional 6 months until the scar softens and loses its contractile potential.

Surgical Management

Following splint therapy, the child is evaluated by a plastic surgeon to assess whether or not any reconstructive surgery is required. Frequently, only minimal surgical intervention is required, and in many cases surgical intervention can be avoided altogether.

The management of oral electrical burns in children requires immediate and long-term management by a multidisciplinary team consisting of a physician, dentist, and plastic surgeon. The dentist plays a major long-term role in the management of oral commissural burns by preventing oral contracture and by minimizing or eliminating the need for cosmetic surgery.

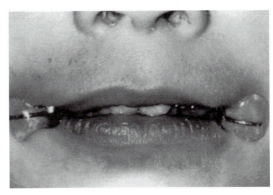

Figure 13–4. Commissural splint in place.

Anticipatory Guidance

Paul S. Casamassimo
Arthur J. Nowak

Dental professionals have always provided direction to parents about their child's dental health, but the major emphasis has always been on caries prevention. The changing patterns of dental caries in children, increasing parental concern about other oral health issues, more single parent families, and dentistry's ability to deal with important issues other than dental caries have broadened the counseling role in dental health care for children.

Anticipatory guidance is a term that describes a proactive, developmentally based counseling system that focuses on the needs of a child at a particular stage of life. The concept of a developmentally relevant, one-on-one intervention between dentist and parent offers a popular alternative to the traditional one-dimensional caries prevention message. Anticipatory guidance gives parents the chance to talk about their child, get age-appropriate information, and look ahead at how growth and the environment will affect their child's oral health in the next few months. It broadens dentistry's reach into areas that have implications for children's oral health. Finally, it gives the dental professional a consistent staged format for counseling and record-keeping and avoids the common humdrum repetition that loses impact rather than motivates.

The accompanying chart suggests one approach to anticipatory guidance in pediatric dentistry. Clinicians can use the chart to formulate practice-specific information for families or to track the information given to parents, or they can modify it into an instrument useful for assessing a child's dental development. In a busy practice, this organized approach allows one clinician to pick up where another has stopped without message duplication.

Suggested Anticipatory Guidance Format

Age	Discussion of Developmental Milestone	Nutrition and Feeding Information	Discussion of Oral Hygiene and Caries Prevention Techniques	Fluoride Information	Trauma Prevention Information	Discussion of Habits and Function, Behaviors, and Problems
Birth through 6 months	Eruption of first tooth and patterns of eruption	Appropriate use of the nursing bottle and danger of bottle caries	Clean teeth daily with soft brush, during bath or after feeding	Fluoride mechanisms and role in caries prevention; cover methods of administration in child's diet		Teething, mouthing objects, non-nutritive sucking, what happens at baby dental visits, *S. mutans* transmission

Age	Discussion of Developmental Milestone	Nutrition and Feeding Information	Discussion of Oral Hygiene and Caries Prevention Techniques	Fluoride Information	Trauma Prevention Information	Discussion of Habits and Function, Behaviors, and Problems
12 months	Review pattern of eruption for next 6 months	Encourage discontinuation of the bottle and use of tippy cup; inquire about sugar consumption; cover food retention issues and caries development	Cover use of toothbrush and dentifrice; demonstrate positioning for brushing	Review and update fluoride dosage and vehicle and ask about compliance problems; check for changes in diet related to fluoride; discuss toxicity and storage issues	Trauma-proofing and signs and management of trauma; confirm emergency access to dental provider	Oral signs of child abuse
18 months	Review anticipated tooth eruption for next 6 months	Cover nutrition and snacking based on child's diet; discuss snacking safety (aspiration)	Ask about problems with child's compliance with oral hygiene procedures	Review and update fluoride status	Discuss oral electrical burns and child-proofing home	Child's normal reaction to a dental visit at this age
2 years	Review occlusion and related concepts of crowding, spacing and space loss, overbite and overjet		Discuss need for parental assistance in oral hygiene; ask about problems	Review fluoride adequacy		Day care instructions for dental emergencies
3 years	Point out that primary dentition is complete; review occlusal wear and bruxing of teeth			Review fluoride status		Separation anxiety at dental visits; role of radiographs in caries diagnosis
4 years					Discuss bike safety	Thumb- and digit-sucking; expected behavior at dental visits
5 years	Exfoliation of teeth; eruption patterns and problems that may occur	Snacking at school			Be sure trauma management plan available at school	Digit-sucking abatement if a problem
6 years	Pivotal nature of 6-year molars; occlusion; orthodontics in scope of child's health; gingival and periodontal disease		Sealants; technique and methods of flossing	Be sure of fluoride availability at school; ask about rinses if supplemental fluoride is needed	Sports safety and mouthguards; review tooth transport media for avulsion	Role of dental caries (pain, lost days to treatment and illness) in school performance

Box continued on following page

Anticipatory Guidance *continued*

Age	Discussion of Developmental Milestone	Nutrition and Feeding Information	Discussion of Oral Hygiene and Caries Prevention Techniques	Fluoride Information	Trauma Prevention Information	Discussion of Habits and Function, Behaviors, and Problems
8 years	"Ugly duckling" stage of development		Weaning child from direct parental supervision of oral hygiene and moving into a periodic intervention and assessment role			
10 years	Cover remaining stages of dental development; talk about facial growth and changes in appearance	Snacking and increased energy needs as they relate to dental health	Sealants for the second molars	Review fluoride status and need for systemics and topicals		Substance abuse and its effect on oral and general health; talk about hormones and their effect on the oral cavity
12 years			Child becomes responsible for own oral hygiene			Consider visits alone as a teenager; encourage knowledge of dental and general health history by the adolescent patient
16 years	Third molars, their development and function					Adolescent's knowledge of oral health issues with emphasis on his or her awareness of long-term consequences of disease
18 years	Generational changes in dentition; TMD					Need for regular visits; review irreversible periodontal disease

From Nowak A, Casamassimo P: Using anticipatory guidance to provide early dental intervention. JADA *126*:1156–1163, 1995.

CLINICAL IMPLICATIONS OF PRETERM AND LOW-BIRTH-WEIGHT INFANTS

Preterm births (gestational age under 37 weeks) account for 7% to 10% of all live births. Prematurely born infants are subjected to a variety of metabolic stresses and exhibit a higher prevalence of oral-dental disturbances than normal full-term infants. Factors such as metabolic disorders, hypoxia, prolonged neonatal jaundice, nutritional deficiencies, and low serum calcium levels have been implicated as causes of the enamel hypoplasia and other mineralization defects in the primary incisors of preterm infants. Preterm, low-birth-weight (LBW) infants appear to have the highest correlation (40%) with enamel hypoplasia and opacities in the primary dentition. Infants weighing less than 2500 g are considered to have a low birth weight. Current evidence suggests that enamel hypoplasias, opacities, and other mineralization defects result from neonatal hypocalcemia during the enamel mineralization process (Melander et al., 1982).

Further evidence has demonstrated a correlation between decreased breast milk intake in LBW infants and enamel hypoplasia, opacities, and other mineralization defects. There is a remarkable association between enamel hypoplasia and mineralization defects in infants with respiratory distress, who also exhibit the least amount of breast milk intake, which is believed to contribute further to the degree of neonatal hypocalcemia.

In addition to transient neonatal hypocalcemia and enamel mineralization defects, preterm infants are more susceptible to the development of abnormalities associated with laryngoscopy and intubation. Traumatic injury caused by laryngoscopy and endotracheal intubation at the critical period of amelogenesis appears to contribute to defects in the primary dentition of LBW infants in whom dental development is already compromised by disturbances in calcium metabolism. Intubated LBW infants exhibit a fourfold increase in primary incisor defects, which occur in approximately 85% of cases. Nearly two thirds of the maxillary incisors affected are located to the left of the midline, corresponding to the greater prevalence of right-handed intubation techniques (Seow et al., 1984).

In addition to injury to the developing incisors during the intubation procedure, prolonged orotracheal intubation of infants is associated with airway damage, palatal groove formation, defective primary incisors, and acquired cleft palate

(Duke et al., 1976). In 1984, Erenberg and Nowak reported a 47.6% incidence of palatal or alveolar ridge groove formation after orotracheal intubation of preterm LBW infants for a period of 1 to 62 days (Erenberg and Nowak, 1984b). They also noted that the incidence of palatal groove formation increased to 87.5% in infants who were intubated for 15 days or more. To help prevent the complications associated with prolonged orotracheal intubation, Nowak and Erenberg developed an intraoral palatal stabilizing appliance to secure the orogastric and orotracheal tubes (Erenberg and Nowak, 1984a). Because they noticed that palatal abnormalities begin to develop as early as 12 hours after intubation, Erenberg and Nowak recommend consideration of a stabilizer for infants who will be intubated for more than 24 hours.

In addition to localized orofacial effects of the intubation process in LBW infants, systemic complications have also been identified. Approximately 30% of LBW infants experience respiratory distress syndrome, and of those infants, 16% develop bronchopulmonary dysplasia (BPD), a chronic lung disease (Koops et al., 1984). BPD places these infants at high risk for respiratory infections, increased airway resistance, and recurrent wheezing, all of which pose potential problems for the child in the dental office.

It is important for the dentist to be aware of the clinical dental implications of preterm LBW infants in order to offer their parents an explanation of the likely causes of any anomalies that may be present (Fadavi et al., 1992). In addition, the dentist may be in a position to act as a resource for information regarding potential dental sequelae in preterm LBW infants or to assist in preventing oral adverse sequelae to prolonged intubation of these infants.

REFERENCES

AAPD: Infant oral health care. Pediatr Dent *19*:70-72, 1997.
Anderson TA, Fomon SJ, Wei SHY: Nutrition counseling and the development of eating habits. *In* Sweeney EA (ed): The Food That Stays: An Update on Nutrition, Diet, Sugar, and Caries. New York, Medcom, 1977, pp 22-27.
Canady JWJ, Thompson S, Bardack J: Oral commissure burns in children. Plast Reconstr Surg *97*:738-744, 1996.
Czerepak CS: Oral splint therapy to manage electrical burns of the mouth of children. Clin Plast Surg *11*(4):685, 1984.
Duke PM, Caulson JD, Santos JI, et al: Cleft palate associated with prolonged orotracheal intubation in infancy. J Pediatr *89*:990, 1976.
Erenberg A, Nowak AJ: Appliance for stabilizing orogastric and orotracheal tubes in infants. Crit Care Med *12*(8):669, 1984a.
Erenberg A, Nowak AJ: Palatal groove formation in neonates

and infants with orotracheal tubes. Am J Dis Child *138:*974, 1984b.

Fadavi S, Adeni S, Dziedzic K, et al: The oral effects of orotracheal intubation in prematurely born children. J Dent Child 59:420–424, 1992.

Goepferd SJ: Infant oral health: A rationale. J Dent Child 53(4):257, 1986a.

Goepferd SJ: Infant oral health: A protocol. J Dent Child 53(4):261, 1986b.

Holt GR, Parel S, Richardson DS, Kittle PE: The prosthetic management of oral commissure burns. Laryngoscope *92:*407, 1982.

Josell SD, Owen D, Kreutzer LW, Goldberg NH: Extraoral management for electrical burns of the mouth. J Dent Child 51(1):47, 1984.

Kaste LM, Selwitz RH, et al: Coronal caries in the primary and permanent dentition of children and adolescents 1–17 years of age: United States, 1988–1991. J Dent Res 75(Spec Iss):631–641, 1996.

Koops BL, Abman SH, Accurso FJ: Outpatient management and follow-up of bronchopulmonary dysplasia. Clin Perinatol *11*(1):101, 1984.

Melander M, Noren JG, Freden H, Kjellmer I: Mineralization defects in deciduous teeth of low birthweight infants. Acta Paediatr Scand *71:*727, 1982.

National Institute of Dental Research (NIDR): Oral Health of United States Children: National and Regional Findings, 1986–1987. NIH Pub. No. 89-2247. Bethesda, MD, National Institutes of Health, September 1989.

Nowak A: Rationale for the timing of the first oral evaluation. Pediatr Dent *19:*8–11, 1997.

Seow WK, Brown JP, Tudehope DI, O'Callaghan M: Developmental defects in the primary dentition of low-birth-weight infants: Adverse effects of laryngoscopy and prolonged endotracheal intubation. Pediatr Dent 6(1):28, 1984.

Silvergrade D, Zacher JB, Ruberg RL: Improved splinting of oral commissure burns: Results in 21 consecutive patients. Ann Plast Surg 9(4):316, 1982.

Swain FR, Pinkham JR: Treatment of lip commissure burns with a commissural stabilizing splint. Quintessence Int 8:789, 1983.

14

Prevention of Dental Disease

Arthur Nowak and James Crall

Chapter Outline

Dental caries and periodontal diseases have been reported to be among the most common bacterial diseases affecting humans. Even though substantial reductions in the levels and severity of these diseases and their sequelae have been reported in most Western nations, millions of children and adults continue to experience caries, periodontal disease, tooth loss, and malocclusions—most of which could be prevented if only they engaged in daily oral hygiene practices, had optimal systemic and topical fluorides, and sought professional care on a scheduled basis. Dental diseases and their sequelae are largely preventable!

The goal of this chapter is to provide clinicians with a plan—a plan that can help infants, children, and young adults to be free from oral disease. The plan involves many participants—not only dental personnel but also children, their parents, and anyone interested and responsible for a child's health and well-being. The plan begins shortly after conception, prior to the initiation of oral disease, and it never ends. It never ends because the mouth and its components with appropriate care can remain healthy for a lifetime.

The mouth plays a major role in the life of a human being. All nutrients must pass through it; expressions of happiness and sadness are developed from the actions of the lips and cheeks; sounds and later speech are produced by the activity of the tongue, lips, and cheeks. Therefore, a healthy mouth with a full complement of teeth, supported by healthy gingiva and bone and having a balanced and stable occlusion, is a goal that we should all promote and seek to achieve for the patients under our care.

PRENATAL COUNSELING

Since the beginning of the twentieth century, the medical profession has recognized the importance of providing prenatal counseling and care to expectant mothers. Through these efforts, infant morbidity and mortality have been greatly reduced. Only recently has the dental profession become involved in this primary preventive effort.

The most common setting for prenatal counseling is in conjunction with programs conducted in community hospitals or neighborhood health centers. Programs also have been developed for office-based settings. Regardless of where the program is conducted, close collaboration among members of the various health professions and community support groups (e.g., dentists, physicians, nurses, nutritionists, social workers) is important to ensure appropriate scheduling of presentations and reinforcement of concepts.

Although many oral health counseling programs have been developed in recent years, the goals of the programs are similar (Table 14–1). Depending on the setting, the time allotted, and staff availability, the program should be individualized to the greatest extent possible and should provide parents with information about the development of oral structures and functions, dental disease processes, and recommended preventive measures. In addition, the program should provide information on the importance of the mother's diet during pregnancy, including the effects of drugs, tobacco, and alcohol, the impor-

TABLE 14–1. A Model of Prenatal Counseling

Purpose

To educate parents about dental development of the child
To educate parents about dental disease and prevention
To provide a suitable environment for the child
To strengthen and prepare the child and dentition for life

Methods

Education concerning development, prevention, and disease
Demonstration of oral hygiene procedures
Counseling to instill preventive attitudes and motivation
Evaluation of learning, acceptance, and needs

Content

External Component (Parents)

Parents' education concerning dental disease and oral hygiene
Parents' motivation for plaque removal program
Changes in mother's oral health
Intake of sweets
Pregnancy gingivitis
Myths and misconceptions about pregnancy and dentition
Parents' dental treatment

Internal Component (Parents and Child)

Parents' education—development of child
Effect of lifestyle on child
Habits (smoking, alcohol consumption)
Intake of sweets
Exposure to disease (e.g., rubella, syphilis)
Effect of drugs on child—e.g., tetracyclines
Nutrition
Calcium
Vitamins
Fluorides
Essential nutrients
Child's needs after birth
Breast feeding versus bottle feeding
Fluoride supplementation
Teething
Hygiene
Non-nutritive sucking
First visit

TABLE 14–2. Dental Treatment for Women During Pregnancy

First Trimester

Consult with woman's physician*
Emergency treatment only

Second Trimester

Elective and emergency treatment
Radiographs can be used with adequate protection

Third Trimester

Emergency treatment only
Avoid supine position
Radiographs can be used with adequate protection

Throughout Pregnancy

Plaque control program for mother and father of child
Local anesthetic is anesthetic of choice
Avoid the use of drugs if at all possible. If drugs are necessary, use only those proved safe for use during pregnancy and use in consultation with a physician
The use of a general anesthetic for dental treatment during pregnancy is contraindicated

---

*The first trimester is most crucial; however, in these litigious times it would probably be good to consult with the woman's physician during the last two trimesters, especially if there is a major problem.

tance of maternal oral health care during pregnancy, and recommended scheduling of dental treatment (Table 14-2).

During prenatal counseling, teething should be mentioned because it most likely will be the first oral event that parents have to deal with. Although the timing of eruption of teeth can usually be predicted, its occurrence frequently surprises new parents, and if the infant experiences difficulties it can create parental anxiety. Teething is a natural phenomenon that usually occurs with no problems. Nevertheless, some infants exhibit signs of systemic distress, including a rise in temperature, diarrhea, dehydration, increased salivation, skin eruptions, and gastrointestinal disturbances (Honig, 1975). Lancing of tissues is usually not indicated. Increased fluid consumption, a nonaspirin analgesic, and palliative care consisting of teething rings to apply cold and pressure to the affected areas generally reduce the symptoms and result in a happier infant (King, 1994). If symptoms persist for more than 24 hours, the infant should be examined by a physician to rule out upper respiratory infection and other common diseases and conditions of infancy.

Prenatal counseling programs also should provide guidelines for the parents about the timing of the first professional dental visit. Historically, asymptomatic children were scheduled for their first dental examination between 3 and 5 years of age. More recently, programs designed to provide comprehensive preventive measures have stressed the importance of initiating professional visits at an earlier age, at or shortly after the time of the eruption of teeth (Nowak, 1997).

Bright Futures—Guidelines for Health Supervision of Infants, Children, and Adolescents (Green, 1994) is a comprehensive and practical resource designed to assist health professionals and families to more effectively promote the health and well-being of all children and adolescents. It recommends an initial dental appointment at around 12 months of age to assess the infant's risk for dental disease, complete a clinical examination, provide anticipatory guidance information, and schedule a follow-up appointment (Nowak and Casamassimo, 1995).

Another innovation in designing preventive programs centers around the concept of risk assessment. The assessing of the child's risk by the dentist allows the practitioner to individualize oral health supervision. All children are not equally affected by dental disease. By determining risk factors, the dentist can individualize a preventive plan with protective factors that promote oral health. Risk factors can change over time. Therefore, the dentist must assess the status periodically and make appropriate modifications (Casamassimo, 1996).

Factors that place the infant at higher risk for dental disease include the following:

1. High-risk pregnancy or complicated delivery
2. Presence of congenital or hereditary defects or developmental disabilities
3. Absence of optimal fluoride therapy
4. Family history of severe to moderate dental disease
5. Presence of feeding disorders (e.g., prolonged use of nursing bottles)
6. High levels of salivary *Streptococcus mutans* (Edelstein and Tinanoff, 1989)
7. Social, ethnic, cultural, and environmental factors (e.g., single-parent households; barriers to access to dental treatment)
8. Low parental interest or involvement in preventive measures

Recommendations for the first dental examination and to establish a "dental home" include the following (Table 14–3):

1. Immediate referral for infants with an apparent dental problem due to trauma, disease, or developmental abnormality
2. Examination at no later than 6 months after eruption of the first tooth for infants at high risk for dental disease
3. Examination at no later than 18 months for infants not at high risk for dental disease

FLUORIDE ADMINISTRATION

Rationale

Significant reductions in the prevalence of dental caries in children were documented in the United States and other countries during the 1990s (Kaste et al., 1996). Although the exact reasons for this decline are unknown, most experts include increased availability of fluorides as one of the primary contributing factors. In spite of these advances, caries remains a relatively common yet largely preventable disease of childhood. Because of the importance of fluoride in this regard, the contemporary dental practitioner should understand the basis for using the many available forms of fluoride.

Mechanisms of Action

Although the precise mechanisms by which fluorides act to prevent dental caries are not fully understood, three general mechanisms are typically considered to be involved. These include (1) increased resistance of the tooth structure to demineralization, (2) enhancement of the process of remineralization, and (3) reduction of the cariogenic potential of dental plaque.

The effects of fluoride are usually classified as either systemic or topical. Systemic effects can be obtained through the ingestion of foods that contain natural levels of fluoride, water that contains natural fluoride or to which fluoride has been added, dietary fluoride supplements, and some forms of fluoride mouth rinses that are meant to be swallowed (most fluoride rinses are intended for topical application only). Topical benefits are available from the previously mentioned sources as a result of their contact with the teeth as well as from fluoride toothpastes and other more concentrated forms that are self-administered or applied professionally.

The indications for administering the various forms of fluoride primarily depend on the age of the child, his or her caries history and perceived susceptibility to develop caries in the future, and whether he or she drinks fluoridated water. For children in the birth-to-age-3 category, the principal concern is that they receive an optimal level of systemic fluoride.

Systemic Fluorides

WATER FLUORIDATION

Water fluoridation remains the cornerstone of any sound caries prevention program. It is not

Dental Home

Arthur Nowak

All infants and toddlers should have a place where they can receive the appropriate health care provided by physicians, dentists, and other allied health professionals. The facility should be accessible, the services comprehensive, and the environment pediatric-oriented. The health provider should know the child and parent and should have established a level of trust and responsibility with the family for optimal cooperation and communications. Most parents have this environment established early for their infants and toddlers because of the Preventive Pediatric Health Care Guidelines established by the American Academy of Pediatrics. To compliment the medical "home," all infants and toddlers should have a dental home. The dental home should be able to provide all of the following services:

1. Schedule early dental visits at approximately 12 to 18 months of age
2. Assess the risk of the infant and toddler for future dental disease
3. Evaluate the fluoride status of the infant and make appropriate recommendations
4. Demonstrate to caretakers the appropriate method for cleaning teeth
5. Discuss the advantages/disadvantages of non-nutritive sucking
6. Be prepared to treat the infant/toddler if early childhood caries is diagnosed or to make the appropriate referral
7. Be available 24 hours a day, 7 days a week to deal with any acute dental problem
8. Be able to recognize the need for specialty consultation and referrals

Whether this dental home is located in a private practice, a community health center, or at the neighborhood hospital, it should be supervised by dentists who are well trained in primary care. Ideally, it should be a pediatric dentist, but not all communities can support a pediatric dentist.

By establishing a dental home early, parents will be appropriately counseled during the early years of the child's life and have a facility to immediately contact in case of orofacial traumatic injuries. The initial infant oral examination not only initiates the preventive oral health care process but supports the concept of the dental home. The time has come for us to join with our colleagues in medicine so that all children have both a medical and a dental home for all their health needs.

BIBLIOGRAPHY

American Academy of Pediatrics: The medical home. Pediatrics *90*:774, 1992.

only the most effective means of reducing caries, it is also the most cost-effective, most convenient, and most reliable method of providing the benefits of fluoride to the population because it does not depend on individual compliance. Historically, studies have documented caries reductions of 40% to 50% in the primary dentition and 50% to 65% in the permanent dentition of children drinking fluoridated water from birth (U.S. Department of Health, Education, and Welfare, 1979). Recent studies have reported on the effects of water fluoridation on caries reduction. The mean DMFS of children with continuous residence in fluoridated areas was about 18% lower than that of children with no exposure. When corrected to remove children that have been exposed to topical or supplemental fluorides, the mean DMFS was 25% lower in the

TABLE 14–3. Recommendations for Preventive Pediatric Dental Care

Because each child is unique, these Recommendations are designed for the care of children who have no important health problems and are developing normally. These Recommendations will need to be modified for children with special health care needs or if disease or trauma manifests variations from normal. The Academy emphasizes the importance of very early professional intervention and the continuity of care based on the individualized needs of the child.

Age[1]	Infancy 6–12 Months	Late Infancy 12–24 Months	Preschool 2–6 Years	School Age 6–12 Years	Adolescence 12–21 Years
Oral hygiene counseling[2]	Parents/ guardians/ caregivers	Parents/ guardians/ caregivers	Child/parent/ caregivers	Child/parent/ caregivers	Patient
Injury prevention counseling[3]	•	•	•	•	•
Dietary counseling[4]	•	•	•	•	•
Counseling for non-nutritive habits[5]	•	•	•		
Fluoride supplementation[6]	•	•	•	•	
Assess oral growth and development[7]	•	•	•	•	•
Clinical oral examination	•	•	•	•	•
Prophylaxis and topical fluoride treatment[8]		•	•	•	•
Radiographic assessment[9]			•	•	•
Pit and fissure sealants			If indicated on primary molars	First permanent molars as soon as possible after eruption	Second permanent molars as soon as possible after eruption
Treatment of dental disease or injury	•	•	•	•	•
Assessment and treatment of developing malocclusion			•	•	•
Substance abuse counseling				•	•
Assessment and removal of 3rd molars					•
Referral for regular and periodic dental care					•
Anticipatory guidance[10]	•	•	•	•	•

[1]First examination at the eruption of the first tooth and no later than 12–18 months.
[2]Initially, responsibility of parent; as child develops, jointly with parents; then when indicated only child.
[3]Initially play objects, pacifiers, car seats; then when learning to walk; and finally sports and routine playing.
[4]At every appointment discuss the role of refined carbohydrates; frequency of snacking.
[5]At first discuss the need for additional sucking; digits vs. pacifiers; then the need to wean from the habit before the eruption of the first permanent front teeth.
[6]As per AAP/ADA *Guidelines* and the water source.
[7]By clinical examination.
[8]Especially for children at high risk for caries and periodontal disease.
[9]As per AAPD Radiographic Guidelines.
[10]Appropriate discussion and counseling should be an integral part of each visit for care.
Reference Manual 1998–1999. American Academy of Pediatric Dentistry. Chicago, 1998. *In* Pediatr Dent *20*:73, 1998.

group exposed continuously to water fluoridation (Brunelle and Carlos, 1990).

Over 50% of the U.S. population currently has access to drinking water containing a significant level of fluoride (>0.7 parts per million). Many of these water supplies contain significant levels of natural fluoride, especially in the midwestern and southwestern sections of the country. Numerous fluoride-deficient community water supplies have been artificially fluoridated at a cost of less than $0.50 per person, depending on the size of the community.

As part of their responsibility in promoting oral health, dentists have the obligation to educate the public about the effectiveness and safety of this proven preventive measure. Involvement at the local level in support of water fluoridation can be one of the major contributions a dentist can make to enhancing the oral health of all children in his or her community.

DIETARY FLUORIDE SUPPLEMENTS

Fluoride supplements provide an alternative source of dietary fluoride for children who do not have access to optimally fluoridated water. Included in this category are children whose public or private water supplies are fluoride-deficient as well as persons who reside in communities with fluoridated water but do not rely on optimally fluoridated water for their primary source of fluid intake.

Dentists also should be aware that, even in areas where the water contains adequate amounts of fluoride, some children may derive substantially less than the average amount of fluid intake from traditional drinking water sources. For example, the use of bottled and processed waters for drinking and cooking has become popular in many communities. Consumers are turning to these water sources as alternatives to tap water that is believed to be contaminated with microorganisms, pesticides, herbicides, industrial waste, and heavy metals. The fluoride content of these bottled waters generally has been found to exhibit wide variability, usually below optimal concentrations (Flaitz et al., 1989; Nowak and Nowak, 1989; Stannard et al., 1990; Tate et al., 1990). Regulations presently do not require bottled water manufacturers to list the fluoride concentration on the label. Hence, dentists need to be aware of the bottled water products readily available in their community and be prepared to obtain fluoride analyses when necessary. Furthermore, all parents, including those who reside in fluoridated areas, should be questioned about the sources of fluid in their

infant's diet and should realize that fluoride supplements are advisable for children who consume very little fluoridated water.

Supplements can be as effective as fluoridated water in preventing caries (Driscoll, 1974; Hargreaves, 1990; Thylstrup, 1990); however, their effectiveness depends largely on the degree of parental compliance. Supplements are commercially available in liquid and tablet forms, both with and without vitamins. The fluoride-vitamin formulations are not inherently superior to supplements without vitamins in terms of reducing caries. The combination of fluoride and vitamins, however, may improve parental compliance, thereby providing greater benefits (Hennon et al., 1966).

Liquid preparations are recommended for younger patients who may have difficulty in chewing or swallowing tablets. Liquid supplements without vitamins are dispensed in preparations that provide a dose of 0.5 mg/ml; liquid supplements with vitamins are dispensed in preparations that provide 0.25 mg/ml and 0.5 mg/ml. Fluoride supplements in tablet form for older patients are available without vitamins in doses of 0.25, 0.5, and 1.0 mg of fluoride, and fluoride-vitamin combinations are available in 0.5- and 1.0-mg doses.

In order to obtain both topical and systemic effects, fluoride supplements should be allowed to contact the teeth prior to being swallowed. With liquid preparations, this can be achieved by placing the drops directly on the child's teeth or by placing the drops in the child's food or drink, although the latter practice may reduce the bioavailability of the fluoride. Older children should be encouraged to "chew and swish" their tablets or allow the tablets to dissolve in the mouth before swallowing to prolong the contact of the fluoride with the outer surfaces of the teeth.

The dosage of fluoride that should be prescribed depends on the age of the child and the fluoride concentration of his or her drinking water. The fluoride concentration of a central community water supply can be determined by contacting the local or state department of health or the local water authority. For persons who do not obtain their drinking water from a central supply, water samples should be tested for fluoride content. This service usually is provided by state health departments, schools of dentistry, or commercially (Omni FluoriCheck Water Analysis Kits, 1-800-445-3386). Alternatively, in-office analyses of water fluoride concentrations can be performed using a relatively inexpensive hand-held colorimeter (e.g., Hach DR 100 Colorimeter, Hach Co., Loveland, CO). Although not as precise as more expensive fluoride electrodes, comparisons have shown that colorimetric assays closely correlate with electrode findings and generally result in comparable supplementation recommendations (Edelstein et al., 1992). When results of electrode findings and colorimetric assays differ, corresponding supplementation recommendations based on colorimetery tend to be lower, thereby minimizing the potential for adverse outcomes (e.g., fluorosis). Because of the potential for considerable variations in fluoride levels in water obtained from different wells in the same area, it is important that each individual noncentral water source be sampled to determine accurately the appropriate level of fluoride supplementation for each patient.

Table 14-4 shows the daily dosage schedule for fluoride supplementation that has been recommended by the American Dental Association and the American Academy of Pediatrics since 1994 (American Dental Association, 1994).

Observations that the increased prevalence of fluorosis has been significantly less in optimally fluoridated areas suggest that additional exposure to traditional sources of ingested fluoride does not seem to be a major etiologic factor. That conclusion is further supported by studies suggesting that fluoride ingestion from dietary sources has remained relatively constant since the 1950s (Pendrys and Stamm, 1990). Notable exceptions in the pediatric population include a lowering of fluoride concentration in most infant formulas (Johnson and Bawden, 1987) and increased availability of fluoridated beverages in nonfluoridated areas (e.g., soft drinks prepared with fluoridated water) (Clovis and Hargreaves, 1988). This latter phenomenon has been called the "halo effect," reflecting the concept of extended water fluoridation benefits beyond fluoridated communities.

The fluoride in most dietary supplements is incorporated as sodium fluoride (NaF). One milligram of fluoride is equivalent to approximately

TABLE 14–5. Sample Supplemental Fluoride Prescriptions

Eight-month-old whose drinking water contains <0.1 ppm fluoride:
Rx: Sodium fluoride solution 0.5 mg/ml (0.25 mg F⁻)
Disp: 50 ml
Sig: Dispense 0.5 ml of liquid in mouth before bedtime

Three-year-old whose drinking water contains 0.2 ppm fluoride:
Rx: Sodium fluoride tablets 0.25 mg fluoride/tablet (0.55 mg NaF/tablet)
Disp: 180 tablets
Sig: Chew one (1) tablet, swish and swallow after brushing at bedtime. Nothing per os (NPO) for 30 minutes.

2.2 mg of sodium fluoride. When prescribing fluoride supplements, the practitioner should clearly specify the dosage that is to be dispensed in terms of fluoride ion, sodium fluoride, or both. Examples of prescriptions for dietary fluoride supplements are given in Table 14-5.

Because it is common for infants and children to experience several contacts with a physician prior to their first dental visit, dentists providing treatment for children should become aware of the prescribing practices of local physicians and be prepared to offer advice about appropriate fluoride supplementation. In addition, dentists can provide input into local prenatal care programs so that expectant parents can be made aware of the benefits and appropriate use of fluorides.

Prescribing systemic fluorides during pregnancy to benefit the developing teeth was once a common practice in the United States. In 1966, however, the U.S. Food and Drug Administration (FDA) banned the promotion of prenatal fluoride supplements in the United States. Safety was not the overriding issue in this decision. Rather, the decision was based on a lack of evidence about the effectiveness of prenatal fluoride supplements in preventing caries in offspring. Data from human studies suggest that the placenta is not an effective barrier to the passage of fluoride to the fetus and that there is a direct relationship between the serum fluoride concentrations of the mother and the fetus (Ekstrand and Whitford, 1988; Shen and Taves, 1974).

A study reported that 5-year-olds whose mothers were provided 1 mg of fluoride daily during prenatal months 4-9 had no statistically significant differences in their caries status than the control group. In addition, the prevalence of very mild fluorosis was low. Therefore, to date, there continues to be little support for prenatal fluoride supplementation (Leverett et al., 1997).

TABLE 14–4. Supplemental Fluoride Dosage Schedule

Age	Concentration of Fluoride in Water		
	<0.3 ppm F	*0.3–0.6 ppm F*	*>0.6 ppm F*
Birth–6 mos	0	0	0
6 mos–3 yrs	0.25 mg	0	0
3 yrs–6 yrs	0.50 mg	0.25 mg	0
6 yrs up to at least 16 yrs	1.00 mg	0.50 mg	0

Issues Involving Fluoride Supplementation

James Bawden

Numerous clinical studies have shown that fluoride supplements (solution and tablets) are effective in preventing dental caries. Such supplements are intended for children who do not have regular access to optimally fluoridated water. They are used widely in the United States, Canada, and some European countries.

In recent years, several issues concerning the use of supplements have been raised. Particular attention has been directed to the guidelines for prescribing supplements currently in use in the United States. These concerns have been expressed in response to documentation that patterns of systemic fluoride intake have changed since the 1980s. The most definitive evidence in that regard is found in studies that show that the prevalence and severity of fluorosis have increased significantly since then. The dose-response relationship between fluoride ingestion and fluorosis has been established. Although most cases of fluorosis are still in the very mild and mild categories and it is not an esthetic problem, a continuing increase in prevalence and severity could cause it to become a matter of public concern and pose a threat to the continued use of systemic fluorides as a major weapon in the prevention of caries. Reports indicate that there are population "pockets" where occurrence of the more severe forms of fluorosis has reached levels of public and professional concern. Studies show that the use of supplements is one of the factors associated with an increased risk of fluorosis. Consequently, authorities in fluoride research and clinical use are seeking means by which the risk of fluorosis can be minimized while the caries-preventive effectiveness of fluoride supplements is maintained. What are the issues involved?

A major problem is that in clinical trials, fluorosis is scored 6 or more years after the biologic response to systemic exposure has occurred. By the time the data are analyzed and published, another year or two has passed. Using the most recently published findings on fluorosis, one can draw conclusions about shifts in systemic exposure that occurred only into the early 1980s. It is not possible to know whether the aspects of exposure that were responsible for increases in fluorosis have intensified, leveled off, or declined in the 1990s. We must turn to other sources of information and make the best judgments possible.

The original supplement dosage schedule was formulated on the assumption that children not drinking fluoridated water consume an insignificant amount of fluoride from fluids. In the late 1970s it became apparent that some infant formulas and baby foods contained relatively high concentrations of fluoride. In response, the supplement schedule was modified by reducing the daily dose from birth to 2 years of age from 0.5 to 0.25 mg. Studies conducted in the mid-1980s showed that fluoride concentrations in formulas had been reduced and are apparently well controlled. The most recent fluorosis data do not tell us whether the changes made in the supplement dosage schedule and the fluoride content of formulas had a significant impact on controlling fluorosis. The time elapsed since the changes in exposure has not been quite long enough to be reflected in the most recent fluorosis studies. In addition, other changes have been made in systemic fluoride exposure that make it difficult to isolate the effect of a single variable.

A major change in fluoride exposure has been brought about by the "halo effect" associated with the fluoridation of municipal water supplies. Many beverages and foods are processed using fluoridated water, and these are distributed to and consumed by children in nonfluoridated areas. A recent nationwide caries study showed that the difference in caries prevalence between nonfluoridated and fluoridated populations is much less than that reported in the original studies by Dean and others. The wide use of topical fluorides is obviously a factor responsible for this change, but the halo effect has apparently had an impact as well. That effect is suggested by the observation that the differences in caries prevalence between nonfluoridated and fluoridated populations are less in regions where water fluoridation is most extensive. In a recent study it was estimated that the mean daily fluoride intake from beverages in a sample of children 2 and 3 years of age was 0.3 mg. The actual impact of the halo effect on fluorosis prevalence is unknown and will be difficult to isolate.

The extensive use of fluoridated dentifrice by young children has introduced an additional source of fluoride ingestion. Studies indicate that significant daily doses of fluoride (0.25 mg) may be ingested from this source. Evidence continues to accumulate associating increased fluorosis prevalence and severity with the use of fluoridated dentifrice at an early age.

If the child's drinking water contains a significant concentration of naturally occurring fluoride, a reduction in the daily supplement dose is indicated. Published reports indicate that most prescriptions for supplements are issued without assaying the home or other contributing water supplies, however. It is also apparent that some dental and medical practitioners are using the original, outdated dose schedule and that some supplements are prescribed for children who are drinking optimally fluoridated water. The extent to which these problems contribute to the general increase in fluorosis is not known.

Children often drink significant amounts of water from more than one source. These sources may contain different fluoride concentrations, which often require adjustment in the supplement dose. The extent to which failure to consider such circumstances leads to supplement overdoses and subsequent fluorosis is not known and would be difficult to determine.

These circumstances have precipitated considerable discussion about the use of fluoride supplements in the United States. Some authorities have questioned whether supplements are needed at all in the presence of declining caries rates and the risk of fluorosis involved. An international workshop report on the use of systemic and topical fluorides, however, agreed that supplements can be of use in certain populations and that they should be used when the child's fluoride intake is less than optimal. The practitioner must be thorough and use good judgment in making that determination. The major issue concerns whether or not the dose schedule should be changed and, if so, in what manner. Uncertainty about the extent to which the circumstances described are individually and collectively responsible for increased fluorosis prevalence and severity has sparked vigorous debate. There is also disagreement about the extent to which these factors can be controlled or corrected.

Fortunately, important progress has been made in our understanding of the biologic mechanisms responsible for fluorosis and their timing. Although there is still much to be learned, some reasonable hypotheses concerning biologic mechanisms have been advanced and are supported by encouraging data. Of most importance are recent epidemiologic studies that indicate clearly that the most sensitive age for inducing fluorosis in the maxillary incisors of the typical child is 22 to 26 months or, at the outer extremes, 18 to 30 months of age.

As in most dimensions of biomedical science, many questions about fluoride supplements cannot be answered using the data available now. Additional studies are urgently needed. The findings will contribute importantly to our understanding and ability to resolve some of the current issues. But some of the questions may never be answered because the required studies are technically impossible to implement or are prohibitively expensive to conduct. The only certainty is that scientific discussion about supplements will continue and that our ability to use them in the most effective and safe manner will improve.

Topical Fluorides

The regular use of a fluoride-containing tooth-paste applied by the parent usually constitutes the only topical application of fluoride in children up to age 3. Children whose teeth contain structural defects or exhibit decalcified areas that are thought to place them at high risk for developing caries, or infants who have previously experienced severe caries (e.g., early childhood caries) may receive additional topical applications in the form of a professionally applied or parentally applied concentrated preparation.

Regardless of whether a toothpaste or a more concentrated form of fluoride is applied, care should be taken to minimize the amount that is used and swallowed. Parents should place only a small dab of dentifrice on the brush and always supervise the brushing session so that the dentifrice and saliva are expectorated.

Examples of concentrated agents for topical application in the home include a 0.5% acidulated phosphate fluoride (APF) and a 0.4% stannous fluoride (SnF_2) gel. SnF_2 gels might be more appropriate for younger children because a 0.4% SnF_2 preparation is only approximately one fourth as concentrated as 0.5% APF. A small amount of the gel should be brushed on the child's teeth daily before bedtime. The child should be encouraged to expectorate following the application but should not be allowed to eat or drink for approximately 30 minutes. Table 14–6 gives a sample prescription for a topical gel intended for home use.

Safety and Toxicity

When used properly, the various forms of fluoride can enhance the oral health status of infants and children. As is true of many other substances, however, when used improperly these same agents have the potential to produce objectionable side effects. Therefore, each member of the dental profession has a responsibility to educate his or her patients about the appropriate storage and administration of these products.

Acute toxicity can result from the accidental ingestion of excessive amounts of fluoride. Acute fluoride toxicity usually produces manifestations that are limited to nausea and vomiting but has on at least one occasion been associated with the death of a child. The amount of ingested fluoride necessary to produce acute symptoms is directly related to the weight of the individual; therefore, precautions should be employed to prevent the accidental ingestion of concentrated forms of fluoride by all children but especially by very young children and infants. The lethal dose of fluoride for a typical 3-year-old child is approximately 500 mg and would be proportionately less for a younger and smaller child.

To avoid the possibility of ingestion of large amounts of fluoride it is recommended that no more than 120 mg of supplemental fluoride be prescribed at any one time (American Academy of Pediatric Dentistry, 1997). Likewise, prescriptions for concentrated topical fluoride preparations intended for home use (e.g., 0.5% fluoride gels that contain 5 mg of fluoride/ml) should be limited to 30–40 ml. Ingestion of moderate volumes of fluoride mouth rinses and toothpastes containing (less than or equal to) 1 mg of fluoride/ml would not be expected to cause severe symptoms, although nausea and vomiting could result.

Parents should be encouraged to store these and all potentially harmful substances out of the reach of small children. Should excessive amounts of fluoride be ingested, vomiting should be induced as quickly as possible following the incident. This can be accomplished by administering 15 ml of Ipecac Syrup (Eli Lilly, Indianapolis, IN) with 6 oz of water for children. If vomiting does not occur within 20 minutes, another dose of Ipecac Syrup should be given. The patient should be referred to a poison control center as soon as possible, where stomach pumping may be considered. The absorption of fluoride can be delayed by administering milk or milk of magnesia, which form complexes with the fluoride.

Repeated ingestion of lesser amounts of fluoride can result in manifestations of chronic fluoride toxicity, the most common of which is dental fluorosis. Infants and young children who cannot fully control their swallowing reflexes or who do not understand that they should expectorate products intended only for topical application may regularly swallow significant amounts of fluoride toothpaste. This amount of fluoride (approximately 0.3 mg at each brushing) may

---

TABLE 14–6. Sample Prescription for Fluoride Gel Intended for Home Use

Three-year-old with prior history of early childhood caries (ECC) and poor parental compliance with oral hygiene:

Rx: 0.4% stannous fluoride gel

Disp: 30 ml

Sig: Brush a small amount of gel on all teeth at bedtime. Allow child to spit out remaining gel after brushing. Do not allow rinsing after gel application.

production and lead to enamel demineralization. Infants who are breast fed truly "on demand" may suckle 10 to 40 times in a 24-hour period. Nevertheless, many feel that the benefits of breast feeding outweigh any harmful effects. Dentists should advise mothers who breast feed on demand to clean their infant's teeth frequently and verify that systemic fluoride intake is optimal.

Although surveys report that most U.S. infants are fed beikost (foods other than milk or formula fed to infants) by 2 months of age, pediatric nutritionists recommend that the infant's total nutritional needs be supplied from milk or formula until 5 to 6 months of age. At 5 to 6 months, iron-fortified dry cereal is recommended followed by one to two new commercially or home-prepared foods each week. Sound eating habits established during infancy assist in the continuation of sound habits later in life. Making an infant drain the last drop from the bottle or finish the last spoonful in the dish is not recommended. Forcing infants to eat when they indicate a desire to stop may contribute to overeating, frequent snacking, and obesity in later life (Fomon, 1993).

By the time the posterior teeth erupt and the infant is sitting in the high chair for meals, the child is usually introduced to a variety of foods. Parents should be advised about appropriate snack foods that are not only nutritious but also "safe for teeth." Finger foods (e.g., soft fruits and vegetables, cereals without sugar coatings, Jell-O cubes, salt-free crackers and cheeses) are all acceptable and should be introduced as the infant develops chewing patterns and swallowing reflexes to handle these new foods. Foods with a high percentage of carbohydrates should be avoided, as should foods that stick to the teeth and are slow to dissolve.

Natural fruit juices and artificially fortified fruit juices are frequently introduced to the infant. Pediatricians recommend that juices not be given to the infant in a bottle. Fruit juices should only be fed by cup. Habitual and prolonged use of juice in the bottle can lead to ECC.

HOME CARE

The initiation of a program to ensure an optimal environment for oral health should begin in infancy. Parents should be made to understand that it is their responsibility to carry out this program, with information and guidance available from the dentist and his or her staff. The preventive program includes many facets—dietary manage-

ment, optimal systemic fluorides, and removal of plaque from the teeth. All are important, but plaque removal in the infant and young child is most often neglected and misunderstood.

Studies have confirmed that the bacteria for dental disease are present at the eruption of the primary teeth (Edwardsson and Mejare, 1978). The source of these bacteria most often is the mother. Studies have shown that there is a well-defined period of infectivity between 19 and 28 months of age, during which bacteria are transmitted from the mother to the child. This interval is a period of active tooth eruption, especially for the first and second primary molars (Caufield et al., 1991). Growth of cariogenic bacteria and components of the infant's diet combine to promote the development of plaque and the subsequent production of acid. This environment around the teeth is conducive to demineralization of enamel and eventually cavitation. In addition, the gingiva are subjected to daily insult from the products of bacterial metabolism, leading to marginal gingivitis.

Daily removal of plaque ensures sound enamel and healthy gingiva. Early initiation of plaque removal helps to establish a lifelong habit of oral care. A disease-free mouth brings happiness and satisfaction not only to the parents and children but also to the dental team, who provided the information, instructions, and reinforcement.

Once the parents have been informed about the dental disease process and have been charged with the responsibility of cleaning the teeth daily, a location for performing the procedure should be selected. Devices for plaque removal should be suggested, the pros and cons of dentifrice use explained, positioning of the infant demonstrated, and a technique for plaque removal described. Initially, oral hygiene for the infant probably should be performed wherever the parent changes the infant's diapers. A changing table is a convenient height and usually has appropriate lighting. As the infant grows, the knee-to-knee position (see Fig. 13–1) becomes preferable. Bathrooms, the usual site for oral hygiene for older children and adults, usually are crowded and are not designed with infant safety in mind.

Once teeth have erupted, a wet, soft-bristled brush can be gently wiped over the teeth. When a number of teeth have erupted, a more thorough and systematic routine should be established in which one makes sure to clean all surfaces of the teeth in both the upper and lower jaws and especially the area near the gingiva. By this time the infant has become stronger and may even object to this activity. The parent should be advised to be persistent. With time, the tooth cleaning activity becomes tolerable and acceptable.

Finding an appropriate time is important. The combination of a tired infant and exhausted parents does not produce a favorable environment for a positive experience. Developmentally, an infant is not prepared to accept or understand the activity. Games may be developed, or music and singing used; the parents must try to create a positive experience. With time, the infant may even become less tolerant, but the parents should be encouraged to be persistent.

A thorough cleaning before bedtime is recommended. Usually the infant is given a bath. Tooth cleaning can follow immediately along with any other personal hygiene. Toward the end of the second year of life, the child will be very mobile, actively involved in play and other "grown up" activities. Parents must remember to save time at the end of a busy day for oral care. Although many 24-month-olds want to clean their own teeth, parents need to understand that fine motor activity remains largely undeveloped at this age. Supervision and removal of plaque from missed areas should be provided by a parent.

Toothbrushes are available in many shapes, colors, sizes, and designs. Brushes with soft rounded nylon bristles are recommended. The size of the head, angle of the head to the handle, and size and shape of the handle all depend on the infant's and parent's preferences. A design that works best in their hands and can get the cleaning and massaging completed is the brush to use. Mechanical or novelty brushes also are available. Although novel, adequate documentation of advantages associated with the use of these devices (e.g., greater likelihood of sustained use) is lacking.

Infants have limited ability to expectorate. Therefore, dentifrices with fluoride should be used sparingly, if at all. Fluoride from the dentifrice can appreciably increase total fluoride intake. If a fluoride dentifrice is used, a very small amount should be placed on the brush and the cleaning completely performed or supervised by the parent. Because spacing usually is present between teeth in the primary dentition, flossing is not necessary until interdental contacts have been established.

Positioning the infant for visibility and control is important. Whether the parent uses the changing table, a bed top, counter top, or the knee-to-knee position, appropriate stabilization, propping of the mouth, and reflection of the lips, tongue, and cheeks are important for a thorough and pleasant hygienic experience.

REFERENCES

American Academy of Pediatric Dentistry: Fluoride guidelines. Pediatr Dent 19:28-29, 1997.

American Dental Association: New fluoride schedule adopted. ADA News May 1994.

Brunelle JA, Carlos JP: Recent trends in dental caries in U.S. children and the effect of water fluoridation. J Dent Res 69 (Special Issue):723-727, 1990.

Casamassimo P (ed): Bright Futures in Practice: Oral Health. Arlington, VA, National Center for Education in Maternal and Child Health, 1996.

Caufield PW, Hagan TW, Cutter GR, Dasanayake AP: Infants acquire mutans streptococci from mothers during a discrete window. J Dent Res 70:814, 1991.

Clovis J, Hargreaves JA: Fluoride intake from beverage consumption. Commun Dent Oral Epidemiol 16:11-15, 1988.

Crall JJ: Biological implications and dietary supplementation. In Pinkham JR (ed): Pediatric Dental Care: An Update for the 90's. Evansville, IN, Bristol-Myers Squibb Company, 1991, pp 25-27.

Driscoll W: The use of fluoride tablets for the prevention of dental caries. In Forrester D, Schultz E (eds): International Workshop on Fluorides and Dental Caries Reductions. Baltimore, University of Maryland, 1974, pp 25-96.

Edelstein BL, Cottrel D, O'Sullivan D, Tinanoff N: Comparison of colorimeter and electrode analysis of water fluoride. Pediatr Dent 14:47-49, 1992.

Edelstein B, Tinanoff N: Screening preschool children for dental caries using a microbial test. Pediatr Dent 11:129-132, 1989.

Edwardsson S, Mejare B: *Streptococcus milleri* (Guthof) and *Streptococcus mutans* in the mouths of infants before and after tooth eruption. Arch Oral Biol 23:811-814, 1978.

Ekstrand J, Whitford GM: Fluoride metabolism. In Ekstrand J, Fejerskow O, Siluentone LM (eds): Fluoride in Dentistry. Copenhagen, Munksgaard, 1988, pp 165-166.

Flaitz CM, Hill EM, Hicks MJ: A survey of bottled water usage by pediatric dental patients: Implications for dental health. Quintessence Int 20:847-852, 1989.

Fomon S: Nutrition of Normal Infants. St. Louis, CV Mosby, 1993.

Food and Drug Administration: Statements of general policy or interpretation, oral prenatal drugs containing fluoride for human use. Fed Reg October 20, 1966.

Green M (ed): Bright Futures: Guidelines for Health Supervision of Infants, Children and Adolescents. Arlington, VA, National Center for Education in Maternal and Child Health, 1994.

Hargreaves JA: Water fluoridation and fluoride supplementation: Considerations for the future. Proceedings of a Joint IADR/ORCA International Symposium on Fluorides: Mechanisms of Action and Recommendations. J Dent Res (Special Issue) 69:765-770, 1990.

Hennon DK, Stookey GK, Muhler JC: The clinical anticariogenic effectiveness of supplementary fluoride-vitamin preparations. Results at the end of three years. J Dent Child 33:3-11, 1966.

Holm AK, Anderson R: Enamel mineralization disturbances in 12-year-old children with known early exposure to fluorides. Commun Dent Oral Epidemiol 10:335-339, 1982.

Honig JJ: Teething: are today's pediatricians using yesterday's notions? J Pediatr 87:415-417, 1975.

Johnson J Jr, Bawden JW: The fluoride content of infant formula available in 1985. Pediatr Dent 9:33-37, 1987.

Kaste LM, Selwitz RH, Oldakowski RJ, et al: Coronal caries in the primary and permanent dentition of children and adolescents 1-17 years of age: United States, 1988-1991. J Dent Res 75(Spec Issue):631-641, February, 1996.

King DL: Teething revisited. Pediatric Dent *16*:179-182, 1994.

Kuthy RA, McTigue DJ: Fluoride prescription practices of Ohio physicians. J Public Health Dent *47*:172-176, 1987.

Leverett DH, Adair SM, Vaughan BW, et al: Randomized clinical trial of the effect of prenatal fluoride supplements in preventing caries. Caries Res *31*:174-179, 1997.

Nowak AJ: Rationale for the timing of the first oral evaluation. Pediatr Dent *19*:8-11, 1997.

Nowak A, Casamassimo P: Using anticipatory guidance to provide early dental intervention. JADA *126*:1155-1163, 1995.

Nowak A, Nowak MV: Fluoride concentration of bottled and processed waters. J Iowa Dent *75*:28, 1989.

Pendrys DG, Stamm JW: Relationship of total fluoride intake to beneficial effects and enamel fluorosis. J Dent Res *69* (Special Issue):529-538, 1990.

Rugg-Gunn AJ, Roberts GJ, Wright WG: Effect of human milk on plaque pH in situ and enamel dissolution in vitro compared with bovine milk, lactose and sucrose. Caries Res *19*:327-334, 1985.

Shen YW, Taves DR: Fluoride concentrations in the human placenta and maternal and cord blood. Am J Obstet Gynecol *119*:205-207, 1974.

Stannard J, Rovero J, Tsamtsouris A, Gavris V: Fluoride content of some bottled waters and recommendations for fluoride supplementation. J Pedodont *14*:103-107, 1990.

Stephan RM: Changes in the hydrogen ion concentration on tooth surfaces and in carious lesions. JADA *27*:718-723, 1940.

Tate WH, Snyder R, Montgomery EH, Chan JT: Impact of source of drinking water on fluoride supplementation. Pediatrics *86*:419-421, 1990.

Thylstrup A: Clinical evidence of the role of pre-eruptive fluoride in caries prevention. J Dent Res *69* (Special Issue):742-750, 1990.

Tinanoff N: Comment on urinary excretion of fluoride following ingestion of MFP toothpastes by infants ages two to six years. Pediatr Dent *7*:345, 1985.

U.S. Department of Health, Education, and Welfare: Evaluatory Surveys of Long-Term Fluoridation Show Improved Dental Health. USPHS Publication No. 84-22647. Atlanta, March 1979.

Woolfolk NW, Faja BW, Bagramian RA: Relation of sources of systemic fluoride to prevalence of dental fluorosis. J Public Health Dent *49*:78-82, 1989.

Non-Nutritive Sucking

John R. Christensen and Henry W. Fields, Jr.

Questions often arise about non-nutritive sucking in infants and its effect on the developing orofacial structures. Is non-nutritive sucking harmful or constructive? Should it be encouraged or discouraged? Non-nutritive sucking, which consists of sucking fingers, pacifiers, or other objects, is considered at several stages of development throughout the book; in this section the discussion is restricted to the infant and toddler.

Non-nutritive sucking is considered a normal part of fetal and neonatal development. As early as 13 to 16 weeks in utero, the fetus has started sucking and swallowing movements. Respiratory-like movements also begin during this stage. These fetal movements are considered to be important precursors of the life-sustaining requirements of respiration and deglutition.

Non-nutritive sucking is intimately related to two reflexes present in the infant at birth. The rooting reflex is the movement of the infant's head and tongue toward an object touching its cheek. The object is usually the mother's breast, but it may also be a finger or pacifier. The rooting reflex disappears in normal infants around 7 months of age. The sucking reflex expresses milk from the nipple and remains intact until 12 months of age. The disappearance of the sucking reflex does not mean that the infant cannot suckle; at this stage of development, the infant has learned to feed and does not need the reflex to obtain nourishment.

During suckling, the infant places the tongue beneath the nipple, in contact with the lower lip, and swallows with the jaws apart and the lips together. This is called the infantile swallow (Fig. 14-1). In contrast, the adult swallows with the teeth together, the tongue tip against the palate and the lips relaxed (Fig. 14-2). The change from an infantile to an adult swallow is gradual. As the diet of the infant changes from liquid to solid foods, there is increased activity of the muscles of mastication and the primary molars are brought into occlusion. This transitional swallow is common in children 3 to 10 years of age, and lip contraction and tongue to lower lip contact during swallowing may or may not be present. The full adult swallow can be observed as early as 3 to 4 years of age and is usually present by age 9 or 10.

To summarize, non-nutritive sucking in infants is nearly universal and is considered normal. The point at which non-nutritive sucking becomes a habit and is not considered normal is unclear. Numerous studies of the prevalence of thumb and digit sucking indicate that a large majority of newborns suck their digits, but the percentage drops steadily with increasing age. These studies indicate that children spontaneously discontinue non-nutritive sucking sometime between 2 and 4 years of age (Nowak et al., 1986; Traisman and Traisman, 1958).

A variety of non-nutritive sucking habits exist, but thumb, digit, and pacifier sucking is most common (Fig. 14-3). Pacifier habits depend on the child's cultural background and may be encouraged in one setting and not in another—children usually have little choice in the matter. Children often combine a non-nutritive habit with another repetitive activity. For example,

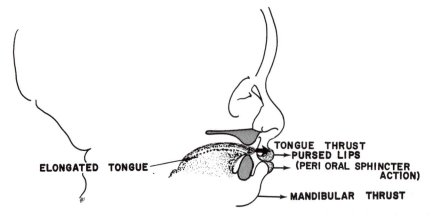

Figure 14–1. The infantile swallow is performed with the lips together, the tongue touching the lower lip, and the jaws apart. (From Graber TM: Orthodontics, Principles and Practice, 3rd ed. Philadelphia, WB Saunders, 1972, p 167.)

they may suck a thumb while carrying a personal blanket, stuffed toy, or favorite doll. Other children play with their hair or rub an article of clothing. In addition, certain situations and times of day influence the habit. Tired children are more likely to suck their thumb, as are children in new or threatening environments. Sucking a digit when entering and exiting sleep is the most common observation.

The effects of non-nutritive sucking on the developing dentition are minor in the child under 3 years of age and are usually limited to changes in incisor position. Some upper incisors become tipped toward the lips, whereas others are prevented from erupting. There is some controversy, however, about the influence one habit

has on the dentition compared with another. At this time, there seems to be no significant difference between digit and pacifier habits in terms of their effects on the dentition after adjusting for the intensity of the sucking habit (Modeer et al., 1982). One study has suggested that arch width in the maxillary canine region is more adversely affected by pacifier habits than by finger- or thumb-sucking habits (Lindner and Modeer, 1989). A conference report on feeding and dentofacial development concluded that children who are given pacifiers discontinue their habit earlier than children who suck their fingers or thumbs (Nowak, 1991).

If parents choose to have their child use a pacifier, some precautions should be taken to

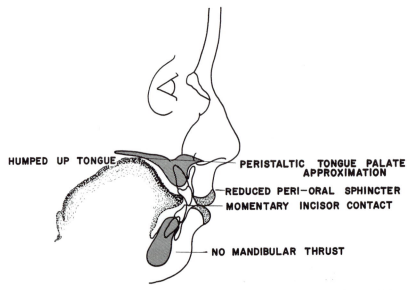

Figure 14–2. The adult swallow is performed with the lips relaxed, the tongue against the palate, and the teeth and jaws together. (From Graber TM: Orthodontics, Principles and Practice, 3rd ed. Philadelphia, WB Saunders, 1972, p 168.)

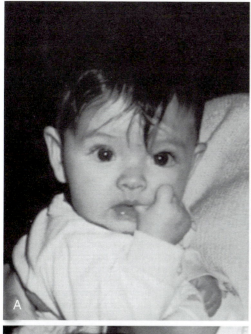

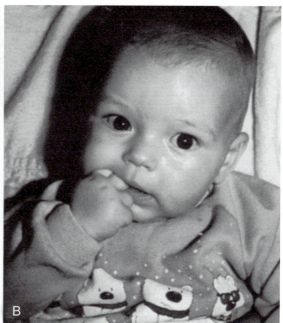

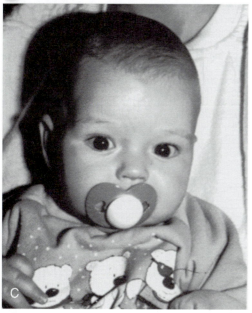

Figure 14–3. Non-nutritive sucking in infants may occur as thumb sucking *(A)*, digit sucking *(B)*, or pacifier sucking *(C)*. The child may engage in one or all three of the habits at one or various stages of development.

ensure their child's safety. The pacifier should never be attached to a ribbon or string around the child's neck because the string may get caught or tangled and cause serious injury or death by strangulation. The United States Consumer Products Safety Commission requires that pacifiers:

1. Be of sturdy, one-piece construction of material that is nontoxic, flexible, and firm but not brittle.
2. Have easily grasped handles.

3. Have inseparable nipples and mouth guards.
4. Have mouth guards of adequate diameter to prevent aspiration and two ventilating holes.
5. Have a label warning against tying the pacifier around the infant's neck (Fig. 14-4).

Additionally, parents should be encouraged to keep the pacifier clean, replace it when worn, and never place honey, sugar, or any sweet syrup on the nipple to encourage sucking. These sweeteners simply increase the risk of caries.

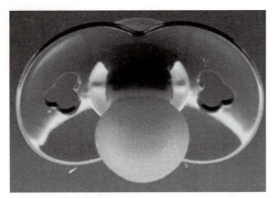

Figure 14–4. This pacifier conforms to the United States Consumer Products Safety Commission standards that require pacifiers to be of sturdy, one-piece construction and to have easily grasped handles, inseparable nipples and mouth guards, and mouth guards with two ventilating holes and adequate diameter to prevent aspiration.

Manufacturers have been quick to develop nipples and pacifiers that "closely resemble the mother's breast." These manufacturers maintain that because the pacifier resembles the breast, it is more natural and therefore best for the infant's growth and development. No long-term controlled studies are available to support these claims. One study found no significant difference in absolute or relative change in maxillary or mandibular arch parameters in infants grouped according to feeding and sucking methods during the first 18 months of life (Bishara et al., 1987).

In the under-3 age group, active intervention to discourage non-nutritive sucking is contraindicated. A period of watchful waiting is ordinarily successful because the majority of children spontaneously abandon the habit between the ages of 2 and 4. In a large percentage of cases, any deleterious tooth movement resulting from the habit tends to resolve if the activity is discontinued prior to eruption of the permanent teeth. Treatment, therefore, is best deferred until the late primary or early mixed dentition stage and is discussed in the next chapter.

REFERENCES

Bishara S, Nowak A, Kohout F, et al: Influence of feeding and non-nutritive sucking methods on the development of the dental arches: Longitudinal study of the first 18 months of life. Pediatr Dent 9:13–21, 1987.

Lindner A, Modeer T: Relation between sucking habits and dental characteristics in preschool children with unilateral crossbite. Scand J Dent Res 97:278–283, 1989.

Modeer T, Odenrick L, Lindner A: Sucking habits and their relation to posterior crossbite in 4 year old children. Scand J Dent Res 90:323–328, 1982.

Nowak A: Conference Report: Feeding and dentofacial development. J Dent Res 70:159–160, 1991.

Nowak A, Bishara S, Lancial L, Heckert A: Changes in nutritive and non-nutritive sucking habits: Birth to two years. J Dent Res 65 (Special Issue): Abstract 1525, 1986.

Traisman AS, Traisman H: Thumb and finger sucking: A study of 2,650 infants and children. J Pediatr 52:566–577, 1958.

15

Introduction to Dental Trauma: Managing Traumatic Injuries in the Primary Dentition

Dennis J. McTigue

Chapter Outline

An injury to the teeth of a young child can have serious and long-term consequences, leading to their discoloration, malformation, or possible loss. The emotional impact of such an injury can be far reaching. It is therefore important that the dentist treating children is

1. Knowledgeable in the techniques for managing traumatic injuries
2. Readily available during and after office hours to provide treatment

If either of the above conditions cannot be met, the child suffering a dental injury should immediately be referred to a specialist.

This chapter provides a straightforward approach to managing dental injuries in the primary dentition. Techniques for diagnosis, treatment, and follow-up care are described. Fundamental issues covered in this chapter, such as classification of injuries, history, examination, and pathologic sequelae of trauma, pertain to both the primary and permanent dentitions.

Chapter 34 focuses on treating injuries to young permanent teeth and refers to this chapter for the information just noted. The principles gleaned from both chapters should enable the dentist to manage the great majority of dental injuries encountered in children.

ETIOLOGY AND EPIDEMIOLOGY OF TRAUMA IN THE PRIMARY DENTITION

Most injuries to primary teeth occur at 1½ to 2½ years of age, the toddler stage. As children begin to walk, they frequently fall forward, landing on their hands and knees. Lack of coordination at this stage of development prevents them from shielding the blow from furniture and other objects they might encounter when falling. Coffee tables are most commonly the culprits, and parents are well advised to remove them from the home until toddlers are walking more confidently. Falls from highchairs and strollers are also frequent causes of dental injury.

The teeth most frequently injured in the primary dentition are the maxillary central incisors. Children with protruding incisors, as in developing Class II malocclusions, are two to three times more likely to suffer dental trauma than children with normal incisal overjets.

Another major cause of dental injuries in young children is automobile accidents. Unrestrained children who are seated or standing often hit the dashboard or windshield when the car is stopped suddenly. Dentists in many states have supported mandatory child restraint laws in automobiles, and it is hoped that the trend for universal adoption of these laws will decrease the incidence of all trauma to children in automobile accidents (Jones et al., 1986).

Children with chronic seizure disorders experience an increased incidence of dental trauma. Frequently, these high-risk children wear protective head gear, and the fabrication of custom mouth guards for them is indicated (see Chapter 40).

Another serious cause of dental injuries to young children is child abuse. Often overlooked by the dental profession, up to 50% of abused children suffer injuries to the head and neck. Cardinal signs of abuse are injuries in various stages of healing, tears of labial frena, repeated injuries, and injuries whose clinical presentation is not consistent with the history presented by the parent (American Dental Association, 1995). Battered children frequently lie to protect their parents or from fear of retaliation. Dentists are required by law to report cases of suspected child abuse (see Chapter 1 for more specific details).

In the primary dentition, teeth are more frequently displaced, or luxated, than they are fractured. This is because the alveolar bone in a young child has large marrow spaces and is relatively pliable. It yields to blows to the primary teeth, allowing these teeth to be moved rather than holding them firmly and thus causing fractures.

CLASSIFICATION OF INJURIES TO TEETH

Tooth fractures may involve the crown, root, or both (Figs. 15-1, 15-2, 15-3, 34-1, 34-2, and 34-3). Fractures of the crown may be limited to the enamel, may involve the dentin, or may include the pulp. Injury to the pulp is the most complicated and demanding to treat.

As just mentioned, the most common types of injuries to primary teeth are luxation (displacement) injuries. These injuries damage supporting structures of the teeth, which include the periodontal ligament (PDL) and the alveolar bone (see Fig. 15-1). The PDL is the physiologic "hammock" that supports the tooth in its socket. Maintaining its vitality is the primary objective in the treatment of all luxation injuries. Several types of luxation injuries occur (Andreasen and Andreasen, 1994):

1. *Concussion*: The tooth is not mobile and is not displaced. The PDL absorbs the injury and is

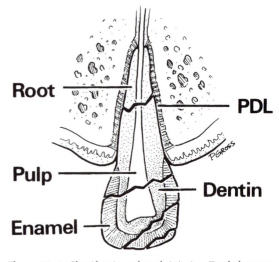

Figure 15–1. Classification of tooth injuries. Tooth fractures may involve enamel, dentin, or pulp and may occur in the crown or the root. PDL = periodontal ligament.

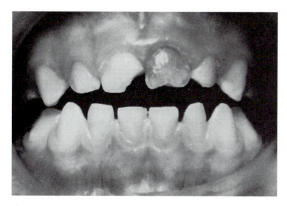

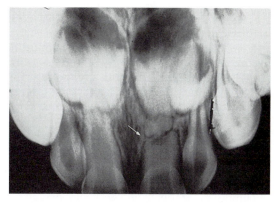

Figure 15–2. Crown fracture of maxillary right primary central incisor involving enamel and dentin. Discolored maxillary left primary central incisor.

Figure 15–3. Root fracture *(arrow)* in apical third of maxillary left primary central incisor.

inflamed, which leaves the tooth tender to biting pressure and percussion.

    2. *Mobility*: The tooth is loosened but is not displaced from its socket.

    3. *Intrusion*: The tooth is driven into its socket. This compresses the PDL and commonly causes a crushing fracture of the alveolar socket. See Figures 15-4A, 15-6, 15-10, and 34-12.

    4. *Extrusion*: This is a central dislocation of the tooth from its socket (Figs. 15-4B and 34-13A). The PDL is usually torn in this injury.

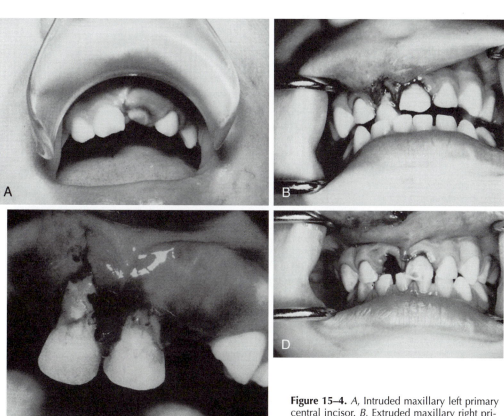

Figure 15–4. *A*, Intruded maxillary left primary central incisor. *B*, Extruded maxillary right primary central incisor. *C*, Lateral luxation of maxillary primary central incisors. *D*, Avulsion of maxillary right primary central incisor.

5. *Lateral luxation*: The tooth is displaced in a labial, lingual, or lateral direction. The PDL is torn, and contusion or fracture of the supporting alveolar bone occurs (Figs. 15-4C and 34-13B).

6. *Avulsion*: The tooth is completely displaced from the alveolus. The PDL is severed, and fractures of the alveolus may occur (Figs. 15-4D and 34-14).

HISTORY

Obtaining an adequate medical and dental history is essential to proper diagnosis and treatment. The medical history should already be on record if the child suffering an injury is brought to his or her regular dentist. Frequently, however, a parent takes an injured child to the closest dentist or to one known to treat children. Thus, with the confusion of a young injured child entering the office for possibly the first time and disrupting the day's schedule, the potential to forget to gather important historical information is great. The use of a trauma assessment form to help record data and organize the management of care is highly recommended (Fig. 15-5).

Medical History

Routine data on the patient's general health should be obtained. Historical information partic-

SCHOOL of DENTISTRY
DEPARTMENT of PEDIATRIC DENTISTRY

Child's Name _____   Student _____

Age _____ Sex _____ Race _____   Faculty _____

Place of Injury _____   Chart No. _____   Date _____

Date of Injury _____

Time of Injury _____

Time Elapsed Since Injury _____

HISTORY

Chief Complaint _____   Previous Trauma _____

Past Medical History _____

Past Dental History _____

How Injury Occurred _____

Tetanus Protection: ☐ No   Yes☐   Date of Last Booster _____

EXTRAORAL ASSESSMENT		INTRAORAL ASSESSMENT	
CNS Status		**Hard Tissue**	
☐ Unconsciousness	☐ Amnesia	☐ Alveolar Fracture	☐ Palatal Fracture
☐ Unequal Pupil Size	☐ Headache	Describe _____	
☐ Fixed Pupils	☐ Nausea		
☐ CSF from Ears	☐ Disorientation	**Soft Tissue**	
☐ CSF from Nose	☐ Loss of Smell	☐ Lips	☐ Frenum
☐ Nystagmus	☐ Seizure	☐ Buccal Mucosa	☐ Tongue
☐ Vertigo		☐ Gingiva	☐ Palate ☐
Describe _____		Describe _____	

Hard Tissue		**Dental Occlusion**	
☐ Cranial Fracture	☐ Zygoma Fracture	Molar _____	Cuspid _____
☐ Mandibular Fracture	☐ Infection	Overjet _____ mm	Overbite _____ %
☐ Maxillary Fracture		Openbite _____	Crossbite _____
Describe _____		Classification deviation induced by trauma _____	
		Describe _____	
Soft Tissue			
☐ Laceration	☐ Abrasion	**RADIOGRAPHS**	
☐ Contusions	☐ Infection	☐ Periapical	☐ Occlusal
☐ Swelling	☐ Embedded Maternal	☐ Lateral Anterior	☐ Panorex
Describe _____		Other _____	
		Pathology _____	

Figure 15–5. Trauma assessment form.

ularly relevant to the dental injury includes the following:

1. Cardiac disease, which may necessitate prophylaxis against subacute bacterial endocarditis
2. Bleeding disorders
3. Allergies to medications
4. Seizure disorders
5. Medications
6. Status of tetanus prophylaxis

The issue of tetanus protection is particularly important when a child has suffered a dirty wound, that is, an avulsion, deep laceration, or intrusion injury in which soil is embedded in the tissues. Wounds containing necrotic tissue, dirt, and foreign material should be cleaned and debrided as an essential part of tetanus prophylaxis. Children acquire active immunity through a series of five injections of adsorbed tetanus toxoid, usually completed by the age of 4 to 6 years. These are normally administered as part of the diphtheria-tetanus-pertussis (DTP) immunizations. Children should then receive a booster of tetanus toxoid at 11 to 12 years of age and every

DENTAL FINDINGS

| Fracture | Class I | Class II | Class III | Class IV |

Draw Injury

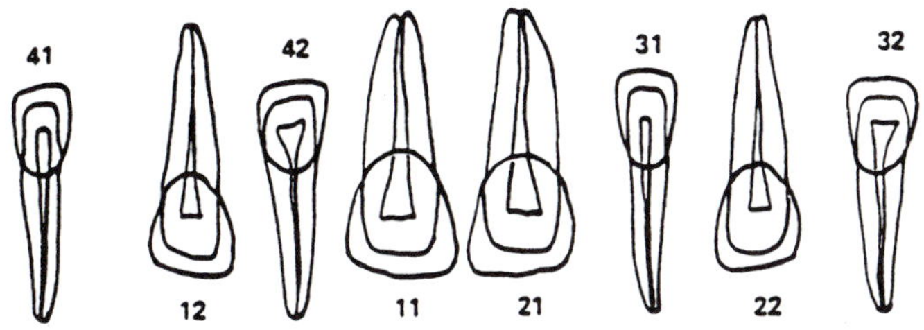

41 42 31 32
12 11 21 22

Involved Teeth _____

Tooth Response — Pulp and PDL

Tooth No.				
Exposure				
Hemorrhage				
Heat				
Cold				
Contamination				
Percussion				
Mobility				
Vitalometer				

Displacement
☐ Intrusion   ☐ Subluxation
☐ Extrusion   ☐ Lateral luxation
☐ Avulsion

Color
☐ Normal   ☐ Dark   ☐ Light

SUMMARY and DIAGNOSIS
Crown _____
Pulp _____
Root _____
Periapical Tissue _____

Alveolar Process _____
Root Displacement _____
Restoration _____
Fragments _____

TREATMENT
Soft Tissues _____
Pulp _____
Restoration _____
Splinting _____
Medication _____

Recall Follow-up
☐ 2 weeks   ☐ 3 weeks   ☐ 6 weeks
☐ 3 months   ☐ 6 months
Other _____

Figure 15–5 *Continued*

10 years thereafter, unless the child suffers a dirty wound as just described. A booster is then indicated if the child has not received one in the last 5 years (American Academy of Pediatrics, 1997, p. 520). Increasing reports indicate that children in the United States are not receiving their childhood immunizations appropriately. If there is any question about the adequacy of a child's tetanus protection, the child's physician should immediately be consulted.

History of the Dental Injury

Three important questions are asked in gathering the dental history: *when, where*, and *how* did the accident occur? The time elapsed since the injury plays a major role in determining the type of treatment to be provided. The dentist should also determine whether the tooth had been injured previously or whether the injury had first been treated elsewhere.

Where the injury occurred sheds light on its severity. Did the toddler slip and hit the coffee table in the living room or did she fall off her parent's bicycle in the park? This information can help determine the need for tetanus prophylaxis as well as signal a need to rule out more serious injury to the child.

How the accident occurred obviously provides the dentist with the most information regarding severity. Serious head injuries should be ruled out by asking if the child lost consciousness, has vomited, or is disoriented as a result of the accident. Positive findings indicate potential central nervous system injury, and medical consultation should be immediately obtained (Davis and Vogel, 1995). Tecklenburg and Wright (1991) note that significant head injuries can lead to symptoms many hours after the initial trauma, and they caution parents to watch for the signs noted earlier for 24 hours, including waking the child every 2 to 3 hours through the night.

As previously discussed, the possibility of child abuse can also be ruled out through a careful dental history. The direction of force to the teeth should be determined. A blow to the underside of the chin frequently causes posterior tooth crown fractures (see Fig. 34-8) and sometimes mandibular symphysis fractures. These injuries have also been correlated with cervical spine fractures (Bertolami and Kaban, 1982).

Directing attention to the specific teeth involved, the dentist should ask the child if there is spontaneous pain from any teeth. Positive findings here may indicate pulp inflammation that is due to a fractured crown or injuries to the supporting structures such as extravasation of

blood into the PDL. Does the child experience a thermal change with sweet or sour foods? If so, dentin or the pulp may be exposed. Are the teeth tender to touch or tender while chewing? Does the child note a change in his or her occlusion? These findings may indicate a luxation injury or an alveolar fracture.

CLINICAL EXAMINATION

Once the medical and dental histories are complete, the dentist is ready to begin the clinical examination. It is tempting to focus immediately on a fractured or displaced tooth and thus miss other important injuries. A disciplined approach to a complete clinical examination should be followed in diagnosing every traumatic injury.

Extraoral Examination

A complete examination should rule out injuries to the child's facial bones (Kaban, 1993). The facial skeleton should be palpated to determine discontinuities of facial bones. Extraoral wounds and bruises should be recorded. The temporomandibular joints should be palpated, and any swelling, clicking, or crepitus should be noted. Mandibular function in all excursive movements should be checked. Any stiffness or pain in the child's neck necessitates immediate referral to a physician to rule out cervical spine injury.

Intraoral Examination

All soft tissues should be examined, and any injuries should be recorded. The presence of foreign matter in lacerations of the lips and cheeks, such as tooth fragments or soil, should be identified. Removal at the initial appointment eliminates chronic infection and disfiguring fibrosis.

Each tooth in the mouth should be examined for fracture, pulp exposure, and dislocation. In some crown fractures, only a very thin layer of dentin remains over the pulp, so that the pulp's outline is visible as a pink tinge on the dentin. The dentist should be careful not to perforate this dentin with an instrument.

Displacement of teeth should be recorded, as should horizontal and vertical tooth mobility. Mobility may be difficult to evaluate clinically in a primary tooth because it increases with normal root resorption. Reaction to palpation and percussion of teeth is recorded. Percussion sensitivity is a good indicator of PDL inflammation.

Pulpal vitality testing is not routinely performed in the primary dentition. This is because primary teeth do not respond to such tests reliably and because the test requires a relaxed and cooperative patient objectively reporting reactions. Many young children lack the ability to report their reactions to pulpal testing objectively.

Radiographic Examination

INDICATIONS FOR RADIOGRAPHS

Radiographs are an important part of the diagnosis and treatment of dental injuries. They allow the clinician to detect root fractures, extent of root development, size of pulp chambers, periapical radiolucencies, resorptions, the degree of displacement of teeth, position of unerupted teeth, jaw fractures, and the presence of tooth fragments and other foreign bodies in soft tissues. Although some radiographs show negative findings at the initial appointment, they are nonetheless important as baseline documentation. Subsequent radiographic evidence can thus be compared with the initial films.

RADIOGRAPHIC TECHNIQUES

There is no "standard series" of radiographs for dental injuries. All films taken should clearly show the apical areas of traumatized teeth (see Chapters 18 and 30). In cases in which root fractures are suspected, a second or third radiograph should be made from slightly different angles both vertically and horizontally to verify the location and extent of the fracture.

A useful film for planning treatment of intruded primary incisors is the lateral anterior view (Fig. 15–6). As is discussed in the part of the chapter dealing with treatment, it is essential to know the precise position of the intruded primary tooth relative to its succeeding incisor. An excellent view can be obtained if the child or parent holds a 3 × 5-inch extraoral film next to the child's cheek and perpendicular to the radiographic beam. For this view, the exposure time for a normal periapical radiograph is doubled.

To determine the presence of foreign bodies such as tooth fragments in the lips or tongue, one fourth of the normal exposure time is used. The film is placed beneath the tissue to be examined, and the radiograph is exposed (Fig. 15–7).

TIMING OF FOLLOW-UP RADIOGRAPHS

As noted previously, many pathologic changes are not immediately apparent in radiographs. After approximately 3 weeks, periapical radiolucencies that are due to pulpal necrosis can usu-

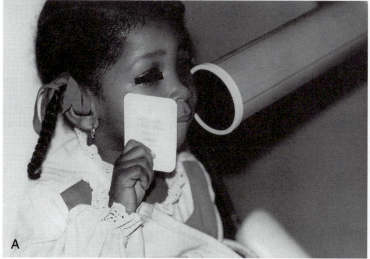
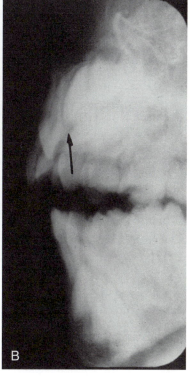

Figure 15–6. *A,* Positioning a child for a lateral anterior radiograph. *B,* Radiograph shows an intruded primary incisor contacting the developing permanent incisor that will succeed it *(arrow).*

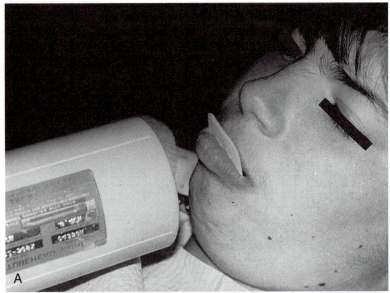

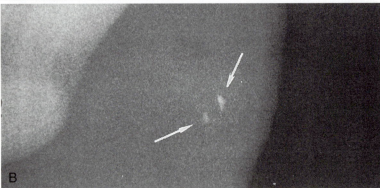

Figure 15–7. *A,* Positioning film to detect presence of tooth fragments in the lip. *B,* Radiograph demonstrating tooth fragments in lip *(arrows).*

ally be detected. Additionally, inflammatory root resorption can be evident at this time. After approximately 6 to 7 weeks, replacement resorption, or ankylosis, becomes visible. Thus, there is adequate rationale to plan postoperative radiographs at 1 month and 2 months after the injury. In the absence of any clinical signs or symptoms, such as development of a fistula, mobility, discoloration, or pain, additional films are not indicated until 6 months after the injury. If changes are to appear radiographically, they usually do so by this time.

PATHOLOGIC SEQUELAE OF TRAUMATIZED TEETH

Traumatized teeth are at substantial risk for pulpal devitalization owing to their lack of collateral circulation. The thin band of neurovascular pulp tissue entering at the root apex can easily be severed by relatively minor blows. It is currently not possible to base accurate identification of the histopathologic condition of a dental pulp on clinical symptoms. The following terms describe a spectrum of clinical signs and symptoms that accompany inflammation and degeneration of the pulp, periodontal ligament, or both.

Reversible Pulpitis

The pulp's initial response to trauma is pulpitis. Capillaries in the tooth become congested, a condition that can be clinically apparent upon transillumination of the crown with a bright light. Teeth with reversible pulpitis may be tender to percussion if the PDL is inflamed (e.g., after a luxation injury). The pulpitis may be totally reversible if the condition causing it is addressed, or it may progress to irreversible pulpitis and necrosis of the pulp.

Pulpal Hemorrhage

As a result of trauma, the capillaries in the pulp occasionally hemorrhage, leaving blood pigments deposited in the dentinal tubules. In mild cases, the blood is resorbed and little discoloration occurs or that which is present becomes lighter in several weeks. In more severe cases, the discoloration persists for the life of the tooth (see Fig. 15-2).

From a diagnostic standpoint, discoloration of primary teeth does not necessarily mean that the tooth is nonvital, particularly when the discoloration occurs within 1 or 2 days after the injury. Color changes that occur weeks or months after the injury are more indicative of a necrotic pulp (Holan and Fuks, 1996). Nevertheless, *in the primary dentition of a healthy child, color change alone does not indicate pulp therapy or extraction of the tooth*. Additional signs and symptoms of necrosis, such as mobility, radiographic radiolucency, or pain, must be evident before further treatment is indicated.

Pulp Canal Obliteration

Pulp canal obliteration is a condition wherein the pulp chamber and canal are gradually obliterated by progressive deposition of dentin (Figs. 15-8A, 34-9, and 34-10B). This is not a normal pulpal reaction, but it represents a pathologic pulpal response to trauma. Ninety percent of primary teeth that have undergone calcific metamorphosis resorb normally (Jacobsen and Sangnes, 1978), and thus treatment in the primary dentition is usually not indicated. These teeth frequently appear somewhat yellowish.

Irreversible Pulpitis

Irreversible pulpitis may be acute or chronic and it may be partial or total. Acute, irreversible pulpitis after a dental injury can be painful if the exudate accompanying the pulpal inflammation is unable to vent. Most frequently in children, however, inflammatory exudates are quickly vented and the pulpitis progresses to a chronic, painless condition.

Pulpal Necrosis

As mentioned previously, a relatively minor blow to the tooth can sever the neurovascular bundle. In the absence of any collateral circulation, the pulp becomes necrotic. Necrosis also occurs when pulpitis progresses untreated. Untreated pulp necrosis may spread beyond the apical foramen, extending the pulp disease into the surrounding supporting tissues. Periapical radiolucencies indicative of a granuloma or cyst are frequently evident radiographically in necrotic anterior teeth (see Fig. 15-8A). Additionally, a parulis is often clinically evident at the level of the involved tooth's root apex (Fig. 15-8B).

Controversy surrounds the most appropriate treatment of primary anterior teeth with necrotic pulps. Some clinicians treat them with a pulpectomy technique similar to that used in permanent teeth. A resorbable paste is packed into the thoroughly cleansed canal (see Chapter 22). Other clinicians choose to extract these teeth owing to the potential for damage to the developing permanent tooth buds. It is generally agreed that pulpectomy is contraindicated in primary teeth with gross loss of root structure, advanced inter-

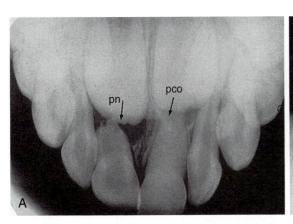
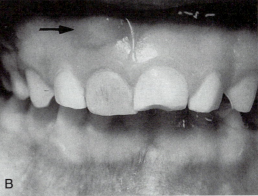

Figure 15–8. *A,* Pulp canal obliteration (pco) in the patient's left primary central incisor and pulp necrosis (pn) in the right primary central incisor. *B,* In the same patient, a parulis is present at the apical level of the necrotic right central incisor *(arrow).*

nal or external resorption, or periapical infection involving the crypt of the succedaneous tooth.

Inflammatory Resorption

Inflammatory resorption can occur either on the external root surface or internally in the pulp chamber or canal (see Fig. 34-10). It occurs subsequent to luxation injuries and is related to a necrotic pulp and an inflamed PDL (Tronstad, 1988). It can progress rapidly, destroying a tooth within months. Clinicians who choose to treat this condition when it occurs in the primary dentition use resorbable zinc oxide paste as an endodontic filling material.

Replacement Resorption

Replacement resorption, also known as ankylosis, results after irreversible injury to the periodontal ligament. Alveolar bone directly contacts and becomes fused with the root surface (Tronstad, 1988). As the alveolar bone undergoes its normal physiologic osteoclastic and osteoblastic activity, the root is resorbed (replaced with bone) (see Fig. 34-11). Ankylosed primary teeth should be extracted if they cause a delay in or ectopic eruption of a developing permanent tooth.

Injuries to Developing Permanent Teeth

The most damaging sequelae of injuries to primary teeth are their effect on the unerupted developing permanent teeth. Anatomically, the permanent anterior teeth develop in close proximity to the apices of primary incisors (see Fig. 15-6B). Thus, periapical pathology that is due to necrotic pulps, intrusion injuries, or over-instrumentation of primary root canals can irreversibly damage the permanent teeth. If the injury occurs during the development of the permanent tooth crown, enamel hypoplasia or hypocalcification may occur (Fig. 15-9). These injuries can also alter the path of the developing permanent tooth crown, causing root dilaceration or ectopic eruption. For these reasons, the clinician should plan treatment for injuries to primary teeth with the ultimate objective of minimizing any damage to the succeeding permanent teeth. Enamel calcification of permanent central incisor crowns is usually completed by age 4, so the risk of injury to them is greater in children under that age.

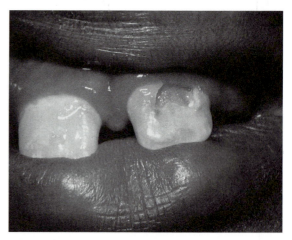

Figure 15–9. Hypoplasia of the patient's maxillary left permanent central incisor as a result of intrusion of a primary incisor.

TREATMENT OF TRAUMATIC INJURIES TO THE PRIMARY DENTITION

No injury to the primary teeth should be considered insignificant. A complete diagnostic work-up as described in this chapter should precede all treatment. Even a blow that causes little, if any, obvious injury to a tooth can lead to pulp necrosis as a result of the severance of the neurovascular bundle at the apex. Any such injury threatens the developing permanent tooth bud; thus, diagnostic follow-up examinations after treatment should occur for all injuries to primary teeth.

Trauma to Teeth

ENAMEL FRACTURES

In small fractures, rough enamel margins can be disked, and no restoration may be necessary. In larger enamel fractures, the tooth can be restored using an acid-etch–composite resin technique (see Chapter 21).

ENAMEL AND DENTIN FRACTURES

Exposed dentin should be covered with an acid-resistant calcium hydroxide paste or with glass ionomer cement to prevent insult to the pulp. The tooth is then restored with an acid-etch–composite resin technique (see Chapter 21).

FRACTURES INVOLVING THE PULP

These injuries are relatively rare in the primary dentition. Their treatment depends on the vitality of the pulpal tissue. A formocresol pulpotomy is completed if the injury has occurred in the last several hours and if the pulp tissue in the canal is judged to be vital (see Chapter 22). If the tissue in the root canal is not vital, pulpectomy with zinc oxide and eugenol or extraction is indicated. Three fourths of the root formation must be present to consider a pulpectomy, and the canals should be instrumented 1 to 2 mm short of the apex. In the primary dentition, a direct pulp cap is not indicated for a crown fracture that exposes the pulp.

Final restoration of the tooth depends on the amount of tooth structure remaining. Some clinicians prefer a composite resin crown using a celluloid crown matrix (see Chapter 21). A stainless steel crown with a composite veneer is an alternative if little crown structure remains.

POSTERIOR CROWN FRACTURES

Fractures of posterior primary crowns usually occur as a result of indirect blows, that is, those that occur to the underside of the chin. Therapy in these cases follows the same principles just described. The only difference is that the final restoration usually has to be a stainless steel crown.

ROOT FRACTURES

Management of root fractures in primary teeth depends on the level of the fracture. The best prognosis is for fractures in the apical one third of the root (see Fig. 15–3). Most of these teeth maintain their vitality and are minimally mobile. The tooth, including the apical fragment, should resorb normally and should be monitored periodically with radiographs.

Fractures that occur in the middle or cervical third of the root indicate extraction. A *gentle* attempt should be made to dislodge the apical root fragment. If it cannot be easily extracted, it should be left and monitored with radiographs. The clinician should make every attempt to avoid disrupting the developing permanent tooth bud.

Trauma to Supporting Structures

CONCUSSION

These injuries are evident clinically because the teeth are tender to percussion or to biting pres-

sure. If the child complains of pain, the tooth can be gently taken out of occlusion. Although the prognosis for concussed primary teeth is usually good, follow-up examination is important.

MOBILITY

Increased mobility is a common reaction of primary teeth to trauma. The child should be instructed to avoid eating with the involved teeth, and follow-up examination should occur in 1 month. No splint should be placed. The prognosis in these cases is usually good.

INTRUSION INJURIES

The intrusion of a primary incisor (see Fig. 15–4A) is potentially one of the most dangerous

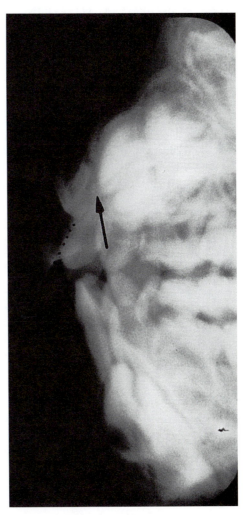

Figure 15–10. An intruded primary incisor not contacting the developing permanent tooth bud *(arrow)* is allowed to re-erupt spontaneously.

injuries to the developing tooth bud. A lateral anterior radiograph, described earlier in the chapter, should be taken (see Fig. 15-6). If the intruded incisor is contacting the permanent tooth bud (see Fig. 15-6B), the primary tooth should be extracted. If it does not contact the tooth bud but is directed more labially (Fig. 15-10), it should be allowed to re-erupt. Ninety percent of these teeth re-erupt in 2 to 6 months, although many undergo pulp canal obliteration. Again, this condition is usually not treated in primary teeth because normal resorption occurs in the great majority of these cases. Follow-up examination should occur each month until the tooth is completely re-erupted. Post-treatment examinations should then occur every 3 months. Extraction of the tooth is indicated if a fistula or a periapical radiolucency develops.

EXTRUSION AND LATERAL LUXATION INJURIES

In these injuries, serious damage to the PDL usually occurs (see Figs. 15-4B and 15-4C). Some clinicians recommend splinting with sutures until periodontal ligament attachment occurs (approximately 2 weeks). I recommend extraction of these teeth, however, because of the potential for aspiration of mobile teeth in young children and because of the potential for subsequent damage to developing permanent tooth buds.

AVULSION INJURIES

Primary teeth that have been avulsed should not be re-implanted (see Fig. 15-4D). The maxillary anterior region is at low risk for space loss unless the avulsion occurs prior to eruption of the primary canines. Either fixed or removable appliances can be fabricated to satisfy parental concerns for esthetics (see Chapter 21), and the risk of injuring developing tooth buds is reduced. Parents should be informed, however, that the permanent teeth may have been injured when the primary teeth were avulsed. Permanent teeth may be delayed in eruption by 1 to 2 years when the primary teeth that they succeed are lost prematurely. This may be due to the development of fibrotic scar tissue in the path of the erupting teeth.

REFERENCES

American Academy of Pediatrics: Tetanus. *In* Peter G (ed): 1997 Red Book: Report of the Committee on Infectious Diseases, 24th ed. Elk Grove Village, IL, American Academy of Pediatrics, 1997, pp 518-523.

American Dental Association: The Dentist's Responsibility in Identifying and Reporting Child Abuse and Neglect. Report of the Council on Dental Practice, 3rd ed. Chicago, American Dental Association, 1995.

Andreasen JO, Andreasen FM: Textbook and Color Atlas of Traumatic Injuries to the Teeth, 3rd ed. Copenhagen, Munksgaard, 1994.

Bertolami CN, Kaban LB: Chin trauma: A clue to associated mandibular and cervical spine injury. Oral Surg 53:122, 1982.

Davis MJ, Vogel BA: Neurological assessment of the child with head trauma. J Dent Child 62:93, 1995.

Holan G, Fuks AB: The diagnostic value of coronal dark-gray discoloration in primary teeth following traumatic injuries. Pediatr Dent 18:3, 1996.

Jacobsen I, Sangnes G: Traumatized primary anterior teeth: Prognosis related to calcific reactions in the pulp cavity. Acta Odontol Scand 36:199, 1978.

Jones JE, Stroup KB, Alley C, Bull MJ: Infant and child passenger restraint systems: The role of pediatric dentistry. Pediatr Dent 8:109, 1986.

Kaban LB: Diagnosis and treatment of fractures of the facial bones in children, 1943-1993. J Oral Maxillofac Surg 51:722, 1993.

Tecklenburg F, Wright M: Minor head trauma in the pediatric patient. Pediatr Emerg Care 7:40, 1991.

Tronstad L: Root resorption—etiology, terminology and clinical manifestations. Endod Dent Traumatol 4:241, 1988.

Chapter 16

Congenital Genetic Disorders and Syndromes

Mary A. Curtis

Chapter Outline

Genetic "disorders" are likely to affect everyone at some time. Some are of more obvious importance than others, depending on the age of onset of the disease, the degree of mental or physical impairment, the numbers of affected persons, and the cost of care. Although many of these disorders are not preventable or curable, early detection may allow significantly improved health care for the affected individual and improved family planning.

The dentist is often in a unique position to pick up a previously unrecognized genetic or birth defect problem in a patient or family. Many "syndromes" affect the oral structures in a unique way, aiding in diagnosis. Also, the dentist is often the only health care provider to see teenagers and young adults. A previously unrecognized genetic condition may first become apparent during this time—for example, Marfan syndrome, Klinefelter syndrome, or neurofibromatosis. Although a "cure" for genetic diseases is generally not yet available, maintenance of good health is important, and prevention of handicapping problems or death may be possible if an appropriate diagnosis is made.

The diagnosis of a genetic or birth defect disorder is most often made by physical evaluation of the patient and laboratory or radiologic investigation in conjunction with careful study of the clinical and family history (pedigree). Many times, review of the pedigree discloses other relatives who have been previously evaluated for a similar clinical problem. Much time, money, and discomfort may be saved by using this information when it is available. For the busy dentist, making use of already available information may give the extra edge in diagnosing a familial disorder. In addition to the family and clinical history, routine use of growth charts, which are readily available, is important in picking up the altered growth patterns that are commonly part of genetic alterations.

Once a genetic disorder is suspected, the question of whether the dentist should proceed with an investigation or refer the patient to a specialist for a diagnostic work-up or other medical care

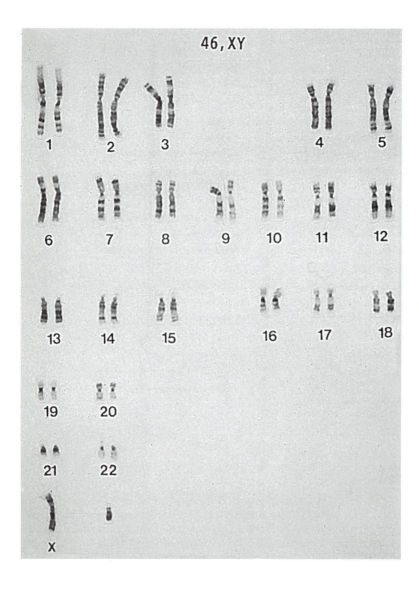

Figure 16–1. Banded chromosomal pattern (karyotype) of a normal male.

depends in part on the interest of the dentist and the availability of consultants and laboratories. Clinical geneticists are prepared to start "from scratch" or to work with others as needed. Names and addresses of such specialists, if not already familiar, can be obtained through the American Society of Human Genetics, 9650 Rockville Pike, Bethesda, Maryland 20814-3998 (telephone 301-571-1825).

A new and useful tool is the web site for McKusick's *Mendelian Inheritance in Man* (OMIM), a complete and monthly updated resource of information regarding human genetic disorders that is available at *http://www3.ncbi. nlm.nih.gov/omim/*. The database, put on line in December of 1995, had 10,000 entries by December 1998. Concise summaries of known clinical, chromosomal, and molecular information for each entry, along with current references and links to Medline, are available. Some photos and video action are in place, with more to be added to this program as it is updated.

Many dental and oral structural problems are known to be genetic. This chapter, however, emphasizes the more common genetic syndromes with which the dentist should also be familiar. Other resources likely to be helpful are listed in the reference section. The textbooks listed are regularly updated.

INHERITANCE PATTERNS

The intricate makeup of the human genetic system is being rapidly unfolded and is more complex than it would appear from the Mendelian inheritance patterns that have been used as models for many years. Germ line mosaicism, gene/chromosome deletion or duplication, imprinting, mitochondrial gene inheritance, and other newly described alterations of genes and chromosomes are detectable by molecular genetic analysis and cytogenetic study. In general, however, the Mendelian hereditary patterns of inheritance are still relied on and are useful in explanations of recurrence risks.

The thousands of nuclear human genes are lined up sequentially and are divided among 23 pairs of gene strands (chromosomes) (Fig. 16-1). One copy of each chromosome (and gene) is inherited from each parent, so that the total normal number of chromosomes in each body cell is 46. One of these pairs is that of the "sex" chromosomes. The X chromosome resembles a middle-sized autosomal chromosome in size, and the Y chromosome resembles one of the smaller and acrocentric (centromere toward one end)

autosomal chromosomes. Cytogenetic banding techniques allow identification of each individual pair of chromosomes. Careful analysis of each of these bands under the microscope is essential to determine whether small chromosomal deletions or duplications are present. The genes are much too small to be seen individually under the microscope but are being studied by molecular and biochemical means.

Location of genes may be noted by identifying the chromosome that the gene is on, followed by further definition of location. The short arm of the chromosome is lettered "p" and the long arm "q." Each of the arms may be divided into two or three subdivisions beginning with 1 toward the centromere of the chromosome and 2 or 3 toward the tip of the short or long arm. Each subdivision may again be similarly divided. Thus, the Treacher Collins gene, for example, is located at 5q32 (5 = chromosome, q = long arm, 3 is the subdivision near the tip of this arm, and 2 is a subdivision of this).

In addition to cytogenetic banding of chromosomes, currently available "genetic" testing includes fluorescence in situ hybridization (FISH) and DNA analysis for an increasingly larger number of human disorders. FISH studies combine cytogenetic and molecular techniques using colored gene probes as chromosome markers to determine minute deletions not detectable by routine cytogenetic banding (microdeletion syndromes such as velo-cardio-facial syndrome and Prader-Willi syndrome). As more and more genes are becoming fully characterized, DNA analyses for specific gene mutations are becoming available, with new tests being offered at a rapid pace.

Dominant

A gene is described as being *dominant* when its effects are generally obvious when it is present in a single dose (a new mutation or inherited from one parent only). A dominantly inherited disorder (Fig. 16-2) should be suspected when vertical transmission of the gene through the pedigree occurs, both sexes are equally affected, variation of expression of the gene is apparent, new mutations are frequent, and altered physical structures seem to be the primary manifesting effects of the gene. The risk for an affected parent to have affected offspring is 50% with each pregnancy.

Recessive

An autosomal gene is said to be *recessive* when its effects are normally not evident unless it is

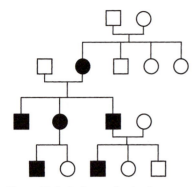

Figure 16–2. Pedigree of a dominant gene.

function. Many conditions are degenerative, with progressive disease leading to increasing health problems, expected retardation in some, and early demise in most. The risk for two carrier parents to have an affected child is 25% with each pregnancy. Fifty percent of offspring are carriers like the parent, and 25% have only normal genes (two thirds of unaffected siblings are carriers). Most recessive disorders are rare with the exception of cystic fibrosis (1 in 20 northern European descendants are carriers) and sickle cell disease (1 in 10 black African descendants are carriers).

present in a double dose (a copy is usually inherited from each parent). It is expected that both parents of an affected individual have a single altered copy of the gene in each body cell and are "carriers" of the gene change without showing any clinical manifestations of its presence. Surprisingly, molecular analysis has recently shown that occasional recessive disease occurs secondary to the presence of the two abnormal gene copies having come from the same parent. This is thought to result from random loss of an initially trisomic chromosome early in the zygote (then providing a normal chromosome count). The remaining chromosomes each have the same altered gene, by chance.

Recessively inherited conditions (Fig. 16–3) have the following characteristics: they generate a horizontal pedigree pattern (primarily affecting siblings and rarely other family members), are often severe and life-threatening, often affect metabolic function more severely than physical characteristics, are relatively rare, affect both sexes equally, and often occur in consanguineous matings. Most recessively inherited conditions cause severe illness, with alteration in physical structure being secondary to abnormal metabolic

X-Linked

Disorders of the sex chromosome genes are nearly always caused by recessive alterations on the X chromosome *(X-linked disease)*. When the individual is heterozygous (e.g., a carrier woman with one affected and one normal copy of the gene), the gene is ordinarily not symptomatic or may cause mild manifestations. A male is hemizygous (he has only one X chromosome and a Y chromosome) for an altered gene. Without a second and unaffected X, a recessive X-linked gene becomes fully manifest. The Y chromosome has relatively few genes, of which those present primarily influence sex determination. X-linked recessive conditions (Fig. 16–4) may seem to skip a generation because carrier women are either mildly affected or clinically unaffected, and the condition tends to be severe in males. X-linked recessive conditions cannot be passed from father to son, whereas all daughters of an affected man are obligate carriers. A carrier woman has a 25% risk with each pregnancy of having an affected son, a 25% risk of having a carrier daughter, and a 50% chance of having an unaffected (noncarrier) son or daughter.

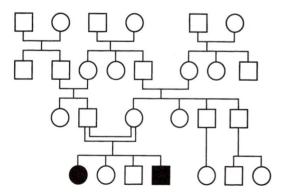

Figure 16–3. Pedigree of an autosomal recessive gene.

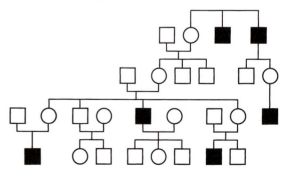

Figure 16–4. Pedigree of an X-linked recessive gene.

Polygenic/Multifactorial

Polygenic/multifactorial inheritance is not well understood. It has been assumed that multiple genes or genetic/environmental factors come together to allow the disorder to become apparent. Birth defects with a polygenic/multifactorial etiology are usually associated with a low recurrence risk for a second affected child to occur in the family (the most frequently quoted recurrence risk is 2–4% for each subsequent pregnancy). This risk generally increases to 10% to 15% for subsequent pregnancies if a couple has had two affected children. Polygenic/multifactorial inheritance has been used as the explanation for some of the most common adult onset familial conditions (e.g., hypertension, cancer, adult-onset diabetes, and allergies). Molecular genetic research has been teasing out some of the multiple and complex gene alterations and interactions that contribute to onset of these disorders. Clinical DNA testing in this arena is becoming available, though it is generally not yet applicable to most family situations and occasionally raises ethical/financial concerns (e.g., BRCA genes for breast cancer).

Chromosomal

In *chromosomal* syndromes, the individual genes are normal in structure but the numbers of copies of the genes present may be altered by deletions or duplications of whole or parts of chromosomes. Because of the many genes on each chromosome segment, chromosomal alterations generally lead to multiple physical anomalies (birth defects), poor growth, and developmental delay or retardation. Such conditions are most often sporadic but may be familial in some cases. Approximately 0.2% of the human population is a carrier of a balanced chromosome rearrangement (Fig. 16-5), which may be deleterious in reproduction. Resulting zygotes from a carrier parent may have extra chromosomal material (trisomy), missing chromosomal material (monosomy), a balanced rearrangement similar to that of the carrier parent, or a normal chromosomal complement. Trisomic or monosomic states may be lethal to the zygote, leading to multiple miscarriages, or they may cause birth defects and delayed growth and development in the newborn. Frequent among the birth defects noted are clefts of the lip or palate. Again, alterations of growth and development, especially when accompanied by birth defects, should alert the dentist to a possible chromosomal alteration.

Nontraditional Inheritance

The previously described inheritance patterns still hold up in explaining most of the inheritable genetic conditions affecting humans. With newer genetic analysis techniques, however, other gene/chromosome alterations have been discovered that may be deleterious and contribute to "genetic" disorders. These include imprinting, triplet repeat expansions, and mitochondrial inheritance.

Imprinting is a normal state for some of our genes and frequently is associated with methylation. A methylated gene is turned off. The ability to turn off activity of a gene may be important for controlling fetal development and for keeping our bodies regulated. Some of our genes are only imprinted on one copy, depending on whether it was passed down from the mother or the father. If a gene that should be present in both states (one imprinted from one parent and one not imprinted from the other parent) is altered by a deletion/duplication or mutation, a resulting imbalance of imprinted and nonimprinted may cause a disorder (several are noted in this chapter). Inheritance is not mendelian and depends on which parent the abnormal inherited gene came from. More and more disease states are being found that relate to imprinting abnormalities.

DNA *triplet repeat expansion* has been identified in several genetic conditions. Most of these, such as Huntington chorea, myotonic dystrophy, spinocerebellar atrophy, and fragile X syndrome, affect the nervous system in some way. The nature of the initial gene alteration leading to the subsequent expansion is unknown. Slight elongation of a gene may be a "premutation" not associated with disease but may lead to a full mutation and disease in offspring of the premutation "carrier." The elongated gene becomes inactivated (and frequently methylated) and unable to produce the expected protein product. Some of these genes are affected by imprinting, with expansion being affected by sex of the parent passing the gene on.

Mitochondrial DNA has been identified, in general, with energy production for our cellular functions. The cytoplasmic location (not nuclear as with the majority of our DNA) of mitochondrial genes is responsible for the interesting inheritance pattern that occurs in affected families. Disease-associated mitochondrial DNA mutations may be passed down in varying degrees to all offspring of carrier mothers but to none of the offspring of affected men. This is because sperm carry little cytoplasm with them, whereas divi-

$$45, XX, \tau (14q21q)$$

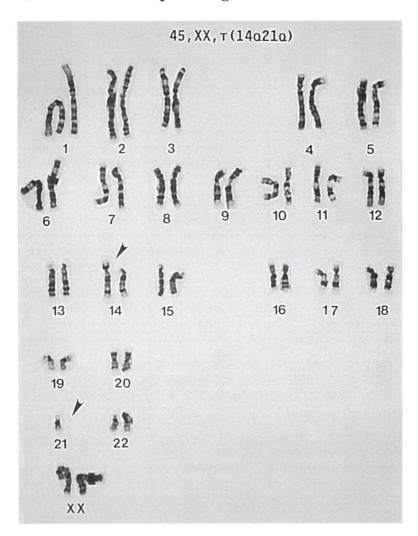

Figure 16–5. Karyotype of a balanced 14/21 translocation.

sion of cytoplasmic content to daughter egg cells is random. Mitochondrial mutations are frequently associated with degenerative diseases and multiple organ involvement. Signs and symptoms may include such entities as progressive myopathy, hypertrophic cardiomyopathy, dementia, seizures, deafness, and blindness.

DOMINANT GENETIC CONDITIONS

Neurofibromatosis I (von Recklinghausen Disease)

Neurofibromatosis I is a dominantly inherited condition with marked variability in expression of the gene and a high rate of new mutation. The incidence is 1 in 2500 to 3000. Because of chronic and progressive physical changes, these patients become a much more prominent group than the actual incidence would indicate. Early intervention may prevent severe disability, severe disfigurement, school drop-out, or potentially life-threatening medical problems.

Further confirmation of neurofibromatosis I should be looked for in persons who have brown birth marks (café-au-lait spots) or more than one neurofibroma (Fig. 16–6). The café-au-lait lesions cannot be distinguished from those in unaffected persons but are present in increased numbers in people with neurofibromatosis I. Although it is extremely rare for unaffected persons to have three or more of these pigmented lesions, persons with neurofibromatosis I typically have six or more café-au-lait lesions. Common "soft signs" of neurofibromatosis I include short stature (average height at the 34th percentile), relative macrocephaly (average head circumference at the 87th percentile), and freckling in intertriginous areas. Learning disabilities or behavior problems are

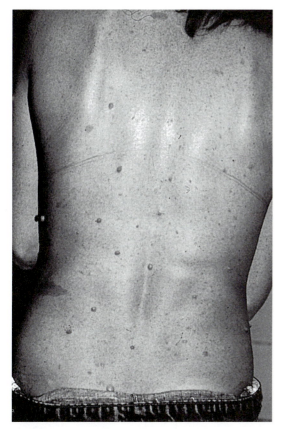

Figure 16–6. Café-au-lait spots and neurofibromas affecting a young woman with neurofibromatosis.

other areas) are common in these patients and may extend into the mouth, affecting tooth alignment and mastication. Unfortunately, these disfiguring tumors, although rarely malignant, may be difficult to treat. Because of their proliferative extension into all surrounding structures, total removal is normally not possible and recurrence of the tumor is usual. Perhaps even more important is the potential for severe bleeding during surgery because these tumors are frequently and surprisingly highly vascular. Spontaneous bleeding is unusual, however. Anesthesia is normally not a problem for patients with neurofibromatosis, although approximately 2% of such persons have a pheochromocytoma, which could lead to a hypertensive crisis during surgery.

The affected gene is on the long arm of chromosome 17 (17q11.2). Though direct DNA testing has become available, such testing currently detects only 70% of affected patients and is usually not necessary for diagnosis. DNA linkage is available for informative, affected families, though rarely necessary.

Tuberous Sclerosis

Tuberous sclerosis is another dominant condition with marked variation of expression. At least

present in nearly half of these patients, and mental retardation occurs in less than 10%. Unexplained hypertension is common in neurofibromatosis I, as are severe headaches (generally not caused by hypertension, brain tumors, pheochromocytomas, renal artery abnormalities, or other apparent physical alterations that may need to be ruled out). "Benign" glial tumors of the brain are present in about 15% of patients and may require treatment if they are symptomatic. In addition to gliomas, about 70% of children with neurofibromatosis I have "bright" areas, especially around the basal ganglia areas on T2 magnetic resonance imaging (MRI). These tend to disappear with time. Malignant tumors, including sarcomas and schwannomas, are thought to occur at a rate of 5% more than in the average population, occur at younger ages in persons with neurofibromatosis, and may occur anywhere in the body.

Oral structures may be affected by the development of neurofibromas anywhere within or outside of the mouth. Plexiform neurofibromas (Fig. 16–7) of the craniofacial structures (and

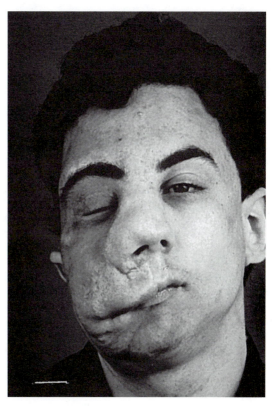

Figure 16–7. A facial plexiform tumor in a patient with neurofibromatosis.

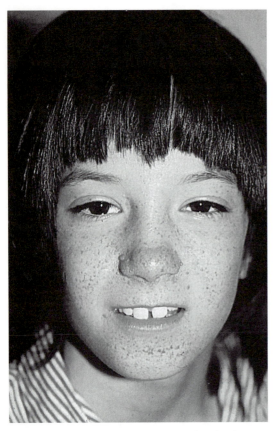

Figure 16–8. Angiofibromas in a young girl with tuberous sclerosis.

three separate genes with indistinguishable clinical features have been identified. New mutations are frequent. Cutaneous lesions are the most common and observable markers of this disorder and are of several types. Facial angiofibromas, although usually not present until the person is 3 or 4 years old, are progressive throughout childhood, may be the first observed alteration of the condition, and may become unsightly (Fig. 16-8). Hypomelanotic macules (ashleaf spots) are present in infancy but may be difficult to see clearly without the use of an ultraviolet light (Wood's lamp). Thickened patches of waxy-appearing skin tissue (shagreen patches and plaques) may become evident within a few years or later in childhood or adolescence. Subungual fibromas may cause grooves and deformities of the nails.

Systemic manifestations of tuberous sclerosis are also variable. Seizures occur in approximately 80% of patients, and mental retardation is present in approximately 48%. "Tubers" of the brain are easily detected on brain imaging. Rhabdomyomas of the heart occur in 40% of patients but are generally asymptomatic after infancy. Cysts of the kidneys and angiomyolipomas are common and may lead to hypertension and other signs of renal dysfunction. The primary dental manifestation of tuberous sclerosis is that of multiple enamel pits, especially in the facial surfaces of incisors and canines. Fibrous nodules may be found on the gingiva, tongue, or palate.

Approximately two thirds of affected persons have a new gene mutation that behaves as a dominant gene, once present. Unlike neurofibromatosis, tuberous sclerosis may be caused by a mutation in any of at least three separate genes that have been identified though not yet fully characterized.

Marfan Syndrome

Marfan syndrome is an autosomal dominant "connective tissue" disorder. Craniofacial features (Fig. 16-9) frequently include a long and narrow face with a high palatal vault. A prominent lower jaw, malocclusion, or both are common. Marked laxity of the joints, lengthening of the long bones

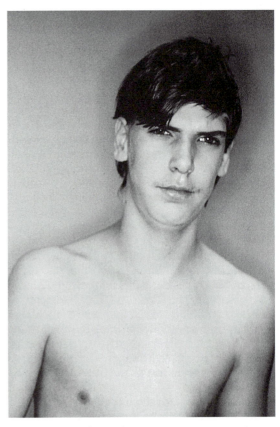

Figure 16–9. Marfan syndrome in a young teenager. Long face and sternal deformity (pectus carinatum) are evident.

leading to disproportionately tall stature and sternal deformity, scoliosis, and a high narrow palate are all part of the bony and ligamentous aspects of this condition. Dislocation of the lens of the eye and severe myopia (frequently a cause of retinal detachment) are the typical ophthalmologic findings. The most serious and life-threatening aspect of Marfan syndrome, however, is the alteration of the connective tissue of the aorta, which may lead to death and is the reason for the reduced life expectancy with this condition. Widening of the aortic root, aneurysm, and subsequent dissection may occur in spite of medical and surgical attempts to correct the problem. New surgical techniques are being used, although their long-range effects are still unknown. Early recognition of Marfan syndrome may allow treatment to prevent loss of vision (especially retinal detachment secondary to severe myopia), prolong life, and prevent sudden death. Although the responsible fibrillin gene on chromosome 15 has been identified, clinical DNA testing is not yet available to families, primarily because so many families have a "private" mutation in the gene, not commonly detected. Clinical gene testing is now available and requires a skin biopsy.

Ehlers-Danlos Syndrome

Ehlers-Danlos syndrome is the overall designation for approximately 10 connective tissue disorders that overlap in clinical symptoms. The common signs of these conditions are marked hyperlaxity of the joints, increased stretchability and velvety softness of the skin, easy bruising, and poor wound healing with marked scarring. Complications of Ehlers-Danlos syndrome vary, depending on the specific type. Spontaneous vascular or bowel rupture leading to death may occur, especially in Ehlers-Danlos syndrome Type IV. Premature loss of teeth (secondary to periodontal disease) is especially noted in Type VIII, and rupture of the cornea is part of Type VI.

At this time a definitive test is clinically available only for Type IV Ehlers-Danlos syndrome in which there is a deficiency in the release of Type III collagen. Such testing is performed on skin fibroblasts obtained by biopsy and culture. More definitive testing by molecular genetic study may become available in the next few years.

Malignant Hyperthermia

Malignant hyperthermia is another potentially life-threatening condition that is thought to be secondary to a dominantly inherited gene. The affected gene leads to alterations in muscle membranes that are triggered by certain anesthetics such as halothane or depolarizing muscle relaxants such as succinylcholine. Mild symptoms such as muscle aches may occur daily but are often overlooked. During surgery, however, the offending agents may trigger tetany-like body tightening and very high body temperatures. If uncontrolled, death may occur immediately or within 1 or 2 days of the surgery.

Attempts to perform tests on family members of patients with malignant hyperthermia have thus far been frustrating. Tests using creatine phosphokinase analysis, muscle biopsy, or both have been inaccurate. Molecular research has demonstrated linked loci on at least six different chromosomes that are involved with the production of skeletal muscle ryanodine receptor proteins and a CACNLIA3 gene, all of which function as calcium release channels. Molecular genetic testing is likely to be available in the near future; however, until such a definitive test becomes available, the family history must be relied on to determine which individuals are at risk. Patients with muscular dystrophy (especially myotonic dystrophy) have a higher than expected incidence of malignant hyperthermia and should also be considered at-risk during surgery.

Precautions to be taken during surgery on family members of affected persons include selection of appropriate anesthetics, temperature monitoring throughout the entire procedure, readily available cooling mechanisms, and availability of dantrolene sodium, which should be administered at the onset of symptoms. At the onset of symptoms, the surgical procedure should be discontinued and the patient stabilized appropriately. Alternative choices for analgesia/sedation include regional anesthesia, nitrous oxide, propofol, opiates, barbiturates, ketamine, benzodiazepines, and nonpolarizing muscle relaxants. Referral to a genetic clinic is helpful in completing a thorough family investigation, preparing family members for possible surgery through counseling, and providing brochure information to be shared with the anesthesiologist. Eventually molecular genetic testing provides the definitive answers as to which family members have inherited the altered gene.

Primary Bone Dysplasias

Bone dysplasias such as achondroplasia, hypochondroplasia, and spondyloepiphyseal dysplasia cause alterations of the oral cavity, leading primarily to problems of space. Orthodontic care may be needed for such conditions. Airway narrowing or collapse may be of concern for the anesthesiologist. Of additional concern for the dentist in caring for such patients is the possibility of atlantoaxial subluxation, which may become symptomatic secondary to spinal cord compression on manipulation of the head and neck. Each such patient should undergo a flexion-extension set of radiographs of the cervical spine prior to such manipulations. Subluxation of more than 3 mm should prompt referral to a neurosurgeon.

Dwarfing or marked shortening of stature is typical of patients with bone dysplasias. Most cause disproportionate shortening (Fig. 16–10), and the specific condition can be classified according to the primary bone structure affected. Dysplasias affecting the spine cause marked vertebral body alterations resulting in shortening of the spine. In chondrodysplasias the trunk length is relatively spared, but there is marked shortening of the limbs.

Other notable health problems may occur with

various bone dysplasias. Chondrodysplasias are noted for marked macrocephaly, occasional hydrocephalus secondary to narrowing of the foramen magnum, lordosis, and bowing of the legs. Severe scoliosis, marked myopia, and hearing loss occur in several of the other bone dysplasia syndromes. Although the appearance of such persons may be striking, normal intelligence is frequent, as is survival beyond middle age.

Many of these conditions are caused by new mutations of a dominant gene that, once present, can be passed on to offspring. DNA testing is now clinically available for several of the primary bone dysplasias, though it is often not necessary for diagnosis of an affected individual. Such testing may, however, help some families considering family planning issues. Achondroplasia, hypochondroplasia, and thanatophoric (lethal) dwarfism have been found to be allelic and caused by a mutation of the fibroblast growth factor receptor, type 3 (FGFR3) on 4p16.

Branchio-Oto-Renal Syndrome

This syndrome (Fig. 16–11) should be considered a potential diagnosis in families or patients with a history of branchial fistulas or cysts. Other outward signs of this condition may include anomalous ear pinnas, preauricular pits, and a long, narrow face with a deep overbite. Of concern, however, are the other significant health problems that may accompany this abnormality. Hearing loss is common, ranging from mild to severe, and may show up at any time into young adulthood. Renal dysplasia, again of varying degrees of severity, may also develop. Hearing evaluations and renal ultrasound investigations should be performed for affected persons and their direct descendants.

Gorlin Syndrome

Gorlin syndrome (basal cell nevus syndrome) causes variations of craniofacial structures (Fig. 16–12) in addition to the increased risk for cancerous changes in skin nevi. Dyskeratotic cysts ("odontogenic keratocysts") of the mandible or maxilla may become symptomatic in childhood or young adult life and frequently require surgical correction. When such cysts are identified, the remainder of the body should be examined for basal cell nevi, which frequently behave malignantly unless removed.

Other physical signs of Gorlin syndrome are typical. These may include a prominent forehead

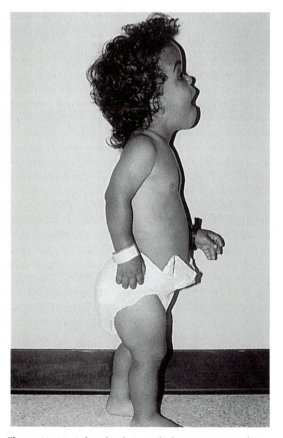

Figure 16–10. Achondroplasia with disproportionate short stature, macrocephaly, midface recession, and so on.

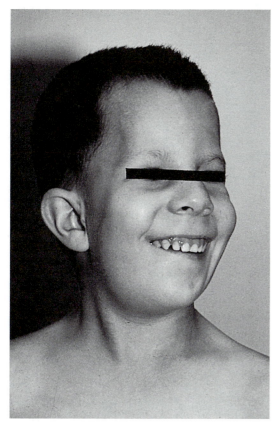

Figure 16–11. Facies of branchio-oto-renal syndrome with hearing aids off. Note preauricular pit.

and eyebrows with deep-set, downslanting, and widely spaced eyes. Teeth may be misshaped or carious, and the jaw prominent. Bifid, fused, or missing ribs are common, as is calcification of the falx cerebri. Medulloblastoma may occur (especially following exposure to radiation), and benign tumors such as lipomas or fibromas of the skin may appear.

This "syndrome" is caused by a mutation of the "patched" (PTC) gene on chromosome 9, most often passed down from a parent. Mutations in somatic cells, however, have been thought to be responsible for sporadic basal cell carcinomas, the most common skin cancer, which is usually not inherited.

Gardner Syndrome

Gardner syndrome (familial polyposis) may be first diagnosed by the dentist, who is likely to note dentigerous cysts, supernumerary teeth, or delayed eruption of teeth. Osteomas of the mandible, face, or other bones are also frequent.

Epidermal inclusion or sebaceous cysts may develop, especially over the trunk, but they may involve the face or scalp.

Unfortunately, the prognosis for untreated persons who have familial polyposis is poor. Malignancy is usual by 30 years of age and may be present by the late teen years. A colectomy is recommended and may provide a cure, although malignancies may occur outside of this area in some patients.

The gene for this condition has been located on chromosome 5 (5q21). DNA testing is now clinically available that allows offspring who do not inherit the mutant gene to avoid unnecessary prophylactic colonoscopic screening examinations.

Single Central Incisor

A single central incisor is an additional but rare condition that can be dominantly inherited, with marked variation of expression (imprinted?) (Figs. 16-13 and 16-14). When fully expressed, this gene causes holoprosencephaly, cebocephaly, and severe mental retardation; death is likely

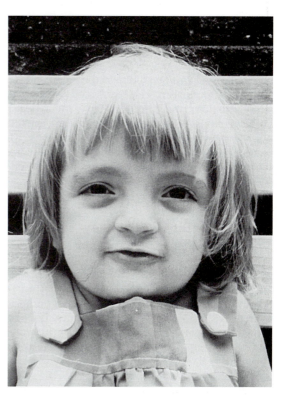

Figure 16–12. Facies of a child with Gorlin syndrome inherited from her father. A prominent forehead, wide-spaced and downslanting palpebral fissures, prominent eyebrows, and deep-set eyes are visible.

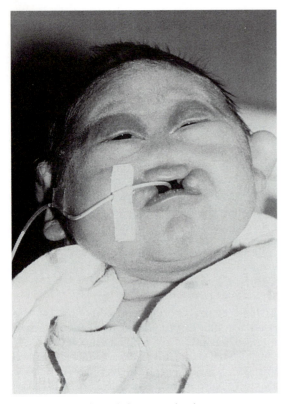

Figure 16–13. Cebocephaly in an infant born to a woman with a single central incisor (shown in Fig. 16–14).

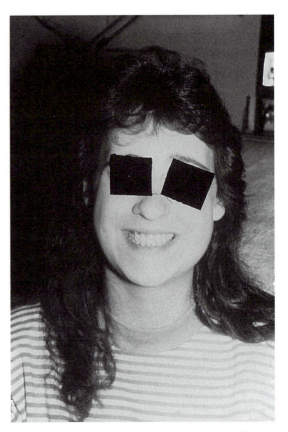

Figure 16–14. Single central incisor in a woman with average intelligence.

in infancy. Milder degrees of expression of this gene are usual and may include the single central incisor, hypotelorism (closely spaced eyes), mental retardation, and microcephaly (small head). Prenatal ultrasound studies may be used to rule out the presence of severe brain alterations. Research has demonstrated that in some families with this condition, this gene is linked to a gene at 7q36.

Treacher Collins Syndrome

Treacher Collins syndrome is an autosomal dominant condition that causes characteristic alterations of the craniofacial structures (Fig. 16–15). Some of the alterations noted in this condition overlap with those of the Pierre-Robin sequence, the facio-auriculo-vertebral spectrum group (also known as Goldenhar syndrome or hemifacial microsomia), Nagar syndrome, Miller syndrome, and Townes syndrome.

Craniofacial characteristics that may be present in all of these syndromes include marked mandibular hypoplasia (micrognathia), cleft palate, macrostomia, malar hypoplasia, down-

slanting palpebral fissures, preauricular tags, microtia or external ear canal defects, anomalies of the middle ear ossicles, and deafness. Treacher Collins syndrome may be distinguished from the others by the presence of a coloboma or ectro-

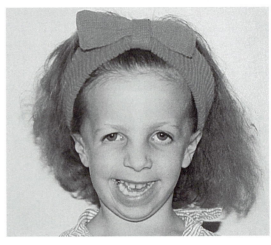

Figure 16–15. Facies of a patient with Treacher Collins syndrome.

pion of the lower eyelid (producing a sagging lower eyelid) and usual dominant inheritance once the gene is present in the family. Abnormal limb development, body asymmetry, other birth defects, or other inheritance patterns suggest an alternative diagnosis.

Severe micrognathia is a medical emergency in the newborn period. Airway obstruction and difficult feeding are usual. A tracheostomy is often required during the first month or two until adequate growth of the jaw occurs. Orthodontic procedures are usual for such patients, and "jaw" surgery is frequently indicated at a later age.

Hearing tests should be performed for all patients with Treacher Collins syndrome. Many require corrective surgery for the abnormal ear structures, and hearing aids may be necessary.

Several types of mutations have been identified in the Treacher Collins gene found on chromosome 5q32.

Cleidocranial Dysostosis and Pyknodysostosis

These two syndromes show some overlapping of features. Both conditions are associated with dental anomalies, including delayed eruption of secondary teeth, supernumerary teeth, more frequent caries, partial anodontia, and malformed teeth or roots. Both of these conditions also cause marked delay in closure of the anterior fontanel, which may be very large (a helmet may be required to protect the brain); Wormian bones of the skull; increased incidence of fractures; reduced stature with relative macrocephaly; mid-

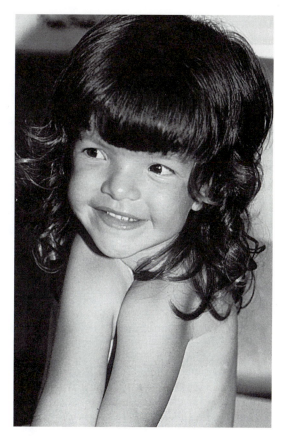

Figure 16–17. Same patient showing absent clavicles.

face hypoplasia with high palate; hearing loss; and hypoplasia of the clavicles.

Cleidocranial dysostosis is usually associated with normal intelligence but may cause marked alterations in appearance. A high, bossed, and broad forehead associated with midfacial and occipital hypoplasia (Figs. 16–16 and 16–17) may be accompanied by severely sloped and hypermobile shoulders. Dental alterations become the major obstacle to a healthy appearance and eating habits as life progresses.

Pyknodysostosis can be distinguished by shortening of the ramus of the mandible, producing a markedly reduced angle (Fig. 16–18), and by an inheritance pattern that suggests possible recessive inheritance. Shortening of the fingers with excessive wrinkling of the overlying skin and an increased incidence of retardation may also be noted.

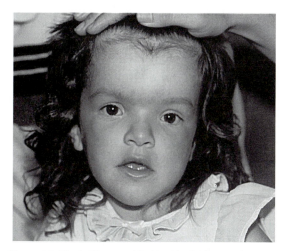

Figure 16–16. A 3½-year-old girl with cleidocranial dysostosis who by history at 10 years of age has only two fully erupted permanent teeth, eight extra permanent teeth, and several horizontally impacted teeth.

Craniosynostosis Syndromes (Apert, Crouzon, Saethre-Chotzen, and Pfeiffer)

The craniosynostosis syndromes (Apert, Crouzon, Saethre-Chotzen, and Pfeiffer syndromes)

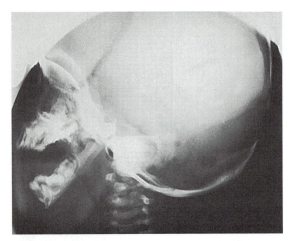

Figure 16–18. Radiograph of a patient with pyknodys-ostosis.

are all generally dominantly inherited once the gene is present in the family. All patients with these abnormalities should be referred at the time of recognition to a neurosurgeon for possible reconstructive surgery. This is especially important in infancy. It is hoped that release of the prematurely closed sutures will allow normal brain growth (and intelligence) and will normalize the shape and appearance of the craniofacial features. Once the brain and skull are fully grown, such surgery is not likely to result in a satisfactory appearance. Mental retardation is an underlying possibility regardless of surgery, although many affected persons are normally intelligent.

Craniofacial alterations noted in patients with craniosynostosis (Fig. 16–19) may be marked and frequently include tall forehead, prominent eyes (shallow orbits), hypertelorism, small and beaked nose, and brachycephaly. The synostosis may be asymmetrical and may cause marked distortion unilaterally if it is not recognized and treated in infancy. Possible hearing and vision loss should be considered in each case with an appropriate referral. Oral cavity variations commonly include impaction, severe crowding, delayed eruption, supernumerary teeth, congenitally missing teeth, thick gingiva, and very high palate (Kaloust et al., 1997). Occasional clefting of the palate is noted.

Limb abnormalities are the primary diagnostic feature distinguishing these various cranio-synostoses from each other. Apert syndrome is associated with "mitten"-like syndactyly of the hands and feet. Saethre-Chotzen syndrome and Pfeiffer syndrome have milder degrees of syndactyly and digital-thumb alterations. No limb abnormalities are associated with Crouzon syndrome.

The Crouzon, Apert, and Pfeiffer syndromes have been found to be caused by different mutations (alleles) within the fibroblast growth factor receptor, type 2 (FGFR2) gene.

Velo-Cardio-Facial Syndrome

Velo-cardio-facial syndrome is another condition that may first be recognized by the dentist. The most common features of this condition include learning disabilities, palatal incompetence, minor facial anomalies (Fig. 16–20), and congenital cardiac defects. Submucous clefts may occur in some cases and, less commonly, a cleft palate with micrognathia (Pierre Robin sequence). Palatal problems are frequently primarily exhibited by altered speech. Typical facial alterations include a prominent nose with squared nasal root and narrow alar base, narrow palpebral fissures, abundant scalp hair, vertical maxillary excess, deficiency malar area, and retruded mandible.

The most common cardiac defect is a ventriculoseptal defect (VSD), though more deleterious changes in this gene may be life-threatening. These include conotruncal cardiac defects and anomalies of thymus and parathyroid leading to immune deficiency/abnormal calcium metabolism. This latter clinical spectrum is often called DiGeorge syndrome.

Velo-cardio-facial syndrome (and DiGeorge syndrome) is secondary to a microdeletion at 22q11.2, which is frequently passed down through a family, appearing as a dominant gene with a 50/50 risk for each offspring to be affected (receive the deleted gene) and with marked variability from one affected family mem-

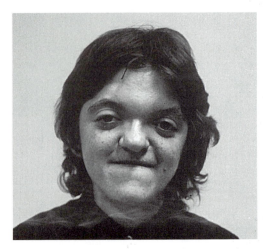

Figure 16–19. Facies of a teenager with Apert syndrome.

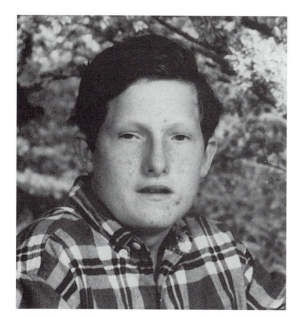

Figure 16–20. A 13-year-old with velo-cardio-facial syndrome confirmed by fluorescence in situ hybridization (FISH). Note palatal incompetence, typical facies with narrow palpebral fissures, prominent nose, small alae, long and flattened midface, and abundant scalp hair.

ber to another. Though direct DNA analysis is not generally available, FISH studies can detect the 85% to 90% of those who have a deletion at 22q11.2. In the past year, it has become apparent that velo-cardio-facial syndrome may be one of the more common identifiable syndromes.

Oculo-Dento-Digital Syndrome

Oculo-dento-digital syndrome is likely more common than previously recognized, though the expression of the dominant gene(s) is variable (Figs. 16–21 and 16–22). Though facial and limb abnormalities may be apparent from birth on, dentists may be the first to recognize this condition in the affected family. Facial variations can include small corneas, small eyes (microphthalmia), epicanthal folds, sparse or abnormally textured hair, a thin nose with small alae nasi, and bent or fused 4th–5th fingers. Common dental anomalies include enamel hypoplasia, wide alveolar ridge, wide mandible, small teeth, and gross dental caries. Intelligence is most often normal. Widening of other bones may be apparent on radiograph. Hearing loss, glaucoma, and occasional neurologic problems may occur. New mutations are common. Studies have linked this condition to chromosome 6q (Gladwin et al., 1997).

AUTOSOMAL RECESSIVE CONDITIONS

Cystic Fibrosis

Cystic fibrosis is the most common recessively inherited disorder in the Caucasian population with a carrier rate of 1 in 22. Cystic fibrosis may become apparent in the newborn, or it may go unrecognized for some time. In the dentist's office, a history of failure to thrive, chronic airway

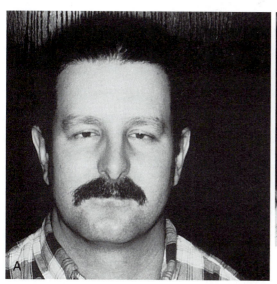
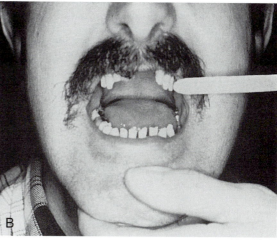

Figure 16–21. *A,* Oculo-dento-digital syndrome in father of the patient shown in Figure 16–22. Note small cornea, small eyes, thin nose with small alae nasi, and abnormal hair texture. *B,* Same patient: note abnormal enamel and small teeth.

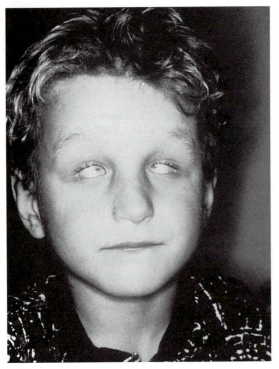

Figure 16–22. Oculo-dento-digital syndrome with more severe ocular anomalies than in the father shown in Figure 16–21A.

disease, or diarrhea should prompt an investigation for possible cystic fibrosis. A sweat test is used to confirm the diagnosis. Over 100 mutations have been described in the CF gene, although deletion of delta 508 is the most common. Currently available clinical DNA tests detect over 90% of mutations. An affected child may have inherited a different mutation from each of the parents. Testing of clinically unaffected family members is being used by some families for pre-implantation diagnosis, prenatal testing, or both.

Good oral hygiene is essential for the well-being of persons with cystic fibrosis because infection control is a constant battle for these patients. Tooth discoloration secondary to tetracycline use is also possible.

Sickle Cell Disease

Sickle cell disease is another recessively inherited chronic disorder that is associated with periods of severe illness (crises). Bone marrow shutdown and sequestered, sickled red blood cells may rapidly lead to shock and subsequent death or brain damage. Sepsis (especially pneumococcal sepsis) is also common if not prevented.

Patients with possible sickle cell trait or disease should be well informed about this disease and should be offered screening (hemoglobin electrophoresis). In persons found to be homologous for the sickle cell gene (i.e., they have sickle cell disease), antibiotic prophylaxis, spleen removal, and good hydration should be routine. Persons who are heterozygous for the sickle cell gene (i.e., they have sickle cell trait) are carriers for the gene but do not ordinarily have illness related to it. Prenatal gene testing is available. Newborn screening in many states includes hemoglobin electrophoresis, although individual patients may not keep appointments for discussion of abnormal test results.

Mucopolysaccharidoses

The mucopolysaccharidoses are all secondary to deficient metabolism of mucopolysaccharides, which are part of the ground substances of the body. The accumulation of byproducts and mucopolysaccharides in various vital organs and tissues accounts for the deterioration in function of these organs and subsequently for the deterioration in the health and life of affected persons. Variations among these disorders depend on which specific enzyme is deficient. With the exception of Hunter syndrome, which has an X-linked recessive inheritance pattern, all are autosomal recessively inherited. The other types include Hurler syndrome, Scheie syndrome, Sanfilippo syndrome, Morquio syndrome, Maroteaux-Lamy syndrome, and beta-glucuronidase deficiency. Multiple allelic forms have been identified for several of these conditions. Although many similarities are present from one type to another, the organs most seriously affected vary according to the importance of the specific deficient enzyme for that organ.

In general, the clinical manifestations (Fig. 16–23) that are most notable are caused by abnormal storage of mucopolysaccharides in the brain, cornea, joints, heart, and liver. Mental retardation, corneal clouding (and reduced vision), joint contractures, and an enlarged heart and liver are noted. Storage in the craniofacial structures also occurs, causing marked "coarsening" of features. Relative macrocephaly with hypertelorism, flat nasal bridge, and short stature may be noted in infancy along with organomegaly. The alterations noted become progressively worse and ultimately cause early demise. Death usually occurs between 10 and 30 years of age, depending on which abnormal gene/allele is present. Inguinal and umbilical hernias may become problematic.

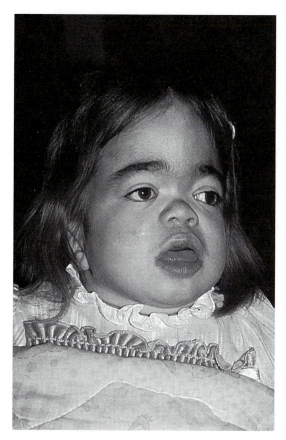

Figure 16–23. Facies of a patient with Hurler syndrome.

Surgical procedures for patients with mucopolysaccharidoses may be more hazardous or difficult than normal. Airway narrowing and instability occur as storage of mucopolysaccharides takes place, so that intubation *and* extubation become problematic. Breathing becomes more labored, and cor pulmonale may result from obstruction as the disease progresses. Heart and liver function should be determined prior to surgery. Fixed contractures of the joints and spinal curvature may cause problems with positioning of such patients.

Dental manifestations of mucopolysaccharidoses may occur early and include prominent lips and tongue, hypertrophied alveolar ridges and gums, and widely spaced teeth.

Carrier and prenatal testing is generally available and should be offered to enhance family planning, as desired.

Treatment for persons affected by a mucopolysaccharidosis condition has generally been unsatisfactory to date. Neither replacement of missing or deficiency enzymes by direct infusion nor bone marrow transplant has consistently slowed the disease process safely. Perhaps better understanding of the genetic alteration will improve treatment in the future.

X-LINKED CONDITIONS

X-Linked Mental Retardation

X chromosome gene mutations are the most common cause of hereditary mental retardation. The most frequent of these is *fragile X* syndrome. Males affected by the fragile X syndrome are usually moderately retarded. The physical appearance of an affected person may not be remarkable, although prognathism, high palate, long face and ears, large head circumference (Fig. 16–24), and large testicles (two to three times normal) are typical. Carrier females may have characteristics such as social anxiety and shyness, and those with a more expanded gene may be mildly retarded.

Clinical DNA testing is available and can be used for confirmation of diagnosis and carrier testing. Named for the fragile-appearing tip of the long arm of chromosome X (when chromosomes are studied with folic acid–deficient media), the newer molecular genetic techniques have cast light on previously confusing clinical observations. The mutated fragile X gene expands (and becomes inactivated) with addition of multiple triplet repeats (CGG) as it is passed down from a female carrier, who may have inherited the gene from her carrier father (he may be the first with the mutation in the family) or mother. Once the gene passes through a female and expands, affected male offspring are usually moderately retarded and females may be mildly retarded. This gene, which is affected differently according to the sex of the parent passing it on,

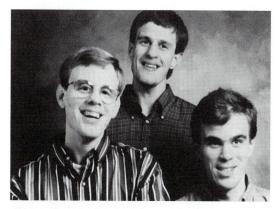

Figure 16–24. Adult brothers, all with fragile X syndrome. Features include long face and ears, prognathism, large head, and retardation (all three require supervised living).

is one of the "imprinted" genes (see discussion earlier in this chapter). A fragile X gene alteration should be suspected and tested for in any retarded male or "slow" female. A number of family members may also be at risk.

Ectodermal Dysplasia

Ectodermal dysplasia is the name given to a large group of syndromes that impair the body structures derived from the ectoderm. The ectodermal structures most commonly affected include hair, nails, teeth, sweat glands, and mucous glands. Some of these syndromes also involve other major body systems that may become the predominant focus of attention (e.g., mental retardation, congenital heart disease, and cleft lip and palate). The best known of the ectodermal dysplasia conditions, and one for which dental care is frequently the most important aspect of treatment, is the anhidrotic X-linked form (Figs. 16–25 and 16–26). Anodontia or hypodontia is usual, as are conical ("peg-shaped") anterior teeth when they are present. Dentures are usu-

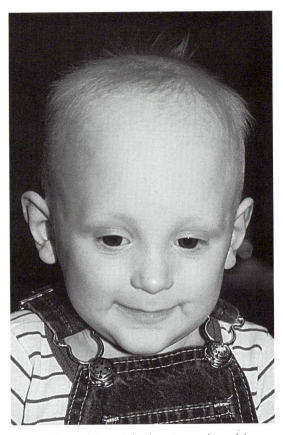

Figure 16–26. Ectodermal dysplasia in grandson of the patient shown in Figure 16–25.

ally needed at an early age but are likely to be more problematic than usual because of poorly developed alveolar ridges. Early dental intervention is important to maintain and improve mastication and facial appearance. Dental implants may be the answer for some.

In X-linked anhidrotic ectodermal dysplasia, intelligence is usually normal and life span good, though both may depend on the availability of high-quality health care. An absence of or sparse placement of sweat glands, sebaceous glands, and mucous glands can lead to deleterious health problems. Of major importance is control of body temperature during hot summer weather, fever, or physical exercise. Without adequate sweating, body temperatures may rise to over 105°F. Such high body temperatures may result in brain damage. Appropriate use of immersion in cool water, wetting of the clothing, air conditioning, and other cooling mechanisms are essential in the care of male children and adults with anhidrotic ectodermal dysplasia. Frequent ear, sinus, and bronchial irritations and secondary infections result from a reduction in mucus pro-

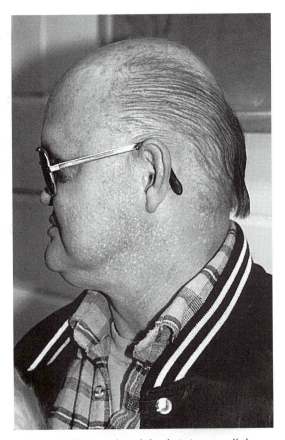

Figure 16–25. Ectodermal dysplasia in a grandfather.

duction. Hydrating nasal sprays or eye drops are occasionally helpful. Antibiotic treatment of ear and respiratory tract problems is frequently necessary in the first few years of life.

In addition to the dental anomalies, other "cosmetic" problems impose a lifelong struggle for the patient. Sparse or absent hair, eyebrows, and eyelashes along with a "saddle" nose, the dental anomalies, and poorly formed nails may create an "old man" or "vampire" appearance in affected persons. Use of a wig is frequently very unsatisfactory; attractive wigs for children are not available, and most acceptable hairpieces for adults are costly. Use of false fingernails has not been generally satisfactory because occlusion may cause fungal infection in the already dystrophic nail. Carrier females may have similar but milder degrees of these anomalies. Absent or hypoplastic mammary glands may be noted. Additional support for the family may be obtained through the National Foundation for Ectodermal Dysplasias, P.O. Box 114, Mascoutah, IL 62258 (telephone 618-566-2020). Prenatal and carrier testing is available for families through linkage analysis of family members. Linkage testing is available to help with genetic counseling.

POLYGENIC CONDITIONS (MULTIFACTORIAL)

Cleft Lip and Cleft Palate

Clefting of the lip or palate most often occurs alone as a polygenic condition. There are, however, many individual syndromes in which a cleft may be noted. Such syndromes may be sporadic (happen only once in a family), may be secondary to teratogenic effects (e.g., maternal diabetes or use of hydantoin or Valium), or may be part of a syndrome with Mendelian inheritance such as the Van der Woude syndrome. The latter condition is dominantly inherited and may manifest as lip pits only (Fig. 16-27), as clefting, or all at once. When polygenic, the incidence of cleft lip or palate is approximately 1 in 800 with a recurrence risk of approximately 4%. The American Indian population, however, has an increased risk of around 7%. As with other polygenic conditions, the risk triples if a couple's second child is born with the defect. Prenatal testing is possible through careful ultrasound study of the fetus.

Care of the patient with cleft lip or palate requires an experienced team including an otolaryngologist, speech pathologist, dentist or orthodontist, and psychologist.

Neural Tube Defects

Neural tube defects seldom affect the oral area directly but may cause changes indirectly because of a resulting hydrocephalus or seizure disorder that requires anticonvulsants. Chronic antibiotic use may be indicated for patients with neural tube defects involving bladder or central nervous system (CNS) alterations.

By the time a dentist sees a patient with a meningomyelocele it is likely that several surgical procedures have taken place. Repair of the primary lesion is performed early to protect the CNS from infection. Because hydrocephalus occurs in approximately 80% of patients with neural tube defects, a shunting procedure may also have been performed. The shunt tubing may be noted readily because it traverses the lateral skull area to the thoracic or abdominal area and lies just under the subcutaneous tissues. It is also likely that an affected patient has been fitted with an indwelling bladder catheter or is being catheterized several times daily to protect the urinary tract from retained urine, which is a good growth medium for bacteria and may reflux upward into the kidneys, causing deterioration. Learning problems may be present in mild or more severe degrees depending on whether a CNS infection or hydrocephalus has been present. Leg bracing or wheelchair use is usual. For the dentist, subacute bacterial endocarditis prophylaxis may be important when a shunt tube or catheter is present, especially if the tip of the distal end of the shunt has been placed within the ventricle of the heart.

The multifactorial recurrence risk of 3% to 5% for subsequent siblings may be reduced to half of this by maternal intake of folic acid supple-

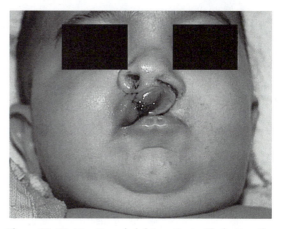

Figure 16–27. Lip pits and cleft in patient with dominantly inherited Van der Woude's syndrome.

ments (0.4 to 4.0 mg) prior to onset of the pregnancy. The exact mechanism of this reduction is not known. Prenatal diagnosis is available by fetal ultrasonography and maternal screening.

CHROMOSOMAL SYNDROMES

Down Syndrome

Down syndrome is most often sporadic in occurrence, although approximately 3% of cases are familial, resulting from a translocated 21 chromosome. This condition is also frequently called trisomy 21. The nondisjunction form (nonfamilial trisomy 21) occurs with increasing frequency with advancing maternal age.

Clinical features of Down syndrome are fairly recognizable (Fig. 16–28) and include moderate mental retardation, short stature, stocky build, hypotonia, a friendly and usually good-natured disposition, stubborn behavior on occasion, and congenital anomalies. These anomalies include a

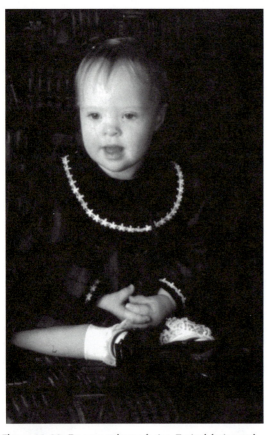

Figure 16–28. Down syndrome facies. Typical facies and habitus for Down syndrome. This includes low tone, short fingers, flat nasal bridge with epicanthic folds, open mouth, upslanting of palpebral fissures, and small ears.

flat nasal bridge, upslanting palpebral fissures, small ears, single palmar creases, shortened fingers and toes with incurving of the fifth finger (clinodactyly), and wide spacing between the first and second toes. The most significant congenital lesion affecting health is a congenital heart defect, which occurs in approximately one third of persons with Down syndrome. Surgical repair is often possible. Thyroid function may become abnormal and should be tested yearly by T4 and thyroid-stimulating hormone analysis. Alzheimer disease is not uncommon with this condition.

Dental characteristics of Down syndrome include a prominent tongue or tongue thrusting, a deeply furrowed tongue ("scrotal" tongue), a low rate of caries, dysplastic enamel, a high prevalence of periodontal disease, and a high prevalence of malocclusion. Subacute bacterial endocarditis (SBE) prophylaxis is required for dental treatments or in those with heart defects. Atlantoaxial instability occurs in approximately one tenth of persons with Down syndrome and should be looked for, although this condition is rarely symptomatic in such persons. Flexion-extension radiographs of the cervical neck are part of the routine care of children with Down syndrome and should be evaluated prior to dental procedures requiring hyperextension or manipulation of the neck.

Prenatal testing is recommended for women who are 35 years of age and older. Such testing is usually reassuring; however, it may allow a couple to plan appropriately should trisomy 21 or another chromosomal variation be identified. Delivery at a tertiary care center may be indicated if a congenital heart lesion is present. Grandparents and significant others can be prepared ahead of time to accept and love the newborn grandchild.

Turner Syndrome

Turner syndrome is caused by a missing X chromosome, deletion of the short arm of the X chromosome, or mosaicism in which some cells have a missing X and some are normal (approximately 20% of cases). In contrast with abnormalities related to autosomal chromosomes, loss of a whole X chromosome is compatible with normal intelligence and a fairly normal lifestyle.

The usual major alterations in affected women are short stature (less than 5 feet), infertility (streak gonads), incomplete or absent secondary sexual changes without estrogen therapy, and coarctation of the aorta in approximately 20% of patients. Minor renal abnormalities, low hairline, webbing or short neck, and visual-spacial perception changes are common. A narrow palate and micrognathia are also common.

Klinefelter Syndrome

Klinefelter syndrome (XXY) is associated with a tall, lanky appearance and problems with secondary sexual characteristics caused by abnormal testicular development. Lack of beard growth may be visible in the dentist's office. Gynecomastia may be present. Intellectual functioning may be less than expected, but mental retardation is unusual.

IMPRINTED GENES

Prader-Willi Syndrome

Prader-Willi syndrome (Fig. 16-29) is often recognized by the extreme obesity noted in untreated children and adults. Affected persons are known

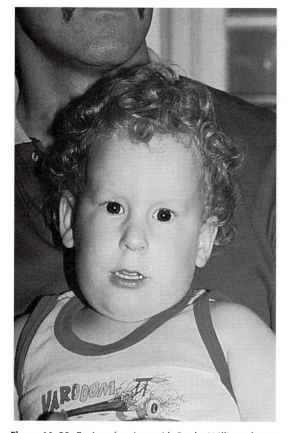

Figure 16–29. Facies of patient with Prader-Willi syndrome.

to need fewer calories to maintain their weight and have other distinct features that separate them from persons with obesity alone.

As newborns, patients generally experience marked hypotonia and difficult feeding. Nasogastric tube feeding is not uncommon. As the months go by, however, feeding improves, hypotonia improves, and weight control becomes increasingly difficult. Good parenting can make a difference in whether the resulting adult is plump or morbidly obese.

Other distinguishing clinical signs include moderate mental retardation, short stature (well below the 5th percentile), small hands and feet compared with height and weight, a tendency toward hypopigmentation (frequent blond or red hair), narrow bifrontal diameter, "almond"-shaped eyes, strabismus, and scoliosis. Chronic regurgitation of food and reduced salivation are common and may contribute to an increased rate of enamel hypoplasia and dental caries.

Prader-Willi syndrome is another condition associated with an imprinted gene. An imbalance of genetic material on the long arm of chromosome 15 (15q11.2) occurs secondary to loss of the paternal genetic material in this area relative to the maternal contribution. This may be visible as a deletion in the paternally derived chromosome (most common) or as two copies of the maternal chromosome (uniparental disomy) and absence of the paternal copy. The latter is thought to have been conceived as a trisomy 15, surviving only because of loss of the third chromosome 15. This is usually a sporadic occurrence (generally only one in a family).

Angelman Syndrome

Angelman syndrome is a distinctly different condition from Prader-Willi syndrome, but it is also associated with a deletion of 15q11.2. In this condition, however, it is the maternal chromosome that is deleted, allowing an abnormal paternal gene on the other chromosome to become active. Physical and mental alterations in Angelman syndrome include severe mental retardation, constant and useless physical activity, outbursts of unprovoked laughter, and seizures. Oral-facial findings in Angelman syndrome include a flatter midface and a prominent jaw with a wide mouth. The tongue is frequently protruding.

Beckwith-Wiedemann Syndrome

Beckwith-Wiedemann syndrome (Fig. 16-30) is thought to be secondary to alteration of the gene

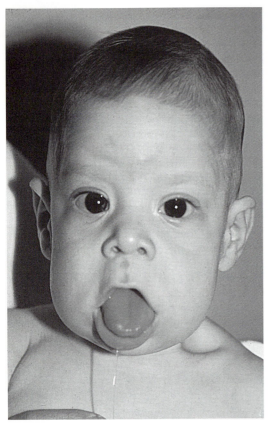

Figure 16–30. Facies of patient with Beckwith-Wiedemann syndrome.

at 11p15.5. Imprinting has been suggested for this condition because of the increased risk of the disease when it is maternally derived and because of the finding of uniparental disomy in some sporadic cases.

Oral-facial alterations in Beckwith-Wiedemann syndrome may be striking in early life but become normal with time. Marked macroglossia in infancy may lead to respiratory and feeding difficulties, although this is not usual. With jaw growth and normal development, the tongue is generally held within the mouth most of the time by school age. Surgical reduction of the tongue is not necessary in most cases. Speech development is usually normal. Primary and secondary dentition may be altered by pressure from the large tongue. Maxillary hypoplasia and prominent eyes (shortened orbits) are common but not usually remarkable, which is also true of the linear ear lobe creases that are common in this condition.

Beckwith-Wiedemann syndrome is also an "overgrowth" syndrome with macrosomia at birth, advanced bone age in many, and proportionate large body size that becomes normal in late childhood. Hemihypertrophy is present in one seventh of cases. Embryonic tumor growth is found in 10% to 12% of affected persons. Of the tumors that develop, half are Wilms tumor of the kidney and the remainder are most often adrenocortical carcinoma, hepatoblastoma, or gonadoblastoma. Upper abdominal ultrasound examinations are performed on a 2- to 4-month basis until the child is about 7 years of age, after which time the risk of tumor is close to that of the average population.

Williams Syndrome

Williams syndrome (Fig. 16–31) is seen regularly by geneticists and dentists. Although retardation and small body size are the most consistent problems, typical facies and behavior allow diagnosis. Other frequent findings include aortic or pulmonic stenosis, hypercalcemia in infancy, and caliectasis.

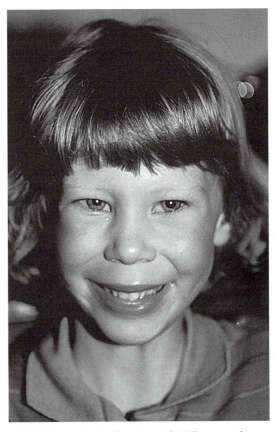

Figure 16–31. Facies of patient with Williams syndrome.

The typical facies includes uncommonly prominent lips with a wide mouth, increased fullness of tissues in the periorbital areas above the eyes, prominent blue eyes with marked whitish, stellate patterning of the iris (not constant), a flatter malar area, and prominent soft ear lobes.

Children with the Williams syndrome are frequently friendly and talkative, seemingly more intelligent than can be tested. They frequently don't relate well to peers but do enjoy contact with adults. Temper tantrums may be a problem.

The gene(s) responsible for Williams syndrome have recently been located at 7q11.23. Most cases are caused by a deletion. "Significantly more severe growth retardation and microcephaly" were detected when the maternal copy was deleted, suggesting "an imprinted locus, silent on the paternal chromosome" (Jurado, 1996).

ADDITIONAL READINGS

Freire-Maia N, Pinheriro M: Ectodermal Dysplasias: A Clinical and Genetic Study. New York, Alan R. Liss, 1984.

Gladwin A, et al: Localization of a gene for oculodentodigital syndrome to human chromosome 6q22-q24. Hum Molec Genet 6(1):123–127, 1997.

Gorlin RJ, Cohen MM, Levin LS: Syndromes of the Head and Neck, 3rd ed. New York, Oxford University Press, 1990.

Jones KL: Smith's Recognizable Patterns of Human Malformation, 5th ed. Philadelphia, WB Saunders, 1997.

Jurado LAP, Peoples R, Kaplan P, et al: Molecular definition of the chromosome 7 deletion in Williams syndrome and parent-of-origin effects on growth. Am J Hum Genet 59:781–792, 1996.

Kaloust S, Ishii K, Vargervik K: Dental development in Apert syndrome. Cleft Palate-Craniofac J 34 (2): 117–121, 1997.

McKusick VA: Mendelian Inheritance in Man, 10th ed. Baltimore, Johns Hopkins University Press, 1992. (This is now on line as noted in the introduction)

Rimoin DL, Connor JM, Pyeritz RE: Emery & Rimoins Principles and Practice of Medical Genetics, 3rd ed. New York, Churchill Livingstone, 1996.

What's in a Face?

Rebecca Slayton

In the textbook *Smith's Recognizable Patterns of Human Malformation* by Kenneth L. Jones, M.D., 12 of the 26 categories of anomalies that are used for differential diagnosis involve features of the head or neck. Of these, three are limited to oral structures. Although many minor malformations involve craniofacial structures, the presence of anomalies in this region is often suggestive of one or more major malformations or of an identifiable genetic syndrome.

The dentist is in a unique situation because he or she often sees children regularly throughout their development, regardless of their health status. Often, physicians are only consulted when a child is ill. In addition, the dentist concentrates their diagnostic expertise on the face and mouth of the child, precisely where many of the minor anomalies will express themselves.

The dentist who looks at a patient's face and is a careful observer can provide a valuable service to the patient by recognizing potential abnormalities and referring the child to the proper medical care provider.

It is important for the dentist to recognize potential genetic conditions for two reasons: First, the condition may result in a medical condition that will affect the way treatment is provided. For example, if a child has Noonan syndrome, he or she could also have a cardiac abnormality that would require the use of subacute bacterial endocarditis prophylaxis prior to dental treatment. Second, you can direct the family to a geneticist who can provide information and counseling to the family and can help them anticipate any potential future health problems related to the genetic condition.

The following list gives various genetic conditions by craniofacial anomaly. This list includes some of the more common syndromes and is not meant to be all-inclusive. For more complete information on these and other syndromes, refer to *Smith's Recognizable Patterns of Human Malformations* or Gorlin's *Syndromes of the Head and Neck*.

Box continued on following page

Oral Region and Mouth

Cleft lip/palate: Van der Woude s., holoprosencephaly, trisomy 13 s., oral-facial-digital s., Rapp-Hodgkin ectodermal dysplasia s.

Cleft palate or bifid uvula without cleft lip: Retinoic acid embryopathy, oral-facial-digital s., Stickler s., Treacher Collins s., Van der Woude s.

Prominent full lips: Autosomal recessive hypohidrotic ectodermal dysplasia, Hunter s., Hurler s., Williams s., Waardenburg s.

Macroglossia: Beckwith-Wiedemann s., Down s., Hurler s., athyrotic hypothyroidism

Larynx: Fraser s., Opitz s., Robin sequence, Treacher Collins s.

Teeth

Anodontia: Autosomal recessive hypohidrotic ectodermal dysplasia s., cleidocranial dysostosis, Rieger s., Van der Woude s., Williams s., Crouzon s., Ehlers-Danlos s.

Hypodontia: Autosomal recessive hypohidrotic ectodermal dysplasia s., chondroectodermal dysplasia, Down s., osteogenesis imperfecta s., tricho-dento-osseous s., Van der Woude s., Williams s., Ehlers-Danlos s.

Enamel hypoplasia: Albright hereditary osteodystrophy, cleidocranial dysostosis, hypophosphatasia, Prader-Willi s., tuberous sclerosis s., X-linked hypophosphatemic rickets, oral-facial-digital s.

Caries: Cleidocranial dysostosis, Cockayne s., Gorlin s., osteogenesis imperfecta, dyskeratosis congenita s., Prader-Willi s.

Irregular placement of teeth: Down s., Goltz s., Gorlin s., Hurler s., Stickler s.

Late eruption of teeth: Aarskog s., Albright hereditary osteodystrophy, chondroectodermal dysplasia, cleidocranial dysostosis, de Lange s., Gardner s.

Dental cysts: Gardner s., Gorlin s.

Maxilla and Mandible

Maxillary hypoplasia: Achondroplasia, Angelman s., Apert s., Bloom s., Crouzon s., fetal alcohol effects, Marfan s., Treacher Collins s.

Micrognathia: Achondrogenesis syndromes, de Lange s., maternal phenylketonuria fetal effects, Moebius sequence, Treacher Collins s., Robin sequence, Turner s.

Prognathism: Angelman s., Beckwith-Wiedemann s., fragile X s., Gorlin s.

Eyes

Hypertelorism: Cat-eye s., DiGeorge s., Noonan s., Opitz s., Pfeiffer s.

Inner epicanthal folds: Down s., Noonan s., Stickler s., Rubinstein-Taybi s., Williams s., Turner s., Gorlin s.

Slanted palpebral fissures: Apert s., cat-eye s., Down s., Treacher Collins s.

Synophrys: de Lange s., Sanfilippo s., Waardenburg s., trisomy 4p s.

Blue sclera: Marshall-Smith s., osteogenesis imperfecta, Russell-Silver s., Marfan s.

Nose

Low nasal bridge: Achondroplasia, Albright hereditary osteodystrophy, fetal warfarin effects, fetal valproate effects, retinoic acid embryopathy, Zellweger s.

Broad nasal bridge: Ehlers-Danlos s., fragile X s., fronto-metaphyseal dysplasia

Ears

Low-set ears: Fibrochondrogenesis, Noonan s., Rubinstein-Taybi s., Smith-Lemli-Opitz s., Treacher Collins s., Down s.

Malformed auricles: DiGeorge s., Down s., Ehlers-Danlos s., Treacher Collins s., Smith-Lemli-Opitz s., fetal alcohol effects, Marfan s., Prader-Willi s.

Preauricular tags or pits: Cat-eye s., facio-auriculo-vertebral spectrum

Facies

"Flat" facies: Achondroplasia, Apert s., Down s., Stickler s., Zellweger s.

"Round" facies: Prader-Willi s., Bardet-Biedl s., cleidocranial dysostosis

Broad facies: Apert s., Crouzon s., Gorlin s., Prader-Willi s.

"Triangular" facies: Turner s., Treacher Collins s.

"Coarse" facies: Hunter s., Hurler s., Fabry s., Williams s.

Brain and Cranium

Microcephaly: Bloom s., fetal alcohol effects, trisomy 13 s., Williams s.

Macrocephaly: Hunter s., Hurler s., Robinow s.

Frontal bossing: Basal cell nevus s., Crouzon s., Hurler s., oto-palato-digital s., Rubinstein-Taybi s.

From this list of anomalies, it is clear that most syndromes have characteristic orofacial manifestations. Although many of the listed syndromes are fairly severe and are likely to have been identified prior to their being seen by a dentist, others have a milder phenotype and may not be apparent until later in the development of the child. This provides the dentist with the opportunity and responsibility to recognize and refer patients in whom they suspect genetic abnormalities.

Summary for Section I

Dentists who have been routinely seeing normal children as infants and having the youngsters recalled before their third birthday have noted that it is rare for children at age 3 to display fears of a dental appointment. This finding is cited as another of the benefits of these early evaluation appointments. The education of the parents of infants in home care, nutrition, and feeding techniques that attend this movement to present children before their third birthday is also a bonus because it is harder to change a diet at age 3 than it is to adopt a good one a year or two earlier.

Unquestionably, dentistry can be important to this age group. Children who are on an appropriate fluoride supplementation regimen who would not have been otherwise definitely benefit. Those who ceased a possibly detrimental nursing habit because of the dentist's urgings also benefit. Also, those children who receive significant improvements in their diet and home care by their parents experience better dental health as a group than would a similar group who did not have any professional intervention before age 3 to 4 and because of this did not benefit from the aforementioned circumstances.

Today's contemporary dentist who treats children must be prevention-oriented. With allegiance to prevention, it only makes sense that a child be seen during infancy. The modest amount of time and the small fee associated with this examination are certainly justified in the long run. The dentist who is concerned with the health of a mother's infant will almost certainly be the dentist of choice the next time that mother seeks dental care for her child and probably for future siblings of that child. Involvement in prenatal classes and with the medical professionals who treat children in one's community is also encouraged. No longer can the dental welfare of the infant and young child be a situation of merely intellectual interest. The infant and young child must be integrated into professional supervision.

In summary, the ultimate responsibility of the dentist to the age group from conception to 3 years is to deliver the child to his or her third birthday as caries-free and gingivally healthy as possible, with effective home care techniques being practiced by the parents. This includes a dietary regimen that encourages good dental health and the appropriate amount of bioavailable fluoride.

II

The Primary Dentition Years: Three to Six Years

This section on the primary dentition years is the largest section of the textbook. The reason is that children between the ages of 3 and 6 have the need for almost the entire range of diagnostic, treatment, and prevention techniques available to today's dentist. The only real exceptions are the treatment of permanent teeth; certain orthodontic, diagnostic, and treatment decisions; and issues such as temporomandibular joint (TMJ) pathology, which could be pertinent at these years but usually does not mainfest problems until later in life. The discussion of acid etching of teeth has been saved for Section III, The Transitional Years, although such techniques are pertinent in the primary dentition also, albeit probably not to the same degree as in the permanent dentition.

Patient management is included along with hospital dentistry in this section because the majority of patient management problems that a dentist will encounter will probably occur in this age group. Along with that, the need for hospitalization of children is probably higher in this age group than in the other three groups that we have defined. This assumes that to some degree, with good prevention, children have escaped ravaging dental disease and the need for hospitalization for treatment before 3 years of age. It is also assumed that most children's gross dental problems are managed well before age 6. Therefore, if a child requires hospitalization for whatever reasons, this will be done before he or she reaches the transitional years.

This is also an age group in which dental needs today, compared with those in past years, are changing or have changed dramatically. The good news is that the caries-free child now exists who, because of fluoride, home care, proper nutrition, and sealants, has no decay at all or, at most, only very modest decay. The bad news is that there are still children who for a variety of reasons need restorative care and sometimes extensive restorative care, including stainless steel crowns and pulp therapy. There are also children who have had extractions and damaging interproximal decay who need space maintenance and, in some instances, space regaining.

The oral habits acquired by children in the first three years, which often were of no concern to the parent or the clinician, become of concern now. Sometimes the possible detrimental effects of these habits are easily discernible even by the untrained eye.

In discussing the dentist's responsibility for the child during infancy and between his first and third birthdays, it was emphasized in Section I that the dentist needed to be able to diagnose the child's prevention needs and to inform and motivate the parents about their responsibilities in making sure that the child has desirable oral health. When discussing the child between ages 3 and 6, the dentist must also address the child's prevention needs but will in many instances have to be able to manage the child in treatment sessions. Some of these treatment sessions will involve the utilization of local anesthesia, the preparation of teeth, the treatment of pulpal tissue, and sometimes the extraction of teeth. In some instances, these treatments will need to be performed with the parents away from the child and out of the operatory. Unquestionably, patient management is a demanding aspect of dentistry for children. Fortunately, dentistry has many useful child management techniques that are quite effective.

Lastly, this age group, with its skills at talking to people and relating to them, is one that many clinicians find delightful. Their efforts with these children feel unusually rewarding. Dentists who enjoy dentistry for children certainly enjoy this age group in particular.

17

The Dynamics of Change

Chapter Outline

Physical Changes

Body

J. R. Pinkham

By the third birthday, the average boy is approximately 38 inches tall and weighs about 33 pounds. The average girl is slightly less than 38 inches (37.6 inches) tall and weighs about a half pound less than a boy. For the next 3 years, children average about 5 pounds of weight gain per year and gain about 4 inches of height per year. Boys are on the whole during this time slightly taller and heavier than girls.

There is a strong tendency for children to maintain their weights and heights compared with other children during the preschool period. Children who are tall or heavy at age 2 are very likely to be regarded as tall or heavy at age 5 also. Similarly, children who are light or short at age 2 are likely to be regarded as light or short at age 5 compared with their peer group (Meredith, 1965). During the preschool period, the correla-

tion between the height of the child and his height in early adulthood is moderately good (Meredith, 1965). It should be pointed out, however, that this is not an absolute correlation, particularly for some short individuals who may later, compared with their peers, become taller. As pointed out earlier in the discussion of growth changes from birth to age 3, the child's developing elongation of body continues to be apparent during the preschool years. During this time, head growth seems slow, whereas limb growth seems extremely rapid. In speed of change, trunk growth can be regarded as intermediate. The protuberant, pudgy abdomen of the toddling 2-year-old gradually disappears between the ages of 3 and 4.

A variety of other body changes take place during these critical years of development. Both the heart rate and the respiration rate slow down. Conversely, blood pressure rises. At around 4 years of age, the growth of the muscular system in relation to the growth of other tissues of the body significantly changes its rate. Before age 4, the growth of the muscular system is roughly the same as the growth of the body as a whole. After age 4, however, because of the change in rate, approximately 75% of the child's acquired weight during his or her fifth year of development is the result of acquisition of muscle (Thompson, 1954).

During this preschool period of ages 3 to 6, it becomes evident to some degree which children have natural athletic ability and which do not. During these years, the cartilage in the skeletal system is increasingly replaced by bone, and all the bones of the body become more calcified and harder. This calcification leads to an increased incidence of fractured and broken bones.

REFERENCES

Meredith HV: Selected anatomic variables analyzed for interage relationships of the size-size, size-gain, and gain-gain varieties. *In* Lipsitt LP, Spiker CC (eds): Advances in Child Development and Behavior, vol 2. New York, Academic Press, 1965, pp 221–256.

Thompson H: Physical growth. *In* Carmichael L (ed): Manual of Child Psychology, 2nd ed. New York, John Wiley, 1954, pp 292–334.

Craniofacial Changes

Jerry Walker

The growth of the head and face remains continuous during the period from 3 to 6 years of age. Figure 17–1 shows that the percentage of increase in facial growth versus cranial growth becomes substantially greater around the age of 3 years (Ranly, 1980). This increased change in growth of the face compared with the cranium has important effects on a child's appearance and craniofacial structures. In 3- to 6-year-olds, in contrast with the newborn, the face becomes larger, wider, longer, and more detailed. During this stage of life, one begins to see the effects of the eruption of permanent teeth.

Vann and colleagues (1978) reported the results of a study reviewing cephalometric analysis of the primary dentition in children. They found no statistical differences between males and females at the .01 significance level (p > .01). Twelve landmarks were identified for this cephalometric analysis. In comparing 17 cephalometric norms established from a sample of 32 Caucasian children of North American ancestry with those of adults, the following conclusions were drawn (Fig. 17–2):

• It seems that the primary incisors are more

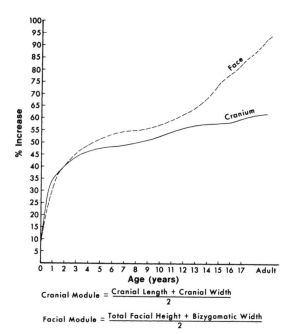

Cranial Module = $\dfrac{\text{Cranial Length + Cranial Width}}{2}$

Facial Module = $\dfrac{\text{Total Facial Height + Bizygomatic Width}}{2}$

Figure 17–1. Comparison of cranial and facial modules (males). Increase in cranial and facial modules during growth. (From Ranly DM: A Synopsis of Craniofacial Growth. New York, Appleton-Century-Crofts, 1980. Data from Scott JH: The growth of the human face. Proc R Soc Med *47*:5, 1954.)

upright than the permanent incisors (in both boys and girls—compare UI-SN and UI-F in Fig. 17–2).

• The similarity of angle SNA in children (82.9) and adults (82.0) supports the concept that the nasion and point A move forward in relation to the sella in such a fashion that angle SNA is no different in preschool children and adults.

• Angles SNB and SNPg in children measure 78.1 and 77.4 degrees, respectively, whereas in adults they measure 80.0 and 83.0 degrees. The ANB angle is greater in children (4.9 degrees) compared with adults (2.0 degrees).

The soft tissue prominence of the nose and to some extent the mandible continue to increase consistently with some reduction in overall facial convexity (Fig. 17–3). It is hard to judge the underlying skeletal configuration from the soft tissue in this age group. Vertically, there is a lowering of the palatal vault with sutural growth and apposition on the oral side of the palate and resorption on the nasal side. There is an even greater lowering of the lowest point of the chin, but the mandibular plane (lower border of the mandible) stays parallel to its original orientation. This occurs because condylar growth exceeds the vertical maxillary growth, which prevents opening of the mandibular plane angle. It is

	Vann (n=32)*	Adult**
SNA	82.9	82.0
SNB	78.1	80.0
SNPg	77.4	83.0
ANB	4.9	2.0
FNA	89.1	88.0
FNB	84.4	87.0
FNPg	85.5	88.0
IMPA	85.2	92.0
FMIA	65.9	65.0
UI-SN	92.4	104.0
UI-F	97.6	110.0
1-1	148.4	130.0
M	67.5	69.0
Y-axis	58.5	59.0
OCC-SN	18.8	14.5
SN-MP	35.3	32.0
FMA	29.2	25.0

Figure 17–2. Cephalometric angles: a comparison between preschoolers (4–5 yr) and adults. (From Vann WF, et al: A cephalometric analysis for the child in the primary dentition. J Dent Child 45:45–52, 1978.)

*All children in this study were between their fourth and fifth birthdays.

**Generally accepted adult norms borrowed from Downs, Steiner, and Tweed.

clearly wrong to think of these as nongrowing years for the face.

There is obviously considerable growth in the transverse direction during this time period as well (Fig. 17-4). Remember that this growth comes to an end earlier than does that in other dimensions, so attention to problems in this dimension is important. Transverse maxillary growth during this time period is largely the result of midpalatal sutural changes, whereas the growth of the body and angles of the mandible are the result of apposition and resorption (Fig. 17-5).

Posterior maxillary and mandibular growth (sutural growth in the maxilla and endochondral growth in the mandible) helps to accommodate the emerging permanent first molars. There is some appositional growth at the dentoalveolar ridges as the permanent anterior teeth erupt.

Consistent with eruption of the new permanent teeth is the continued eruption of the primary teeth (Fig. 17-6). Often the magnitude of this vertical change is unappreciated. It is also obvious that the permanent anterior teeth will occupy a more anterior and protrusive position in the face.

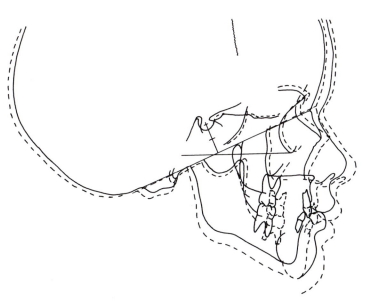

Figure 17–3. This anterior cranial base superimposition of the Bolton Standard for 3- and 6-year-olds demonstrates the magnitude of anteroposterior and vertical skeletal growth during this period as well as the soft tissue change. (Redrawn from Broadbent BH, Sr, Broadbent BH, Jr, Golden WH: Bolton Standards of Developmental Growth. St. Louis, CV Mosby, 1975.)

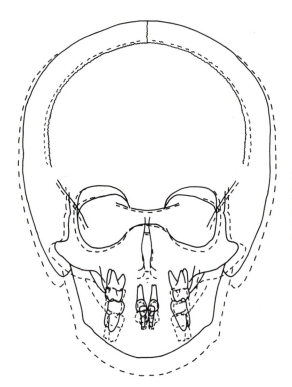

Figure 17–4. This anterior cranial base superimposition of the Bolton Standard for 3- and 6-year-olds demonstrates the magnitude of transverse and vertical skeletal growth during this period. (Redrawn from Broadbent BH, Sr, Broadbent BH, Jr, Golden WH: Bolton Standards of Developmental Growth. St. Louis, CV Mosby, 1975.)

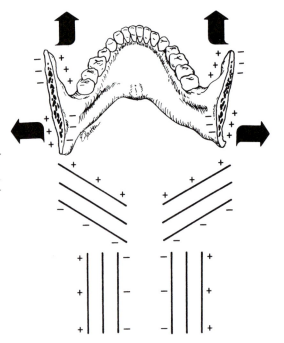

Figure 17–5. Cross-section through the rami and coronoid processes, illustrating how these areas of the mandible can be visualized as following the V principle. (From Ranly DM: A Synopsis of Craniofacial Growth. New York, Appleton-Century-Crofts, 1980. Adapted from Enlow DH, Harris DB: A study of the postnatal growth of the human mandible. Am J Orthod *50*:25, 1964.)

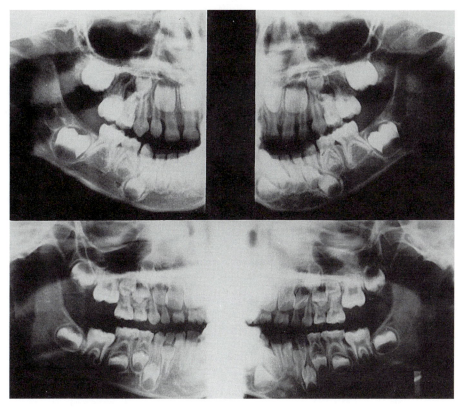

Figure 17–6. These two panoramic radiographs show the transition of the dentition beginning and the alteration in arch length required for accommodation of the permanent teeth.

REFERENCES

Broadbent BH Sr, Broadbent BH Jr, Golden WH: Bolton Standards of Developmental Growth. St. Louis, CV Mosby Co, 1975.

Ranly DM: A Synopsis of Craniofacial Growth. New York, Appleton-Century-Crofts, 1980.

Vann WF, Gilley GJ, Nelson RM: A cephalometric analysis for the child in the primary dentition. J Dent Child 45:1, 1978.

Dental Changes

C. A. Full

Table 12-5 of Chapter 12 presents a chronology of human dentition. This table demonstrates that the entire primary dentition has completed root development by 3 years of age. This is a relatively stable period clinically for the primary dentition, which was very active before its eruption was completed by 24 to 36 months and before root formation was completed by age 3 years. This is a significant period of time for the development of the clinical crowns of the permanent dentition and their subsequent eruptions, however. There will also be some root resorption of the primary incisors for most children during the last 6 months of this period.

As the permanent dentition develops, some obvious differences in morphologic appearance become apparent compared with the primary dentition (Fig. 17-7). Wheeler (1958) described the following essential differences:

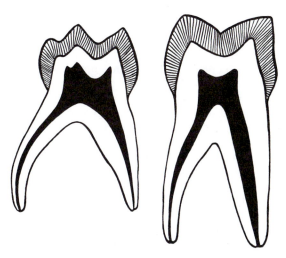

Figure 17–7. Comparison of maxillary second primary and permanent molars, linguobuccal cross-section. (From Finn SB: Clinical Pedodontics, 4th ed. Philadelphia, WB Saunders, 1973.)

1. The crowns of primary anterior teeth are wider mesiodistally compared with their cervicoincisal length than are the crowns of the permanent teeth.

2. The roots of the primary anterior teeth are narrower mesiodistally. Narrow roots with wide crowns present a morphologic appearance at the cervical third of crown and root that differs markedly from that of the permanent anterior teeth. When the teeth are examined from the mesial or distal aspects, somewhat the same situation in the root and crown measurement at the cervix is observed. The cervical ridge of enamel at the cervical third of the crown, labially and lingually, is much more prominent in the primary teeth than in the permanent teeth.

3. The crowns and roots of the primary molars are more slender mesiodistally at the cervical third than those of the permanent molars.

4. The cervical ridge buccally on the primary molars is much more pronounced, especially on both the maxillary and mandibular first molars.

5. The roots of the primary molars are relatively more slender and longer than the roots of the permanent teeth. They also flare out more apically, extending out beyond the projected outlines of the crowns. This flaring allows more room between the roots for the development of permanent tooth crowns before it is time for the primary molars to lose their anchorage.

6. The buccal and lingual surfaces of the primary molars are flatter above the cervical curvatures than those of the permanent molars.

7. The primary teeth are usually lighter in color than the permanent teeth.

REFERENCE

Wheeler RC: Dental Anatomy and Physiology. Philadelphia, WB Saunders, 1958.

Cognitive Changes

J. R. Pinkham

In our society, the years between ages 3 and 6 are often referred to as the preschool years and the children are called preschoolers. Cognitively, these years represent an enormous change. The child's power of reasoning grows substantially. The simplistic "why" questions of the 2-year-old are replaced by more sophisticated and specific inquiries, such as "How did it get so big?" and "Where did it come from?"

In Piaget's categorization of cognitive intelligence, the years between the ages of 3 and 6 are called preoperational. The preoperational phase of cognitive development begins at the end of stage six of the sensorimotor period, somewhere around 18 to 24 months of age, and lasts until age 6 or 7 years. Piaget further labeled the first part of the preoperational phase preconceptual and concluded that it lasted until about the age of 4 years. During the preconceptual phase the child's mind and mental prowess develop at a rapid rate. The child's mind acquires the ability to think symbolically with mental imagery. In the sensorimotor period, the child was restricted to actions with real objects. By the preconceptual phase, the child can play and fantasize using mental symbols.

Although the child is increasing his or her cognitive abilities almost immeasurably, the child in the preconceptual stage must still be regarded as unsophisticated in thinking. The child still generalizes all entities. For example, a bird is *any* bird or, better yet, any bird is *a* bird. Use of more specific nouns like robin, quail, or heron must await a later level of development. If a child of this age masters both the word chicken and the word bird, he or she will not understand that a chicken is also a bird.

The preconceptual mind is also *centered*. Centration was defined by Piaget as the process of focusing all thought and reasoning of any mental problem on only one aspect of the whole of the structure and disregarding all other features. Piaget used a dramatic experiment to prove this assumption. He found that children who watched him pour water from one of two identically filled tall, thin vases into a short, wide vase often asserted that the tall vase had more water in it than the short one. Children who made that assertion centered on the height of the water. Furthermore, the child's thought during these years is irreversible. The child cannot mentally pour the water back from the short vase to the tall one to see that it would be at the same level as the water in the other tall vase.

After the preconceptual stage comes a stage labeled the period of intuitive thought. This stage starts at around age 4 and lasts until age 7 or 8. This is a period of sophistication of the child's abilities to group objects according to class, using more complex thoughts and images, and outgrowing the tendency toward centration. Late in this period the child can begin to acquire reading and writing skills. All of this, combined with an increased vocabulary, longer attention span, control over impulses, and toleration of separation from parents, demonstrates that the child is ready for school.

Emotional Changes

J. R. Pinkham

As discussed in the introduction to Section II, the fear of most children of strangers, separation from parents, and new experiences has diminished by the third birthday to the point where these youngsters can take on new social situations without emotional consequences. The process of self-control and control of emotions, such as frustration and fear, develops dramatically between the ages of 3 and 6 and is paralleled by an equally dramatic socialization process. During these years, a child's sense of sexual identity emerges, and a certain degree of masculine or feminine qualities is adopted by the child. A sense of identity and a concept of self-esteem also emerge during these years.

One dramatic difference between the child from birth to age 3 and the child from age 3 to age 6 is the development of self-control. Preschool children can be taught methods of self control, such as distracting themselves when they become impatient or when they are receiving a local anesthetic from a dentist. They can be taught to monitor their own behavior. During the preschool years, the conscience of the child develops, and he or she becomes capable of feeling guilty or anxious if and when he or she violates a moral norm.

An understanding of aggression is important for parents of preschool children and for other adults who deal with preschool children. Aggression is often caused by a child's inability to exert self-control. There are two kinds of aggression. One is called instrumental aggression and is designed for achieving a goal such as taking a piece of candy from a sibling. The other is hostile aggression, and this type is intended to cause hurt or pain to another person. During the preschool years the frequency of instrumental aggression should decline. Children who remain hostilely aggressive during the preschool years are children who come from families in which parents and other children are also overtly aggressive. A parenting philosophy that is inconsistent and unclear in the enforcement of rules has also been linked with aggression in children (Mussen et al., 1984).

In summary, at the sixth birthday a child is certainly not emotionally mature but is emotionally complex. He or she is capable now of feeling friendship and hostility, acting out aggression, and experiencing guilt and anxiety. This is a child who is susceptible to praise and can suffer hurt feelings. Much of the literature available in bookstores for children in this age group covers "how people feel about things." Obviously, these children can relate to the emotions of other people.

REFERENCE

Mussen PH, Conger JJ, Kagan J, et al: Child Development and Personality, 6th ed. New York, Harper & Row, 1984.

Social Changes

J. R. Pinkham

Ages 3 to 6 are a time of enormous social growth in the child. Two-year-olds, for instance, cannot for the most part play with a peer. Their play is at best separate but parallel. For example, a pair of 2-year-olds may play in the same sandbox, but there is no relationship between the project of one and the project of the other. By age 3 a child can understand taking turns, and by age 4 cooperative play is possible. By age 6, a child is capable of simple team games.

Between ages 3 and 6, children need to gain an understanding of their own personal identification and how they are to relate to other people, including nurturing parents, siblings, peers, and authority figures. During these years, a value system develops, self-discipline is imposed upon basic urges, and a consciousness that is capable of feeling guilt emerges. The social transformations of preschoolers ensure that their lives will never be the same.

Many theories seek to explain the reasons for the dramatic psychosocial transitions that take place in this age group. The medical-psychoanalytical theory asserts that sexual fantasies and the guilt associated with these fantasies, which at first take the form of an unusual feeling for the parent of the opposite sex (Oedipus or Electra complex), are the underlying reasons for personality changes. As a child seeks a way to resolve these problems, he or she is forced into identification with the parent of the same sex and into the adoption of a system of morality, complete with its code of values. This code of moral values has been labeled the *superego*. Behaviorists ascribe the assumption of sex-appropriate roles and social values to the effects of reinforcement, both positive and negative, during this period.

Social learning theories explain the changes during this period as the product of the influences of parenting and parental behavior. Some theorists believe that as the child becomes conscious of the reasons behind systems of things, she or he is better able to recognize and be allegiant to the reasoning that underlies social order and values.

Regardless of the theoretical position one may subscribe to, it cannot be argued that the role of parents is extremely powerful in the preschooler's life. In 1983, Shonkoff pointed out that anyone observing the play of preschoolers will note that the fantasies they enact are rich in relation to sexual and adult values. He further noted that many parents have often been embarrassed by their children acting out realistic domestic situations that have occurred in the home.

There continues to be considerable debate in the literature about where stereotypical sex roles merge and how much they are controlled biologically or culturally. Data do exist that suggest that boys are inherently more aggressive than girls. Conversely, preferences for activities such as active sports and playing with dolls are certainly influenced by reinforcement. It can also be argued that media such as television may in a given situation provide information that stereotypes a child's behavior and that media may have more influence than the parents in some situations.

REFERENCE

Shonkoff JP: Patterns of variation over time: Preschool. *In* Levine MD, Carey WB, Crocker AC, et al (eds): Developmental-Behavioral Pediatrics. Philadelphia, WB Saunders, 1983, pp 97–107.

Epidemiology and Mechanisms of Dental Disease

Steven M. Adair

Development of a full complement of healthy primary teeth is important for proper oral function and general health. Aside from the specific early caries patterns discussed in Chapter 12, primary teeth are benefitting from the general reduction in dental caries that has taken place in many industrialized nations in recent decades. Still, primary teeth are susceptible to caries, especially as posterior contacts develop, and comparatively little data exist to document caries prevalence at this age. This chapter part discusses the epidemiology of caries in the primary dentition and etiologic factors in the caries process at this age.

EPIDEMIOLOGY OF CARIES IN THE PRIMARY DENTITION

Data regarding the prevalence of caries in the primary dentition have not been systematically collected on populations as large as those surveyed in permanent dentition studies. There is, however, a body of worldwide literature spanning several decades from which trends can be ascertained. Table 17–1 illustrates a selected number of these reports. Direct comparisons cannot be drawn because of the various ways (e.g., dmfs, deft) in which the data are reported, the variety of populations studied, the fluoridation status of the communities, and a host of other variables that are not consistent across studies. Inspection of Table 17–1 reveals that caries in the primary dentition remains a problem, at least for certain segments of the population. Three surveys of 3- to 6-year-old children enrolled in Head Start Programs found mean caries experiences ranging from 2.37 to almost 10 decayed, extracted, and filled primary tooth surfaces (defs) or 4.8 to 11.07 decayed, missing, and filled primary tooth surfaces (dmfs) (Johnsen et al., 1986; Louie et al., 1990; Trubman et al., 1989). Caries levels in other populations around the world show similar levels of primary tooth involvement.

Some rough comparisons are possible. Hennon and associates (1969) found a mean defs of 6.16 in fluoride-deficient areas of Indiana in 1969 among 36- to 39-month-olds. Johnsen and colleagues (1986) reported a mean defs of 4.7 among 3½- to 5-year-old subjects in fluoride-deficient areas of Ohio almost 20 years later. Two studies conducted in Philadelphia demonstrate the effects of fluoridation in that city. The subjects in the first study (Wisan et al., 1957) were born when Philadelphia was a fluoride-deficient community, although the city had become fluoridated by the time of the survey. The second survey 12 years later (Bronstein, 1969) demonstrated lower mean defs rates among the 3- to 5-year-old children. The several studies of South African children also demonstrated a trend toward caries reductions over time in that country that is not clearly related to community water fluoridation (Cleaton-Jones et al., 1978; Chosack et al., 1988; Williams et al., 1985). The surveys of Stecklin-Blicks and co-workers (1989) over a 20-year period in Umea, Sweden clearly documented reductions of dmfs and dmft among the 4-year-olds of that city, with concomitant increases in the prevalence of caries-free children.

More recent surveys, although demonstrating a trend for caries reductions in the primary dentition, indicate that by age 3 perhaps 25% to 65% of children have been affected by dental caries. The population distribution of caries in the primary dentition demonstrates a higher prevalence in economically disadvantaged groups. Data (Speechley and Johnston, 1996) indicate that the general decline in dental caries may be reversing in the primary dentition, at least in some parts of the world.

LOCATION OF CARIES IN THE PRIMARY DENTITION

The distribution of caries among occlusal, facial-lingual, and proximal surfaces as illustrated in Table 17–2 clearly demonstrates the differential effect of fluoride on the various surfaces of primary teeth. In optimally fluoridated communities, caries reductions on proximal and facial-lingual surfaces lead to 41% of the caries occurring on the occlusal surfaces. In fluoride-deficient communities, the distribution is somewhat more uniform with a higher proportion of proximal lesions and proportionately fewer occlusal

TABLE 17–1. Selected Surveys of Caries in the Primary Dentition

Study	Subject Age	defs	deft	dmfs	dmft	dfs	dft	Percent Caries-Free	Remarks
Savara et al. 1954	1 year		0.67					78	Portland, OR
	2		0.83					77	
	3		2.72					38	Fluoridation status
	4		4.05					39	not given
	5		4.76					22	
	6		5.13					17	
Wisan 1957	2 years	0.6							Philadelphia FD*
	3	2.2							when subjects
	4	3.6							were born
	5	3.5							
Halikis 1963	2 years	3.79						37	Australia;
	3	8.87						2	Fluoridation status
	4	10.45						3	not given
	5	10.95						0	
	6	11.17						2	
Bronstein 1969	3 years	0.47	0.38					85	Philadelphia OF†
	4	1.57	1.13					71	
	5	2.27	1.60					58	
Hennon et al. 1969	18–23 mo	1.75							FD areas, Indiana
	36–39 mo	6.16							
Winter et al. 1971	12–23 mo		0.4					98	England
	24–35		0.76					82	
	36–47		3.07					64	
	48–60		0.4					42	
Bruszt et al. 1977	3 years				3.4			36	Hungary
	4				5.2			17	
	5				6.3			11	
	6				7.3			9	
Sutcliffe et al. 1977	3 years			2.74	1.88				Scotland
	4			5.43	2.98				
Cleaton-Jones et al. 1978	1 year				0.6			88	Rural South Africa
	2				1.5			70	
	3				1.0			57	
	4				1.9			58	
	5				3.0			49	
	1				1.0			83	Urban South Africa
	2				1.3			79	
	3				2.7			56	
	4				4.1			29	
	5				4.4			28	
Schwarz et al. 1979	2 years	1.2							Denmark
	3	2.1							
	4	4.1							
	5	7.3							
Salem and Holm 1985	3–5 years				1.2			67	Saudi Arabia
Williams et al. 1985									
1981 data	2 years				0.9			71	
	3				1.8			48	
	4				2.3			45	
	5				3.9			27	
1983 data	2 years				0.7			75	South Africa
	3				1.5			60	
	4				2.4			47	
	5				2.8			41	
Johnsen et al. 1986	3½–5	3.3	2.3						Ohio: Urban OF
		4.7	2.8						Urban FD
		3.3	2.0						Rural OF
		4.7	2.8						Rural FD
Chosock et al. 1988	3 years				1.64				South Africa, low
	4				3.13				salivary Strep
	5				2.09				groups
Cleaton-Jones et al. 1989	1 year				0.3–1.8			82–99	South Africa,
	2				0.83–5.06			43–85	disparate
	3				1.54–7.38			27–70	populations
	4				2.28–8.04			29–53	

TABLE 17–1. Selected Surveys of Caries in the Primary Dentition *Continued*

Study	Subject Age	defs	deft	dmfs	dmft	dfs	dft	Percent Caries-Free	Remarks
Holbrook et al. 1989	4 years			3.3	2.4				Iceland
Stecklin-Blicks et al. 1989	4 years								Umea, Sweden
1967 data				7.8	5.3			17	
1971 data				4.5	3.2			33	
1976 data				2.9	2.4			36	
1981 data				2.0	2.0			50	
1987 data				2.0	1.6			58	
Trubman et al. 1989	3 years	2.37	1.34						Mississippi Head Start Program
	4	4.91	2.58						
	5	7.33	3.53						
	6	9.99	4.32						
									California:
Louie et al. 1990	3½–5½					4.8	2.97	36	OF
						7.44	4.03	30	FD
						11.74	5.13		Hawaii
						11.07	5.4		Micronesia
Fujiwara et al. 1991	0–2 years	2.4						72	Low *Strep*
		7.71						56	High *Strep*
Wendt et al. 1991	1 year							99	Sweden,
	2							92	longitudinal study
Grindefjork et al. 1995	3½ years					1.7		63.3	Sweden; second year of a 2-year longitudinal study

*FD = fluoride-deficient community water supply.
†OF = optimally fluoridated community water supply.

lesions (Louie et al., 1990). The prevalence of proximal lesions is higher than that reported for permanent teeth by a factor of 3 to 4.

Within the primary dentition, individual tooth susceptibility is determined to a large extent by tooth and dental arch morphology. Primary first molars in both arches are less susceptible to occlusal caries because of the relative lack of deep pits and fissures on that tooth as compared with primary second molars. The broad contact area between primary first and second molars contributes to a high proportion of proximal caries occurring at those surfaces. The distal surface of the primary second molar has no approximating tooth until the permanent first molar

erupts. Thus, it is relatively unaffected by caries until age 6 or 7, after which it becomes more susceptible. The caries susceptibility of the distal surface of the primary canine and the mesial surface of the primary first molar is similar, and both are less affected than the first molar–second molar contact area. The canine–first molar contact area is less broad. In the mandibular arch this contact area serves as the primate space and thus is often free-cleansing.

ETIOLOGIC FACTORS

The etiologic factors discussed in Chapter 12 apply to primary as well as permanent teeth. Studies have indicated that differences may exist between younger and older children for some of the factors, however. Saliva, one of the host factors, differs among preschool children in its levels of lysozyme activity and IgA concentration (Camling and Kohler, 1987; Tweetman et al., 1981). Salivary flow rate is lower among younger children and lower among females than males (Andersson et al., 1974). The concentrations of certain salivary solutes, notably amylase and phosphate, increase during the first year, whereas others (potassium, sodium, protein) decrease during the same time. The net effect of these changes is unclear at this time.

TABLE 17–2. Distribution of Dental Caries in the Primary Dentition by Tooth Surface

	Fluoridation Status of Community		
Tooth Surface	Optimally Fluoridated	Fluoride Deficient	Both
Facial-lingual	26.3%	25.0%	25.9%
Proximal	32.7%	39.5%	34.9%
Occlusal	41.0%	35.3%	39.2%

Data derived from Louie R, Brunelle JA, Maggiore ED, Beck RW: Caries prevalence in Head Start children, 1986-87. J Public Health Dent *50*:299-305, 1990.

The increased use of antibiotics, especially in young children, has been suggested as another possible reason for the decline in caries in the primary dentition. Administration of antibiotics during the eruption of teeth may delay colonization by *Streptococcus mutans* and allow the establishment of other bacteria in the occlusal pits and fissures (Loesche, 1986). Early establishment of *S. mutans* in the mouth of infants may lead to a greater caries experience by age 4 (Alaluusua and Renkonen, 1983).

Sugar consumption in early childhood has been linked to caries levels, as might be expected. Primary dmft scores above 3 have been correlated with intakes of more than 95 g/day, whereas scores below 3 are associated with daily sugar consumption of less than 50 g (Sreebny, 1982). Pacifiers dipped in honey and other sweeteners have been shown to be detrimental to the dentition. Rampant caries is not uncommon among 3- and 4-year-olds who practice this habit (Holt et al., 1988). Another contributing factor for children who are continuously on medication is the high sugar content of some formulations (Roberts and Roberts, 1979).

Many other factors contribute to the risk of caries in children. Such predisposing factors include oral hygiene, socioeconomic status, and nutrition, but the major interactions occur among a susceptible host, dietary sucrose, and the presence of cariogenic microflora.

REFERENCES

Alaluusua S, Renkonen O-L: *Streptococcus mutans* establishment and dental caries experience in children from 2 to 4 years old. Scand J Dent Res *14*:453-457, 1983.

Andersson R, Arvidsson E, Crossner C-G, et al: The flow rate, pH and buffer effect of mixed saliva in children. J Int Assoc Dent Child *5*:5-12, 1974.

Bronstein E: A survey of caries-experience among the preschool children of Philadelphia. J Public Health Dent *29*:24-26, 1969.

Bruszt P, Bánóczy J Esztáry I, et al: Caries prevalence of preschoolchildren in Baja, Hungary in 1955 and 1975. Comm Dent Oral Epidemiol *5*:136-139, 1977.

Camling E, Kohler B: Infection with the bacterium *Streptococcus mutans* and salivary IgA antibodies in mothers and their children. Arch Oral Biol *32*:817-823, 1987.

Chosack A, Cleaton-Jones P, Woods A, Matejka J: Caries prevalence and severity in the primary dentition and *Streptococcus mutans* levels in the saliva of preschoolchildren in South Africa. Comm Dent Oral Epidemiol *16*:289-291, 1988.

Cleaton-Jones P, Richardson BD, Rantsho JM: Dental caries in rural and urban black preschoolchildren. Comm Dent Oral Epidemiol *6*:135-138, 1978.

Cleaton-Jones PE, Hargreaves JA, Roberts G, Williams SD: The dmfs and dmft of young South African children. Comm Dent Oral Epidemiol *17*:38-40, 1989.

Fujiwara T, Sasada E, Mima N, Ooshima T: Caries prevalence and salivary mutans streptococci in 0-2-year-old children of Japan. Comm Dent Oral Epidemiol *19*:151-154, 1991.

Grindefjord M, Dahllof G, Modeer T: Caries development in children from 2.5 to 3.5 years of age: a longitudinal study. Caries Res *29*:449-454, 1995.

Halikis SE: A study of dental caries in a group of Western Australian children: Part II. The incidence of dental caries in children aged 2-6 years. Aust Dent J *8*:114-122, 1963.

Hennon DK, Stookey GK, Muhler JC: Prevalence and distribution of dental caries in preschool children. JADA *79*:1405-1409, 1969.

Holbrook WP, Kristinsson MJ, Gunnarsdóttir S, Briem B: Caries prevalence, *Streptococcus mutans* and sugar intake among 4-year-old urban children in Iceland. Comm Dent Oral Epidemiol *17*:292-295, 1989.

Holt RD, Joels D, Bulman J, et al: A third study of caries in preschool aged children in Camden. Br Dent J *165*:87-91, 1988.

Johnsen DC, Bhat M, Kim MT, et al: Caries levels and patterns in Head Start children in fluoridated and non-fluoridated, urban and non-urban sites in Ohio, USA. Comm Dent Oral Epidemiol *14*:206-210, 1986.

Loesche WJ: Decline in *Streptococcus mutans*-associated caries secondary to medical usage of antibiotics. *In* Hamada S, et al. (eds): Molecular Microbiology and Immunology of *Streptococcus mutans*. Amsterdam, Elsevier Science (Biomedical Division), 1986, pp 371-379.

Louie R, Brunelle JA, Maggiore ED, Beck RW: Caries prevalence in Head Start children, 1986-87. J Public Health Dent *50*:299-305, 1990.

Roberts IJ, Roberts GJ: Relation between medicines sweetened with sucrose and dental disease. Br Med J *2*:14-16, 1979.

Savara BS, Suher T: Incidence of dental caries in children 1 to 6 years of age. J Dent Res *33*:808-823, 1954.

Salem GM, Holm SA: Dental caries in preschoolchildren in Gizan, Saudi Arabia. Comm Dent Oral Epidemiol *13*:176, 1985.

Schwarz E, Hansen ER: Caries experience of Danish children evaluated by the child dental health recording system. Comm Dent Oral Epidemiol 7:107-114, 1979.

Speechley M, Johnston DW: Some evidence from Ontario, Canada, of a reversal in the dental caries decline. Caries Res *30*:423-427, 1996.

Sreebny LM: Sugar availability, sugar consumption and dental caries. Comm Dent Oral Epidemiol *10*:1-7, 1982.

Stecklin-Blicks C, Holm AK, Mayanagi H: Dental caries in Swedish 4-year-old children: Changes between 1967 and 1987. Swed Dent J *13*:39-44, 1989.

Sutcliffe P: Caries experience and oral cleanliness of 3- and 4-year-old children from deprived and non-deprived areas in Edinburgh, Scotland. Comm Dent Oral Epidemiol *5*:213-219, 1977.

Trubman A, Silberman SL, Meydrech EF: Dental caries assessment of Mississippi Head Start children. J Public Health Dent *49*:167-169, 1989.

Tweetman S, Lindner A, Modeer T: Lysozyme and salivary immunoglobulin A in caries free and caries susceptible preschool children. Swed Dent J *5*:9-14, 1981.

Wendt LK, Hallonsten AL, Koch G: Dental caries in one- and two-year-old children living in Sweden. Part I—a longitudinal study. Swed Dent J *15*:1-6, 1991.

Williams SD, Cleaton-Jones PE, Richardson BD, Smith C: Dental caries and dental treatment in the primary dentition in an industrialized South African community. Comm Dent Oral Epidemiol *13*:173-175, 1985.

Winter GB, Rule DC, Mailer GP, et al: The prevalence of dental caries in pre-school children aged 1 to 4 years. Br Dent J *130*:271-277, 1971.

Wisan JM, Lavell M, Colwell FH: Dental survey of Philadelphia preschool children by income, age and treatment status. JADA *55*:1-10, 1957.

Examination, Diagnosis, and Treatment Planning

Paul S. Casamassimo, John R. Christensen, and Henry W. Fields, Jr.

Chapter Outline

DIAGNOSIS AND TREATMENT PLANNING FOR NONORTHODONTIC PROBLEMS

The examination of the 3-year-old child often represents a youngster's first dental experience, although earlier examinations are advocated by most pediatric dentists and the American Academy of Pediatric Dentistry for diagnostic, preventive, and treatment purposes. For a child who has not had a dental examination previously, the new environment, new people, and manipulation of tissues can be difficult or overwhelming.

An initial examination of a child this age can also be stressful for the dentist, who is faced with a potential behavior problem, no clinical baseline, and the challenge of providing both immediate and long-term planning and treatment.

The initial examination is a first experience for both dentist and patient and provides an opportunity to establish a course of dental health for years to come. Of particular interest in the examination of the 3- to 6-year-old are the following factors:

1. Lack of an existing history
2. No clinical baseline data
3. Behavioral unknowns
4. A primary dentition occlusion with limited predictive value
5. Preventive needs that must be assessed

All of the above need to be addressed in evaluating a child this age, especially if this is the child's initial dental visit.

PATIENT RECORDS

The nature of health care record-keeping in dentistry has evolved from a historical or financial repository to a vital working document. The bare essentials for a pediatric dental record are a health history, examination record, treatment plan, and series of visit notes. Parental or guardian consent should be obtained and recorded at the initial visit. Adjunctive records such as study casts and preventive and dietary forms or analyses also should be kept with the record, if indicated. The history form should permit updating and summary.

The possibilities for a dental examination record for children are endless.

Many practitioners opt for a standard form or use the one they employed in dental school. No clear-cut guidelines exist for choice of a pediatric dental tooth chart, but there are some basic requirements from a medicolegal standpoint and from the standpoint of providing a developmental history. The examination record should do the following:

1. Adequately record both developmental status and existing pathosis of teeth
2. Provide a record of each examination or procedure including recalls, periodic examinations, and radiographs
3. Record facial and occlusal status
4. Record oral hygiene, periodontal, and intraoral soft tissue status

The tooth chart need not be anatomically correct, and, in many cases, a diagram of teeth is of more value. It is critical that the charting system address both primary and permanent teeth so that each record entry provides an up-to-date developmental profile. In addition to a notation of the presence or absence of a tooth, as is done with adults, the mobility of primary teeth and clinically evident eruption of teeth are noted in the pediatric dental chart. Current child safety concerns strongly suggest making an initial charting of the dentition, including restorations and abnormalities. For many children the absence of restorations or caries makes this an academic exercise.

Periodontal probing of all teeth is not routine, but the dental chart should provide an area for noting deep pocketing or loss of attachment in some manner. The nature of this notation requires simply adequate baseline data to accomplish treatment and follow-up.

A diagnosis or diagnostic code will soon be essential for all conditions and pathology. This diagnostic code combined with a treatment code, which is already in common use, allows evaluation of treatment outcomes.

Many practitioners develop individual approaches to prevention that can be efficiently addressed on the examination record. A serial chart of oral hygiene performance or gingival scores can be helpful. Other helpful items on the examination record are vital signs, medical alerts, behavior notes, and unusual findings. Reasons for deferring radiographic examination need to be noted in the record. These data provide quick reference for the dentist at chairside.

The treatment plan should indicate the sequence of care and permit notation of the date of completion of individual procedures. Each visit's progress note indicates what was done and any notable occurrences.

THE HISTORY

The parent or guardian is the historian for the child. The dentist needs to address both real and perceived problems. Parents may provide erroneous and unverified information simply because the information has not been tested by the health system. Two such examples are reported heart murmurs and allergies. Parents may have been informed of a murmur but are unaware of its seriousness. Parents also may confuse nausea with a true allergic reaction. The dentist may be required to address these concerns directly with a physician to obtain accurate information. In other situations, a long-established or past problem may have been forgotten or dismissed as unimportant.

A general health history form can be used to determine a child's health background if attention is given to specific elements that relate to children. The dentist should be well versed in conditions that relate specifically to children. Table 18-1 provides a list of health items that are particularly common in the 3- to 6-year-old age group.

A short and noncontributory history was unusual in this age group in the past, but with the improvement in infant health practices and home care, immunization, and early intervention, many routine problems and illnesses have been reduced. On the other hand, a growing number of infants survive who would have perished previously. Although some develop normally, a substantial number are physically or mentally compromised and require alternative and more complex health care approaches. The dentist's review of a check list with annotations can be used to complete an accurate medical history. Significant findings should be explained in the record. Any health history should be finalized by a summary of the status of the child, especially in the areas of drug allergies, surgical procedures and related problems, cardiac abnormalities, and developmental status.

The dental history should be comprehensive. Many parents have not thought to characterize their child's dental history other than the eruption of the first tooth. The dental history should cover, at a minimum, past problems and care, fluoride experience, current hygiene habits, and an eruption-developmental profile. Table 18-1 addresses the essential elements of the dental history.

THE EXAMINATION

The examination encompasses six major sections: behavioral assessment; general appraisal;

TABLE 18–1. Selected Health History Considerations with Common Findings in the 3- to 6-Year-Old Group

Area of Concern	Common Findings
General Health	
Allergies	Probably related to food and other environmental allergens; may have allergy to medications such as antibiotics; rash is common manifestation; false allergies often reported
Asthma	May be reported; triggering factors usually known; medications also well known; impact of dental intervention usually not known
Bleeding	Parent may suggest excessive bruising without real problem
Blood transfusion	May have been performed at birth
Childhood infections	Immunizations will have occurred, or there is a clear history of having had a specific illness such as measles or chickenpox
Development	Poor parental knowledge for normal children; for those with developmental delays, a good history of diagnostic procedures and status
Heart	Functional murmur may exist, or parent may have been told of a murmur
Hypertension	Usually unknown, unless child has chronic problem
Illnesses	Probable history of upper respiratory infections
Jaundice	Possible at birth
Medications	Probably has taken acetaminophen (Tylenol) as necessary; may have received amoxicillin or other antibiotic
Surgical procedures	Possible tonsillectomy or adenoidectomy; possible ear tubes; circumcision seldom noted as procedure
Seizures	Possibly febrile; may be on seizure medication for only one seizure
Dental Health	
Bottle use	Probably considered not to contribute to decay
Developmental/eruption	Knowledge may be limited to eruption dates of first teeth, unless consistently very early or late
Fluoride	May know water status; possible vitamin with fluoride supplementation
Habits (thumb sucking)	Will be well known to parent if present
Home care	Usually confined to tooth brushing; may be largely left to child
Previous care	Possibly none; no dentist or care rendered
Reaction to care (behavior)	Possibly none; likely poor or tentative
Trauma to teeth and chin	Possible, but usually left untreated unless serious; commonly upper teeth and chin

This table suggests usual or common responses to questions put to parents of this age group for the average child, but it does not suggest a norm or most frequent response for all children.

and head and neck, facial, intraoral, and radiographic examinations.

Behavioral Assessment

A complete behavioral assessment is discussed in Chapter 21. The general appraisal and chairside examination provide two opportunities to observe behavior and initially assess potential cooperation.

General Appraisal

The general appraisal addresses the child's physical and behavioral status. The classic areas of this appraisal include gait, stature, and presence of gross signs and symptoms of disease. The normal 3- to 6-year-old is ambulatory, well coordinated in basic tasks, engaging, and physically healthy in appearance. Table 18–2 lists physical and be-

havioral milestones for the 3- to 6-year-old child. The dentist should incorporate these markers mentally into a profile for evaluation of the child. The general appraisal of the child is best accomplished in the waiting room or similar nonthreatening environment. This appraisal should be followed by clarification of any abnormal findings and discussion of potential behavior problems with the parent.

The role of vital signs in the general appraisal is twofold. The first purpose is to identify abnormalities, and the second is to satisfy the medicolegal role of providing baseline health data for emergency situations. Vital signs may be distorted if the child is upset or anxious. Taking vital signs of blood pressure, pulse, and respiration may be put off until the child has become accustomed to the environment, but these data must be obtained before any drugs are administered. Weight should be obtained and recorded in a conspicuous location on the chart so that the information is available in an emergency. Height

TABLE 18–2. Selected Developmental Characteristics of the 3- to 6-Year-Old Child

3-Year-Old	4-Year-Old	5-Year-Old
Intellectual Development		
Gives first and last name	Recognizes colors	Names four colors
Counts three objects	Counts four objects	Counts 10 objects
States own age and sex	Tells a story	Asks about the meaning of words
Gross/Fine Motor Skills		
Puts on shoes	Dresses without supervision	Dresses and undresses
Pedals tricycle	Balances on one foot	Hops on one foot
Copies a circle	Copies cross and square	Draws a triangle
Psychological		
The 3- to 6-year-old is in the *phallic* stage of development. During this period, the child undergoes *oedipal* conflicts, which may lead to opposite-sex parental preference. The child may exhibit some aggression to siblings. By age 6, the child may be ready to surrender some dependency toward parents.		
Dental Implications		
Needs maternal presence, especially during stress	May be difficult and aggressive	Should leave parent for treatment
	Responds to verbal direction	Proud of possessions
Fear of separation	Auditory fear	Bodily harm fear
Visual fear		
Physiological Height (75th percentile)		
Boys = 97.5 cm	Boys = 106 cm	Boys = 113 cm
Girls = 97 cm	Girls = 104.5 cm	Girls = 111.5 cm
(Growth rate for this period is approximately 6–8 cm/yr)		
Weight (75th percentile)		
Boys = 15.5 kg	Boys = 18 kg	Boys = 20 kg
Girls = 15.5 kg	Girls = 17.5 kg	Girls = 19.5 kg
(Growth rate for this period is approximately 2 kg/yr)		
Pulse (90th percentile)		
105/min	100/min	100/min
Respiration (90th percentile)		
30/min	28/min	26/min
Blood Pressure		
100/60	100/60	100/60

should also be recorded and, together with weight, should serve as an index of physical development.

Head and Neck Examination

Examining a 3-year-old requires attention to both clinical findings and the patient's behavior in the dental setting. Said differently, the product (dental findings) cannot be separated from the process (patient's behavior) of the examination. The examination provides a moderately threatening environment for development of behavioral interactions between dentist and child.

Table 18–3 outlines the elements and expectations for a thorough head and neck examination. The process begins with an orientation about what is to occur. What will take place at each step in the examination should be described by the dentist. The tell-show-do technique, which involves explanation, demonstration, and finally completion of a step, is usually the way the diagnostic process is handled. Positive or negative responses from the child should be encouraged. Children also should be warned and supported prior to making positional changes or beginning intraoral manipulation.

Parental presence is always a matter of controversy. Initial parental involvement may be encouraged to allow a transition to be made from a dentist-parent to a more direct dentist-child relationship. This supported transition is important for children under 3 years of age but is less threatening for children near school age. Each child reacts differently to having a parent in the operatory, and the dentist must assess the benefit of that presence on the developing relationship he or she has with that child. It is within the parent's purview to request to be present during the examination and treatment, but it is within the practitioner's purview to

TABLE 18–3. Elements of Head and Neck Examination

Structure	Diagnostic Technique	Normal Characteristics	Selected Abnormal Findings/Possible Causes
Head			
Hair	Visualization	Quality Thickness Color	Dryness/malnutrition, ectodermal dysplasia Baldness/child abuse, self-abuse, chemotherapy Infestation/neglect
Scalp	Visualization	Skin color Dryness Ulceration	Scaling/dermatitis Sores/abuse, infection, neglect
Ears	Visualization Palpation Assessment of hearing	Intact and normally formed external ear and auditory canal Gross normal hearing	Malformed ears and canals/genetic malformation syndrome (e.g., Treacher Collins) Conductive and neurologic hearing loss/trauma, developmental disability
Eyes	Visualization Assessment of vision	Position and orientation in fact Movement of eyes Vision Reaction to light	Variation in separation and orientation/genetic malformation syndromes Cranial nerve damage/trauma, developmental disability
Nose	Visualization	Normal size, shape, function, and location	Malposition/genetic malformation syndrome (e.g., median facial cleft) Misshapen/ectodermal dysplasia, congenital syphilis, achondroplasia Discharge/upper respiratory infection (URI), asthma, allergy Poor smell, cranial nerve damage
Lip	Visualization Assessment of function	Speech, closure Integrity Absence of lesions	Poor closure/lip incompetence Clefting/genetic clefting syndrome Asymmetry/Bell's palsy or cranial nerve damage Ulceration/herpes infection
Temporomandibular joint	Visualization Palpation Auscultation	Symmetry in function Smooth movement Absence of pain Range of motion (maximum)	Deviation/trauma Crepitus, pain/temporomandibular joint disorder Limitation/arthritis, trauma
Skin	Visualization	Color Tone Moisture Absence of lesions	Edema/cellulitis, renal disorder Redness/allergic response Dryness/dehydration, ectodermal dysplasia Ulceration/infectious disease, abuse
Chin	Visualization	Absence of scar	Scar indicates previous mandibular trauma
Neck			
Lymph nodes	Palpation	Normal size, mobility	Increased size/infection, neoplasia Fixation/neoplasia
Thyroid	Palpation	Normal size	Increased size/goiter, tumor
Oral Cavity			
Palates	Visualization Palpation Assessment of function	Integrity Absence of lesion Normal function	Cleft/genetic syndrome Ulceration/herpes, mononucleosis, or other infection, abuse Petechiae/sexual abuse Deviation/cranial nerve damage
Pharynx	Visualization	Normal color Normal size of tonsils	Redness/URI, tonsillitis
Tongue	Visualization Palpation Assessment of function	Normal color Range of motion Absence of lesions	Redness/glossitis Ulceration/herpes, aphthous, or other infection, trauma Deviation/cranial nerve damage Limited movement/cerebral palsy
Floor of mouth	Visualization Palpation	Salivary function Absence of swelling Absence of lesions	Swelling/mucocele, sialolith Ulceration/aphthous ulceration or other infection, abuse
Buccal mucosa	Visualization Palpation	Absence of lesions Absence of swelling Salivary function	Ulceration/cheek bite, abuse Swelling/salivary gland Infection, mumps

Table continued on following page

TABLE 18–3. Elements of Head and Neck Examination *Continued*

Structure	Diagnostic Technique	Normal Characteristics	Selected Abnormal Findings/Possible Causes
Teeth	Visualization Palpation Percussion	Normal development Morphologic appearance Occlusion Color Integrity Mobility Hygiene	Absence/delayed eruption/congenital absence, genetic syndromes Extra teeth/supernumerary, cleidocranial dysplasia Abnormal morphologic appearance/microdontia, macrodontia, fusion Abnormal color/amelogenesis, dentinogenesis imperfecta, staining, pulpal necrosis, caries Fracture/trauma, abuse, caries Mobility/periapical infection, trauma, bone loss conditions, exfoliation Malposition/malocclusion, trauma Pain/periapical involvement

choose not to treat the child under those circumstances. Growing numbers of practitioners allow parents in the treatment setting, and most data indicate that parents are neutral factors (Pfefferle et al., 1982).

The examination must involve evaluation of the head and neck. Palpation to identify enlarged and fixed lymph nodes or other swellings is critical. Many children of this age have swollen nodes, but they are usually movable and confined to the lower face and jaws and indicate minor infections. Nodes in the neck and clavicular region are more rare and may indicate more serious ailments.

Critical to a thorough examination of the head and neck is evaluation of form and function. The cranial nerves, speech, and mandibular function should be evaluated. A complete cranial nerve examination need not be performed, however, because careful observation of sensory and motor function and the child's responses can indicate nerve status to a significant degree. Normal conversation can be used to identify gross speech pathosis. While palpating the craniofacial structures, the dentist should talk with the child and observe his or her responses. Asking the child to open and demonstrate maximum opening and maximum intercuspation allows the child to perform simple tasks. Mandibular movements should be observed for deviation and restriction of range of movement. The child should also be asked to move the mandible from side to side and to protrude it. Restriction of these movements may identify functional and morphologic problems that are developmental or the result of trauma.

Verbal responses also serve as behavioral signals of the child's adaptation. A child's cooperation, nonverbal communication, and physiologic responses often suggest stable, improving, or deteriorating behavior. Because the examination setting is only moderately threatening, it provides a good opportunity to develop cooperation.

The manual examination should address any physical variations as well as the strength and mobility of structures. The visual aspect of the process should address color changes, asymmetry, and marked physiologic responses such as sweating or trembling.

Facial Examination

A systematic facial examination should be undertaken to ensure that relevant information is not omitted. A systematic facial examination is one portion of a complete orthodontic evaluation that describes skeletal and dental relationships in three spatial planes: anteroposterior, vertical, and transverse. The steps include a description of the overall facial pattern, the positions of the maxilla and mandible, and then the vertical relationships. Next, the position of the lips is determined. Finally, facial symmetry is assessed and the maxillary dental midline is located relative to the facial midline.

First, the facial profile is evaluated in the anteroposterior plane. An assumption is made that the soft tissue profile reflects the underlying skeletal relationship. To begin the examination, the child should be seated in an upright position, looking at a distant point. Three points on the face are identified: the bridge of the nose, the base of the upper lip, and the chin.

Line segments connecting these points form an angle that describes the profile as convex, straight, or concave. A well-balanced profile in this age group is slightly convex. A well-balanced profile in the anteroposterior dimension has an underlying skeletal relationship that is labeled

Class I (Fig. 18-1*A*). This terminology is used because most Class I skeletal relationships also have Angle Class I or end-to-end permanent first molar dental relationships and flush terminal plane or mesial step second primary molar relationships. Further, the canine relationships will be Class I and there will be overjet of 2 to 5 mm. The Angle dental classification is described in a later section.

Most profiles, skeletal relationships, and dental relationships (molar, canine, and overjet) are consistent. If they are not, the reason for the inconsistency should be determined. It may be due to missing and subsequently drifted teeth, protrusion of incisors due to non-nutritive sucking habits, or dental drift to compensate for skeletal problems.

Some children in this age group have extremely convex profiles (Fig. 18-1*B*). This is consistent with a Class II skeletal relationship, and these patients usually have Class II permanent first molar relationships and distal step second primary molar relationships, Class II canine relationships, and increased overjet.

Other children have straight or concave profiles (Fig 18-1*C*). These are usually found with Class III permanent first molar relationships and mesial step second primary molar relationships, Class III canine relationships, and negative overjet.

If the profile is excessively convex or concave, the clinician can try to determine which skeletal component is contributing to the problem. This is a necessary step if orthodontic treatment is being considered. When one knows the problem, one can direct treatment to appropriately address the problem.

Specifically, in this diagnostic step, the anteroposterior position of the maxilla and mandible are determined. This can be accomplished by extending a vertical reference line from the bridge of the nose (the anterior aspect of the cranial base) and noting where other soft tissue points are located relative to the reference line (Fig. 18-2). If the maxilla is properly oriented relative to other skeletal structures, the base of the upper lip will be on or near the vertical line. The soft tissue chin will be slightly behind the reference line if the mandible is of proper size and in the correct position. If the maxilla is positioned significantly in front of the vertical reference line, the patient is said to exhibit maxillary protrusion. If the maxilla is substantially behind the line, the patient exhibits maxillary retrusion. The position of the mandible is described in the same way.

So, if the overall skeletal pattern is significantly convex (Class II), the reason is a maxilla positioned in front of the line (maxillary protrusion), a mandible positioned behind the line (mandibular retrusion), or both. Class II skeletal relationships are sometimes caused by one jaw alone but are often the result of some combination of maxillary protrusion and mandibular retrusion.

Conversely, if the facial pattern is straight or extremely concave (Class III), the reason is a

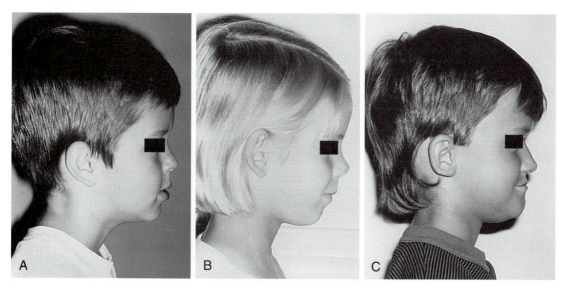

Figure 18–1. *A,* A Class I skeletal relationship is characterized by a well-balanced profile in the anteroposterior dimension. These relationships can be judged by mentally connecting the points of the bridge of the nose, the base of the upper lip (maxilla) and the soft tissue chin (mandible). This line should be slightly convex. *B,* A Class II skeletal relationship is characterized by a truly convex profile. *C,* A Class III skeletal relationship is characterized by a straight or concave profile.

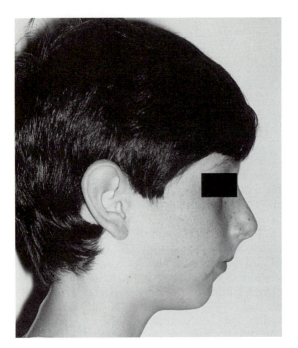

Figure 18–2. The contributions to the skeletal malocclusion can be estimated extraorally by determining the positions of the maxilla and mandible. A perpendicular reference line is established beginning at the soft tissue bridge of the nose. The position of the maxilla and mandible are related to this line. If the base of the upper lip and nose are anterior to this line, the maxilla is protrusive. If these points are posterior to this line, the maxilla is retrusive. Similarly, the soft tissue chin is determined to be anterior (protrusive) or posterior (retrusive) to this line. This patient has a significantly convex facial profile (Class II), which is contributed to by a near normal maxilla that is near the line and a clearly retrusive mandible that is posterior to the line.

maxilla positioned behind the line (maxillary retrusion), a mandible positioned in front of the line (mandibular protrusion), or both. Again, both jaws usually contribute to the skeletal dysplasia.

Some caution must be exercised because soft tissue profile relationships do not always accurately reflect the underlying skeletal relationships. Research has shown that the 3- to 6-year-old age group is especially difficult to classify

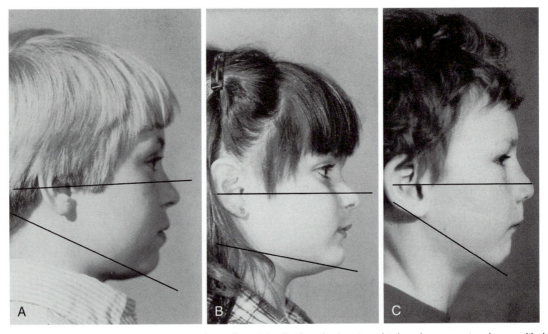

Figure 18–3. *A,* Vertical facial proportions can be evaluated by dividing the face into thirds or by comparing the mandibular plane with a horizontal reference line. In a well-proportioned face, the facial thirds are equal in size. *B,* A child with short vertical facial dimensions has a proportionately smaller lower facial third and a flat mandibular plane. *C,* A child with long vertical facial dimensions has a proportionately larger lower facial third and a steep mandibular plane.

accurately from a profile analysis (Fields and Vann, 1979). In addition, vertical facial relationships influence the anteroposterior relationships. This interaction between the horizontal and vertical planes of space and its effect on the profile is discussed later.

The third portion of the facial examination is an evaluation of the vertical relationships. Proportionality is judged by dividing the face into thirds, the upper third extends from approximately the hair line to the bridge of the nose, the middle third from the bridge of the nose to the base of the upper lip, and the lower third from the base of the upper lip to the bottom of the chin (Fig. 18-3*A*). These thirds are approximately equal in well-proportioned faces. Vertical facial height also can be evaluated by comparing the mandibular plane, a line tangent to the lower border of the mandible, to a horizontal reference line such as the Frankfort Horizontal Plane (the line connecting the upper extent of the auditory meatus and the lower rim of the orbit). These two lines form an internal angle that grows larger the steeper the mandibular plane relative to the horizontal reference line.

Vertical problems tend to be manifest below the palate in the lower third of the face (Fields et al., 1984). The short-faced person tends to have a lower facial third that is smaller than the other thirds and have a flat or low mandibular plane angle (Fig. 18-3*B*). The long-faced patient has a lower facial third that is larger than the other thirds and a steep or high mandibular plane angle (Fig. 18-3*C*).

Next we advocate an evaluation of the anteroposterior lip position to give an estimation of the anteroposterior incisor position. Incisor position is grossly reflected in lip contour and posture. Lip posture is assessed by drawing an imaginary line from the tip of the nose to the most anterior point on the soft tissue chin. The lips normally lie slightly behind this line; however, in the 3- to 6-year-old child, the lower lip is generally 1 mm anterior to the line (Fig. 18-4). Two facts must be kept in mind. First, lip protrusion is characteristic of different ethnic groups, and lips that are considered protrusive in one group may not be considered protrusive in another. For example, African-Americans and Asians tend to have more lip protrusion than do people of northern European descent. Second, the lips are evaluated in the context of the nose and chin. A large nose and chin can accommodate more protrusive lips, whereas a small nose and chin require less protrusive lips to be proportional.

Transverse facial dimensions are examined to rule out true facial asymmetry. Facial symmetry

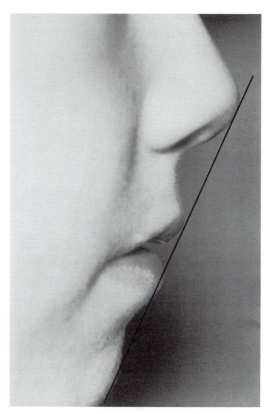

Figure 18–4. The anteroposterior position of the lips is determined by drawing a line from the tip of the nose to the most anterior point on the soft tissue chin. The upper lip normally should lie slightly behind the line, whereas the lower lip should lie slightly in front of this line in the 3- to 6-year-old child.

is best evaluated with the patient reclined in the dental chair and the dentist seated in the 12 o'clock position (Fig. 18-5). Hair is pulled away from the face, and a piece of dental floss can be stretched down the middle of the upper face to aid in judging lower face symmetry. The mandible should be either at rest or in centric relation position. Maximum intercuspation or centric occlusion positions can be affected by dental interferences during closing.

All faces show a minor degree of asymmetry, but marked asymmetry is not normal (Fig. 18-6). Deviations or asymmetric positioning of the eyes, ears, or nose may be symptoms of cranial synostosis, an undiagnosed syndrome, or severe trauma. A child with these findings should be referred to appropriate professionals for a complete evaluation.

Asymmetry usually manifests in the lower facial third, whereas upper facial asymmetry is extremely rare. In this age group, a deviation of the midpoint of the mandible to one side or

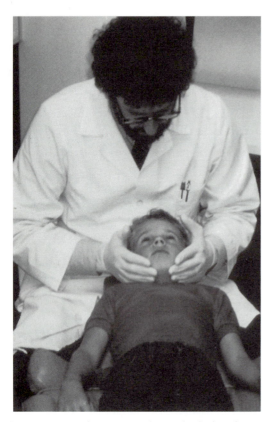

Figure 18–5. Facial symmetry is best judged when the patient is reclining and the dentist is seated in the 12 o'clock position.

mouth. Children in this age group often permit oral inspection with "just fingers," and the dentist can use this technique as a springboard to obtain cooperation for the use of mirror and explorer. The mirror should be the first instrument introduced. This is usually readily accepted by the child owing to its familiarity and nonthreatening shape.

Young children are sometimes uncooperative. If they are, a decision must be made early about how to manage the behavior. Parental assistance can be used to obtain an examination of the oral cavity. Use of physical restraint by the dentist without parental consent is risky and is not advisable. Parents are more likely to accept restraint in conjunction with an emergency examination than with a routine examination.

An important portion of the intraoral examination is directed toward the teeth. Each of the 20 primary teeth should be explored and scrutinized visually. Selective periodontal probing may be performed, but the yield is likely to be minimal because of the infrequency of irreversible attachment loss in the primary dentition.

Occlusal Evaluation. Another portion of the intraoral examination is the systematic analysis of the occlusion in three spatial planes. In addition, each dental arch is analyzed individually to

another may be due to true asymmetry, but it is most often indicative of a posterior crossbite and mandibular shift due to a dental interference. Posterior crossbites and mandibular shifts are two findings that are discussed later in the chapter.

The maxillary dental midline should be compared with the upper facial midline. This helps determine where the midline of the mandibular teeth is relative to the face when it is compared with the upper dental midline.

Intraoral Examination

The armamentarium for the intraoral examination includes mirror, explorer, gauze, and periodontal probe. Additional materials are disclosing solution, dental floss, toothbrush, and scaler.

The intraoral examination begins with an excursion around the oral cavity, noting its general architecture and function. The fingers should be used to identify soft tissue abnormalities of the cheeks, lips, tongue, palate, and floor of the mouth before instruments are placed in the

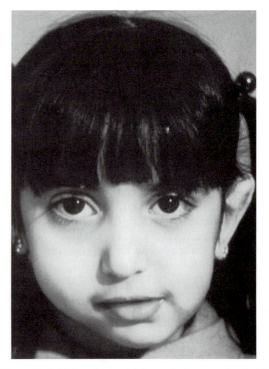

Figure 18–6. This patient exhibits marked asymmetry that is the result of a congenital fusion of the left condyle and coronoid process to the temporal bone.

describe arch form and symmetry, spacing and crowding, and the presence or absence of teeth. Arch analysis is best performed on diagnostic study models; however, diagnostic casts are usually not indicated in this age group unless there is some need to further study the intraoral findings or if tooth movement is contemplated.

If diagnostic casts are necessary, an appropriate impression tray must be chosen. Properly fitted trays seat comfortably in the mouth and extend far enough posteriorly to cover the most distal tooth and either the maxillary tuberosity or the mandibular retromolar pad. The trays should be of a nonperforated variety that hold the impression material in the tray and express the excess material into the vestibule. Expression of the excess material into the vestibule is desirable because it displaces the soft tissues, which allows the dentoalveolar morphology to be clearly viewed on the cast. The trays also can be lined with wax that aids in tissue displacement and makes seating the tray into position more comfortable.

After the appropriate tray has been selected, the alginate is mixed and placed in one tray. For either arch, the tray should be rotated laterally into the mouth and firmly seated, first posteriorly against the palate or the retromolar pad. This technique limits the posterior flow of alginate and forces excess alginate anteriorly and laterally. The tray is then rotated and seated over the anterior teeth. Finally, the tray is held in place until the alginate has set. After the upper and lower impressions are obtained, a wax bite is made by placing a softened piece of baseplate wax between the teeth and having the patient close in centric occlusion. The wax is cooled with air and serves to orient the casts properly during trimming.

Impressions should be wrapped in moist paper towels and stored in sealed plastic bags or poured soon in white plaster because the alginate will dehydrate and distort if it is left exposed for more than a few minutes. The plaster is thoroughly mixed usually using a vacuum spatulator to reduce bubbles and then vibrated into the impression and flowed from one tooth to another to prevent air entrapment, which results in holes in the models. Separate plaster bases are poured, and the impressions are inverted on the bases when the plaster is partially set. After the plaster has set, the trays are separated carefully from the casts to prevent breaking the teeth.

The maxillary cast is trimmed so that the top of the base is parallel to the occlusal plane. The back of the upper cast is trimmed perpendicular to its top and the midpalatal raphe. The maxillary and mandibular casts are occluded, and the back of the mandibular base is trimmed parallel to the top of the maxillary cast. Finally, the sides of the casts are trimmed symmetrically, which allows the clinician to judge arch symmetry.

Alignment. Dental arches can be categorized as either U-shaped or V-shaped. The mandibular arch is normally U-shaped, whereas the maxillary arch can be either shape. The dental arch should be symmetrical in the anteroposterior and transverse dimensions. Individual teeth are compared with their antimeres to determine if there is anteroposterior or transverse symmetry (Fig. 18-7).

The ideal arch in the primary dentition has spacing between the teeth. Two types of spaces are identified. The first type, primate space, is located mesial to the maxillary canine and distal to the mandibular canine. Developmental space is the space present between the remaining teeth (Fig. 18-8). Anterior spacing is desirable in the primary dentition because the permanent incisors are larger than their primary precursors. Although the presence of primate and developmental spacing does not ensure that the permanent dentition will erupt without crowding, these spaces usually alleviate some crowding. Crowding or overlapped teeth in the primary dentition may occur, although it is rare. True crowding in the primary dentition almost always guarantees a crowded permanent dentition. Crowding of isolated teeth, however, is sometimes due to space loss or indicative of a sucking habit. Lower anterior teeth can be tipped lingually into a crowded position as a result of constant pressure from a finger (active digit habit).

Although it seems elementary, the clinician should carefully count the number of teeth in the mouth. Children in this age group should have all their primary teeth present. Those with delayed dental eruption may have either a very slow but normal sequence of eruption or some isolated eruption problem. To distinguish the two, the eruption sequence of the child is compared with the normal sequence of eruption, and the eruption pattern on the right side is compared with that on the left. If the sequence seems to be appropriate, dental development is probably slow. If, however, the patient's eruption pattern deviates from the normal sequence and there are differences between the contralateral sides of the mouth, further investigation is warranted to determine whether teeth are missing or are impeded from erupting. The maxillary lateral incisor is the most common missing tooth

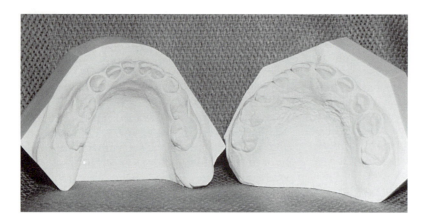

Figure 18–7. These casts illustrate marked dental arch asymmetry in the transverse dimensions. Asymmetry of this magnitude is not in the normal range.

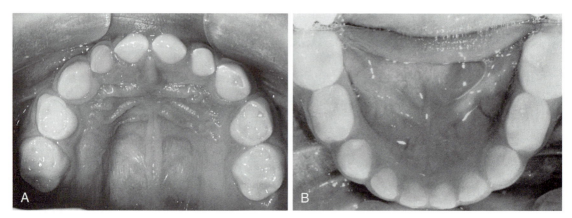

Figure 18–8. These maxillary *(A)* and mandibular *(B)* arches show primate spaces (mesial to the maxillary canines and distal to the mandibular canines) and developmental spacing (space between the remaining teeth).

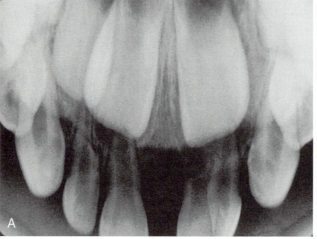

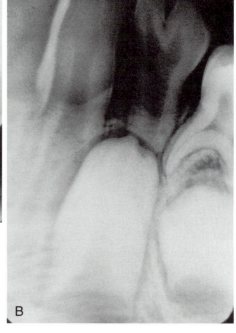

Figure 18–9. Supporting radiographs such as these are often necessary to distinguish fusion from gemination. *A,* These fused primary teeth are joined only at the dentin and have independent pulp chambers and canals. *B,* This geminated primary tooth has a large crown and a common pulp canal. (Photos courtesy of Dr. W.F. Vann.)

in the primary dentition (Valachovic and Lurie, 1980).

Counting the teeth also reveals the presence of supernumerary or extra teeth. Approximately 0.3% of children have supernumerary teeth in the primary dentition. The prevalence of fused and geminated teeth is approximately 0.1% to 0.5% (Valachovic and Lurie, 1980). One can usually distinguish fusion of two primary teeth from gemination without the aid of radiographs by counting the number of teeth. If two teeth are fused, there should be 9 teeth in the arch, one of which is very large, rather than 10 teeth. If gemination has occurred, there should be 10 teeth in the arch and one will be very large. A radiograph may be necessary to confirm the preliminary diagnosis of fusion or gemination. Fused primary teeth show two distinct and independent pulp chambers and canals with union of the dentin. Geminated primary teeth show two crowns and two pulp chambers connected to a single root and pulp canal (Fig. 18-9).

Anteroposterior Dimension. After the maxillary and mandibular arches have been examined for symmetry, spacing, and tooth number, the relationship of the two arches to each other is examined. In the anteroposterior dimension, primary molar and canine relationships are determined and compared with the skeletal classification. In the primary dentition, molars are called flush terminal plane, mesial step, or distal step (Fig. 18-10). Primary canines are classified as Class I, Class II, Class III, or end-to-end. These dental classifications generally reflect the skeletal classification.

Primary molar relationships, as described by

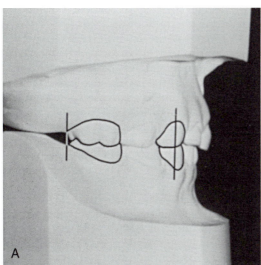

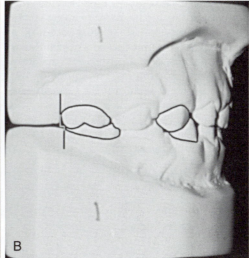

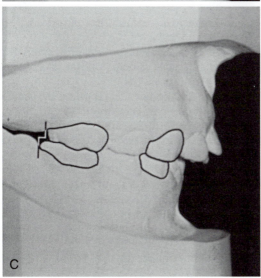

Figure 18–10. *A*, In the primary dentition, an occlusion is classified according to the relationship of the mandibular second molars and canines to the maxillary second molars and canines. In this example, the distal surface of the mandibular second molar is flush with the distal surface of the maxillary second molar. This primary molar relationship is called flush terminal plane. The long axis of the mandibular canine is coincident with the long axis of the maxillary canine. This is described as an end-to-end canine relationship. *B*, In this example, the distal surface of the mandibular molar is mesial to the distal surface of the maxillary molar. This primary molar relationship is termed mesial step. The maxillary canine is positioned in the embrasure between the mandibular canine and the first molar. This is described as a Class I canine relationship. *C*, In this example, the distal surface of the mandibular molar is distal to the distal surface of the maxillary molar. This primary molar relationship is called distal step. The maxillary canine is positioned in the embrasure between the mandibular canine and the lateral incisor. This is described as a Class II canine relationship.

the distal surfaces of the primary second molar, are worthy of attention not only because they describe the relationship of the primary mandibular teeth to the primary maxillary teeth but also because these surfaces guide the permanent molars into occlusion and determine the permanent molar relationships. Documenting primary molar relationships also allows one to follow the effects of growth or treatment.

Overjet, the horizontal overlap of the maxillary and mandibular incisors, is measured in millimeters (Fig. 18-11). It may be more helpful to describe overjet as ideal, excessive, or deficient rather than as a millimetric measure.

Transverse Relationship. The transverse relationship of the arches is examined for midline discrepancies and posterior crossbites. The midline of each arch is compared with the other and with the midsagittal plane. Remember that the upper midline was evaluated to the facial midline during the facial evaluation. A large midline discrepancy is unusual in the early primary dentition, and clinicians should be suspicious of a mandibular shift. The presence of a mandibular shift is often indicative of a posterior crossbite.

If a posterior crossbite is encountered, the clinician should try to determine its cause. The majority of posterior crossbites are due to constriction of the maxillary arch. This is one situation in which diagnostic casts are helpful to aid in or confirm the diagnosis. After the arch at fault

is identified, an attempt is made to determine whether the crossbite is bilateral or unilateral. If models are available, they can be measured to see whether teeth are equidistant from the midpalatal raphe. If models are not available, the determination must be made clinically. The first step is to guide the mandible into centric relation. If teeth are in crossbite on both sides of the arch when the mandible is in centric relation, the child has a bilateral crossbite. If the teeth are in crossbite on only one side of the arch when the mandible is in centric relation, the crossbite is unilateral (Fig. 18-12). It is important to check that the mandible is in centric relation because a bilateral crossbite appears to be unilateral if the mandible shifts laterally into maximum intercuspation (Fig. 18-13). The child shifts the jaw because the teeth do not fit well together, and the bite is uncomfortable because of dental interferences. A true unilateral crossbite that is due to a unilateral maxillary constriction in the primary dentition is rare but can occur.

Vertical Dimension. Overbite, the vertical overlap of the primary incisors, is measured and recorded in millimeters or as a percentage of the total height of the mandibular incisor crown (see Fig. 18-11) and is approximately 2 mm in the primary dentition. Deepbite is the complete or nearly complete overlap of the primary incisors. Anterior open bite, the absence of vertical overlap, is usually indicative of a sucking habit in this age group (Fig. 18-14). If the patient and parent deny the existence of a sucking habit, further investigation into the cause of open bite is needed. Skeletal malocclusion, condylar fracture or the sequela of trauma, and degenerative diseases such as juvenile rheumatoid arthritis may account for the open bite and should be investigated.

Ankylosis, the fusion of tooth to bone, is common in the primary dentition (Fig. 18-15). Although an ankylosed tooth cannot erupt further, the unaffected adjacent teeth will continue to erupt. This creates the illusion that the ankylosed tooth is submerged in the bone. The prevalence of ankylosed teeth is between 7% and 14% in the primary dentition (Brearly and McKibben, 1973; Kurol and Koch, 1985). In addition, 50% of patients with an ankylosed tooth have more than one ankylosis. The following is a list of the most commonly ankylosed teeth in the primary dentition (Brearly and McKibben, 1973):

1. Mandibular primary first molar
2. Mandibular primary second molar
3. Maxillary primary first molar
4. Maxillary primary second molar

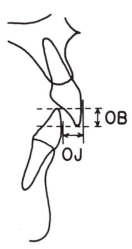

Figure 18–11. Overjet (OJ) is the horizontal overlap of the maxillary and mandibular central incisors and is measured from the most anterior point on the facial surfaces of these teeth. Overbite (OB) is the vertical overlap of the incisors and is measured from the incisal edge of one incisor to the other. Overbite can be recorded in millimeters or as a percentage overlap of the total length of the mandibular incisor.

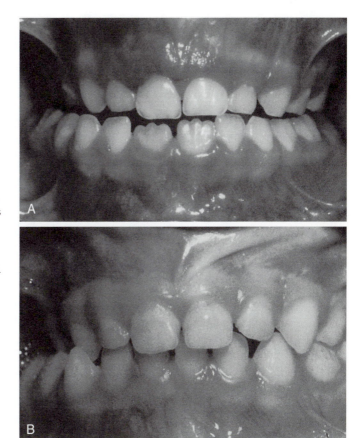

Figure 18–12. It is important to determine the patient's centric relation to identify the etiology of the problem and the treatment needs. *A,* This patient has a bilateral posterior crossbite when the teeth are positioned in centric relation. *B,* This patient has a unilateral posterior crossbite when the teeth are positioned in centric relation. These two patients will be approached differently.

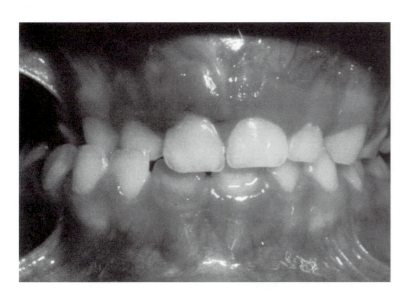

Figure 18–13. The same patient pictured in Figure 18–12*A,* with the teeth in centric occlusion. This emphasizes the importance of determining centric relation occlusion because it is the basis for most treatment decisions. Although this looks remarkably similar to the occlusion in 18–12*B,* the differences disclosed by the centric relation occlusion will result in different treatment.

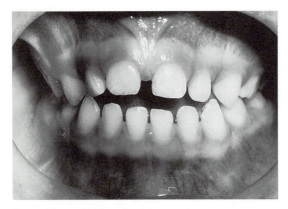

Figure 18–14. This patient exhibits an anterior open bite, the absence of vertical overlap. Anterior open bite is most commonly caused by a sucking habit in this age group.

A number of eruption and exfoliation problems have been blamed on ankylosed teeth. Longitudinal studies, however, indicate that ankylosed primary teeth exfoliate normally and allow normal eruption of succedaneous teeth (Kurol and Koch, 1985; Messer and Cline, 1980). An ankylosed tooth should not be removed routinely unless a large marginal ridge discrepancy develops between it and the unaffected adjacent teeth. If a marginal ridge discrepancy develops, the adjacent teeth may tip into the space occupied by the ankylosed tooth and cause space loss.

Radiographic Evaluation

The dentist requires radiographs to make a thorough diagnosis or problem list in the 3- to 6-year-old child. Children in this age range may find it difficult to cooperate with the radiographic procedures, in which case the radiographic examination should be deferred until behavior improves or can be managed. Introduction of the child to intraoral radiography can be managed as follows:

1. Use a tell-show-do introduction with a camera analogy. It helps to do a dry run, showing an unexposed packet of film and an exposed radiograph to explain the process. By positioning the film and the x-ray machine, the dentist can also determine whether a child will cooperate for an exposure, preventing unproductive irradiation.

2. Match film size to comfort. Many children have difficulty with the film impinging on the lingual soft tissue of the mandible. In some cases, bending the anterior corners helps, but this may lower the diagnostic quality of the radiograph. Another technique is to place the film vertically to minimize anteroposterior size (Fig. 18–16).

3. Obtain the least difficult radiograph first to acquaint the child with the procedures. Anterior occlusal films are usually easiest.

4. Be certain that all settings are made on the machine and that the apparatus is positioned before positioning the film. Some children can hold a film for only a short period because of the gag reflex, discomfort, or a short attention span.

For the primary dentition, no radiographs are indicated when all proximal surfaces can be visualized and examined clinically. When the proximal surfaces cannot be visualized and clinically examined, bitewing radiographs are indicated to

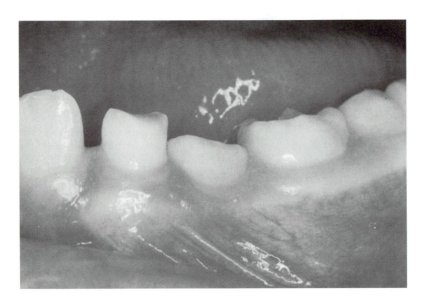

Figure 18–15. Ankylosis, the fusion of tooth to bone, is common in the primary dentition. This patient has an ankylosed primary mandibular first molar that is below the plane of occlusion.

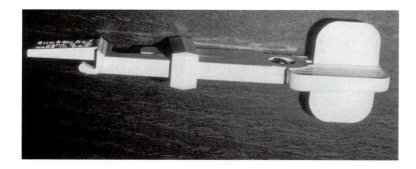

Figure 18–16. Decreasing antero-posterior size by rotating a size 0 film 90 degrees often makes a film easier for the patient to tolerate. Care must be taken to obtain views of all contacting posterior tooth surfaces.

determine the presence of interproximal caries (Fig. 18-17). Other projections are indicated in the following circumstances: history of pain, swelling, trauma, mobility of teeth, unexplained bleeding, disrupted eruption pattern, or deep carious lesions (University of Texas, 1987). These views include the maxillary (Fig. 18-18*A*) and mandibular (Fig. 18-18*B*) periapical views and the maxillary (Fig. 18-18*C*) and mandibular (Fig. 18-18*D*) occlusal views.

An occlusal-size film can be used to obtain a lateral jaw radiograph in children of this age if needed to identify pathosis and if a panoramic film isn't obtainable. The lateral jaw film can be

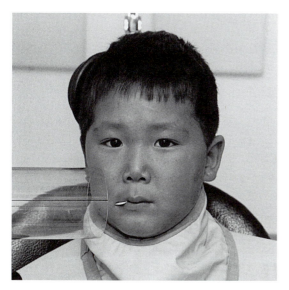

Figure 18–17. The proper technique for obtaining a posterior bitewing radiograph (No. 0 film) is critical because it is used frequently. The tube head should have a vertical angulation of +10 degrees and a horizontal angulation such that the face of the cone is parallel to the film packet with the beam directed to the open embrasures. The film packet should be placed lingual to the teeth with the child biting on the tab. The film should be placed anteriorly to obtain a view of the distal surfaces of the canines. Asking the child to smile to show the teeth often helps to orient the beam and prevents overlap.

made by having the child hold the film or lie on his or her side, as shown in Figure 18-19.

Pediatric (0 size) films should be used most often, with the exception of the occlusal films, which are No. 2 size. The Snap-A-Ray (Rinn Corporation, Elgin, IL) device has been used for film positioning in this age group with great success because of its small size and light weight. Other positioning instruments can be used, but some thought should be given to the size and weight of the instrument that must be placed intraorally. The patient should be adequately protected from unnecessary radiation. A lead apron and collar are necessary to provide thyroid and gonadal protection. A 16-inch or longer cone further reduces skin exposure. Ideally, rectangular collimation should be used, but patient movement by children of this age may yield less than ideal radiographs with an extremely truncated beam. Prior to exposure of the radiographs, the ability of the child to cooperate must be assessed to prevent unnecessary radiation exposure. When parents assist, they must be adequately shielded, pregnancy must be ruled out, and the parent must demonstrate the ability to stabilize the film and patient before exposure (White, 1982).

A concerned parent may ask about frequency of films. The American Academy of Pediatric Dentistry (1985) advises the use of radiographic exposure at a rate necessary to maximize detection of abnormalities yet minimize exposure to ionizing radiation. Table 18-4 lists selection criteria for pediatric radiographs in the 3- to 6-year-old child. All radiographs should be made only after a clinical examination and history have been completed.

DIAGNOSIS AND TREATMENT PLANNING FOR NONORTHODONTIC PROBLEMS

The process of diagnosis of disease is a complicated one based on clinical, historical, and sup-

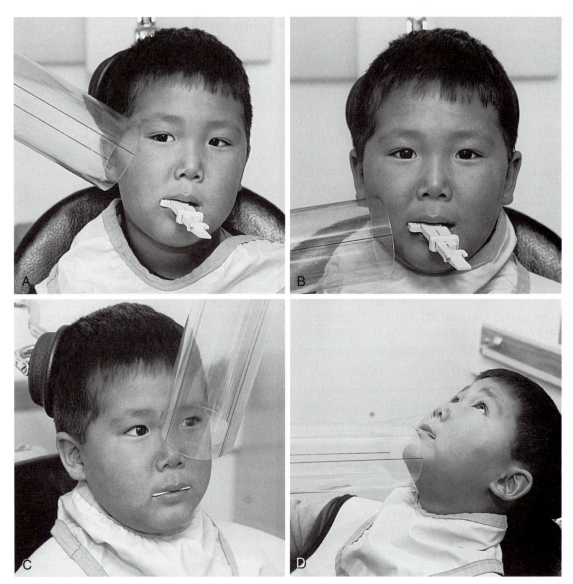

Figure 18–18. The following techniques are commonly used to obtain supplementary views. *A,* Maxillary periapical view (No. 0 film). Vertical angulation: Beam at right angle to film; starting angle of +30 degrees. Horizontal angulation: Face of cone parallel to facial surface of teeth. Film placement: With film in jaw of holder, holder is placed between the maxillary and mandibular teeth with dimpled surface of film against the lingual surfaces of teeth. Child bites on larger sides of jaws. *B,* Mandibular periapical view (No. 0 film). Vertical angulation: Beam at right angle to film; starting angle of −5 degrees. Horizontal angulation: Face of cone parallel to facial surface of teeth. Film placement: With film in jaws of holder, holder is placed between the maxillary and mandibular teeth with dimpled surface of film against the lingual surfaces of teeth. Child bites on larger sides of jaws. *C,* Maxillary occlusal view (No. 2 film). Vertical angulation: +60 degrees, with beam directed downward. Horizontal angulation: Beam directed along midsagittal plane. Film placement: Film packet is placed between maxillary and mandibular teeth so that it is parallel to floor. Film is oriented so that the long dimension extends to the right and left. The child bites gently on the film while seated upright. *D,* Mandibular occlusal view (No. 2 film). Vertical angulation: −15 degrees, with beam directed upward. Horizontal angulation: Beam directed along midsagittal plane. Film placement: Film packet is placed between the maxillary and mandibular teeth, and child is instructed to bite gently on the film. Patient is reclining so that the chin is extended. Bisecting angle technique is used.

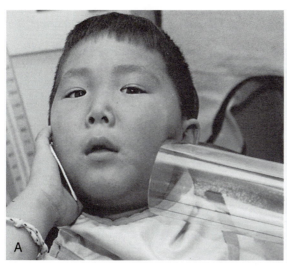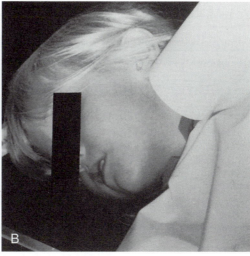

Figure 18–19. Lateral jaw techniques. *A,* Child is seated upright with head tilted approximately 20 degrees. Film packet is held or taped across area to be exposed. Beam is directed from side opposite film through the tissues at about −10 degrees. The central beam is directed perpendicular to the film and is aimed at the center of the film. *B,* This technique can be used for an active child or a patient with cerebral palsy. The dental chair is reclined, and the patient lies on one side with the head tilted. Pillows can be used to stabilize the body and head. The film is placed between the child and the chair, and the beam angulation is adjusted accordingly.

portive data. A problem list may be preferable to a series of diagnoses because the list presumes that treatment will be provided. A synthesis of all data is required. The practical portions of the diagnostic process consider the following:

1. Existence of an abnormal state
2. Determination of cause
3. Alternatives or options to correct the problem
4. Anticipated benefits, immediate and long-term
5. Problems or requirements for accomplishing treatment

A primary consideration is denoting an abnormal state, such as caries or a nonvital pulp. A problem list helps to separate those abnormalities that are in need of treatment from those that are simply identified. For example, a carious primary molar in a 6-year-old is a problem; a loose carious mandibular incisor may not be if it is about to exfoliate. Identification of the cause of the abnormality is critical to determine short- and long-term treatment. A manageable cause most often results in both short- and long-term success. Caries is a largely environmental condition that can be managed with great likelihood of success in both the short and long term. On the other hand, dentinogenesis imperfecta is genetic and has a guarded and limited prognosis.

For most patients, no single treatment plan is ideal. A variety of alternatives must be consid-

ered and based on the child's health, cooperation, parental finances, and the anticipated benefits to be derived from the treatment. These issues are shared by dentist and parent. For example, extraction of decayed primary teeth may be preferred to restoration if pulpal therapy is likely to be unsuccessful. Another example is the choice of a stainless steel crown rather than a three-surface amalgam restoration in a decay-prone person because fewer surfaces will be left exposed to recurrent decay.

Finally, a frank assessment of the cooperation and involvement in the child's treatment by the family must be considered. Dental treatment is necessarily a cooperative effort, with success resting on both personal and professional maintenance. The behavioral plan is critical to the success of the treatment plan in general. For the 3- to 6-year-old child, the methods of behavior management to be used must be included in the treatment plan. The sequencing of behavior management, obtainment of consent for medications, and reasonable alternatives to recommended procedures should be covered in discussion of the behavioral plan with the parents.

Generally, acute infection and pain are treated first. Hopelessly involved teeth should be extracted, although this is a rude introduction to dental care for the young child. If numerous large lesions are present, they may be excavated and interim restorations placed. This reduces the chance of the decay's progressing with resultant

TABLE 18–4. Selection Criteria and Guidelines for Pediatric Radiographs in the 3- to 6-Year-Old Child

Projection	Criteria	Frequency
Posterior bitewing	Proximal surfaces of posterior teeth cannot be examined clinically Child is cooperative	*At initial examination* if contacts closed *Semi-annually* if interproximal surfaces have been restored, until child achieves low-risk status* or is caries-free; also semi-annually if child is at high risk* *Annually* to 24-month interval if child is caries-free at initial bitewing examination
Posterior periapical	Suspected pathosis Confirmed pathosis Child is cooperative	As needed to diagnose and monitor treatment or patient condition
Anterior occlusal	Suspected pathosis Confirmed pathosis Child is cooperative	Same as above

*High risk for dental caries may be associated with (1) poor oral hygiene, (2) fluoride deficiency, (3) prolonged or inappropriate nursing, (4) high-carbohydrate diet, (5) poor family dental health, (6) developmental enamel defects, (7) developmental disability or acute medical problem, or (8) genetic abnormality.

Excerpted from The Selection of Patients for X-Ray Examinations: Dental Radiographic Examinations. VSDHHS, PHS, FDA (HHS Publication FDA 88-8273), U.S. Government Printing Office: Washington, DC, 1988.

pain and reduces the difficulty in cleaning while reducing the deleterious oral flora. If deep lesions and chronically pulpally involved teeth are not painful, they can be incorporated in a treatment plan that proceeds by quadrant or sextant.

All things being equal, restorative care often is easiest in the maxillary posterior areas. The infiltration injections are easiest for the patients to tolerate. One can then move to the mandibular posterior sextants. Seldom are the mandibular anterior teeth involved unless rampant decay is present.

Finally, the maxillary anterior teeth can be approached. This is a good final selection because the injections are uncomfortable, and some families will not pursue necessary care if the maxillary anterior teeth are restored first and esthetics are good.

When restorative care is complete and the patient and parent demonstrate that they can maintain good oral health, orthodontic care—active or space maintenance—can be considered. It is best if space maintenance can be implemented in the first 6 months after necessary extractions because space loss is most common during this period.

Patients with Special Health Care Needs

Paul Casamassimo

Care of special needs patients is a responsibility shared by general dentists and pediatric dental specialists. By definition, pediatric dentistry is the specialty charged with care of the special child. As is the case with dentistry for all children, however, the general dentist cares for the vast majority of persons with disabilities and chronic illnesses.

A basic skill set for the dentist who wants to commit to care of special patients includes the following:

1. Knowledge of the medical elements of conditions in order to understand the biologic processes and therapies that may affect oral health delivery, such as congenital heart disease
2. Knowledge of oral health implications of conditions, such as precocious periodontal disease in Down syndrome or gingival overgrowth in transplant patients

3. Essential management skills to communicate with, stabilize, and manage patients in the care setting

4. Awareness of the social, therapeutic, and cultural milieu of those with special health care needs

A functional or problem-oriented view of dental care for the special patient offers a way for dentists to organize education, staff training, and integration of these patients into a practice. The functional view establishes a number of problem areas or obstacles to care that must be addressed before the special patient can be treated successfully. These problem areas are not unique to patients with special health care needs but occur more often and in constellations with persons with disabilities and chronic illnesses. For example, many patients, whether disabled or not, experience fear or difficulty in paying for care. Many patients bring with them chronic or short-term medical problems that are acquired during their life with a practice. The disabled patient may cluster a number of problem areas, some of which may be severe, and challenge the practice's ability to keep that patient in the practice family. On the other hand, in today's world, with aging baby boom and burgeoning elderly populations, with the Americans with Disabilities Act, and with continuing advances in medical care, the black-and-white concept of disabled versus nondisabled is blurring. Every dentist can count those fragile elderly persons, children with learning disabilities or asthma, and adults with acquired heart disease on multiple medications in their practice family.

The specific terminology of problem areas or obstacles may vary by author, but the following summary should suffice to explain the basic concepts and give the motivated clinician a start in developing a practice philosophy and method.

1. *Accessibility*: The person with a disability experiences physical, mental, and system-wide obstacles to access. The most overt would be an architectural barrier. More subtle are attitudes of staff, community transportation limits, and office decoration that blocks access, confuses the poorly sighted, or inhibits wheelchairs, walkers, or canes. An office "accessibility audit," perhaps conducted by a person who is disabled, can point out overt and hidden obstacles.

2. *Psychosocial*: The person with special care needs may develop in an environment of chronic care, painful procedures, and emphasis on aspects of health other than dentistry. Families may be preoccupied with a disability, ignoring oral health. The clinician may be faced with a high-anxiety, low-dental-IQ patient and family.

3. *Financial*: Cost of dental care is an issue for many patients. Persons with special health care needs may not have incomes yet be beset with competing medical costs. They may qualify for public assistance, yet these programs often reimburse at rates that discourage dentist participation. The practice committed to care of special-needs patients will learn about public and private programs, work with families, and develop realistic treatment plans.

4. *Communication*: The dentist-patient chairside relationship demands a functional communication cycle of both parties—input, processing, and output. The patient with special needs may have compromised senses (input), have intellectual limitations (processing), or have speech difficulties (output). Less obvious may be the compromises the dentist owns such as equipment noise (input), preoccupation with a dental procedure (processing), and use of dental terminology (output). Effective chairside communication may require the sophistication of a signing interpreter or the simplicity of a pad and pencil.

5. *Medical*: Special health needs often translate into chronic illness and polypharmacy. Dentists are faced with pathology and therapy that present risks for the patient and complicate treatment. Congenital heart disease, drug interactions, and susceptibility to infection are just a few of the overlying concerns this population brings to dental practice.

6. *Mobility and stability*: Dental offices are designed for fully functional humans, but many of those who would describe themselves as such have difficulty in positioning, reclining for long periods, or even fitting in the contours of the chair. Some patients with special needs require stabilization, support, and assistance entering or leaving the dental chair.

Box continued on following page

Patients with Special Health Care Needs *continued*

7. *Preventive*: Basic oral hygiene home care may need to be supplemented with fluoride rinses, antimicrobials, saliva substitutes, and other adjunctives. Special-needs patients may need special instruction for self-care, and the dentist's problem-solving skills are called into play. Again, the continuum of "special need" brings in the child with cerebral palsy as well as the healthy adult on saliva-reducing medication.

8. *Treatment planning*: The ideal treatment plan is the one that is right for that patient. The special needs patient may need and want treatment that balances cost, longevity, difficulty of achievement, esthetics, and function. These principles are common to all patients, but with special needs patients the combination often challenges conventional thinking.

9. *Continuity of care*: Crises often bring the special needs patient to the dentist, and the myriad of problems they experience can force them into oral neglect. The culture of special needs care brings together a variety of professionals concerned with the health of these patients, and dentistry must sit at this table. Similarly, dentists must expand outside the cottage-care concept and utilize the physical therapist, psychologist, medical subspecialist, and other nondental professionals in achieving dental treatment goals.

Dentistry as a health science community must be available for all patients no matter how dramatic their special needs are. In the development of the specialist in pediatric dentistry it is implied that an essential feature of that educational growth be directed toward understanding and giving care to special children. Generalists find this domain of dentistry to be challenging and one that requires additional knowledge and skills over and beyond their dental education.

Although the work is challenging, the gratifying emotional rewards of taking care of patients with special needs are difficult to describe. The dentistry rendered is also received by the caretakers of these patients with vast appreciation for the dentist and the dental staff.

REFERENCES

American Academy of Pediatric Dentistry: Oral Health Policies: Dental Radiographs in Children. Chicago, American Academy of Pediatric Dentistry, 1985.

Brearly IL, McKibben DH: Ankylosis of primary molar teeth: Parts I and II. ASDC J Dent Child 40:54–63, 1973.

Fields HW, Vann WF: Prediction of dental and skeletal relationships from facial profiles in preschool children. Pediatr Dent 1:7–15, 1979.

Fields HW, Proffit WR, Nixon WL, et al: Facial pattern differences in long-faced children and adults. Am J Orthod 85:217–223, 1984.

Kurol J, Koch G: The effect of extraction on infraoccluded deciduous molars: A longitudinal study. Am J Orthod 87:46–55, 1985.

Messer LB, Cline JT: Ankylosed primary molars: Results and treatment recommendations from an eight-year longitudinal study. Pediatr Dent 2:37–47, 1980.

Pfefferle JC, Machen JB, Fields HW, Posnick WR: Child behavior in the dental setting relative to parental presence. Pediatr Dent 4:311–316, 1982.

University of Texas Dental School at San Antonio: Pediatric Dentistry Radiography: Early Eruptive Stage (5 Years and Under). San Antonio, University of Texas Dental School at San Antonio, 1987.

Valachovic RW, Lurie AG: Risk-benefit considerations in pedodontic radiology. Pediatr Dent 2:128–146, 1980.

White SC: Radiation exposure in pediatric dentistry: Current standards in pedodontic radiology with suggestions for alternatives. Pediatr Dent 3:441–447, 1982.

Chapter 19

Prevention of Dental Disease

Arthur Nowak and James Crall

Chapter Outline

FLUORIDE ADMINISTRATION

Dietary Fluoride Supplementation

Topical Fluoride Therapy

Professional Applications of Fluoride
Indications for Professional Topical Fluoride
   Applications
Cost-Benefit Considerations
Need for Prophylaxis Prior to Topical
   Fluoride Treatment
Methods of Application
Considerations for Special Patients

DIETARY MANAGEMENT

DIETARY COUNSELING

HOME CARE

With the complete eruption of all primary teeth, the preschool child enters a relatively short period of stabilization in preparation for the loss of the first primary tooth and the lengthy process of eruption of the permanent teeth. Historically, the preschooler's first dental examination occurs during this period. Instructions are provided for appropriate oral hygiene techniques. Adjustments in optimal systemic fluoride supplementation should be considered if the child is not living in a fluoridated community.

Dietary management may now become a problem. This is the period of development of favorite foods and dislikes for other foods. The effect of commercials from television, radio, and the press begins to take its toll. Children are frequently sent to a preschool educational environment for either a quasi-educational experience, a babysitting service, or a true preschool developmental experience. Meals may be prepared by surrogate parents, lunches may be packed by parents to be consumed later, snacks may be provided by peers or care providers, and control of the quality and quantity of the diet is sometimes greatly sacrificed.

With the end of the day in sight and the "I want to watch just one more TV program" routine common, the daily supervised oral hygiene routine is sacrificed for the quick 30-second unsupervised brushing. It is amazing how quickly parents assume that 4-year-old children can be responsible for their own oral hygiene when they cannot even comb their hair or clearly print their name.

FLUORIDE ADMINISTRATION

Dietary Fluoride Supplementation

Steps to ensure an optimal dietary intake of fluoride should continue to be a primary concern with children 3 to 6 years of age. For children who do not have access to fluoridated drinking water, this means continuing to provide adequate fluoride supplementation. By age 3 most children are able to chew and swallow tablets; therefore, prescriptions for supplemental fluoride should be changed accordingly to reflect this change in developmental status. The recommended supplemental fluoride dosage schedule also requires an increase in the amount of fluoride prescribed after a child reaches 3 years of age. The recommended daily dosage of supplemental fluoride for children aged 3 to 6 is 0.5 mg for children whose drinking water contains less than 0.3 ppm of fluoride and 0.25 mg for children whose water contains between 0.3 and 0.6 ppm. Children whose drinking water contains more than 0.6 ppm of fluoride do not require any supplementation. Although the potential for producing dental fluorosis on anterior teeth has diminished in this age group owing to substantial crown formation, the practice of analyzing samples of each child's drinking water prior to prescribing supplemental fluoride should continue. Analysis can be requested from the local public health department, through the family's dentist, or by commercial laboratories.

Because parental compliance continues to play a key role in determining the effectiveness of these supplements, efforts to reinforce parental motivation should be made. One method of assessing parental compliance is to monitor the need to rewrite supplemental fluoride prescriptions at recall visits. The dosage and amount of fluoride prescribed should be noted in each patient's record whenever a prescription is written. Parents who indicate no need for an additional prescription when the patient's record suggests that the previously prescribed amount of supplement should have been consumed should be questioned about the number of tablets remaining. A large existing supply suggests poor compliance during the period prior to the recall visit.

Topical Fluoride Therapy

Topical fluorides play an increasing role in the 3- to 6-year-old group. The child's ability to use fluoride dentifrices increases throughout this period, although restraint in the amount of toothpaste used at each brushing should continue to be exercised. Professional topical applications are often initiated during this interval. One mode of topical application that is generally not recommended for the younger members of this age group is the use of fluoride mouth rinses because most preschoolers are unable to avoid swallowing some of these solutions.

Professional Applications of Fluoride

Topical applications of highly concentrated forms of fluoride have been provided in clinical settings for 50 years. The most commonly used agents have included 8% to 10% solutions of stannous fluoride as well as 2% sodium fluoride and 1.23% acidulated phosphate fluoride (APF), the latter two compounds being available in solution, gel, and foam formulations. Numerous studies conducted prior to 1980 reported caries reductions averaging approximately 30% for these agents (Brudevold and Naujoks, 1978; Ripa, 1982). Several more recent studies, however, including a large-scale national demonstration program (Bell et al., 1984), have reported a more limited effect from semiannual applications of these agents (i.e., caries reductions of 15% or less), especially in fluoridated areas (Wefel, 1985).

More recently, fluoride varnish has been suggested for conditions in which decalcified enamel secondary to poor plaque removal or prolonged use of the nursing bottle or breast has been practiced (see the Fluoride Varnish Box in Chapter 14) (Seppa et al., 1995; Weinstein et al., 1994).

INDICATIONS FOR PROFESSIONAL TOPICAL FLUORIDE APPLICATIONS

The questions of when and for whom topical applications of fluoride should be provided in the dental office are the source of some controversy. One school of thought invokes the argument that professional fluoride applications are a primary preventive measure and should be provided to all children to minimize the potential for development of new carious lesions. This argument seems to have some merit in the absence of methods that predict whether an individual patient is likely to develop caries. Advocates of this philosophy tend to focus only on the potential benefits that might be achieved from topical fluoride applications while ignoring the costs associated with providing the service.

Others feel that the decision to provide topical fluoride therapy should be based on the factors that have been shown to be associated with the risk of developing caries in groups or in individuals (e.g., access to fluoridated drinking water, use of other forms of topical fluoride, degree of spacing between teeth). Their approach is to consider the likelihood that each patient develops disease according to these factors and then to recommend professional topical fluoride therapy for those who are deemed to be at significant risk for developing caries. Proponents of this philosophy tend to consider the costs associated with providing the service as well as the potential benefits to be gained.

The validity of the second approach obviously depends on the degree of accuracy with which one is able to predict which persons are more likely to experience caries. Several approaches aimed at differentiating high-risk from low-risk patients are currently being developed and evaluated. As methods of caries prediction are refined over time, the argument for individualizing preventive treatments is likely to become increasingly more compelling.

COST-BENEFIT CONSIDERATIONS

In a private practice setting the patient's willingness to pay for different forms of treatment usually is an important factor in determining what types of services are provided. In the case of public programs or private third-party payors, the decision to provide reimbursement for various services may be based on a more formal analysis of the relationship between the costs and benefits associated with those services. The ratio of costs to benefits has historically been higher for topical fluoride applications provided in dental offices than for other types of preventive services or for the same services provided in other settings. Consequently, professional topical fluoride treatments have not been justifiable as a public health measure because of their unfavorable cost-benefit ratio. Documented changes in caries levels and patterns of decay in children in the United States have pushed these ratios even higher. Specifically, four large-scale studies (Bell et al., 1984; Kaste et al., 1996; National Institute of Dental Research, 1981, 1989). have reported that a substantial proportion of schoolage children in the United States are caries-free and that a relatively small percentage of children account for a large percentage of all decay. Also, in addition to the overall decline in the level of caries, there has been a decrease in the proportion of smooth-surface caries and a corresponding increase in the proportion of pit and fissure caries. The combination of these factors seems to be associated with a reduction in the effectiveness of concentrated topical fluoride therapy in terms of the actual number of surfaces saved from becoming carious during a given period of time (Bell et al., 1984).

Changes of this nature have led some investigators to call for a re-examination of the manner in which various preventive measures are provided. In an era when increased attention is being focused on measures for controlling all types of health care costs, some have proposed that consideration be given to making preventive dental services more cost-effective. One means of improving the cost-benefit ratio of topical fluoride therapy would be to provide this therapy in settings other than dental offices (i.e., at school or in the home) via self-application techniques. Another previously mentioned method that could also apply to preventive services provided in dental offices would be to identify patients who are more likely to develop caries and target preventive services to those individuals.

One factor that has been repeatedly demonstrated to be associated with a reduction in both the risk of developing caries and the relative effectiveness of topical fluoride therapy is the availability of drinking water containing fluoride. Studies have shown that topical fluorides are considerably less effective in reducing the incidence of decay in fluoridated areas compared with nonfluoridated areas (Bell et al., 1984; Wei, 1974). Therefore, the cost of preventing a carious lesion in a fluoridated area by means of professional topical fluoride therapy is significantly greater than the cost of preventing a lesion in a nonfluoridated area. From a cost-benefit perspective, this suggests that in fluoridated areas topical fluoride treatments should be reserved for patients who have a history of moderate to high caries development or who belong to proven high-risk categories. Those who do not seem to be particularly prone to developing caries, especially smooth surface decay, would probably benefit more from other forms of prevention such as occlusal sealants.

The question of which preventive services should be provided for a particular child in the dental office remains a private matter between the dentist and the patient (or his or her parents). Thus, the final decision about the costs and benefits of professional preventive services must be made by the child's parents. The influence of third-party coverage for different types of services, however, can significantly affect this decision and ultimately the care received by the child.

NEED FOR PROPHYLAXIS PRIOR TO TOPICAL FLUORIDE TREATMENT

Another issue related to the effectiveness of professional topical fluoride therapy, which also has implications for lowering the cost-benefit ratio, concerns the need for the prophylaxis that has traditionally been provided prior to fluoride application. Research in both laboratory and clinical settings has shown that the ability of a variety of topical fluoride agents to penetrate dental plaque and deposit fluoride in the enamel is not significantly reduced by the presence of an organic layer on the tooth surface (Joyston-Bechal et al., 1976; Klimek et al., 1982; Tinanoff et al., 1974). This concept has been tested further in a 3-year clinical study that demonstrated that the ability of a professionally administered APF gel treatment to prevent caries was not influenced by whether prior prophylaxis had been performed (Ripa et al., 1984).

It has been pointed out that elimination of the prophylaxis could significantly reduce the labor cost of delivering topical fluoride treatments (Heifetz, 1978). The practical implications of these findings in terms of a dental office are (1) that the decision to provide thorough prophylaxis, less rigorous cleaning (i.e., toothbrushing prior to fluoride treatment), or no cleaning prior to fluoride treatment can be made individually, depending on the condition of the patient, and (2) that several children could be treated simultaneously, thereby reducing the time and cost of the procedure (Ripa, 1982).

Some persons insist that prophylaxis is an excellent way to introduce children to the sensations associated with the use of a handpiece in the mouth. Although this may be true, the practitioner should realize that elimination of this step does not appear to affect adversely the caries protection provided by topical fluoride therapy in most cases.

METHODS OF APPLICATION

The most popular professional topical fluoride agents in use today are APF and sodium fluoride. APF was developed as a solution containing 1.23% fluoride at pH 3.2 (Wefel, 1985). For decades, fluoride varnish has been used in Europe and Scandanavia for topical application. Recent studies show that fluoride varnish is as effective as a gel in preventing approximal lesions (Seppa et al., 1995). Less time is required to place the varnish, and therefore the treatment is more cost-effective when compared with gel use.

Applications of APF or sodium fluoride should be provided to at-risk patients semiannually in disposable polystyrene trays via a gel or foam as a vehicle. The recommended application time for both APF and sodium fluoride is 4 minutes. Manufacturers of foam products suggest a 1-minute application. Most studies report the use of 4-minute applications of topical fluoride gel or foam. Enamel uptake is similar with both types at 4 minutes, but when foam is used, about one fifth the amount is used. This reduces fluoride retention by the patient and subsequent postapplication complications (Whitford et al., 1995).

The advantages of the foam or gel-tray systems include (1) generally good patient acceptance, (2) a relatively long shelf-life of the agents, (3) control over the areas to which fluoride is applied, and (4) minimization of personnel time because the application process usually involves treating both arches simultaneously. Occasionally a child is not able to tolerate the use of two trays at once; in these instances, each arch may have to be treated separately.

The usual procedure involves (1) selecting an appropriately sized tray, (2) dispensing a small amount of gel (approximately 1.5 ml per tray) or foam into each tray, (3) drying the teeth in the maxillary and mandibular arches with gauze or a stream of air prior to placing the trays, (4) inserting the trays and checking for proper coverage, (5) inserting a saliva ejector, and (6) asking the child to bite down and close his or her lips around the saliva ejector. A saliva ejector should always be used during topical fluoride applications with trays to minimize swallowing of these highly concentrated agents. Following the topical application, the saliva ejector should be used for at least 30 seconds to remove any excess fluoride that may have remained.

CONSIDERATIONS FOR SPECIAL PATIENTS

As in any age group, some children require special consideration with respect to their need for fluoride therapy or the manner in which this therapy must be provided. Specifically, alternative approaches should be available for children with developmental disabilities or medical conditions that either place them at higher risk for caries or limit their ability to obtain fluoride in the usual manner.

For example, patients with cerebral palsy may find it difficult to tolerate the trays used for topical fluoride applications. Topical fluorides may have to be applied with a brush or cotton swab in these persons. Fluoride varnishes can be applied quickly to dried interproximal surfaces. Children who are being treated with irradiation or chemotherapy often experience ulcerative degeneration of the soft tissues, causing them to be extremely sensitive to preparations having a low pH (i.e., APF) or to certain flavoring agents. A diluted, neutral, nonirritating formulation should be provided for these patients. Children with chronic renal failure may experience elevated serum fluoride levels for prolonged periods following ingestion of concentrated fluoride preparations owing to their kidney impairment. Because they also have been noted to have a lower incidence of caries than matched controls, systemic or professional topical fluorides are not recommended for these patients (Crall and No-wak, 1985). These are just a few of the many types of patients who require modification of the usual preventive practices. The National Foundation of Dentistry for the Handicapped has prepared a manual that outlines recommendations for conventional as well as alternative preventive regimens for individuals with handicapping conditions (National Foundation of Dentistry for the Handicapped, 1981).

DIETARY MANAGEMENT

A number of factors begin to emerge during the preschool period that can have a profound effect on the growth and development of children as well as on their dental health. Following the large gains in growth during the first 3 years of life, the preschool child's rate of growth slows markedly. Therefore, caloric requirements need to be reduced accordingly, but a balanced diet need not be sacrificed. Because it is becoming common for both parents to be employed once the child reaches 3 years of age, the management and control of the child's diet that was maintained during the first 3 years of life may become threatened. When preschoolers are sent off to a baby-sitter, grandparents, or day care center, children are introduced to new environments, food selections, and management styles. It is no wonder that they become confused, begin to question routine dietary practices, and may even stop eating foods that were once favorites.

By this time the effect of television begins to be felt. The preschooler may be exposed to 2-8 (or more) hours of television on any one day. Advertisements during this period are numerous, and unfortunately most are for food items, all of which the preschooler seems to want when he or she accompanies the parents to the market to do the weekly shopping.

Fortunately, during this period children are still willing to try new foods. Parents need to experiment not only with new foods but also with the preparation of these foods. In addition, the presentation of foods is most important. Appropriate amounts of a variety of colorful foods go a long way toward increasing their consumption at meal time.

Although preschoolers seem to be always busy, they have an increasing amount of "idle" time because of their decreasing willingness to take a morning or afternoon nap. With more time available, reinforcement from the comments heard on television, and the encouragement of peers, snacking increases during this period. Appropriate snacking is encouraged. It is only when snacks are restricted to foods heavy with salt, fats, or refined carbohydrates of a consistency that adheres to the teeth and oral tissues or dissolves slowly that there will be a problem. Parents, teachers, and caretakers must be educated or told by parents or guardians about the kinds of snacks that are best for their children. On special occasions—for example, birthday parties, Halloween, or Valentine's Day—a special treat of sweets can be suggested. At all other times snacks should be selected from a list of foods that have been shown to be "friendly to teeth."

Fortunately, preschoolers are highly impressionable and can be greatly influenced by experiences within the family. Therefore, meal times are important "classrooms" in which they learn and observe the feeding practices of older siblings and their parents. A friendly, congenial atmosphere at meal time without threats ("You'd better eat all your food or you'll get no dessert") or badgering from siblings goes a long way toward establishing positive dietary practices.

It is because of these factors that the dentist may find it difficult to encourage parents to modify dietary practices when they are implicated in dental disease. Although many approaches are available to the dental team, no one approach is successful all the time. The approach used must be individualized to the personality of the practice, the willingness of the family to learn, and the specific dental problems encountered. Although many studies on the effect of diet and dietary practices on dental disease have been and continue to be conducted, there continues to be considerable reluctance as well as controversy about the approach to be used by the dental team.

Although historically sucrose has been implicated as the major carbohydrate necessary for acid production, we now know that other simple carbohydrates can produce acid—for example, corn sweeteners, commonly used in processed and convenience foods, and fructose and glucose, which occur naturally in honey, fruits, and vegetables. Therefore, it is no longer a simple matter of recommending that the patient reduce his or her sucrose intake. Over the years, sucrose has been appreciably replaced in the food industry with fructose and other sweeteners. The critical factor that remains is the ability of food to produce acid that lowers the pH in and around the tooth in the presence of plaque. Many foods have been tested and found to lower pH to 5.5 or lower (Schachtele and Jensen, 1984) (Table 19-1).

TABLE 19–1. Foods That Cause the pH of Interproximal Plaque to Fall Below 5.5

Apples, dried	Doughnuts
Apples, fresh	Gelatin-flavored dessert
Apple drink	Grapes
Apricots, dried	Milk, whole
Bananas	Milk, 2%
Beans, baked	Oatmeal
Beans, green canned	Oranges
White bread	Orange juice
Whole wheat bread	Pasta
Caramels	Peanut butter
Cooked carrots	Potato, boiled
Cereals, presweetened and	Potato chips
regular	Raisins
Chocolate milk	Rice
Cola	Sponge cake, cream-filled
Crackers, soda	Tomato, fresh
Cream cheese	Wheat flakes

Other critical factors are the ability of food to adhere to the teeth, the rate at which food dissolves, the ability of food to stimulate saliva production, and the ability of food to buffer the production of acid. It has been suggested (Schachtele, 1982) that a food with a low cariogenic potential would have the following attributes:

1. A relatively high protein content
2. A moderate fat content to facilitate oral clearance
3. A minimal concentration of fermentable carbohydrates
4. A strong buffering capacity
5. A high mineral content, especially of calcium and phosphorus
6. A pH greater than 6.0
7. The ability to stimulate saliva flow

Although foods have been identified with these characteristics, it continues to be difficult to assist parents in the selection of a diet and dietary practices that are best for the individual family.

DIETARY COUNSELING

Although the dental profession recognizes the role of good nutrition and appropriate dietary practices in achieving and maintaining good oral health, the execution of the process has been difficult to promote. Fortunately, in recent years the profession has been greatly assisted by the popularity of the promotion of physical fitness, dietary practices, and professional health supervision. Parents appear to be more aware of these

issues, they are willing to listen, and many are even ready to make some changes. The Dietary Guidelines for Americans provides information for families' nutritional requirements, promoting health, supporting active lives, and reducing major risk factors. When used in conjunction with the Food Guide Pyramid, parents have practical information on making choices from the food groups and the number of servings from each group each day (U.S. Department of Agriculture, 1995). How can the dentist and his or her staff help them?

In families with a preschool child and no dental disease, the approach would be quite different than that recommended for families with a preschool child with dental disease. For all children, the dentist should ask the parents the following questions during the initial interview to develop a baseline for further dietary assessment:

1. At what age was the child weaned from the breast or bottle?
2. If he or she was still on the breast or bottle after 1 year of age, what was the frequency and duration of use?
3. When were solids introduced?
4. Were baby foods commercially prepared or homemade?
5. How many meals are served presently? Does the family eat together?
6. Who selects the menu and prepares the food?
7. Are snacks provided? Are they given at home, in nursery school, or by a babysitter? As a parent do you choose the snacks? If not, do you know what they are?
8. Is the child a good eater? Does he or she eat a balanced diet? If not, what are the problem areas?
9. Does the child have any grandparents living at home? Or does the child spend appreciable time at the grandparents' home?
10. Are there any religious or ethnic preferences that would limit dietary choices?
11. What is the source of the water used for drinking and preparation of foods?
12. What is the child's daily liquid intake? How much of that liquid is derived from drinking water in your community?

If the child has a disability, additional questions are indicated:

1. What dietary practices are modified because of the child's disability?
2. Are there additional nutritional requirements because of the disability?
3. Does the child feed herself or himself or does she or he require assistance?

4. What medications are taken by mouth and how often are they taken?

5. Does the child have difficulty with chewing and swallowing?

6. Does the child hold (ruminate) food in his or her mouth for long periods? Does he or she regurgitate his or her food?

The answers to these questions should provide the dentist with basic background information on the nutritional requirements and dietary practices of the patient and his or her family.

In families with a preschool child with no dental disease and evidence of sound dietary management, a word of positive reinforcement from the dentist is indicated. Dietary histories and counseling would seem to be counterproductive in this situation.

In families with preschool children with caries or who appear to be at high risk for caries, further assessment by the dentist is indicated. A dietary history should be obtained, either by means of a 24-hour recall or by keeping a record for 3 to 7 days. Although the reliability of dietary histories is often questioned, in a spirit of trust and respect much can be learned. Attempts to embarrass or reprimand the parents should be avoided.

Many dietary history forms are available commercially, or they can be easily made. Parents need to be instructed on how to complete the history, making sure to list all foods eaten at each meal, the amounts eaten by the child, the types and quantities of food consumed between meals, and the liquid intake. Dietary or vitamin supplements as well as oral medications should also be listed.

Although the primary purpose of the dietary assessment in the dental office is to identify dietary patterns that are or may be potentially deleterious to oral health, the dentist should be aware of dietary intake and patterns that may also greatly influence overall growth and development. If these problems are noted, the parents should be referred for further assessment and counseling by the primary health provider.

With the dietary history available, the dentist can review the findings alone or in conjunction with the parent:

1. How many times a day does the child eat?
2. Is there a good diversified selection of foods? Are the meals well balanced?
3. Are the four basic food groups being satisfied daily?
4. What is the frequency of snacking?
5. Are foods high in (refined) carbohydrates consumed frequently? Are they consumed during, after, or between meals?

6. Are snack foods of the kind that dissolve slowly or that adhere to the teeth?

Once the problem areas have been identified, recommendations can be offered. Sweeping modifications of the family diet and dietary practices will be met with resentment, poor compliance, and negative results. It is recommended that the practitioner select one area, make a recommendation for change, wait a few weeks, and then evaluate the results. If these are positive, another area can be modified, and the family can then build on its successes.

Follow-up histories are indicated depending on the oral health status. Dietary counseling is only part of a comprehensive preventive program, although at times it is the most obvious area in need of adjustment. It can also be the most difficult area in which to obtain success.

A number of electronic nutrition analysis programs are available for purchase or can be accessed through the Internet (World Wide Web). After a dietary history is entered, a number of analyses become available, including meal planning. To date none is specific for evaluating diets that may contribute to oral disease in pediatric patients.

HOME CARE

With the changes in the child's knowledge base, socialization, and maturation in growth and development taking place during this period, daily home care should be less difficult. Unfortunately, that usually is not the case. Parents tend to assume that children can be more independent than they actually are. They also assume that their motor coordination has progressed to a point where manipulation of the toothbrush and floss is within their reach. Meanwhile, children want to be independent; they like to go to the bathroom themselves and don't need help from mom and dad.

A negotiated settlement has to be reached. For example, after meals the child can *brush* the teeth with minimal or no supervision, but at bedtime, the parents will *clean* the teeth and massage the gums. Working together as a team, the parent and child can each carry out their identified responsibilities, developing a successful program that can be further monitored and modified by the dentist.

During this period all the primary teeth are present. Spaces that were visible earlier may begin to close. Cleaning the mouth includes brushing the teeth and cleaning the areas where the gingiva touch the teeth. This is a fine motor activity that most 3- to 6-year-olds cannot perform completely without assistance. In addition, the lingual surfaces of the mandibular posterior teeth and the buccal surfaces of the maxillary posterior teeth are the most difficult to reach and to see if all the plaque has been removed.

As spaces are closing, the use of dental floss is indicated. Children 3 to 6 years old are unable to floss. Parents are responsible for this activity. A commercially available floss holder helps greatly. Care should be taken not to snap the floss into the interproximal gingiva, causing injury.

Visibility and accessibility can be greatly enhanced by correct positioning. Although most preschoolers want to stand at the sink, this is a difficult position from which parents can assist comfortably. Placing the child in a supine position periodically to improve visibility is recommended. A wet soft-bristled brush cleans the teeth and massages the gums. Once cleaning is completed, the child can be directed to the bathroom for additional brushing with a dentifrice added to the brush.

A fluoride-containing dentifrice is recommended, although with parental supervision. A small amount of dentifrice should be wiped on the brush and the child instructed to expectorate when brushing is completed. Large amounts of dentifrice are not indicated, and studies have shown that preschoolers swallow large amounts of dentifrice that may contribute to causing fluorosis (Barnhart et al., 1974; Levy and Zarei, 1991).

Good hygiene practices suggest that mouth care be performed after meals. Children should establish this habit early in life. When they are unable to, a thorough swishing of the mouth with water is recommended. At bedtime mouth care is especially important because of the reduction in saliva production at night with an increase in acid production. Therefore, parental supervision and assistance are important. Toward the end of this period the preschool child begins to lose the primary teeth. The areas of exfoliation may be painful and the gingiva may be swollen, leading to discomfort. During these times the parent must assist the child daily to maintain the habits established earlier and to eliminate additional inflammation around exfoliating teeth.

Children with disabilities may require additional assistance. Depending on the disability and its severity, various positioning methods may be helpful for increasing visibility into the mouth and reducing excessive movements. Mouth props help to keep the mouth open for thorough cleaning. Brushes can be modified to increase handle size for improving grip. Minimal dentifrice should be used to reduce the potential for gagging.

REFERENCES

Barnhart WE, Hilles HL, Leonard GJ, Michaels SE: Dentifrice usage and ingestion among four age groups. J Dent Res 53:1317, 1974.

Bell RM, Klein SO, Bohannan HM, et al: III. Analysis of DMFS increments. *In* Treatment Effects in the National Preventive Dentistry Demonstration Program. Santa Monica, Rand Corporation, 1984, pp 19–41.

Brudevold F, Naujoks R: Caries-preventive fluoride treatment of the individual. Caries Res 12(Suppl 1):52–64, 1978.

Crall JJ, Nowak AJ: Clinical uses of fluoride for the special patient. *In* Wei SHY (ed): Clinical Uses of Fluorides. Philadelphia, Lea & Febiger, 1985, pp 193–201.

Heifetz SB: Cost effectiveness of topically applied fluorides. *In* Burt B (ed): The Relative Efficiency of Methods of Caries Prevention in Dental Public Health. Ann Arbor, University of Michigan Press, 1978, pp 69–104.

Joyston-Bechal S, Duckworth R, Braden M: The effect of artificially produced pellicle and plaque on the uptake of 18F by human enamel in vitro. Arch Oral Biol 21:73–78, 1976.

Kaste L, Selwitz R, et al: Coronal caries in the primary and permanent dentition of children and adolescents 1–17 years of age: United States 1988–1991. J Dent Res (Special Issue) 75:631–641, 1996.

Klimek J, Hellwig E, Ahrens G: Fluoride taken up by plaque, by the underlying enamel and by clean enamel from three compounds in vitro. Caries Res 16:156–161, 1982.

Levy SM, Zarei MZ: Evaluation of fluoride exposure in children. J Dent Child 58:467–473, 1991.

National Foundation of Dentistry for the Handicapped: A Guide to the Use of Fluorides. Denver, National Foundation of Dentistry for the Handicapped, 1981.

National Institute of Dental Research: Summary of findings. *In* The Prevalence of Dental Caries in United States Children, 1979–1980. NIH Publication No. 82-2245, December 1981, pp 5–8.

National Institute of Dental Research: Oral Health of United States Children: The National Survey of Dental Caries in U.S. School Children: 1986–1987. NIH Publication No. 89-2247, 1989, pp 6–8.

Ripa LW: Professionally (operator) applied topical fluoride therapy: A critique. Clin Prev Dent 4:3–10, 1982.

Ripa LW, Leske GS, Sposato A, Varma A: Effect of prior toothcleaning on bi-annual professional acidulated phosphate fluoride topical fluoride gel-tray treatments: Results after three years. Caries Res 18:457–464, 1984.

Schachtele CF: Changing perspectives on the role of diet in dental caries information. Nutr News 45:13–15, 1982.

Schachtele CF, Jensen ME: Can foods be ranked according to their cariogenic potential? *In* Guggenheim B (ed): Cariology Today. Basel, Karger, 1984, pp 136–146.

Seppa L, Leppönen T, et al: Fluoride varnish versus acidulated phosphate fluoride gel: A 3 year clinical trial. Caries Res 28:327–330, 1995.

Tinanoff N, Wei SHY, Parkins FM: Effect of a pumice prophylaxis on fluoride uptake in tooth enamel. JADA 88:385–389, 1974.

U.S. Department of Agriculture and US Department of Health

and Human Services: Nutrition and your health: Dietary Guidelines for Americans, 4th ed. Hyattsville, MD, US Department of Agriculture, 1995.

Wefel JS: Critical assessment of professional application of topical fluorides. *In* Wei SHY (ed): Clinical Uses of Fluorides. Philadelphia, Lea & Febiger, 1985, p 20.

Wei SHY: The potential benefits to be derived from topical fluorides in fluoridated communities. *In* Forrester DJ, Schultz EM Jr (eds): International Workshop on Fluorides and Dental Caries Prevention. Baltimore, University of Maryland, 1974.

Weinstein P, Domota P, et al: Results of a promising open trial to prevent Baby bottle tooth decay: A fluoride varnish study. J Dent Child *61*:338–341, 1994.

Whitford G, Adair S, et al: Enamel uptake and patient exposure to fluoride: Comparison of APF gel and foam. Pediatr Dent *17*:199–203, 1995.

20

Dental Materials

Kevin James Donly and Adriana Segura

Chapter Outline

Restorative materials used in pediatric restorative dentistry are commonly the same as those used in restorative dentistry in general. This chapter identifies commonly used materials in pediatric dentistry and provides information that applies specifically to their use. Many materials are available, and in many cases clinical considerations dictate the choice of the appropriate material. Table 20-1 identifies the most commonly used materials in pediatric restorative dentistry and the relevant clinical considerations. Chapters 21, 32, and 39 discuss the specific clinical uses of dental restorative materials.

BASES AND LINERS

The use of bases and liners is important in pediatric dentistry. Bases and liners are available to reduce marginal microleakage from the restoration and to prevent sensitivity to the underlying tooth structure. Traditionally, preparations of calcium hydroxide, zinc oxide-eugenol, and zinc phosphate were the materials of choice. Presently, glass ionomer cement is also a common base.

Calcium Hydroxide

Calcium hydroxide cements are supplied in a visible light–cured system and a two-paste system. A catalyst paste containing calcium hydroxide, zinc oxide, and zinc stearate in ethylene toluene sulfonamide reacts with a base paste containing calcium tungstate, calcium phosphate, and zinc oxide in glycol salicylate to form an amorphous calcium disalicylate. The alkaline pH aids in preventing bacterial invasion. Studies have shown that calcium hydroxide "softens" under amalgam and composite resin restorations (Donly et al., 1990; Pereira et al., 1990). The results are attributed to hydrolysis of the calcium hydroxide by fluid contamination from dentinal tubules and microleakage. As hydrolysis occurs, occlusal forces cause gingival displacement of the restoration, leading to discrepancies and breakdown at the restoration margin. Calcium hydroxide remains the material of choice for direct pulp caps in permanent teeth and for areas that are within 0.5 to 1.0 mm of the pulp following tooth preparation. Visible light–cured calcium hydroxide preparations have demonstrated clinical success (Straffon et al., 1991) and may

TABLE 20–1. Commonly Used Biomaterials in Pediatric Dentistry

Materials	Types Available	Composition	Clinical Considerations
Varnish	—	Natural gums such as copal, dissolved in an organic solvent	Two coats applied to amalgam cavity preparations Applied to vital teeth prior to use of zinc phosphate cement Not placed under composite resins
Intermediary bases	Calcium hydroxide Zinc oxide-eugenol*	Thin pastes of calcium hydroxide or zinc oxide and eugenol suspended in resins	Placed on small areas of cavity preparation deeper than ideal depth Placed on exposed dentin of preparations undergoing acid etching Used for direct pulp capping of permanent teeth Must not be left on enamel of preparations
Amalgam	Lathe-cut Spherical Admixed Unicompositional*	Silver (40-74%) Tin (25-30%) Copper (2-30%) Zinc (0-2%) Mercury (0-3%)	A high copper (>6%) admixed or unicompositional, precapsulated alloy is recommended for restoration of pit and fissure and interproximal caries in posterior teeth
Stainless steel crowns	Straight sides Precontoured* Pretrimmed*	Iron (65-73%) Chromium (17-20%) Nickel (8-13%) Manganese, silicon, and carbon (<2%)	Restoration of badly broken down teeth, usually posterior must be well trimmed, contoured, polished, and cemented to ensure optimum gingival health
Filled composite resin	(Based on filler size) Traditional, 5-30 μm Microfill, .04-1 μm* Hybrids, .04-100 μm* (Available as auto-cure or visible light-activated)*	Dimethacrylate (BIS-GMA) resin or urethane matrix with filler particles of quartz, silicates, or glass	Esthetic restoration of anterior teeth Available for use in class I and II restorations in posterior teeth Microfills provide most polishable surfaces and have excellent esthetics Hybrids demonstrate least shrinkage and wear and have good polishability and esthetics Visible light activation provides better polymerization control, better color stability, and less porosity than auto-polymerized resins
Cements	Zinc phosphate*	Zinc oxide and phosphoric acid	Primary use is cementation of stainless steel crowns
	Polycarboxylate*	Zinc oxide and polycarboxylic acid	May be used as a base
	Glass ionomer*	Silicate glass containing Ca, Al, F, polycarboxylic acid	Glass ionomer may be used as a liner for resins and conservative restorations in primary teeth
	Reinforced zinc oxide and eugenol* Zinc silicophosphate Zinc oxide-eugenol	Zinc oxide reinforced with EBA or alumina or polymer, eugenol Zinc oxide and silicate phosphoric acid Zinc oxide, eugenol	Reinforced zinc oxide and eugenol most frequently used for obliterating primary pulp chambers following pulpotomy

*Denotes types most frequently used.

be less susceptible to hydrolysis. When calcium hydroxide is used, a less soluble high-strength base may be placed to overlay the calcium hydroxide.

Zinc Oxide–Eugenol

Zinc oxide-eugenol cement contains zinc oxide, rosin, and zinc acetate in the powder. The rosin increases fracture resistance, and the zinc acetate is effective in accelerating the reaction rate. The liquid is a preparation of eugenol, which reacts with the powder to form an amorphous chelate of zinc eugenolate. The zinc oxide-eugenol cements are used to provide a sedative effect, but their low compressive strength presents clinical limitations. To strengthen zinc oxide-eugenol cements, acrylic resin and alumina reinforcers have been added. Although these cements are stronger, they remain weaker than the zinc phosphate and glass ionomer cements. When evaluated as a base, zinc oxide–eugenol demonstrated significant microleakage compared with glass ionomer cement (Manders et al., 1990). Because of its sedative effects and years of clinical success, zinc oxide–eugenol remains the material of choice for the pulp chamber filling material after pulpotomies or pulpectomies in the primary dentition. Zinc oxide–eugenol cements should not be used under composite resin restorations: The eugenol inhibits the polymerization of the resin.

Zinc Phosphate

Zinc phosphate cement is composed of zinc oxide and magnesium oxide powder that is mixed with a solution of phosphoric acid and water. The zinc oxide alkaline surface reacts with the phosphoric acid to form a cement of zinc phosphate surrounding particles of zinc oxide. The addition of aluminum and zinc ions buffers the solution to slow the setting reaction. Mixing the cement on a cooled slab minimizes heat production during the chemical setting and increases the working time. When using zinc phosphate cement as a base, additional zinc oxide powder is placed in the mixture to provide a thick consistency, increasing the strength and decreasing the hardening time of the cement.

Glass Ionomer Cement

Glass ionomer cement has become a commonly used basing agent. It has the ability to create a physicochemical bond to tooth structure and to release fluoride. Glass ionomer cement consists of calcium aluminosilicate glass particles mixed with polyacrylic acid. The initial reaction stage involves the ionization of polyacrylic acid, which leads to a change in the polymer chains from a coiled to linear form. The hydrogen ions produced by ionization attack the calcium aluminosilicate glass, which also contains fluoride, and causes the release of metal and fluoride ions. The majority of the metal cations (Ca^{+2}, Al^{+3}), divalent or trivalent, respectively, are bound by the ionized polymer to form cross-linked salt bridges. Calcium and aluminum ions bind to polyacrylic acid at the carboxyl groups, and a gel phase is precipitated to form a matrix of the hardening cement. Calcium carboxylates are formed first as a firm gel because of the rapid binding of calcium to the polyacrylic acid chains. This initial set has the property of being carvable,

but at this stage the ionomer is susceptible to water absorption. Likewise, the free aluminum ions are susceptible to diffusion from moisture contamination and thus are lost from the cement because they are unable to cross-link with the polyacrylic acid chains. Isolation of prepared teeth with a rubber dam is recommended. Aluminum salt bridges are then formed with the polyacrylic acid matrix, and the cement hardens. The trivalent aluminum ions ensure a much stronger cross-linking than is possible with the calcium divalent bonds alone. The slower reaction of aluminum ions is attributed to the more stringent steric requirements imposed by a trivalent ion on polyanion chain configuration.

Glass ionomer is able to bond to dentin by free hydrophilic carboxyl groups in the cement, promoting surface wetting to form hydrogen bonds at the tooth interface. At the same time, an ionic exchange occurs at the interface, with calcium ions being displaced by phosphate ions. Some manufacturers recommend removing the smear layer, created during cavity preparation, with polyacrylic acid. This tooth "conditioning" provides an uncontaminated tooth surface for bonding.

Tartaric acid is added to the glass ionomer cement to accelerate the rate of hardening without decreasing the working time. Itaconic acid may be placed in glass ionomer mixtures to increase the reactivity of the polyacrylic acid to the glass, and polymaleic acid may be added to modify the reaction.

Studies have shown that glass ionomer bases and liners exhibit less marginal microleakage than zinc oxide–eugenol, zinc phosphate, and calcium hydroxide (Heys and Fitzgerald, 1991; Manders et al., 1990), thereby preventing bacterial penetration. Fluoride is released from glass ionomer cement by diffusion. Glass ionomer bases and liners have demonstrated the inhibition of secondary caries formation (Garcia-Godoy and Jensen, 1990; Hicks et al., 1986; Jensen et al., 1991). The fluoride released is taken up by both the enamel and dentin adjacent to the material (Skartveit et al., 1990). This fluoride aids in creating an inhibition zone that is not susceptible to demineralization compared with areas adjacent to non–fluoride-releasing materials.

Glass ionomer cements are supplied in anhydrous and hydrous forms. Because of the viscosity of the hydrous form, mixing the cement may be difficult. The anhydrous form has a longer shelf-life because the polyacrylic acid is dehydrated and placed in the powder. It is critical that glass ionomer be mixed according to the manufacturer's instructions. If the cement is mixed too thick, the thickness of zinc phosphate cement, it will not provide sufficient water to complete the reaction and dentin sensitivity may be encountered; the necessary water will be obtained from the dentin, causing sensitivity due to hydraulic pressures created within the dentin.

Resin-modified glass ionomer cement preparations are available and can be light-cured (Mitra, 1989). Photoinitiated polymers have been placed into the glass ionomer cement formulation to provide light polymerization. Although these resin-modified glass ionomer cements can be light-cured, the material sets as a true cement, an acid-base reaction taking place; therefore, the material chemically sets without light-curing.

A glass ionomer cement has a coefficient of thermal expansion similar to that of tooth structure, can protect an underlying base and dentin, and has the advantages of bonding to composite resin and releasing fluoride to inhibit secondary decay.

CAVITY VARNISHES

Cavity varnishes are resins that are insoluble in oral fluids. Varnish is to be used with amalgam restorations; it inhibits surface bonding of composite resin systems, dentin bonding systems, and glass ionomer systems as well as prevents the fluoride release of glass ionomer from gaining access to the restoration or tooth interface. The purpose of cavity varnishes is to reduce microleakage at restoration margins and inhibit penetration of corrosion products from amalgam into dentin, thereby preventing tooth discoloration adjacent to restorations. The varnishes do not prevent thermal sensitivity.

DENTIN BONDING AGENTS

Dentin bonding agents have been incorporated into the restorative dentistry armamentarium. Previously, dentin or enamel bonding agents fell into two groups. The first was halophosphorous esters of BIS-GMA. The second group was categorized as polyurethanes. The polyurethanes are halophosphorous esters of hydroxyethyl methacrylate (HEMA). Both of these dentin bonding agents relied on a phosphate-calcium bond for retention.

Removing the smear layer was found to increase the effectiveness of the dentin bonding agents. The newer bonding agents include conditioning or primer components that remove or alter the smear layer over the dentin. This results in the creation of a mechanical bond by the infiltration of monomers into a zone of demineralized dentin, where the monomers polymerize and interlock with the dentin matrix (Erickson, 1989). A majority of the contemporary dentin bonding agents are similar to those previously discussed or composed of 4-methacryloxyethyl trimellitic anhydride (4-META).

RESTORATIVE MATERIALS

Amalgam

Traditionally, amalgam was the material of choice for Class I and Class II restorations. Today, amalgam continues to be an effective restorative material. A 3-year study of the clinical performance of 260 amalgam restorations (86.4% Class II) demonstrated 254 to be successful (Osborne, 1990). It is important to understand the clinical make-up and setting reaction of amalgam to correlate restoration successes and failures with the basic fundamental properties of the material.

AMALGAMATION

Dental amalgam consists of an alloy mix of silver, copper, tin, and, in some cases, zinc particles combined with mercury. The alloy particles have either a spherical or comminuted (lathe-cut) configuration. The unreacted alloy particles are called the silver-tin (gamma) phase. These particles are combined with mercury, the mercury actually acting as a "wetting" agent of the alloy particles to initiate the setting reaction termed amalgamation. The particle surfaces react with mercury to form a cementing matrix, consisting of the gamma-1 and gamma-2 phases. The gamma-1 phase employs the binding of silver and mercury ($Ag_2 Hg_3$). The gamma-2 phase involves the binding of tin and mercury ($Sn_7 Hg$). The gamma-2 phase is held responsible for early fracture and failure of the comminuted particle amalgam restorations. Tin cannot be eliminated from the alloy because of its importance in the setting reaction and control of dimensional change of amalgam. To avoid the detrimental gamma-2 phase, copper was introduced into the amalgamation reaction. The copper replaced the tin-mercury phase with a copper-tin phase (Cu_5Sn_5). The copper-tin matrix decreases the corrosion of tin, preventing secondary weakening with subsequent fracture of the restoration.

The amount of mercury necessary to complete the amalgamation reaction depends on the alloy composition and particle configuration but usu-

Pediatric Dentistry Restorative Materials: 1990–2000 . . . What a Difference a Decade Makes

Theodore P. Croll

Remarkable advances in dental restorative materials in the 1980s and 1990s are irrevocably changing pediatric restorative dentistry. The children of the 21st century will probably learn about "silver fillings" from history books, the Internet, and their parents' stories.

The ideal direct-application dental restorative material would have the following properties and characteristics:

- Biocompatible with the dental pulp and nontoxic in the mouth
- Adhesively bonds to dentin and enamel, and the bonded interface is impervious to oral fluids
- Has fracture strengths, wear resistance, and compressive strength at least equivalent to that of enamel, and its physical properties should not diminish in the oral environment over time
- Should be dimensionally stable during application and throughout the hardening reaction and have a coefficient of thermal expansion compatible with that of surrounding tooth structure
- Should be virtually insoluble in the mouth
- Should strengthen residual tooth structure by its adhesive properties
- Should be tooth-colored
- Has easy handling characteristics, ideal working time, and hardens significantly, on command
- Can be placed quickly, easily, and comfortably
- Would be of reasonable cost for the dentist and patient (parent)

It is apparent that the ideal restorative material for children's teeth has not yet been developed. Today's dentist, however, has more options than ever before when considering how to restore carious, malformed, or traumatically injured primary and permanent teeth. With the "ideal" in mind, the chief types of dental restorative materials for children, as we approach the 21st century, are as follows:

1. Silver amalgam
2. Traditional glass ionomer cements (self-hardening)
3. Glass-ionomer silver-cermet cement
4. Stainless steel crowns (primary molars and canine teeth)
5. Stainless steel crowns with prefabricated resin veneer facings (incisors)
6. Resin composites
7. Resin-modified glass-ionomer cements
8. Polyacid modified resin composites

The use of *silver amalgams, traditional glass ionomer cements*, and *glass-ionomer silver cement* (Ketac-Silver [ESPE]) is declining in the United States. Silver amalgams have served dentists treating children very well in the 19th and 20th centuries, but now adhesive tooth-colored materials are proving themselves so durable and reliable that silver amalgam is becoming a less desirable alternative. The traditional glass ionomer restorative cements, including the cermet cement, harden initially in about 4 to 5 minutes. The light-hardened resin-modified glass ionomers have a hard initial set after 40 seconds of light curing. In addition, fracture strengths and wear resistance are improved in the resin-modified materials, so if a polymerizing light is available there are no advantages to use of the self-hardening materials.

Stainless steel crowns for primary canines (Croll and Blum, 1982) and molars (Full et al., 1974) and permanent molars (Croll, 1987; Croll and Castaldi, 1978) are strong, durable, and can remain in place for 5 to 10 years or more with no additional treatment. They can also be repaired if worn through. Modern steel crown forms are pre-contoured and have excellent anatomic form, so dentists have a much easier time adapting these crowns to properly prepared teeth. The new self-hardening resin-modified glass ionomer luting cements, with their improved physical properties, will undoubtedly make stainless steel crown recementation a rare occurrence.

A most welcome addition to pediatric dentistry restorative material inventories has been the *pre-veneered stainless steel crown for primary anterior teeth* (Croll and Helpin, 1996). Certain dental laboratories supply anterior stainless steel crowns with resin veneer facings covering the labial, incisal, mesial, and distal aspects. When severely diseased primary incisors or canines are prepared correctly, such pre-veneered crowns can be cemented into place, imperceptibly restoring the child's smile. Full crown restorations for primary incisors have always been a difficult challenge for dentists treating children, and now a new, and perhaps best, option is available. Two carious primary central incisors (Fig. 20–4A) are shown with crown restorations in place (Fig. 20–4B).

Resin composites are the best direct application *enamel replacement* currently available to dentists. Via the acid-etch method, they adhesively bond to enamel and dentin and have excellent physical strength. They also can imperceptibly restore cosmetically prominent anterior teeth and have the great advantage of curing on command with light activation. The chief disadvantages of the resin composites are the need for perfect handling, material shrinkage during the polymerization reaction, and eventual marginal leakage due to forces that can open the resin–tooth structure interface. Improvements in techniques and materials and continuing developments of improved dentin and enamel bonding agents are making resin composite more attractive to clinicians. Starting in the late 1970s (Simonsen, 1978a, 1978b, 1987), resin composites completely revolutionized treatment of enamel pits and fissures in permanent teeth to the point that silver amalgam should now be considered an inferior alternative as a first restorative material for a Class I lesion (Personal communication, Dr. R.J. Simonsen).

Polyacid-modified resin composite materials (often called *compomers*) are resin composites made with a fluoride containing glass filler and polyacid components, similar to acids used in glass ionomer materials (Albers, 1996). These materials do not undergo a significant acid/base hardening reaction and therefore must be light-cured. They cannot be classified as glass ionomer systems. Dentists treating children have been using the polyacid-modified resins for primary teeth primarily because of ease of use. At this time (January 1998), durability and reliability of such restorative materials are not yet known but look promising. Examples of this class of materials include Dyract [Caulk], Compoglass (Vivadent), Hytac (ESPE), and F2000 (3M).

In 1992, *resin-modified glass-ionomer restorative cements* were first marketed. The three chief products were Fuji II LC (GC), Vitremer Tri-Cure (3M), and Photac-Fil (ESPE). These cements have the favorable properties of the glass ionomer class of materials as well as a resin component that provides initial light-cure hardening in only 40 seconds. Furthermore, the resin component gives these materials improved wear resistance and fracture strengths. The resin-modified glass-ionomer restorative cements are causing a veritable renaissance in pediatric restorative dentistry (Croll, 1995; Croll et al., 1993), and improvements in the materials, or improved related materials, are inevitable. This class of materials is perhaps the most ideal *dentin replacement* material ever produced.

Box continued on following page

Conclusion

Even though prevention of dental caries has improved the oral health of many children, the caries problem, especially in those receiving no fluoride protection, will continue to challenge dentists well into the 21st century. Malformed and traumatically injured teeth will also continue to command much of the clinical dentist's time. Treatment planning for our youngest patients has become much more complex. Dentists need to be perpetual students, continuing to discover the advantages and disadvantages of each class of restorative material and the subtle nuances of each brand supplied by the manufacturers. Only then will such materials be able to be scientifically understood and artistically applied to benefit the children.

REFERENCES

Albers HR: Tooth-Colored Restoratives. Santa Rosa, CA, Alto Books, 1996, pp 4a–3.

Croll TP: Restorative dentistry for preschool children. *In* Dental Care for the Preschool Child. Dent Clin North Am *39*(4):737–770, 1995.

Croll TP: Permanent molar stainless steel crown restoration. Quintess Int *18*:313–321, 1987.

Croll TP, Blum JR: The stainless steel crown for a primary canine tooth: A pictorial essay. J Pedodont *6*:301–314, 1982.

Croll TP, Castaldi CR: The preformed stainless steel crown for permanent posterior teeth in special cases. JADA *97*:644–699, 1978.

Croll TP, Helpin ML: Preformed resin-veneered stainless steel crowns for restoration of primary incisors. Quintess Int *27*:309–313, 1996.

Croll TP, Killian CM, Helpin ML: A restorative dentistry renaissance for children: Light-hardened glass ionomer/resin cement. J Dent Child *60*:89–94, 1993.

Full CA, Walker JD, Pinkham JR: Stainless steel crowns for deciduous molars. JADA *89*:360–364, 1974.

Simonsen RJ: Preventive resin restorations (I). Quintess Int *9*:69–76, 1978a.

Simonsen RJ: Preventive resin restorations (II). Quintess Int *9*:95–102, 1978b.

Simonsen RJ: The preventive resin restoration: A minimally invasive, nonmetallic restoration. Compend Contin Educ Dent *8*:428–432, 1987.

ally falls between 42% and 54% of the amalgam mix. When mercury exceeds 55%, there is a detrimental reduction in amalgam strength. Spherical alloy particles, with the addition of copper, require less mercury than comminuted particles to complete the amalgamation process. It is important to point out that once amalgamation occurs, unreacted mercury is not available; the mercury is alloyed with silver, tin, or copper. Although it has been brought to the attention of the public that mercury is present in the amalgam restoration, no controlled clinical research indicates that mercury from amalgams has any toxic effects (American Dental Association, 1990). Zinc is present in some alloy mixes to act as a scavenger for oxygen, which inhibits the formation of copper, silver, or tin oxides that weaken the amalgam restoration. Using pre-encapsulated amalgam or strictly following the manufacturer's recommendations for dispensing, trituration, and manipulation is critical to achieving a successful restoration.

PROPERTIES

Hardening amalgam may expand or contract depending on the type and manipulation of the material. The American Dental Association (Council on Dental Materials and Devices, 1977) requires that there be no more than 20 μm/cm of expansion or contraction after 24 hours.

The compressive strength required by the Council on Dental Materials and Devices (Council on Dental Materials and Devices, 1977) for amalgam is 11,600 psi (88 MN/m^2) after 1 hour. Tensile strength is substantially lower; therefore, cavity preparation design becomes critical. The preparation should have a design that allows the amalgam to be condensed as a "bulk" of material, avoiding shallow depths and a thin isthmus where fracture may occur. Comminuted and spherical low-copper amalgam demonstrates decreased marginal fracture resistance. This is partially due to the increased creep of these amalgams. *Creep* is the dimensional change that occurs when amalgam sustains a load during mastication, a result of the viscoelastic property of amalgam. The ADA requires that an amalgam have a maximum of 5% creep to be certified.

Corrosion, a chemical or electrochemical deterioration of amalgam, occurs at the surface or subsurface. Deterioration may be due to pitting or scratching secondary to poor condensation, carving, or finishing of amalgam, which allows food or saliva components to attack the chemical matrix. Dissimilar metals in contact can also cause corrosion, a galvanic action that encourages the materials to go into solution. Pitting occurs and food entrapment within the pits subsequently causes further corrosion. The gamma-2 phase (tin-mercury) is most susceptible to corrosion; therefore, the spherical high-copper amalgams are the least susceptible. Although extensive corrosion can lead to restoration failure, minimal corrosion in conjunction with creep allows open restoration margins to be packed full enough with corrosion byproducts to significantly close these margins.

CONDENSATION

Amalgam should be placed and condensed immediately after trituration according to the manufacturer's recommendations. Placement of amalgam in small increments is appropriate. Condensation allows force to be applied for material adaptation with a minimum of excess mercury. Use of small condensers with firm pressure on small increments of amalgam minimizes voids within the final restoration. A delay in condensation should be avoided; the effective removal of excess mercury becomes more difficult owing to the initial hardening that occurs before initiating condensation. This in turn decreases restoration strength and increases the creep in the material. Moisture contamination should also be controlled because excess moisture causes delayed expansion, particularly in zinc-containing alloys. The use of a rubber dam can prevent moisture contamination and isolate the working field effectively.

FINISHING AND POLISHING

Finishing and polishing of the amalgam surface is highly recommended. Small scratches and pits can be removed with finishing burs, and abrasive stones and rubber points impregnated with abrasives. The final polish can be accomplished with a tin oxide compound. Care should be taken to use water when polishing to avoid the vaporization of mercury from the amalgam. Most amalgam restorations should not be polished for 24 hours, although the spherical high-copper amalgam can be polished almost immediately because its strength is obtained rapidly.

Composite Resin

Composite resin has become one of the most widely used contemporary restorative materials in recent years. Currently, composite resin is used for sealants and for Class I, II, III, IV, and V restorations in primary and permanent teeth. Composite resin restorations have been accepted primarily because of their excellent esthetic qualities. Other advantages include relatively low thermal conductivity, preservation of tooth structure in cavity preparation, and advances in the stability of compositional properties of the material.

Conventional composite resins are viscous fluid involatile monomers (BIS-GMA) that have filler particles incorporated into the resin. Bowen (1962) formulated the BIS-GMA resin by synthesizing a dimethacrylate monomer, the product of the reaction between bisphenol-A and glycidyl methacrylate. Many contemporary composite restorative materials contain dimethacrylate monomers (BIS-GMA) as the major component of the matrix phase. A relatively low-viscosity monomer triethyleneglycol dimethacrylate (TEGDMA), which helps produce the desired handling qualities of the material, is an important component of the matrix phase. Figure 20-1 schematically illustrates the chemical structure of BIS-GMA, and Figure 20-2 illustrates the chemical structure of TEGDMA.

Incorporated into the monomer matrix are filler particles. A small number of available products contain urethane dimethacrylates rather than the BIS-GMA matrix. Initially, fused quartz and various glasses were incorporated into the BIS-GMA monomer as filler particles, providing a reinforced resin composite. The fillers were coated with a vinyl silane coupling agent, the silane chemically bonding with the polymer matrix (Phillips et al., 1969). These particles were usually irregularly shaped to provide mechanical retention within the resin.

Composites available today contain quartz, colloidal silica, borosilicate glasses, and glasses containing barium, strontium, and zinc. Excluding quartz and colloidal silica, these filler particles

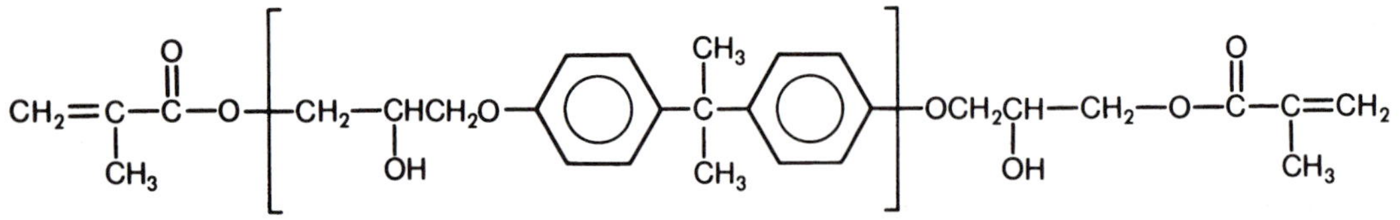

Figure 20–1. Chemical composition of 2,2-bis [4-(2 hydroxy-3-methacryloyloxy-propyloxy)-phenyl] propane (BIS-GMA).

give the material radiopacity, which is clinically advantageous during radiographic examination. Contemporary posterior composite resins contain a high percentage of filler particles by volume. This composition provides wear resistance and more stability. Thermal expansion and polymerization contraction are both reduced by increasing the volume percentage of filler particles. The increased filler content, needed for wear resistance, requires a decrease in matrix resin polymer, therefore allowing for a reduction in the amount of shrinkage that occurs upon polymerization. As the concentration of filler particles increases, the modulus of elasticity increases and tends to minimize shrinkage (Ruyter, 1982).

Composite resins absorb water, yet hygroscopic expansion is infrequently sufficient to compensate for polymerization shrinkage. Therefore, the incremental placement and polymerization of composite resin is critical during restorative care.

Glass ceramic inserts have been developed to act as fillers in composite resin restorations (Bowen et al., 1991). The inserts are available in various shapes and sizes and are intended to be inserted into composite resin restorations to create a larger volume of the restoration (Fig. 20–3). The silane-treated glass ceramic inserts have the advantages of mechanical and chemical bonding to composite resin, increased stiffness and strength of the restoration, increased durability, reduced polymerization shrinkage and cuspal deflection, and reduction of microleakage.

CHEMICALLY POLYMERIZED COMPOSITE RESIN

The traditional chemically activated composite resins form cross-links during copolymerization of methyl methacrylate and ethyleneglycol di-

methacrylate. The dimethacrylate monomers polymerize, by means of a free radical–initiated polymerization, to form the organic matrix of a three-dimensional network. This highly viscous monomer can undergo free radical addition polymerization to provide a rigid cross-linked polymer. Usually the benzoyl peroxide present in one paste acts as the initiator, whereas a tertiary amine (dihydroxyethyl-p-toluidine) acts as the catalyst in the other paste (Craig, 1981).

VISIBLE-LIGHT–POLYMERIZED COMPOSITE RESIN

Today, most composite resins are visible-light–activated materials. This allows for more control in the placement of the composite resin into a cavity preparation; the application can easily be done in increments. The visible light–activated composite resins usually contain a diketone initiator (camphorquinone) and an amine catalyst (dimethylaminoethyl methacrylate). The diketone absorbs light at a wavelength of approximately 470 nm to form an excited state, which, together with the amine, results in ion radicals to initiate free radical polymerization (Ruyter, 1985; Smith, 1985).

Problems that may be associated with light-activated composite resins include polymerization toward the light source, sensitivity of composite to ambient light, and variability in the depth of polymerization due to the intensity of light penetration. Polymerization toward the light source may cause the composite resin to pull away from the preparation. Sensitivity of composite resin to ambient light may cause initial polymerization before placement of the material into the preparation. Variability in the depth of light penetration, differences in light intensity, light source active diameter, and time of light

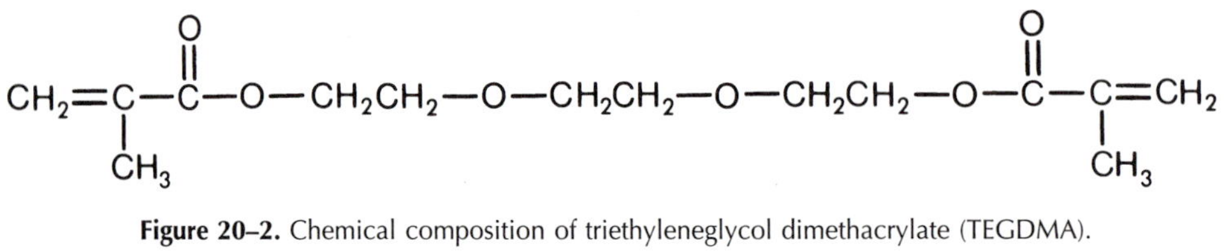

Figure 20–2. Chemical composition of triethyleneglycol dimethacrylate (TEGDMA).

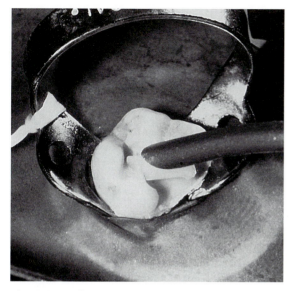

Figure 20–3. Glass ceramic insert being placed into a cavity preparation to consume a large portion of the preparation dimensions. Composite resin is then placed to fill the remainder of the preparation and chemically bonds to the silane-treated insert.

exposure can result in variations of polymerization. The benefits of light-activated composite resins include ease of manipulation, control of polymerization, and lack of need for mixing. Because mixing is not required with light-activated composite resins, there is less chance of air being incorporated into the material and therefore fewer voids.

COMPOSITE RESIN WEAR

Early composite resins, used for posterior restorations, exhibited excessive occlusal wear. Studies have shown that when conventional composites are placed in high stress concentration areas,

excessive wear occurs (Eames, 1974; Leinfelder et al., 1980; Osborne et al., 1973; Phillips, 1972). Further investigation pursued factors that might influence the rate of wear, such as the size and hardness of the filler particles, the amount of porosity within the material, and the method of polymerization (Leinfelder and Roberson, 1983). It was found that the ceramic filler particles nearly always remained intact. There was no evidence of wear on the particles: They were found to be hard enough to cause wear of the unfilled resin during mastication until the resin matrix was gradually worn from the particles. Once a critical portion of the filler particle was exposed, it was easily dislodged. Although there seemed to be a correlation between the size of the filler particle and its hardness (larger particles possessing a more critical hardness), substantially larger particles were found to accelerate the wear. Therefore, the hardness of particle is not necessarily the most significant factor affecting wear; particles that have adequate hardness, are distributed within minimal unfilled resin, and have the least abrasion potential during mastication are ideal.

Porosity has been shown to play a major role in the wear rate of posterior composite resins (Leinfelder and Roberson, 1983; Philips and Lutz, 1983). All resin restorations have a certain degree of porosity. These porosity defects, the occurrence of voids, can be minimized by careful insertion and polishing of the material. The use of light-cured composites avoids the mixing process, which creates fewer voids and increases abrasion resistance. Problems of wear appear to be improved with newer composites. Composite resins are vacuum-packed to decrease porosity. It is important to note that mixing shades for esthetics may cause an increase in porosity. This problem is due to the incorporation of air during

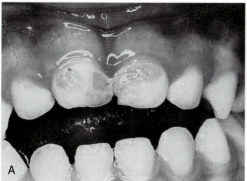
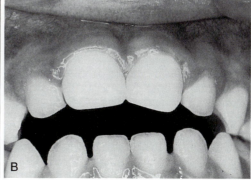

Figure 20–4. *A,* 28-month-old child with severe nursing-related caries of the central incisors. *B,* Stainless steel crowns with prefabricated resin veneer facings, 12 months after placement.

the mixing process. Current posterior composite resins show minimal wear. This has been achieved by incorporating a variety of particle sizes into the polymer matrix. The increased filler content results in a decrease of matrix resin polymer. The mechanism of wear is hypothesized to be due to the loss of the resin matrix. Increasing wear resistance is believed to be possible because the filler particles are situated in close proximity, thereby leaving little unfilled resin exposed.

MARGINAL ADAPTATION

The use of composite resins for restoring posterior teeth has historically presented the problem of marginal leakage at the resin-tooth interface (Derkson et al., 1983; Phillips, 1972). This marginal leakage caused teeth with posterior composite resin restorations to be more prone to secondary caries than teeth with amalgam restorations. Failure of the composite to bond to the cavity preparation walls and voids in the restorative material have been identified as the cause of inadequate marginal adaptation. This problem has been reduced by (1) using contemporary posterior composite resins, which contain a high volume of filler that decreases polymerization shrinkage, (2) using an enamel bevel, (3) using newer dentin bonding agents and glass ionomer cements, and (4) acid-etching the enamel.

FORMULATIONS

Enamel-Bonding Agents. The use of phosphoric acid (35–50%) has demonstrated an acid-etch pattern on enamel that creates an effective mechanical bond with the BIS-GMA enamel bonding agent. Enamel-bonding agents are placed over the acid-etched enamel prior to composite resin placement. The bonding agents are merely unfilled dimethacrylates and are used because they can easily penetrate the etched enamel surface because of the low viscosity. The resin matrix of the composite resin then chemically bonds to the bonding agent.

Sealants. The use of pit and fissure sealants has been effective in preventing occlusal caries for over two decades (Ripa, 1993; Simonsen, 1991). Sealants are composed of a BIS-GMA resin structure used in composite resin. The BIS-GMA monomer is diluted with low-weight dimethacrylate monomer to make the sealant material a fluid that can easily penetrate the pits and fissures of occlusal surfaces. Sealants are available in two-component systems that self-polymerize when mixed and light-polymerized systems.

Although the use of sealants is an excellent preventive technique, there remained at first the concern that caries could occur at sealant margins or where the sealant had partially broken away. The concept of adding fluoride-releasing resins was examined for caries inhibition and found to be effective (Hicks and Flaitz, 1992; Jensen et al., 1990).

Microfilled Composite Resin. Microfilled composite resin has silane-treated colloidal silica filler particles (approximately 30–50% by weight) in a BIS-GMA resin matrix. Because of the high percentage of resin matrix, the particle configuration, and the small particle size (less than 1 μm in diameter), this composite resin is easily polishable and reaches a high lustrous appearance. Microfilled composite resins are recommended for restorations that are highly visible yet encounter minimal stress during mastication. The low percentage of filler results in a decrease in strength and increase in wear. To compensate for polymerization shrinkage, some of the BIS-GMA resin in the composite resin is pre-polymerized by the manufacturer.

Macrofilled Composite Resin. Macrofilled composite resin has silane-treated filler particles (approximately 80% by volume) in a BIS-GMA resin. The particle sizes are much larger than those found in microfilled systems. Although these particles are larger than those found in the microfilled composite resin, they are smaller than the conventional composite resin particles. The high filler particle percentage increases wear resistance. Because most of these composite resins are used for posterior restorations, the material is usually radiopaque from the filler type.

Hybrid Composite Resin. Hybrid composite resins have a combination of small and large particles, representing the size of the particles found in microfilled and macrofilled composite resins, respectively. The high percentage of filler particles provides strength and wear resistance, yet the smaller filler particles allow for particles to arrange in close proximity to each other, which can provide minimal polymerization shrinkage and improved polishability compared with macrofilled composite resin. These composite resins are considered for restorations that may have stress-bearing areas during mastication but need to have a well-polished surface; Class IV restorations fall into this category.

Glass Ionomer

ANTERIOR RESTORATIONS

Preparations of glass ionomer are available in various shades that can be used for anterior restorations. The use of glass ionomer for anterior restorations is limited to Class III and Class V preparations. The low fracture resistance and mechanical bonding strength to enamel make its use impractical for Class IV restorations. Retention of glass ionomer restorations in Class V restorations, when the gingival margin is not in enamel, may carry advantages. The fluoride release from glass ionomer restorations has been shown to inhibit secondary caries.

POSTERIOR RESTORATIONS

The major disadvantage of glass ionomer cement as a posterior restorative material is its susceptibility to fracture and wear. Metal particles have been added to glass ionomer cement to increase the strength and wear resistance for posterior restorations. Fracture resistance remains a concern, and critical decisions should be made when using the material for posterior restorations. Investigation has demonstrated the clinical success of a resin-modified glass ionomer cement as a posterior restorative material in the primary dentition (Donly et al., 1997). Again, the fluoride release and bonding capabilities are advantages of the glass ionomer cement.

Compomers

Compomers have become available more recently and are recommended for use as a pediat-ric dental restorative material (Peters and Roeters, 1994). Compomers are actually a cross between composite resin and glass ionomer cement.

The compomers are expected to bring the favorable properties of composite resin, such as wear resistance, color stability, and polishability, to the material. An acid-base reaction takes place within the compomer material, but is not the primary setting reaction; therefore, visible-light polymerization is necessary to complete the setting reaction. Compomers are used in conjunction with methyl methacrylate primers that bond to enamel, dentin, and compomer restorative material; therefore, manufacturers consider the etching of tooth structure prior to restoration placement optional.

CEMENTS

Cements are frequently used in the practice of pediatric dentistry. Their primary use is for the cementation of stainless steel crowns and orthodontic bands. Zinc phosphate, polycarboxylate, zinc oxide–eugenol, and glass ionomer are the cements most commonly used. These cements were touched on earlier in the discussion of bases and liners. When they are used as luting cements, adjustments may be made in the mix of the cement to provide properties needed for

TABLE 20–2. Comparison of Dental Cements

Cement	Composition	Working Time	Setting Time	Compressive Strength	Bond Strength to Dentin	Release of Fluoride	Pulpal Response	Removal of Excess
Ideal	—	Medium	Short-medium	Very high	High	Yes	None	Easy
Zinc phosphate	Zinc oxide Phosphoric acid	Medium	Medium	Medium	None	No	Low-medium	Easy
Polycarboxylate	Zinc oxide Polycarboxylic acid	Short	Short	Low-medium	Low-medium	No	None	Medium-difficult
Glass ionomer	Silicate glass containing Ca, Al, F Polycarboxylic acid	Short-medium	Short	High	Medium	Yes	Low	Moderate
Zinc silicophos-phate	Zinc oxide and silicate Phosphoric acid	Medium	Medium	High	None	Yes	Medium	Easy
Zinc oxide and eugenol	Zinc oxide Eugenol	Long	Medium	Low-medium	None	No	None	Easy
Reinforced zinc oxide and eugenol	Zinc oxide reinforced with EBA or alumina or polymer Eugenol	Long	Medium-long	Low-medium	None	No	None	Easy

Adapted from Farah JW, Powers JM: Rating permanent cements. Dental Advisor 2(1):3, 1985.

cementation. For example, less powder is placed in zinc phosphate cement when it is being used as a luting cement than when it is being used as a base or liner. The particles in glass ionomer cement are usually larger than those found in glass ionomer bases. There is less particle surface area available for reaction in the cement, and therefore the cement sets slower than the base and allows more working time. The importance of the accuracy in liquid-powder ratio of glass ionomer cement has been discussed. Encapsulated, premeasured cement is available and may be considered for clinical use.

The various cements most commonly used in pediatric dentistry and their clinical considerations are noted in Tables 20–1 and 20–2.

REFERENCES

American Dental Association Divisions of Communication and Scientific Affairs and Department of State Government Affairs: When your patients ask about mercury in amalgam. JADA *120*:395-398, 1990.

Bowen RL: Dental filling material comprising vinyl-silane treated fused silica and a binder consisting of the reaction product of bisphenol and glycidyl methacrylate. U.S. Patent 3,066,112, 1962.

Bowen RL, Eichmiller FC, Marjenhoff WA: Glass-ceramic inserts anticipated for "megafilled" composite restoration. JADA *122*:71-75, 1991.

Council on Dental Materials and Devices: Revised American Dental Association Specification No. 1 for alloy for dental amalgam. JADA *95*:614-617, 1977.

Craig RG: Chemistry, composition and properties of composite resins—Symposium on Composite Resins in Dentistry. Dent Clin North Am *25*:219-239, 1981.

Derkson GD, Richardson AS, Waldman RJ: Clinical evaluation of composite resin and amalgam posterior restorations: Two year results. J Can Dent Assoc *4*:277-279, 1983.

Donly KJ, Kanellis M, Segura A: Glass ionomer restorations in primary molars: Three-year clinical results. J Dent Res *76*(A): Abst. #1454, 1997.

Donly KJ, Wild TW, Jensen ME: Posterior composite Class II restorations: In vitro comparison of preparation designs and restoration techniques. Dent Mater *6*:88-93, 1990.

Eames WB: Clinical comparison of composite, amalgam, and silicate restorative materials. JADA *89*:1111-1117, 1974.

Erickson RL: Mechanism and clinical implications of bond formation for two dentin bonding agents. Am J Dent *2*:117-123, 1989.

Garcia-Godoy F, Jensen ME: Artificial recurrent caries in glass ionomer-lined amalgam restorations. Am J Dent *3*:89-93, 1990.

Heys RJ, Fitzgerald M: Microleakage of three cement bases. J Dent Res *70*:55-58, 1991.

Hicks MJ, Flaitz CM: Caries-like lesion formation around fluo-ride-releasing sealant and glass ionomer. Am J Dent *5*:329-334, 1992.

Hicks MJ, Flaitz CM, Silverstone LM: Secondary caries formation in vitro around glass ionomer restoration. Quintessence Int *17*:527-532, 1986.

Jensen ME, Wefel JS, Hammesfahr PD: Fluoride-releasing liners: In vitro recurrent caries. Gen Dent *39*:12-17, 1991.

Jensen ME, Wefel JS, Triolo PT, Hammesfahr PD: Effect of a fluoride-releasing fissure sealant on artificial enamel caries. Am J Dent *3*:75-78, 1990.

Leinfelder KF, Roberson TM: Clinical evaluation of posterior composite resins. Gen Dent *31*:276-280, 1983.

Leinfelder KF, Sluder TB, Santos JF, Wall JT: Five year clinical evaluation of anterior and posterior restorations of composite resin. Oper Dent *5*(2):57-65, 1980.

Manders CA, Garcia-Godoy F, Barnwell GM: Effect of a Copal varnish, ZOE or glass ionomer cement bases on microleakage of amalgam restorations. Am J Dent *3*:63-66, 1990.

Mitra SB: Property comparisons of a light-cure and a self-cure glass ionomer liner. J Dent Res *68*(A):Abst #740, 1989.

Osborne JW: Three-year clinical performance of eight amalgam alloys. Am J Dent *3*:157-159, 1990.

Osborne JW, Gale EN, Ferguson GW: One-year and two-year clinical evaluation of composite resin vs. amalgam. J Prosthet Dent *30*:795-800, 1973.

Pereira JC, Manfio AP, Franco EB, Lopes ES: Clinical evaluation of Dycal under amalgam restorations. Am J Dent *3*:67-70, 1990.

Peters MCRB, Roeters FJM: Clinical performance of a new compomer restorative in pediatric dentistry. J Dent Res *73*(A):Abst. #34, 1994.

Phillips RW: Observations on a composite resin for Class II restorations: Two year report. J Prosthet Dent *28*:164-169, 1972.

Phillips RW, Lutz F: Status reports on posterior composites: Council on Dental Materials, Instruments and Equipment. JADA *107*:74-76, 1983.

Phillips RW, Swartz ML, Norman RD: Materials for the Practicing Dentist. St. Louis, CV Mosby, 1969, pp 182-191.

Ripa LW: Sealants revisited: An update of the effectiveness of pit-and-fissure sealants. Caries Res *27*(Suppl 1):77-82, 1993.

Ruyter IE: Monomer systems and polymerization. *In* Vanherle C, Smith DC (eds): Posterior Composite Resin Dental Restorative Materials. Utrecht, Peter Szulc, 1985, pp 109-135.

Ruyter IE: Polymerization and conversion in composite resins. *In* Taylor DF (ed): Proceedings of the International Symposium on Posterior Composite Resins, Chapel Hill, North Carolina, October 1982.

Simonsen RJ: Retention and effectiveness of dental sealants after fifteen years. JADA *122*:34-42, 1991.

Skartveit L, Tveit AB, Totdal B, et al: In vivo fluoride uptake in enamel and dentin from fluoride-containing materials. J Dent Child *58*:97-100, 1990.

Smith DC: Posterior composite dental restorative material: Materials development. *In* Vanherle G, Smith DC (eds): Posterior Composite Resin Dental Restorative Materials. Utrecht, Peter Szulc, 1985, pp 47-60.

Straffon LH, Corpron RL, Bruner FW, Daprai F: Twenty-four-month clinical trial of visible-light–activated cavity liner in young permanent teeth. J Dent Child *58*:124-128, 1991.

Chapter 21

Restorative Dentistry for the Primary Dentition

William F. Waggoner

Chapter Outline

Pediatric restorative dentistry is a dynamic combination of ever-improving materials and tried and true techniques. Many aspects of restoring primary teeth have not changed for decades. In 1924, G. V. Black outlined several steps for the preparation of carious permanent teeth to receive an amalgam restoration. These steps have been adopted, though slightly modified, for the restoration of primary teeth. Restorative techniques for the primary dentition that use amalgam and stainless steel crowns have remained relatively consistent for many years (Fig. 21-1). With an increased use of composite resins and bonding systems, however, there has been a shift toward more conservative preparations and res-

torations. Materials such as glass ionomers, resin-ionomer products, and amalgam bonding systems have been developed that may ultimately have a profound impact on the restoration of primary teeth. Unfortunately, long-term clinical data regarding these new materials are limited: even so, many clinicians are using these new materials with increasing frequency. Hence, we find ourselves in a transitional age.

The clinician can stay with the proven, successful materials of the past, such as amalgam and stainless steel, or move to newer but not yet fully proven materials that offer advantages such as bonding to tooth structure, fluoride release, improved esthetics, reduction of mercury expo-

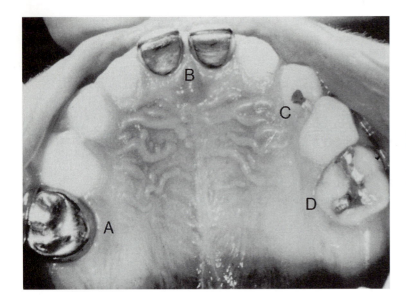

Figure 21–1. Restored primary dentition demonstrating stainless steel crown (*A*), open-face steel crowns (*B*), class III amalgam (*C*), and class II amalgam (*D*).

sure, and conservation of tooth structure. This chapter provides information on both the new and the old restorative techniques. A more detailed discussion of dental materials used in pediatric restorative dentistry can be found in Chapter 20.

INSTRUMENTATION

Nearly all instrumentation for restorative procedures is carried out with the high-speed air turbine handpiece (100,000–300,000 rpm) combined with coolant. The coolant may be water spray or air alone. A water spray coolant is often recommended for high-speed instrumentation; however, there is some evidence that air coolant alone may be used without the creation of irreversible pulpal damage (Bhaskar and Lilly, 1965; Bouschor and Matthews, 1966). There are some instances when a water spray coolant is absolutely necessary. This is especially true when removing old amalgam restorations or using diamond burs. Regardless of the coolant used, intermittent cutting at intervals of a few seconds with light, brushing strokes should be used to prevent excessive heat generation. Protective masks and eyewear should always be worn when one uses the high-speed air turbine handpiece.

The slow-speed handpiece (500–15,000 rpm) is most frequently used for caries removal and for polishing and finishing procedures. As with high-speed instrumentation, light pressure and brushing strokes should be used when one employs the slow-speed handpiece. Hand instrumentation is minimal in most operative prepara-

tions in the primary dentition. It is usually limited to final caries removal or planing of enamel walls.

In recent years one other method of instrumentation for preparing teeth has become somewhat popular. This technique, known as air abrasion, uses a stream of purified aluminum oxide particles (27–50 μm), which are forced under pressure (40–120 psi) through a fine-focused nozzle onto the tooth surface. This cuts through enamel and dentin quickly or can also abrade or roughen a tooth surface (Goldstein and Parkins, 1994). Originally introduced in dentistry by Black in 1945 (Black, 1945), air abrasion virtually disappeared from the dental environment by the early 1960s until reintroduced in the early 1990s. Air abrasion offers several advantages over conventional handpieces. There is an absence of vibration and noise, caries excavation can often be performed without the need for local anesthesia, and tooth preparation can be very fast. It is best suited for use with composite resin restorations that require minimal tooth preparation and less rigid classic cavity design than does amalgam. The cost of the air abrasion unit (several thousand dollars) and the fact that it does not totally eliminate the need for conventional handpieces are two disadvantages of the system that will probably keep it from gaining widespread use quickly.

ANATOMIC CONSIDERATIONS OF PRIMARY TEETH

Although some primary teeth resemble their permanent successors, they are not miniature per-

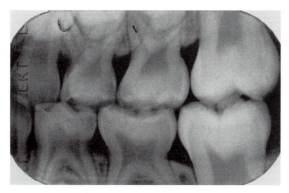

Figure 21–2. Note the difference in enamel thickness. The enamel of the primary molars is approximately half the thickness of the enamel of the first permanent molars. Also note the interproximal caries requiring restoration on the distal surface of the mandibular first primary molar and between the maxillary first and second primary molars.

manent teeth. Several anatomic differences must be distinguished before restorative procedures are begun.

1. Primary teeth have thinner enamel and dentin than permanent teeth (Fig. 21-2).
2. The pulps of primary teeth are larger in relation to crown size than permanent pulps.
3. The pulp horns of primary teeth are closer to the outer surface of the tooth than permanent pulps. The mesio-buccal pulp horn is the most prominent.
4. In primary teeth, the enamel rods of the gingival third of the crown extend in an occlusal direction from the dentino-enamel junction. This is in contrast to the permanent dentition, in which the rods extend in a cervical direction.
5. Primary teeth demonstrate greater constriction of the crown and have a more prominent cervical contour than permanent teeth.
6. Primary teeth have broad, flat proximal contact areas.
7. Primary teeth are whiter than their permanent successors.
8. Primary teeth have relatively narrow occlusal surfaces compared with their permanent successors.

USE OF THE RUBBER DAM IN PEDIATRIC RESTORATIVE DENTISTRY

The rubber dam is indispensable in pediatric restorative dentistry. Numerous advantages have been listed for its use, all allowing for provision of the highest quality of care:

1. Better access and visualization are gained by retracting soft tissues and providing a dark contrasting background to the teeth.
2. Moisture control is superior to other forms of isolation.
3. The safety of the child is improved by preventing aspiration or swallowing of foreign bodies and by protecting the soft tissues.
4. Placement generally results in decreased operating time.
5. Many children tend to become more quiet and relaxed with a rubber dam in place. The dam seems to act as a separating barrier, so that movements in and out of the oral cavity are perceived by the child as being less invasive than without the dam in place.
6. With a rubber dam in place, a child becomes primarily a nasal breather. This enhances nitrous oxide administration, when it has been deemed necessary from a behavioral standpoint.

Almost all pediatric restorative procedures can be completed with the rubber dam in place. The few instances in which it may not be used include (1) the presence of some fixed orthodontic appliances, (2) a very recently erupted tooth that will not retain a clamp, and (3) a child with an upper respiratory infection, congested nasal passages, or other nasal obstruction. Even poor nasal breathers may tolerate the rubber dam, however, if a small (2-3 cm) hole is cut in the dam in an area away from the operative quadrant. This allows for some mouth breathing.

Preparing for Placement of the Rubber Dam

The rubber dam is available in an assortment of colors and may even be scented or flavored. Virtually all rubber dams are made of latex, although a latex-free rubber dam material is available (Hygienic Corporation, Akron, OH) for use in latex-sensitive patients. A 5 × 5 inch medium-gauge rubber dam is best suited for use in children. Rubber dams are available in which a disposable rubber dam frame is manufactured already attached to the dam (Handidam, Aseptico, Kirkland, WA), eliminating the need for a separate dam frame. The darker the color of the dam, the better the contrast between the teeth and dam. The holes should be punched so that the rubber dam is centered horizontally on the face and the upper lip is covered by the upper border of the dam but the dam does not cover the nostrils. One method of proper hole placement is shown in Figure 21-3A. Figure 21-3B

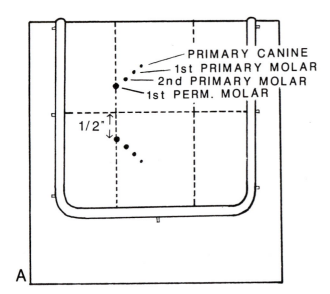
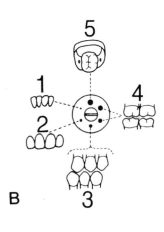

Figure 21–3. Preparation of the rubber dam. *A,* The Young's frame is applied to the rubber dam. The upper limit of the frame coincides with the upper edge of the rubber dam material. The dam is divided vertically into thirds, and the area inside the frame is divided in half horizontally. The holes for each tooth are placed as indicated, at a 45 degree angle 3–4 mm apart. *B,* The rubber dam punch table with corresponding teeth and hole sizes. (*B* reprinted by permission of the publisher from The DAE Project: Instructional Materials for the Dental Health Professions: Rubber Dam. New York, Teachers College Press, © 1982, Teachers College, Columbia University. All rights reserved. p. 42.)

demonstrates proper hole size selection for different teeth.

The minimum number of holes necessary for good isolation of all tooth surfaces to be restored is punched in the dam. For single Class I or V restorations, only the tooth being restored need be isolated. If interproximal lesions are being restored, at least one tooth anterior and one tooth posterior to the tooth being restored should be isolated. This allows better access, more ease in placing a matrix, and visualization of adjacent marginal ridges for appropriate carving of the restoration.

When isolating several teeth, instead of punching numerous holes in the dam, some clinicians simply punch two holes approximately 1/2 inch apart and cut the rubber dam with scissors connecting the two holes. This is called the slit technique and allows for quick placement of the rubber dam. Because there is no rubber dam material interproximally, moisture control is not as dependable with this placement technique, but it is often still adequate, especially for isolation of maxillary quadrants.

Proper clamp selection is one of the most critical aspects of good rubber dam application. Table 21-1 lists the most frequently used clamps and their areas of use. Incisors usually require ligation with dental floss for stabilization instead of a clamp.

After selecting an appropriate clamp, place a

12-18 inch piece of dental floss on the bow of the clamp as a safety measure (Fig. 21-4). This is necessary for easy retrieval of the clamp if it is dislodged from the tooth and falls into the posterior pharyngeal area.

Before trying the clamp on the tooth, floss the contacts through which the rubber dam will be taken. If floss is unable to pass through the contact because of defective restorations or other reasons, modification of the contacts or rubber dam is necessary before placement. Next, using the rubber dam forceps, place the clamp on

TABLE 21–1. Common Rubber Dam Clamps for Pediatric Restorative Dentistry

Teeth	Clamp No.
Partially erupted permanent molars	14A, 8A*,†,‡
Fully erupted permanent molars	14, 8*,†,‡
Second primary molars	26, 27‡, 3*,†
First primary molars/bicuspids/ permanent canines	2, 2A*,†
	207, 208‡
Primary incisors and canines	0*
	00†
	209‡

"A" clamps have jaws angled gingivally to seat below subgingival heights of contour.
*Ivory, Miles Inc., Dental Products, South Bend, IN.
†Hygienic Corp, Akron, OH.
‡HuFriedy, Chicago, IL.

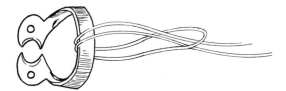

Figure 21–4. A floss safety through the bow of the rubber dam clamp allows for easy retrieval of the clamp, should it become dislodged from the tooth. (Reprinted by permission of the publisher from The DAE Project: Instructional Materials for the Dental Health Professions: Rubber Dam. New York, Teachers College Press, © 1982, Teachers College, Columbia University. All rights reserved. p. 66.)

the tooth, seating it from a lingual to a buccal direction. Be certain that the jaws of the clamp are placed below the height of contour and are not impinging on the gingival tissues. After seating the clamp, remove the forceps and place a finger on the buccal and lingual jaws of the clamp and apply gingival pressure to ensure that the clamp is stable and has been seated as far gingivally as possible.

Placement of the Rubber Dam

The punched rubber dam should be lightly stretched onto the rubber dam frame prior to placement of the clamp. This holds the corners of the dam out of the line of the operator's vision during placement. If the material is stretched too tightly, tension is too great and the clamp may be dislodged when the material is stretched over the bow of the clamp. Next, pull the floss attached to the clamp through the most posterior hole in the dam that has been punched for the clamped tooth. Instruct the child to open the mouth widely, and with the index fingers, stretch the most posterior hole of the rubber dam over the bow and wings of the clamp. Sometimes when isolating the most posterior maxillary molars, the bow of the clamp rests very close to the anterior border of the ramus when the mouth is opened wide. This makes slipping the dam material over the bow difficult, but when one simply asks the child to close the mouth slightly, the ramus moves posteriorly and allows the material to slide between the bow and the ramus.

If necessary, adjust the tension of the rubber dam on the frame. Next, stabilize the rubber dam around the most anterior tooth. This may be done by placing a wooden wedge interproximally, by stretching a small piece of rubber dam through the contact, or by ligating with dental floss. To ligate, place floss (12–18 inches) around the cervical aspect of the tooth and have the

dental assistant hold the floss gingivally on the lingual aspect with a blunt instrument. Draw the floss tightly around the tooth from the buccal aspect and tie a surgical knot below the cervical bulge. Do not cut the ends of the ligature tie because the long ends remind the operator that the ligature is present. After anterior stabilization, all other teeth can be isolated for which holes have been punched. A blunt hand instrument can be used to invert the rubber dam into the gingival sulcus around each isolated tooth.

Removing the Rubber Dam

To remove the rubber dam, first rinse away all debris and cut and remove any ligatures used for stabilization. Next, stretch the rubber dam so that the dam's interproximal septa may be cut with a pair of scissors. The clamp, frame, and dam are then removed as a unit with the rubber dam forceps. Inspect the dam and the mouth to see that no small pieces of dam material have been left interproximally. Gently massage the tissue around the previously clamped tooth, and rinse and evacuate the oral cavity.

RESTORATION OF PRIMARY MOLARS

The anatomy of the primary molars, with their fissured occlusal surfaces and broad, flat interproximal contact areas, makes them the most caries-susceptible primary teeth. The importance of primary molars in mastication and as maintainers of space for the succedaneous teeth, coupled with the development of suitable economic restorative materials, has shaped a philosophy of restoring and conserving primary molars. Stainless steel crowns, amalgam, and, most recently, composite resins, glass ionomers, and resin-ionomers, are the materials used in the restoration of primary molars. Although use of composite resin for restoring posterior teeth is increasing in frequency, amalgam remains the restorative material of choice for many clinicians. Concerns about the mercury in amalgam and the exposure of dentists, patients, and the environment to mercury have been raised, however. This has brought the use of amalgam under recent attack. Current scientific information continues to support the use of amalgam as a restorative material, but for a more detailed discussion of the controversy the reader is referred to Chapter 20.

Class I Amalgam Restorations

GENERAL CONSIDERATIONS

The outline form for Class I restorations in primary molars is shown in Figure 21–5. The outline form should include all retentive fissures and carious areas but should be as conservative as possible. Ideal pulpal floor depth is 0.5 mm into dentin (approximately 1.5 mm from the enamel surface). The length of the cutting end of the No. 330 bur is 1.5 mm, so this becomes a good tool for gauging cavity depth. The cavosurface margin should be placed out of stress-bearing areas and should have no bevel. To help prevent stress concentration, the outline form should be composed of smooth flowing arcs and curves and all internal angles should be rounded slightly. When a dovetail is placed in the second primary molars, its buccolingual width should be greater than the width of the isthmus to produce a locking form to provide resistance against occlusal torque, which may displace the restoration mesially or distally. The isthmus should be one third of the intercuspal width, and the buccolingual walls should converge slightly in an occlusal di-

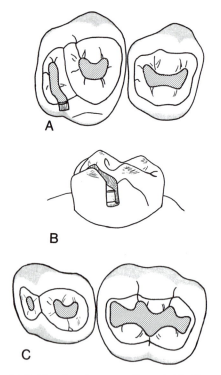

Figure 21–5. Class I cavity preparations. *A,* Maxillary right second and first primary molars (occlusal view). *B,* Maxillary second primary molar, lingual view of distolingual groove preparation. *C,* Mandibular right first and second primary molars (occlusal view).

rection. The mesial and distal walls should flare at the marginal ridge so as not to undercut ridges. Oblique ridges should not be crossed unless they are undermined with caries or are deeply fissured. Primary mandibular second molars often have buccal developmental pits. When carious, these should be restored with a small teardrop or oval shaped restoration, including all the adjacent susceptible pits and fissures.

Neither liners nor bases are very widely used for restoring primary teeth, but various bases and liners are discussed in Chapter 20. Thin liners such as calcium hydroxide do not provide thermal insulation, and recent evidence suggests that calcium hydroxide may hydrolyze over time (Pereira et al., 1990), leaving a small void underneath the restoration and ultimately weakening the restoration (Donly et al., 1990). Therefore, use of calcium hydroxide is discouraged. Cavity varnish, though widely used in the past to prevent microleakage, is no longer considered useful. Small amalgam restorations can be placed directly into prepared cavities without any varnish or, if desired, a self-curing bonding agent applied to primed dentin prior to amalgam placement can be used. The amalgam and bonding agent will intermix, mechanically forming an amalgam attachment to the cavity wall (Lacy and Young, 1996). Placement of bases in primary teeth is also uncommon. Because the pulp chamber in primary teeth is relatively large, preparations that are deep enough to require bases are generally found to be into the pulp and hence require other treatment.

STEPS OF PREPARATION AND RESTORATION OF CLASS I AMALGAM RESTORATIONS

1. Administer appropriate anesthesia and place the rubber dam.

2. Using a No. 330 bur in the high-speed turbine handpiece, penetrate into the tooth parallel to its long axis in the central pit region and extend into all susceptible fissures and pits to a depth 0.5 mm into dentin.

3. Remove all carious dentin. Use a large, round bur in the slow-speed handpiece or a sharp spoon excavator.

4. Smooth the enamel walls, and refine the final outline form with the No. 330 bur.

5. Rinse and dry the preparation, and inspect for (1) caries removal, (2) sharp cavosurface margins, and (3) removal of all unsupported enamel with hand instruments, as necessary.

6. (*Optional*) Apply self-curing dentin bonding agent to primed dentin.

7. Triturate the amalgam, and place one carrier load of amalgam into the preparation.

8. Using a small condenser, immediately begin condensation of the amalgam into the preparation, condensing small overlapping increments with a firm pressure until the cavity is slightly overfilled.

9. Following condensation, carving of most of the newer alloys can begin almost immediately. A small cleoid-discoid carver works very well for carving primary restorations. Always keep part of the carving edge of the instrument on tooth structure so that over-carving of the cavosurface margin does not occur. Remove all amalgam flash from cavosurface margins. Keep the carved anatomy shallow. Placing deep anatomy in primary teeth (i.e., grooves) can weaken the restoration by creating a thin shelf of amalgam at the cavosurface margin and by reducing the bulk of amalgam in the central stress-bearing areas, both of which lead to fracture.

10. Burnish the carved amalgam when the amalgam has begun its initial set and resists deformation. Burnishing is done with a small, round burnisher, which is lightly rubbed across the carved amalgam surface to produce a satin-like appearance. Besides smoothing, burnishing creates a substructure with fewer voids and reduces finishing time.

11. A wet cotton pellet can be wiped across the burnished amalgam for a final smoothing (*optional*).

12. Remove the rubber dam, and check the occlusion. Before the rubber dam is completely removed, children must be cautioned that they must not close their teeth into occlusion until instructed to do so. With articulating paper, check the restoration for occlusal irregularities, instructing the child to close gently. Make necessary adjustments with the carver.

13. Rinse the oral cavity, and massage the soft tissue around the previously clamped tooth.

COMMON ERRORS WITH CLASS I AMALGAM RESTORATIONS

Some frequent errors made in Class I amalgam restorations are (1) not including all susceptible fissures, (2) preparing the cavity too deep, (3) undercutting the marginal ridges, (4) carving the anatomy of the amalgam too deep, (5) not removing amalgam flash from cavosurface margins, and (6) under-carving, which leads to subsequent fracture of amalgam from hyperocclusion.

Class II Amalgam Restorations

GENERAL CONSIDERATIONS

The outline form for several Class II amalgam preparations is shown in Figure 21–6. The guide-

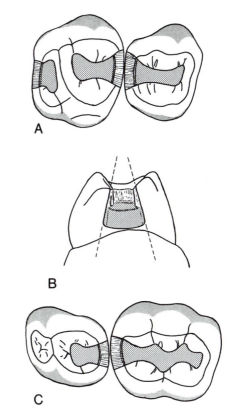

Figure 21–6. Class II cavity preparations. *A*, Maxillary right second and first primary molars (occlusal view). *B*, Mandibular second primary molar (proximal view)—note occlusal convergence of proximal walls. *C*, Mandibular right first and second primary molars (occlusal view).

lines given for the Class I preparation should be followed during the preparation of the occlusal portion of the Class II preparation; additionally, there are several recommendations for the proximal box preparation. The proximal box should be broader at the cervical than at the occlusal aspect. The buccal, lingual, and gingival walls should all break contact with the adjacent tooth, just enough to allow the tip of an explorer to pass. The buccal and lingual walls should create a 90-degree angle with the enamel. The gingival wall should be flat, not beveled, and all unsupported enamel should be removed. Ideally, the axial wall of the proximal box should be 0.5 mm into dentin and should follow the same contour as the outer proximal contour of the tooth. Because occlusal forces may permit a concentration of stress within the amalgam around sharp angles, the axiopulpal line angle is routinely beveled or rounded. No buccal or lingual retentive grooves should be placed in the proximal box. The mesiodistal width of the gingival seat should be 1 mm, which is approximately equal to the width of a No. 330 bur.

In primary teeth, many practitioners limit Class II amalgam restorations to relatively small two-surface restorations. Three-surface (mesio-occlusodistal—MOD) restorations may be done, but studies have shown that stainless steel crowns are a more durable and predictable resto-ration for large multiple-surface restorations in primary teeth (Dawson et al., 1981). Messer and Levering (1988) reported that stainless steel crowns placed in 4-year-old and younger children yielded a success rate that was approximately twice that of Class II amalgams for each year up to 10 years of service. Roberts and Sherriff (1990) reported that after 5 years, one third of Class II amalgams placed in primary teeth had failed or required replacement, whereas only 8% of stainless steel crowns required retreatment. In the preschool child with large proximal carious lesions, stainless steel crowns are preferred to amalgams because of their durability. Similar-sized lesions in teeth that are within 2 to 3 years of exfoliation may be restored with amalgam be-cause the anticipated lifespan is fairly short. Pins for retention of amalgam in primary teeth are contraindicated. Because of the large relative size of the primary pulp, the thin dentin thickness, and the marked cervical constriction of the pri-mary crown, successful placement of the pin is difficult without pulp exposure or a perforation into the gingival sulcus.

MATRIX APPLICATION

Matrices must be placed for interproximal resto-rations to aid in restoring normal contour and normal contact areas and to prevent extrusion of restorative materials into gingival tissues. Many types of matrix bands are available for use in pediatric dentistry:

1. *T-band:* allows for multiple matrices; no special equipment is needed
2. *Sectional matrices* (Strip Ts, DENOVO, Baldwin Park, CA): allow for multiple matrix placement, easy to use, not circumferential, must be held in place by a wedge
3. *Tofflemire matrix:* used infrequently be-cause it does not fit primary tooth contour well and is difficult to place as multiple matrices
4. *Spot-welded matrix:* allows for multiple ma-trix placement; a spot welder is required at chair-side

T-bands are available in different sizes, con-tours, and materials. A straight, narrow, brass T-band works in almost all pediatric restorative procedures. The T-band matrix (Fig. 21-7) is formed by folding the band back on itself in the

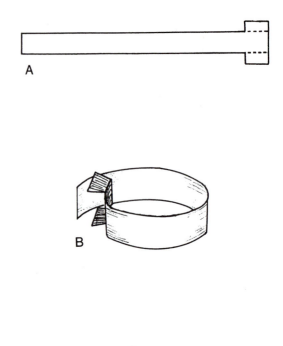

Figure 21–7. *A,* The T-band matrix. *B,* The T-band is formed into a circle, and the extension wings are folded down to secure the band. *C,* The T-band is adapted to fit the tooth tightly and is trimmed with scissors, and the free end is bent back.

form of a circle and by folding over the extension wings of the T to make an adjustable loop. The band is contoured and positioned onto the tooth with the folded extension wings on the buccal surface. The free end of the band is drawn mesi-ally to pull the band snugly against the tooth. The extension folds are then grasped firmly with a pair of Howe No. 110 pliers and removed from the tooth. The band should then be tightened an additional 0.5 to 1.0 mm, and the free end should be bent back over the vertical folds and cut with scissors to a length of 5 to 6 mm. The band is then reseated onto the tooth and wedged. It must fit below the gingival margin of the prepara-tion and must be at least 1 mm higher than the marginal ridge of the adjacent tooth.

The T-band is removed by opening the exten-sion wings with an explorer or spoon excavator and allowing the band to open. Scissors are then used to cut one end of the band close to the restored proximal surface, the wedge is removed, and the band is then drawn buccally or lingually through the contact.

The sectional matrices or "matrix pieces" (Strip Ts, DENOVO) are stainless steel matrix strips approximately 1/2 inch long that do not encircle the prepared tooth but only fit in the prepared proximal area. For small Class II preparations, they are simple to place and use. After placement they must be firmly wedged to be held in place. They are not recommended for proximal preparations that extend beyond the line angles; a circumferential matrix (or stainless steel crown) is more appropriate in that instance.

Figure 21-8 demonstrates the fabrication and placement of a spot-welded matrix retainer. Steel matrix material of various widths is available in spools. A piece of matrix material approximately 2 inches in length is cut from the spool, and the ends of the band are welded together in one spot (Fig. 21-8A). This loop is then placed around the tooth and adapted snugly by grasping the band with the Howe No. 110 pliers from the buccal surface (Fig. 21-8B). The band is removed, and two spot welds are placed at the seam where the band was pinched together on the buccal surface (Fig. 21-8C). Excess band material is cut away with scissors. Contouring pliers may be used to contour the cervical and contact areas. The welded band is then placed back onto the tooth, and wooden wedges are placed (Fig. 21-8D). After the amalgam has been placed, the band may be removed by placing a flat-bladed hand instrument between the tooth's buccal surface and the band and applying a rotational force to the instrument (Fig. 21-8E). This should break the spot welds and allow for easy removal of the band.

STEPS OF PREPARATION AND RESTORATION FOR CLASS II AMALGAM RESTORATIONS

1. Administer appropriate anesthesia, and place the rubber dam.

2. Place a wooden wedge in the interproximal area being restored (*optional*). This acts to retract the gingival papilla during instrumentation, keeps the operator from cutting the interseptal rubber dam material and underlying gingiva, and creates some prewedging, which helps ensure a tight proximal contact of the final restoration.

3. Using a No. 330 bur in the high-speed turbine handpiece with a light, brushing motion, prepare the occlusal outline form at ideal depth.

4. To prepare the proximal box, begin at the marginal ridge by brushing the bur buccolin-

gually in a pendulum motion and in a gingival direction at the dentino-enamel junction. Continue until contact is just broken between the adjacent tooth and the gingival wall and the wedge is seen. If the gingival wall is made too deep, the cervical constriction of the primary molar will create a very narrow gingival seat. The widest buccolingual width of the box will be at the gingival margin. Care must be taken not to damage the adjacent proximal surface.

5. Remove any remaining caries with a sharp spoon excavator or with a round bur in the slow-speed handpiece.

6. Round the axiopulpal line angle slightly. Because of the shape of the No. 330 bur, all other internal line angles are automatically gently rounded.

7. Remove any unsupported enamel of the buccal, lingual, or gingival walls with a small enamel hatchet.

8. Remove the wedge placed at the beginning of the treatment, and place a matrix band.

9. While holding the matrix band in place, forcefully reinsert the wedge between the matrix band and the adjacent tooth, beneath the gingival seat of the preparation. The wedge is placed with a pair of Howe pliers or cotton forceps from the widest embrasure. The wedge should hold the band tightly against the tooth but should not push the band into the proximal box. It may be necessary to trim the wedge slightly to achieve a proper fit.

10. (*Optional*) Apply a self-curing dentin bonding agent to primed dentin.

11. Triturate the amalgam, and with the amalgam carrier, add the amalgam to the preparation in single increments, beginning in the proximal box.

12. Using a small condenser, condense the amalgam into the corners of the proximal box and against the matrix band to ensure the reestablishment of a tight proximal contact. Continue filling and condensing until the entire cavity is overfilled.

13. Carving of the occlusal portion is performed with a small cleoid-discoid carver, as in Class I restorations. The marginal ridge can be carved with the tip of an explorer or with a Hollenback carver.

14. Carefully remove the wedge and the matrix band.

15. Remove excess amalgam at the buccal, lingual, and gingival margins with an explorer or Hollenback carver. Check to see that the height of the newly restored marginal ridge is approximately equal to the adjacent marginal ridge.

16. Gently floss the interproximal contact to

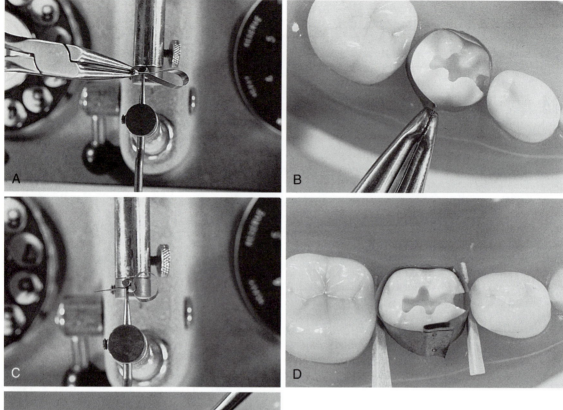

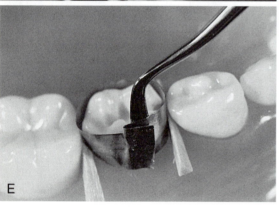

Figure 21–8. *A,* A piece of matrix material approximately 1.5 inches long is formed into a loop, and the ends are spot welded together. *B,* The looped matrix material is adapted around the tooth with the Howe pliers. *C,* The band is returned to the spot welder, and two welds are placed at the seams. *D,* The excess matrix material is cut away, and the welded matrix is replaced on the tooth. Wooden wedges help to secure the band and restore an appropriate proximal contour. *E,* To remove the spot-welded matrix, a flat-bladed instrument is placed between the tooth and the matrix band, and a rotational force is exerted against the band in the area of the spot weld. This will break the weld and allow easy removal of the band.

check the tightness of the contact, to check for gingival overhang, and to remove any loose amalgam particles from the interproximal region.

17. Burnish the restoration, and use a wet cotton pellet held with the cotton pliers for final smoothing if this is needed.

18. Remove the rubber dam carefully.

19. Check the occlusion for irregularities with articulating paper, and adjust as needed.

ADJACENT OR BACK-TO-BACK CLASS II AMALGAM RESTORATIONS

Adjacent interproximal lesions are not uncommon in the primary dentition. From the stand-

point of time and patient management, it is desirable to restore these lesions simultaneously. Preparation for adjacent proximal restorations is identical to those previously described. A matrix is placed on each tooth and is properly wedged. T-band, sectional, or spot-welded matrices are preferable because multiple matrix holders are difficult to place side by side. Condensation of the amalgam should be done in small increments, alternately in each preparation, so that the restorations are filled simultaneously (Fig. 21–9). Condensation pressure toward the matrix helps ensure a tight interproximal contact. Carve the marginal ridges to an equal height, and carefully remove the wedge and matrix bands one at a

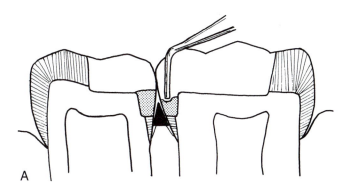

Figure 21–9. "Back-to-back" amalgam preparations. *A,* After wedging, begin condensing the adjacent proximal boxes alternately. *B,* Continue condensing the amalgams alternately until both preparations are slightly overfilled.

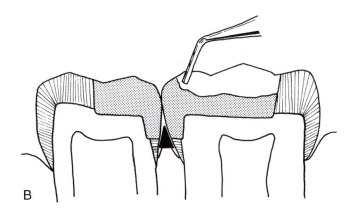

time. Final carving is similar to that described for solitary Class II restorations.

Problems with Amalgam Restorations

Most restorative problems in pediatric dentistry result from a failure to prepare and restore the teeth in a way that accounts for their anatomic or morphologic structural characteristics and limitations (Fig. 21-10). Fracture of the isthmus of a Class II amalgam restoration is a frequent problem that may result from the restoration being left high in occlusion or from insufficient bulk of amalgam in the isthmus because the preparation is too shallow or because the amalgam has been over-carved. Marginal failure in the proximal box, usually owing to an excessive flare of the cavo-surface margin, is another frequent problem with Class II amalgam restorations. Failure to remove all caries or to extend preparations into caries-susceptible fissures is another common reason for failure of restorations (Myers, 1977).

Finishing of Amalgam Restorations

Historically, polishing of amalgams has been advocated to (1) eliminate surface scratches and blemishes, which act as centers of corrosion, (2) remove any remaining amalgam flash not carved away, and (3) refine the anatomy and occlusion. Amalgam polishing is described in a number of textbooks and taught in most, if not all, dental schools. Anecdotal surveys of practitioners, however, reveal that few dentists routinely polish their amalgams after graduating from dental school. A study by Straffon and associates (1984) compared the clinical performance of polished and unpolished amalgams after 3 years. This blinded study demonstrated that there was no significant difference in marginal integrity between carved and burnished-only and polished restorations through 3 years. Polishing of Class I amalgam restorations did not result in better-adapted margins after 36 months of function. The surface texture of the polished amalgams was significantly smoother than the burnished-only amalgams; however, by 36 months a significant number of the burnished-only restorations had exhibited improvement in surface texture over baseline.

If polishing of amalgam is not going to be done it is important that the amalgam at least be well burnished and all excess amalgam marginal flash be removed at the time of placement. Burnishing is best accomplished with a rounded

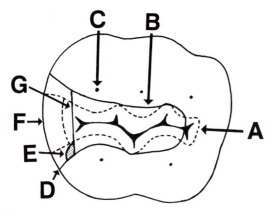

Figure 21–10. Common errors with class II cavity preparations. *A,* Failure to extend occlusal outline into all susceptible pits and fissures. *B,* Failure to follow the outline of the cusps. *C,* Isthmus cut too wide. *D,* Flare of proximal walls too great. *E,* Angle formed by the axial, buccal, and lingual walls too great. *F,* Gingival contact with adjacent tooth not broken. *G,* Axial wall not conforming to the proximal contour of the tooth, and the mesio-distal width of the gingival floor is greater than 1 mm. (From Forrester DJ, Wagner M, and Fleming J: Restorative procedures. In Sheldon P: Pediatric Dental Medicine. Philadelphia, Lea and Febiger, 1981.)

instrument. The surface of the amalgam is smoothed by rubbing the burnisher in back-and-forth motion. Burnishing should be done after the amalgam has reached its initial set and is resistant to deformation. Burnishing 10 minutes after the onset of trituration produces the smoothest surface. After burnishing, care should be taken to see that all amalgam flash is removed with either a small carver or an explorer. When small overhangs of marginal flash are left, they may fracture under occlusal forces. The fracture may then create a marginal discrepancy.

There are no contraindications to polishing amalgams. Many clinicians do not polish because they feel that it is a time-consuming procedure for which most patients do not care to return or reimburse. An alternative to a separate polishing appointment exists, however. Many restorations could be polished at subsequent restorative visits. Because amalgam polishing does not require anesthesia, a practitioner could anesthetize a child in the area that he or she will be restoring that day and then polish previously placed restorations while allowing the anesthesia to take effect. A polishing technique with a simple armamentarium and a low potential for heat production is most desirable. Such a technique is outlined here. Polishing should be delayed for at least 24 hours following amalgam placement.

1. If needed, gross contouring of the amalgam or flash removal is carried out with a tapered green stone.

2. Multiple fluted amalgam finishing burs brushed lightly across the restoration at high speeds smooth and shine the surface. For primary teeth, three sizes of round finishing burs, together with a pear-shaped and flame finishing bur, are sufficient to polish any amalgam restoration.

3. A final polish can be placed on the restoration via a rotary bristle brush with a pumice slurry to remove small scratches, followed by a polishing agent such as tin oxide for the finish luster. Rubber abrasives may be used for final polishing, but great care should be taken not to generate excessive heat.

4. Proximally, small sandpaper disks will polish the enamel-amalgam margins. A well-polished amalgam restoration should allow the explorer to pass easily from enamel to amalgam and back again.

Resin Materials in Primary Molars

As early as the mid-1960s, composite resins were suggested as esthetic replacements for Class I and Class II amalgam restorations in molars. Initial results were promising, but clinical failures of the resin restorations began to occur after approximately 2 years, the greatest problem being occlusal wear (Leinfelder et al., 1980). Recent improvements in composite materials, however, such as smaller filler particles, increases in material strength, and improvement of dentin bonding agents, have led to much improved clinical results. For example, two studies using composite resin for restoration of posterior permanent teeth both demonstrated very good clinical results. In a 5-year study comparing posterior composites and amalgams, Norman and colleagues (1990) reported that both materials were satisfactory over the time period studied and the only significant statistical differences were a poorer marginal integrity for the amalgam and a greater wear rate for the resin. The wear rate for the composite, however, was well within the acceptable limits established by the American Dental Association (ADA) Council on Dental Materials. Roberts and associates (1992) also found no significant difference in clinical performance of Class II amalgam and composite resin restorations evaluated for 3 years. After 3 years, they found no significant differences in wear between the amalgam and composite.

Resin restorations in primary molars offer the advantages of improved esthetics, elimination of mercury, low thermal conductivity, more conservation of tooth structure, and bonding of the restorative material to the tooth. Disadvantages include an exacting technique, increased operator time, potential marginal leakage, postoperative sensitivity, and a tendency toward open or loose contacts (ADA Council of Dental Materials, Instruments, and Equipment, 1986a, 1986b; Leinfelder and Vann; 1982; Waggoner; 1984). The ADA has approved several composite resins for use in posterior teeth, and there is no doubt that several more will be approved in the future. Because the use of amalgam will likely continue to be challenged (as mentioned previously in this chapter and in Chapter 20), composite resins and resin-ionomer products will undoubtedly become more widely used in posterior teeth; therefore, a brief discussion of their use in primary molars is included in this discussion.

GENERAL PRINCIPLES FOR RESTORING PRIMARY POSTERIOR TEETH WITH COMPOSITE RESINS

Composite resins and glass ionomers have been used in restorative dentistry for several years. For occlusal and occlusoproximal restorations, composite resins tend to be more predictable restorations than glass ionomers. New dental materials that are hybrids of glass ionomers and composites, however, have become available and also show promise as a posterior restorative material (Christensen, 1996). For the sake of simplicity, only the use of composite resins is discussed in this chapter. The resin-modified ionomers can be used similarly but are not covered here.

Some general principles must be remembered when using composite resins for restoring posterior primary teeth. (1) Placement of composite resin is technique-sensitive, and the final restoration is negatively affected by any moisture contamination. If a dry field cannot be maintained, composite resin is probably the worst choice of restorative material. (2) In general, preparations for composite resin restorations in primary teeth are more conservative than preparations for amalgam. Composite resin does not require as much volume to resist clinical fracture as does amalgam, allowing for smaller, more shallow preparations. Noncarious pits and fissures adjacent to caries do not need to be included in the preparation as "extension for prevention"; instead they can simply be sealed as part of the restorative process (Leinfelder, 1996). (3) Because composite resin bonds to tooth structure, the need for mechanical retention in the preparation is lessened. Remember that the bond strengths of resin to enamel are consistently higher than

those of resin to dentin, however, and that reducing mechanical retention in the preparation means a greater reliance on the micromechanical retention of resin to etched enamel. Because primary enamel is approximately one half the thickness of permanent enamel, retention gained solely from acid etching will be similarly reduced, and therefore it is still prudent to include some minor mechanical retention in the preparations. (4) Occlusal wear is the most common problem with posterior composite. Wear will be minimized if the preparation can be kept small and out of heavy occlusion. (5) Common sense and knowledge of the dental materials being used dictate final cavity preparation. No clinical studies since the 1980s have evaluated a conservative, modified preparation for composite resins in primary molars (Oldenburg et al., 1987; Pagrette et al., 1983). The results from these studies were discouraging for the modified resin preparations. Since those studies were published, however, dentin bonding agents have improved dramatically; calcium hydroxide is no longer used to cover all of the dentin, resulting in a larger surface area to bond to; and the resin materials themselves are significantly improved. All of these improvements coupled with documented success of modified preparations in permanent teeth, provide for some level of confidence for successful application in primary teeth.

SEALANTS AND PREVENTIVE RESIN RESTORATIONS FOR PRIMARY TEETH

A thorough discussion of sealants and preventive resin restorations (PRRs) for permanent teeth is found in Chapter 32; however, a brief discussion of their use and placement in primary teeth is included here. Pit and fissure sealants are defined as the application and mechanical bonding of a resin material to an acid-etched enamel surface, thereby sealing existing pits and fissures from the oral environment. This prevents bacteria from colonizing in the pits and fissures and nutrients from reaching the bacteria already present. Although sealants are used for the most part on permanent molars and bicuspids, they may be used in primary teeth as well. The indications for sealing a primary molar are essentially the same as those for permanent teeth. They include (1) deep, retentive pits and fissures that may cause wedging of the explorer, (2) stained pits and fissures with minimal decalcified or opacified appearances, (3) pit and fissure caries or restorations in other primary teeth, (4) no radiographic or clinical evidence of interproximal decay, (5) a patient who is receiving other preventive treatment, such as systemic or topical fluoride to inhibit interproximal caries formation, and (6) situations in which adequate isolation from salivary contamination is possible (Siegal and Kumar, 1995).

Sealants are not widely used on primary teeth for a few reasons. One of the main reasons is moisture control. Teeth must be kept absolutely dry during etching and sealant application. Because sealants alone are usually used without anesthesia and preschool children have a low tolerance for the discomfort of a rubber dam clamp on nonanesthetized gingiva, however, rubber dam placement on primary teeth solely for sealant placement is often avoided. Cotton roll isolation can provide adequate dryness of the tooth in cooperative patients, but poor cooperation makes this isolation extremely difficult. A second reason that sealants are not widely used on primary teeth is the limited lifespan of the tooth. If a second primary molar reaches age 6 without caries, it need only go another 4 to 6 years before it is lost to exfoliation. The cost-effectiveness of sealant placement here needs to be considered. If a child has caries on the occlusal surface of one second primary molar, however, sealing the contralateral molar to prevent caries is probably a prudent decision.

It must be noted that sealant retention on primary molars is similar to that of retention on permanent first molars: 95% after 1 year and 93% after 3 years (Hardison et al., 1987). Additionally, as with permanent molars, when the sealant is retained, caries development in the pits and fissures is virtually eliminated.

Briefly, the technique involves the following steps: (1) isolate the tooth from salivary contamination, (2) clean the tooth surface, (3) acid-etch for 15 to 20 seconds, (4) rinse and dry the surface, (5) apply the sealant to the etched surface, (6) polymerize the sealant, (7) evaluate the sealant with an explorer, and (8) evaluate and adjust the occlusion.

The PRR is a logical extension of sealant philosophy and technique. The preventive approach of sealing susceptible pits and fissures is combined with conservative cavity preparation of caries occurring on the same occlusal surface. Instead of the traditional amalgam cavity preparation's "extension for prevention" beyond the area of decay into the adjacent pits and fissures, the PRR limits cavity preparation to the discrete areas of decay. These preparations are filled with a posterior composite resin and then the entire occlusal surface is sealed. This results in a restoration that conserves tooth structure and is both therapeutic and preventive. A detailed discussion

of PRRs is presented in Chapter 32. Simonsen and Stallard (1977) first described the PRR technique using autopolymerizing resins and identified three types of PRRs: Types A, B, and C. More recently, with wear-resistant posterior composite resins and visible-light polymerization, three similar types of PRRs have been described: Types 1, 2, and 3 (Simonsen, 1985). Although there are minor differences, many use the PRR designations A, B, C and 1, 2, 3 interchangeably. In both classification systems, the first type (A or 1) is the most conservative tooth preparation, progressing to the more involved (B or 2, and C or 3).

The teeth that are suitable for PRRs are those that demonstrate small, discrete regions of decay often limited to a single pit (Fig. 21–11A). As with sealants, the ability to isolate the tooth and keep it dry throughout the procedure is the single most important indication. Amalgam, being less technique- and moisture-sensitive, is the restorative material of choice if the tooth cannot be kept dry. Many PRRs do not require anesthesia because of the minimal tooth preparation, although soft tissue anesthesia may be necessary for comfort in placing the rubber dam.

The Type 1 PRR technique is used when pit and fissure decay is minimal or when the operator is in doubt about the presence of decay and does not want to simply place a pit and fissure sealant. A very small round bur (No. ¼ or ½) is used to widen the fissures and remove the areas of questionable decay (Fig. 21–11B, C). The preparation is confined to enamel. After selective enameloplasty of the fissures, the tooth is etched and a pit and fissure sealant is applied and polymerized.

The Type 2 PRR technique involves a similar ultraconservative preparation with a small round bur in the area of the decay but is used when the preparation extends into dentin (Fig. 21–11D). After caries removal, the entire preparation and occlusal surface is etched, rinsed, and dried, and a bonding agent placed. Then a wear-resistant posterior composite resin material is placed into the cavity preparation with a brush or plastic instrument. Excess resin is gently agitated into the adjacent pits and fissures to act as a pit and fissure sealant. The entire surface is then polymerized.

The Type 3 PRR technique is similar to the Type 2 PRR, except that a sealant layer forms an integral part of the restoration (Fig. 21–11E). As with the Type 2 PRR, the preparation extends into dentin, but in a Type 3 PRR the wear-resistant resin is used only to restore the cavity preparation. Pit and fissure sealant is then applied to seal the adjacent pits and fissures.

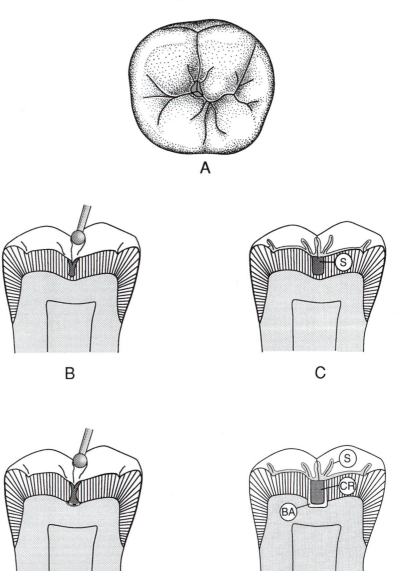

Figure 21–11. *A,* The occlusal surface of a mandibular second primary molar with a small, discrete area of decay in the central pit. *B,* A small round bur (No. ½, No. 1) is used to remove the decay, which is confined to the enamel. *C,* A preventive resin restoration (PRR), Type 1, is placed. A filled sealant (S) is applied into the preparation and over all susceptible pits and fissures. *D,* In this diagram the caries extends into the dentin. Again, a small round bur is used to conservatively remove the decay. *E,* A PRR, Type 3. A bonding agent (BA) and posterior composite resin (CR) material are placed into the preparation. Then, a sealant (S) is applied over all the remaining susceptible pits and fissures.

The PRR is ideally suited for minimal carious lesions in teeth that would otherwise lose a considerable amount of tooth structure if the "extension for prevention" treatment were followed (Simonsen, 1987). Houpt and colleagues (1994) reported 79% retention of PRRs in permanent molars after 9 years and concluded that the PRR was a successful conservative alternative to treatment of minimal occlusal caries. Although long-term retention studies of PRRs in primary teeth are lacking, with retention rates of PRRs and sealants in permanent teeth being similar it is not unreasonable to believe that retention rates of PRRs in primary teeth would also be similar to sealant rates. Retention studies of primary

PRRs would be a welcome addition to the existing literature, however.

CLASS I AND II PREPARATION AND RESTORATION OF PRIMARY MOLARS WITH RESIN

The steps in preparation and restoration of a primary or permanent molar with composite resin are similar to those followed for restoration with amalgam but with a few alterations (Christensen, 1992). Absolute moisture control is a must, making a rubber dam almost mandatory. Tooth preparations for Class II resins have been through a tremendous evolution over the years, with many peculiar shapes and designs suggested. Unlike amalgam preparations, which have been well defined for years, there is no current consensus about the precise design of a Class II resin preparation for a primary molar. Some recommend a G.V. Black Class II amalgam preparation that is modified to be slightly more shallow and narrow, but Leinfelder (1996) recommends that a Class II preparation be primarily restricted to the region of the caries, with little to no occlusal extensions. He also states that extending the proximal box line angles in "self-cleansing" areas is not necessary and in fact creates a larger restoration that is more prone to occlusal wear. The gingival floor of the proximal box should be prepared to preserve as much enamel as possible and have a modest bevel extending cervically. Pre-wedging of teeth is highly desirable to achieve a slight separation of teeth and consequently a tighter interproximal contact of the final restoration. The wedge also protects the interproximal gingival tissue during instrumentation and thereby reduces the likelihood of hemorrhage into the proximal box. The preparation should be etched for 15 to 20 seconds with an acid gel. A dentin-bonding agent or glass ionomer liner is placed before placement of a matrix band and the composite material. Clear plastic or thin steel matrices may be used. Both may provide acceptable results, but the steel bands or strips are easier to use and more reliable in producing adequate contact areas. Circumferential matrix bands that are tightly constricted around the tooth may leave open proximal contacts because there will be minimal condensation force against the band to create a tight contact. Circumferential bands should thus be avoided.

Many composites are pre-packaged in small ampules that can be injected directly into the preparation. A plastic instrument or a condenser can be used to pack or condense the composite into the preparation. No more than a 2 mm depth of composite should be polymerized at one time. Placement of the resin into the preparations should be done incrementally. Donly and associates (1987) found that when the resin was placed in small buccolingual increments, the polymerization shrinkage was significantly less than when the composite was placed in gingivo-occlusal increments or as one complete unit. Complete curing or polymerization of the composite is important to the success of the restoration. Under-curing of the resin may lead to a weakened restoration prone to failure under masticatory forces. Finishing can begin immediately following polymerization. The occlusal surface is grossly contoured with round, high-speed car-

bide finishing burs or fine finishing diamond burs. Gross contouring of proximal surfaces is accomplished with flame-shaped, high-speed carbide finishing burs and with garnet disks, where accessible. Final finishing can be completed with a white stone or with rubber abrasive points to eliminate surface irregularities and final polishing with a composite polish. Fine abrasive disks or strips are used for final polishing of accessible proximal margins. The application of a surface sealant after polishing may serve to reduce occlusal wear and contraction gaps (Lacy and Young, 1996).

Use of Stainless Steel Crowns

Pre-formed or stainless steel crowns were introduced to pediatric dentistry by Humphrey in 1950. Since then they have become an invaluable restorative material in the treatment of badly broken-down primary teeth. As mentioned previously, they are generally considered superior to large multisurface amalgam restorations and have a longer clinical lifespan than two- or three-surface amalgam restorations (Dawson et al., 1981; Einwag and Dunninger, 1996; Messer and Levering, 1988). The crowns are manufactured in different sizes as a metal shell with some pre-formed anatomy and are trimmed and contoured as necessary to fit individual teeth.

There are two commonly used types of stainless steel crowns (Fig. 21–12):

1. Pre-trimmed crowns (Unitek Stainless Steel Crowns, 3M Co., St. Paul, MN; and Denovo

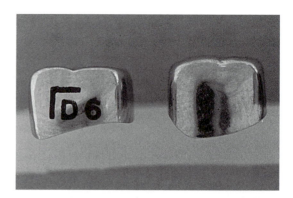

Figure 21–12. This is a buccal view of two types of stainless steel crowns for a mandibular first primary molar. On the left is a Ni-Chro Ion Crown (3M Co., St. Paul, MN). It is a pretrimmed, precontoured crown. On the right is a pretrimmed Unitek (3M Co., St. Paul, MN) crown. Note how much longer the Unitek crown appears. Also note the straight, noncontoured proximal surfaces of the Unitek device. The lettering on the crown identifies it as a left mandibular first molar, size 6.

Crowns, Denovo Co., Arcadia, CA): These crowns have straight, noncontoured sides but are festooned to follow a line parallel to the gingival crest. They still require contouring and some trimming.

2. Precontoured crowns (Ni-Chro Ion Crowns and Unitek Stainless Steel Crowns, 3M Co, St. Paul, MN). These crowns are festooned and are also precontoured. Some trimming and contouring may be necessary but usually are minimal. If trimming of these crowns becomes necessary, the precontour is lost and the crown fits more loosely than before trimming.

INDICATIONS FOR USE OF STAINLESS STEEL CROWNS

1. Restoration of primary or young permanent teeth with extensive carious lesions. These include primary teeth that have caries on three or more surfaces or where the caries extends beyond the anatomic line angles. First primary molars with mesial interproximal lesions are included in this category because the morphologic appearance of the tooth results in inadequate support for mesial interproximal restoration.

2. Restoration of hypoplastic primary or permanent teeth.

3. Restoration of primary teeth after pulpotomy or pulpectomy procedures.

4. Restoration of teeth with hereditary anomalies such as dentinogenesis imperfecta or amelogenesis imperfecta.

5. Restorations in disabled persons or others in whom oral hygiene is extremely poor and failure of other materials is likely.

6. As an abutment for space maintainers or prosthetic appliances.

STEPS OF PREPARATION AND PLACEMENT OF STAINLESS STEEL CROWNS

Several different preparation designs have been advocated over the years. Only one such preparation, requiring minimal tooth reduction, is discussed here. Either Unitek or Ni-Chro Ion crowns may be used following these steps.

1. Evaluate the preoperative occlusion. Note the dental midline and the cusp-fossa relationship bilaterally.

2. Administer appropriate local anesthesia, ensuring that all soft tissues surrounding the tooth to be crowned are well anesthetized, and place a rubber dam. Because gingival tissues all around the tooth may be manipulated during crown placement, it is important to obtain lin-

gual or palatal anesthesia as well as buccal or facial anesthesia.

3. Establish access with a No. 330 or 169L bur in the high-speed handpiece, then remove decay with a large, round bur in the slow-speed handpiece or with a spoon excavator.

4. Reduction of the occlusal surface is carried out with a No. 169L taper fissure bur or a football diamond in the high-speed handpiece. Make depth cuts by cutting the occlusal grooves to a depth of 1.0 to 1.5 mm and extend through the buccal, lingual, and proximal surfaces. Next, place the bur on its side and uniformly reduce the remaining occlusal surface by 1.5 mm, maintaining the cuspal inclines of the crown (Fig. 21-13).

5. Proximal reduction is also accomplished with the taper fissure bur or thin, tapered diamond. Contact with the adjacent tooth must be broken gingivally and buccolingually, maintaining vertical walls with only a slight convergence in an occlusal direction. The gingival proximal margin should have a feather-edge finish line. Care must be taken not to damage adjacent tooth structure. Ledges formed by deep caries should not be removed.

6. Round all line angles, using the side of the bur or diamond. The occlusobuccal and occlusolingual line angles are rounded by holding the bur at a 30- to 45-degree angle to the occlusal surface and sweeping it in a mesiodistal direction. Buccolingual reduction for the stainless steel crown preparation is generally limited to this beveling and is confined to the occlusal one third of the crown. If problems are later encountered in selecting an appropriate crown size or in fitting a crown over a large mesiobuccal bulge, more reduction of the buccal and lingual tooth structure may become necessary. The buccal and lingual proximal line angles are rounded by holding the bur parallel to the tooth's long axis and blending the surfaces together. All of the angles of the preparation should be rounded to remove corners but not so much as to create a round preparation.

7. Selection of a crown begins as a trial-and-error procedure. The goal is to place the smallest crown that can be seated on the tooth and to establish pre-existing proximal contacts. (*Helpful hint:* A size 4 is the most frequently used crown size for molars.) The selected crown is tried onto the preparation by seating the lingual first and applying pressure in a buccal direction so that the crown slides over the buccal surface into the gingival sulcus. Friction should be felt as the crown slips over the buccal bulge. Some teeth are an "in-between" size, so that one crown size

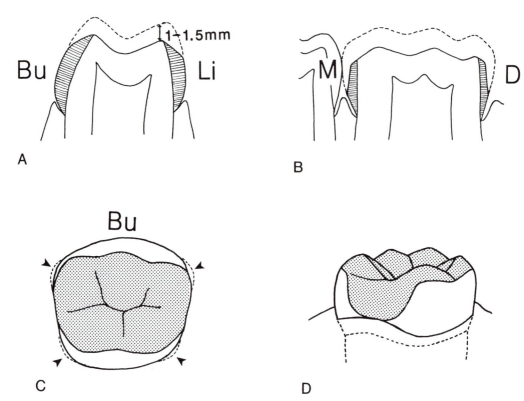

Figure 21–13. Stainless steel crown preparation. Mandibular second primary molar. *A,* Proximal view (Bu = buccal; Li = lingual). *B,* Buccal view. Note feather edge gingival margins. *C,* Occlusal view. Note rounded line angles. *D,* Mesio-lingual view. Note that lingual and buccal reduction is limited to the bevelling of the occlusal one third. (From Stainless Steel Crown Preparation and Restoration, Project TAPP, Quercus Corporation, © 1977.)

is too small to seat and the next larger size fits loosely, even after contouring. Further tooth reduction may be necessary in these cases to seat the smaller crown size.

After seating a crown, establish a preliminary occlusal relationship by comparing adjacent marginal ridge heights. If the crown does not seat to the same level as the adjacent teeth, the occlusal reduction may be inadequate; the crown may be too long; a gingival proximal ledge may exist; or contact may not have been broken with the adjacent tooth, preventing a complete seating of the crown. If an extensive area of gingival blanching occurs around the crown, this indicates that the crown is too long or is grossly overcontoured. Crowns are manufactured longer than necessary for the average tooth, and hence many require some trimming. A properly trimmed crown extends approximately 1 mm into the gingival sulcus. The Ni-Chro Ion precontoured crowns usually require the least trimming. Before trimming, place the crown onto the preparation and lightly mark the level of the gingival crest on the crown with a sharp instrument such as a scaler. The crowns are removed and are

trimmed 1 mm below the mark with crown and bridge scissors or with a heatless wheel on the slow-speed straight handpiece. The crown margins should be trimmed to lie parallel to the contour of the gingival tissue around the tooth and should consist of a series of curves without straight lines or sharp angles.

8. Contour and crimp the crown to form a tightly fitting crown. Contouring involves bending the gingival one third of the crown's margins inward to restore anatomic features of the natural crown and to reduce the marginal circumference of the crown, ensuring a good fit. Contouring is accomplished circumferentially with No. 114 ball and socket pliers (Fig. 21-14A) or with No. 137 Gordon pliers. Final close adaptation of the crown is achieved by crimping the cervical margin 1 mm circumferentially. The No. 137 pliers may be used for this; special crimping pliers, No. 800-417 (Unitek, 3M Co., St. Paul, MN) (Fig. 21-14B), are also available. A tight marginal fit aids in (1) mechanical retention of the crown, (2) protection of the cement from exposure to oral fluids, and (3) maintenance of gingival health. After contouring and crimping, firm resis-

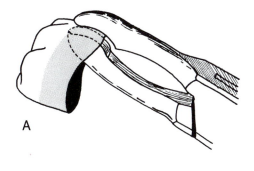

A

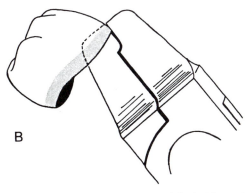

B

Figure 21–14. *A,* Contouring is accomplished with a pair of No. 114 pliers. *B,* Final crimping is accomplished with a pair of No. 800-417 pliers. (From Stainless Steel Crown Preparation and Restoration, Project TAPP, Quercus Corporation, © 1977.)

tance should be encountered when the crown is seated. After seating the crown, examine the gingival margins with an explorer for areas of poor fit. Observe the gingival tissue for blanching, and examine the proximal contacts. If proximal contact needs to be established, it can be done with ball and socket pliers after removal of the crown.

When removing the crown, one can use a scaler or amalgam carver to engage the gingival margin and dislodge the crown. A thumb or finger should be kept over the crown during removal so that the movement of the crown is controlled.

9. The rubber dam is removed and the crown replaced so that the occlusion may be checked. Examine the occlusion bilaterally with the patient in centric occlusion. Look for movement of the crown occlusogingivally with biting pressure, and check for excessive gingival blanching.

After the rubber dam is removed, special care must be taken when handling the crown in the mouth. A 2 × 2 inch gauze pad should be placed

posterior to the tooth being crowned to act as a safety net to prevent the crown from dropping into the oropharynx.

10. Final smoothing and polishing of the crown margin should be performed before final cementation. Smoothing is begun with the heatless stone to create smooth, flowing curves and to thin the margin of the crown slightly. Rotation of the stone should be toward and at a 45-degree angle to the edge of the crown. A rubber wheel is used to remove surface scratches, using light, brushing strokes. A wire brush can be used to polish the margins to a high shine.

11. Rinse and dry the crown inside and out, and prepare to cement it. A zinc phosphate, polycarboxylate, glass ionomer, or self-curing resin-ionomer cement can be used. The crown is filled approximately two thirds with cement, with all inner surfaces covered.

12. Dry the tooth with compressed air, and seat the crown completely. Cement should be expressed from all margins. The handle of a mirror or the flat end of a band pusher may be used to ensure complete seating, or the patient may be instructed to bite on a tongue blade. Before the cement sets, have the patient close into centric occlusion and confirm that the occlusion has not been altered.

13. Cement must be removed from the gingival sulcus. Zinc phosphate cement can be easily removed with an explorer or scaler. Polycarboxylate cement, after it has partially set, reaches a rubbery consistency. Excess cement should be removed at this stage with an explorer tip. The interproximal areas can be cleaned by tying a knot in a piece of dental floss and drawing the floss through the interproximal region.

14. Rinse the oral cavity well, and reexamine the occlusion and the soft tissues before dismissing the patient.

TWO PRINCIPLES FOR OBTAINING OPTIMAL ADAPTATION OF STAINLESS STEEL CROWNS TO PRIMARY MOLARS (Spedding, 1984)

With few exceptions, most stainless steel crowns look good in the mouth. Except in cases of bruxism when crowns may be worn and flattened down, the crowns continue to appear clinically acceptable for many years. The radiographic appearance of the crowns is usually not as encouraging. Radiographically, margins are noted to be poorly adapted to proximal tooth surfaces. Often they are too long. Proximal contours of crowns are not well reproduced. Fortunately, these deficiencies seen to have little adverse effects on the supporting periodontal tissues. The deficiencies

Stainless Steel Crowns in Pediatric Dentistry

N. Sue Seale

The stainless steel crown (SSC) is an often underused and underappreciated restoration for the primary dentition. It is durable, inexpensive, and easily and quickly placed. Because it is frequently lumped with cast crowns in the minds of many dentists, however, it is viewed as an aggressive restorative approach and its indications for use in the primary dentition are poorly understood. For many practitioners, the decision to restore a tooth with a crown denotes excessive tooth removal, great expense, and a general feeling of having compromised the tooth. The weightiness of condemning a permanent tooth to a crown is often transferred to the use of SSCs for the primary teeth. Rarely do dental students have time to assimilate the differences in treatment planning for the developing, changing primary dentition compared with the more static nature of the permanent dentition.

Restorative decisions for the primary dentition are driven by different goals and expectations than for the permanent dentition. The primary teeth are a temporary dentition with known life expectancies of each tooth. By matching the "right" restoration with the expected life span of the tooth, we can succeed in providing a "permanent" restoration that will never have to be replaced. This is essentially impossible in the permanent dentition because the life expectancies of the restorations are much shorter than the life expectancies of the teeth. Picking that "right" restoration involves understanding the limitations of the primary dentition to hold certain types of restorations over time and the durability of the restorative options available. The most commonly used restorative materials available are amalgam, composite, and stainless steel crowns.

The strength of the primary tooth itself, rather than the size of the lesion being restored, is often the major limiting factor in the choice of a successful restoration. Primary teeth are small, with correspondingly thin layers of enamel and dentin, and are intended to fit the face and jaws of the 2-year-old child. The removal of even small carious lesions often compromises the structural integrity of the anterior teeth and first molars. In the primary molars, the contact area is broad, and a relatively large truncated box is required to place the margins of an amalgam or composite in self-cleansing areas. The first primary molar is small, and the buccal and lingual retaining walls become thin and weak with little remaining supporting dentin. Therefore, if the restoration is required to last over 2 years in the first primary molar, shallow preparations combined with weak walls often doom Class II restorations to failure.

Studies evaluating the durability and life span of SSCs and Class II amalgams demonstrate the superiority of crowns for both parameters (Levering and Messer, 1988). Crowns placed in children 4 years of age and younger have a success rate approximately twice that of amalgams for each year up to 10 years of service (Levering and Messer, 1988). This trend is also apparent in children older than 4 years, with the success rate of crowns almost twice that of Class II amalgams for each year up to 10 years of service. When a choice exists between a Class II amalgam and a crown in a child younger than 4 years, the likelihood of failure of the amalgam is approximately twice that of the crown (Levering and Messer, 1988). Where durability is concerned, the SSC is the clear choice.

Two other factors that weigh heavily in the decision to use SSCs are the potential for long-term follow-up and parental compliance in home care. If you will not see the child regularly or home care will not be sufficiently supervised to ensure compliance, an additional advantage of crowns is the preventive aspect that full coverage provides. In the caries-prone child or the child for whom recall and long-term follow-up will be lacking, this restoration provides protection from recurrent caries. Additionally, when a Class II restoration fractures and the proximal box is lost before or during active stages of eruption, mesial drifting results in space loss. The SSC is not subject to failure through fracture and improves the chances of successful restoration even without supervision.

The dental school experience rarely prepares the young general dentist to feel confident in placing SSCs. Therefore, even when the Class II is not the ideal restoration, many choose it because they are most comfortable with it and are confident they can do it well. When these restorations fail, replacement with another amalgam/composite is usually impossible because recurrent caries removal and redefinition of the preparation further weaken the tooth. A crown (and many times a pulpotomy, depending on recurrent caries involvement) is required for retreatment. Cost-comparison studies of restorations in primary teeth have shown that amalgam replaced by a crown is the most costly (Messer and Levering, 1988). Third-party payers are requiring increased accountability for the cost-effectiveness of the outcomes of our treatment. This then becomes part of the multifactorial decision-making process we use to select a restoration, and the expectation for long-term success must be considered. The dentist treating children should recognize the durability, preventive aspect, and cost-effectiveness of the SSC as a restorative choice for the primary dentition.

REFERENCES

Levering NJ, Messer LB: The durability of primary molar restorations: III. Costs associated with placement and replacement. Pediatr Dent *10:*86–93, 1988.
Messer LB, Levering NJ: The durability of primary molar restorations: II. Observations and predictions of success of stainless steel crowns. Pediatr Dent *10:*81–85, 1988.

though can be largely avoided when attention is paid to two key principles: (1) crown length and (2) shape of the crown's gingival margins.

The length of a stainless steel crown should allow the crown to fit just into the gingival sulcus, engaging the natural undercuts. But more importantly, the crown length should extend just slightly apical to the tooth's height of contour. For primary teeth the buccal, lingual, and proximal heights of contour happen to be just above the gingival crest. As a stainless steel crown is trimmed in length such that its gingival margins come closer to the greatest diameters (heights of contour) of the tooth crown, the spaces between the margins of the crown and tooth surfaces lessen. Thus, when the margins of the metal crown nearly approximate the greatest diameter of the tooth, the spaces are small enough so that the metal can be adapted closely to the tooth. In other words, crowns that extend well beyond a tooth's height of contour are difficult to adapt closely to the tooth surface.

The shape or contour of the gingival margins differs from first to second primary molar as well as from buccal to lingual to proximal. The margins of the trimmed crown should approximate the shape of the gingival crest around the tooth. Figure 21–15A demonstrates the different gingival contours. As you look at the marginal gingiva around the second primary molar you will note that the occlusogingival heights gradually become shorter along the crests of the gingival margins toward both the mesial and distal surfaces. The outlines of buccal and lingual gingiva around second primary molars resemble *smiles.* The buccal gingiva of the first primary molar has a different outline. Because of the mesiobuccal cervical bulge, the gingival margin dips down as it is traced from distal to mesial. If you can picture the letter S on its side and stretched out somewhat, and if a tooth crown is placed on top of this curved line, the term *stretched-out S* can be used to describe the contour. The contours of the lingual marginal gingiva of all first primary molars resemble *smiles,* however. The proximal contours of almost all primary teeth *frown* (Fig. 21–15B) because the shortest occlusocervical heights are about midpoint buccolingually. If one keeps these shapes in mind when trimming the stainless steel crowns, the close adaptation to the tooth is made much easier.

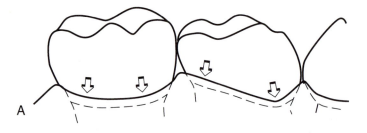

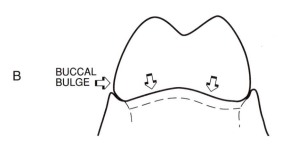

Figure 21–15. *A,* The buccal gingival contour of the second primary molar (on left) has been described as a *smile,* and the buccal gingival contour of the first primary molar has been described as a *stretched-out S.* Note the contour in the region of the mesial buccal bulge of the first primary molar. The gingival contour of all of the lingual surfaces (not pictured) is a smile. *B,* The proximal gingival contour of primary molars has been described as a *frown* because the shortest occlusocervical heights are about midpoint buccolingually.

The margins of the finished, trimmed steel crown consist of a series of curves or arcs as determined by the marginal gingivae of the tooth being restored. There are no corners, jagged angles, right angles, or straight lines on these margins. As described in an earlier section, crown and bridge trimming scissors, a heatless stone mounted on the slow-speed straight handpiece, and a rubber wheel can be used to neatly trim and smooth a stainless steel crown. Contouring and crimping pliers are necessary to apply the appropriate gingival adaptation. Keeping the principles of crown length and marginal shape in mind ensures optimal adaptation and clinical success of the crown.

SPECIAL CONSIDERATIONS FOR STAINLESS STEEL CROWNS (Nash, 1981)

Placement of Adjacent Crowns. When quadrant dentistry is practiced, it often is necessary to place stainless steel crowns on adjacent teeth. The tooth preparation and crown selection for placing multiple crowns are similar to that previously described for single crowns, but a few areas of consideration need to be discussed.

1. Prepare the occlusal reduction of one tooth completely before beginning the occlusal reduction of the other tooth. When reduction of two teeth is performed simultaneously, the tendency is to under-reduce both.

2. Insufficient proximal reduction is a common problem when adjacent crowns are placed.

Contact between adjacent proximal surfaces should be broken, producing an approximately 1.5-mm space at the gingival level.

3. Both crowns should be trimmed, contoured, and prepared for cementation simultaneously. It is generally best to begin placement and cementation of the more distal tooth first. Most importantly, however, the sequence of placement of crowns for cementation should follow the same sequence as that when the crowns were placed for final fitting. Sometimes crowns seat quite easily in one placement sequence and seat with great difficulty if the sequence is altered.

Preparing Crowns in Areas of Space Loss. Frequently, when the tooth structure is lost as a result of caries, a loss of contact and drifting of adjacent teeth into space normally occupied by the tooth to be restored occur. When this happens, the crown required to fit over the buccolingual dimension is too wide mesiodistally to be placed and a crown selected to fit the mesiodistal space is too small in circumference. The larger crown, which fits over the tooth's greatest convexity, is selected, and an adjustment is made to reduce mesiodistal width. One accomplishes this adjustment by grasping the marginal ridges of the crown with Howe utility pliers and squeezing the crown, thereby reducing the mesiodistal dimension. Considerable recontouring of proximal, buccal, and lingual walls of the crown with No. 137 or No. 114 pliers is necessary. If difficulty is still encountered in crown placement, this may necessitate additional tooth reduction of the buccal and lingual surfaces and selection of another, smaller crown.

When the area of space loss is in the region of the distal surface of a mandibular first primary molar and difficulty is encountered as one is finding the appropriately sized crown because of the space loss, an alternative exists. Select a maxillary first primary molar crown for the opposite side of the mouth and try it on the mandibular tooth. Owing to the space loss, the mandibular tooth preparation often more resembles a maxillary tooth and therefore is more suited for placement of the maxillary crown. By selecting the maxillary crown for the opposite side of the mouth, the crown's gingival margin contour in the area of the mesiobuccal cervical bulge fits the mandibular mesiobuccal cervical bulge. If several millimeters of space loss have occurred, it may be necessary to extract the tooth and place a space maintainer, rather than struggle with a crown on a compromised tooth preparation.

RESTORATION OF PRIMARY INCISORS AND CANINES

Indications for restoration of primary incisors and canines are generally based on the presence of (1) caries, (2) trauma, or (3) developmental defects of the tooth's hard tissue. Class III and Class V composite resins are frequently placed in primary anterior teeth. Class IV resins may be used also; however, if a great deal of tooth structure has been lost, full coverage with a crown provides a superior restoration.

Class III Resin Restorations (Fig. 21-16)

Class III resin restorations on primary incisors are challenging to do well. Caries often extends subgingivally, making good isolation and hemorrhage control difficult. Because of the large size of the pulps of these teeth, the preparations must be kept very small. But in spite of one's attempts to keep the restoration small and conservative, experience shows that retention of Class III resins solely with acid etching is often inadequate and that additional mechanical retention is required. Retention can be gained with retentive locks on the facial or lingual surface and by beveling the cavosurface margin to increase the surface area of the enamel etched.

Restoring the distal surface of primary canines (Fig. 21-17) requires a preparation slightly different from the preparation for incisors. The proximal box is directed at a different angle toward the gingiva. Either amalgam or resin may be used as the restorative material in this location. The preparation, with the exception of a short cavosurface bevel for the resin, is identical regardless of the restorative material chosen. A dovetail may be placed on the facial surface, except when amalgam is chosen for a maxillary canine; in that

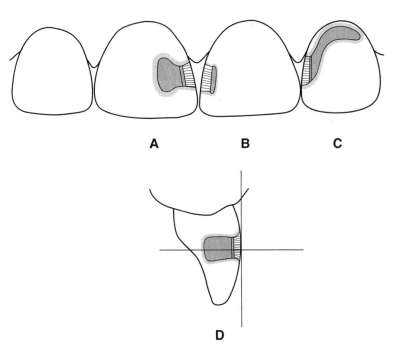

Figure 21–16. Class III cavity preparations (*A, B, C*—labial view). Note that a short bevel is placed on the cavosurface margin of all three preparations. *A,* Slot preparation with a dovetail—the most frequently used class III preparation. The dovetail provides additional retention. *B,* Slot preparation—used for very small class III carious lesions. *C,* Modified slot preparation—used when extensive gingival decalcification is evident adjacent to interproximal caries. *D,* The interproximal box is placed perpendicular to a line tangent to the labial surface.

A   B   C

D

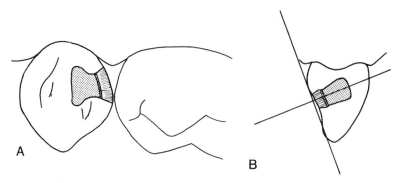

Figure 21–17. Class III preparation for primary canines. *A,* The dovetail is usually placed on the lingual surface of maxillary canines and on the labial surface of mandibular canines. A short bevel (not shown) is placed on the cavosurface margin of preparations to be restored with composite resin. *B,* The proximal box is placed perpendicular to a line tangent to the surface on which the dovetail is placed.

situation, the dovetail is placed on the palatal surface.

STEPS IN PREPARATION AND PLACEMENT OF A CLASS III COMPOSITE RESTORATION

1. Administer appropriate anesthesia, and place the rubber dam. Ligation of individual teeth with dental floss provides the best stability.

2. Create access, and remove caries with a No. 330 bur or a No. 2 round bur in the high-speed handpiece using a facial access. The axial wall is ideally placed 0.5 mm into dentin. A round bur in the slow-speed handpiece can be used to remove deep decay. The gingival and lingual walls should just break contact with the adjacent tooth. Contact with the incisal wall of the preparation need not be broken to ensure adequate remaining tooth structure.

3. To enhance retention, a dovetail or lock is placed on the labial surface. The lock should not extend more than halfway across the labial surface and is kept in the middle horizontal third of the tooth.

4. Place a short bevel (0.5 mm) at the cavosurface margin. This may be accomplished with a fine, tapered diamond or with a flame-shaped composite finishing bur.

5. Clean and dry the preparation with water and compressed air.

6. Etch the preparation for 15 to 20 seconds. An acid gel is preferable. Etching aids in retention and ensures improved marginal integrity and reduced marginal leakage. After etching, rinse and dry the preparation well.

7. Place a plastic matrix. Most matrices first need to be cut in half horizontally because they are manufactured for permanent teeth and are too wide for primary teeth. The matrix is placed interproximally, and a wedge is inserted.

8. Place a dentin bonding agent into the preparation with a small brush. Gently blow compressed air into the preparation to disperse a thin layer of bonding agent evenly over both dentin and enamel.

9. With a plastic instrument or a pressure syringe, place the composite into the preparation and pull the matrix tight around the cavity preparation with finger pressure and hold until cured. Visible light–cured composites provide a controlled polymerization time and are recommended over autopolymerizing materials. Hold the visible light as closely as possible to the composite, and polymerize according to the manufacturer's instructions. The light should be directed from both the facial and the lingual aspects to ensure complete polymerization. Avoid looking directly at the polymerization light when it is turned on.

10. Finishing and polishing can be performed immediately after polymerization. The smoothest and most desirable surface of a composite is that which remains after a properly adapted matrix is removed; however, it is difficult to adapt a matrix so accurately that additional adjustment to the margins is unnecessary. Gross finishing or contouring can be performed with fine grit diamonds or with carbide finishing burs. A flame carbide finishing bur (12–20 flutes) is excellent for finishing the facial and interproximal surfaces. A scalpel with a curved blade may be used to remove gingival flash. The lingual surface is best finished with a round or pear-shaped carbide finishing bur. A lubricated, pointed white stone may also be used for smoothing.

Final interproximal polishing of the restoration is completed with sandpaper strips. These strips are best used if they are cut into thin strips 2 to 3 mm in width. Mounted abrasive disks can be used to finish the facial and lingual surfaces.

After polishing is completed, an unfilled resin glaze may be added to the polished restoration. The glaze helps provide a better marginal seal and a smooth, finished surface. Before adding the glaze, the restoration and surrounding enamel should first be etched for 15 to 20 seconds to remove surface debris. After rinsing and drying, the resin is painted onto the restoration and is polymerized. Care should be taken not to bond adjacent teeth together with the resin glaze.

11. When finishing is completed, remove the rubber dam and floss the interproximal areas to check for overhangs and to remove excess glaze material.

Class V Restorations for Incisors and Canines

Class V restorations may be resins (most frequently) or amalgams. They are most often needed on the facial surface of canines. To prepare these restorations, penetrate the tooth in the area of caries with a No. 330 bur until dentin is reached (approximately 1 mm from the outer enamel surface). Move the bur laterally into sound dentin and enamel, thus establishing the walls of the cavity. The pulpal wall should be convex, parallel to the outer enamel surface. The lateral walls are slightly flared near the proximal surfaces to prevent undermining of enamel. The final external outline is determined by the extent of caries. Mechanical retention in the preparation can be achieved with a No. 35 inverted cone bur or a No. 1/2 round bur, creating small undercuts in the gingivoaxial and incisoaxial line angles. For resins, a short bevel is placed around the entire cavosurface margin. Etching, resin placement, and finishing are similar to that described for Class III composite placement, except that no matrix is used.

Full Coronal Coverage of Incisors
(Fig. 21–18)

INDICATIONS

1. Incisors with large interproximal lesions
2. Incisors that have undergone pulp therapy
3. Incisors that have been fractured and have lost an appreciable amount of tooth structure
4. Incisors with multiple hypoplastic defects or developmental disturbances (e.g., ectodermal dysplasia)
5. Discolored incisors that are esthetically unpleasing
6. Incisors with small interproximal lesions that also have large areas of cervical decalcification

It is a challenging task to repair extensively destroyed anterior teeth with restorations that

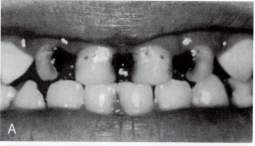
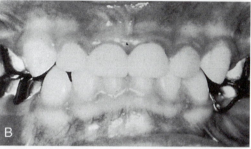
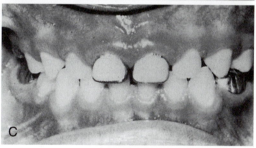

Figure 21–18. Full coronal coverage of primary incisors. *A,* Extensive caries in primary incisors. *B,* Same incisors after restoration with acid-etched composite crowns. *C,* Open-face stainless steel crowns on maxillary central incisors (see Fig. 21–1 for lingual view).

are durable, retentive, and esthetic. There are several methods of providing full coronal coverage to primary incisors; acid-etched resin crowns (Fig. 21–18B), stainless steel crowns, and veneered or open-face stainless steel crowns (Fig. 21–18C). Each has shortcomings (Table 21–2), but each may be used at some time. The most esthetic, and a frequently placed crown, is the acid-etched resin crown. Open-face crowns are popular with many operators because their retention is superior to resin crowns; however, esthetic results are compromised. Plain stainless steel crowns provide a durable restoration but are esthetically unpleasing to most parents. Stainless steel crowns with a resin veneer prebonded to the facial surface are commercially available. These crowns provide a one-step esthetic restoration that, unlike resin or open-face crowns, can be placed in the presence of hemorrhage without affecting the final esthetics.

TABLE 21–2. Comparison of Full-Coverage Techniques for Primary Incisors

Technique	Esthetics	Durability	Time for Placement	Selection Criteria
Resin (Strip) crowns*	Very good initially; may discolor over time	Retention depends on amount of tooth structure present and quality of acid etch. Can be dislodged fairly easily if traumatized	Time required for optimal isolation, etching, placement, finishing	When esthetics are a great concern. Adequate tooth structure remains for etching/bonding. Child is not highly trauma-prone. Gingival hemorrhage is controllable
Steel crowns	Poor	Very good; a well-crimped, cemented crown is very retentive and wears well	Fastest crown to place	Severely decayed teeth. Esthetics of little concern. Unable to adequately control gingival hemorrhage. Need to place a restoration quickly because of inadequate cooperation or time
Open-face steel crowns	Good; however, usually some metal is showing	Good—like steel crowns, are very retentive; however, facings may be dislodged	Takes longest to place because of two-step procedure: • Crown placement • Composite placement	Severely decayed teeth. Durability needed—active, accident-prone child or severe bruxism evident
Prefabricated veneered steel crowns	Good	Good, although facings occasionally break	Not as fast as the plain steel crown; must make tooth fit the crown	Esthetics are a concern. Hemorrhage difficult to control

*Restoration of choice esthetically.

PREPARATION AND PLACEMENT OF RESIN CROWNS

1. Administer appropriate anesthesia.
2. Select the shade of composite resin to be used, then place and ligate the rubber dam.
3. Select a primary incisor celluloid crown form (Unitek Strip Crown, 3M Co., St. Paul, MN) with a mesiodistal width approximately equal to the tooth to be restored.
4. Remove decay with a large round bur in the slow-speed handpiece. If pulp therapy is required, do it at this time.
5. Reduce the incisal edge 1.5 mm, using a fine, tapered diamond or a No. 169L bur.
6. Reduce the interproximal surfaces 0.5 to 1.0 mm (Fig. 21-19). This reduction should allow a crown form to slip over the tooth. The interproximal walls should be parallel, and the gingival margin should have a feather edge.
7. Reduce the facial surface at least 1.0 mm

and the lingual surface 0.5 mm. Create a feather-edge gingival margin. Round all line angles.

8. Place a small undercut on the facial surface in the gingival one third of the tooth with a No. 330 bur or a No. 35 inverted cone. When the resin material polymerizes, engaging the undercut, this serves as a mechanical lock.
9. Trim the selected crown form by cutting away excess material gingivally with crown and bridge scissors, and trial-fit the crown form. A properly trimmed crown form should fit 1 mm below the gingival crest and should be of comparable height to adjacent teeth. Remember that maxillary lateral incisor crowns are usually 0.5 to 1.0 mm shorter than those of central incisors.
10. After the celluloid crown is adequately trimmed, punch a small hole in the lingual surface with an explorer to act as a vent for the escape of trapped air as the crown is placed with resin onto the preparation.
11. Etch the tooth for 15 to 20 seconds using

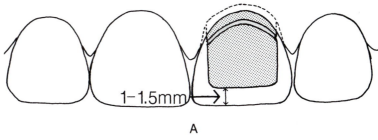

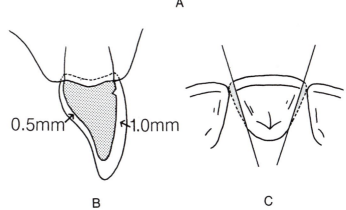

Figure 21–19. Acid-etched (strip) composite crown preparation. *A,* Labial view. *B,* Proximal view. *C,* Incisal view. The proximal slice should be parallel to the natural external contours of the tooth.

an acid gel. Rinse and dry the tooth thoroughly, then apply a dentin bonding agent to the entire tooth.

12. Fill the crown form approximately two-thirds full with a resin material, and seat it onto the tooth. Excess material should flow from the gingival margin and the vent hole. While holding the crown in place, remove the gingival excess with an explorer.

13. Allow the material to polymerize. If using a light-cured material, be certain to direct the light from both the facial and lingual directions.

14. Remove the celluloid form by using a composite finishing bur or a curved scalpel blade to cut the material on the lingual aspect, and then peel the form from the tooth.

15. Remove the rubber dam and evaluate the occlusion.

16. Little finishing should be required on the facial surface. A flame carbide finishing bur can be used to finish the gingival margin should any irregularities be noted on a tactile examination with an explorer. A round or pear-shaped finishing bur may be used for final contouring of the lingual surface. Abrasive disks are used for final polishing of the areas of the crown that require contouring.

PREPARATION AND PLACEMENT OF AN OPEN-FACE (CHAIRSIDE-VENEERED) STEEL CROWN

Nonveneered stainless steel crowns are not frequently used on maxillary primary incisors be-

cause of the poor esthetics. They are often used on severely decayed canines and mandibular incisors, however, where esthetics are less noticeable. Steps for preparation and placement of both veneered (Helpin, 1983) and nonveneered crowns are discussed in this part of the chapter.

The preparation for a steel crown is identical to that of a resin crown, except no facial undercut is made for the steel crown. After the preparation is completed, select a crown and try it on the tooth. Anterior steel crowns often need to have their cervical shapes changed before placement. When manufactured, the crowns have an ovoid shape with a small faciolingual dimension. This must often be changed to allow the crown to slip onto the tooth. This is done by simply squeezing the crown slightly mesiodistally with a pair of Howe No. 110 utility pliers, thereby increasing the faciolingual dimension. The fit of the crown should be snug, and difficulty may be encountered seating the crown with finger pressure only. A gentle rocking of the crown faciolingually facilitates its seating. An orthodontic band pusher or tongue blade may be used to aid in seating, but care should be used not to apply too much pressure. Anterior steel crowns do not generally require much trimming. If trimming is necessary, it is best done with a heatless stone on a straight slow-speed handpiece.

Contouring and crimping are necessary to ensure a good marginal fit. No. 137 Gordon pliers are best suited for this task. Check the final marginal adaptation with an explorer. Polishing and cementation procedures are identical to those for posterior steel crowns. These procedures complete the nonveneered stainless steel crown placement. For placement of the open-face or veneered steel crown, the cement must be allowed to set completely, then a labial window is cut in the crown using a No. 330 or No. 35 bur. The window extends just short of the incisal edge—gingivally, to the height of the gingival crest, and mesiodistally, to the line angles. It is desirable that little metal be seen from the facial aspect. With a No. 35 inverted cone bur (Fig. 21–20), remove the cement to a depth of 1 mm. Undercuts must be placed at each margin. This can be performed with the No. 35 bur or with a No. ½ round bur. Mechanical retention is necessary because there is usually little enamel to etch. Smooth the cut margins of the crown with a fine green or white finishing stone.

A thin layer of dentin bonding agent and then composite is placed into the cut window, engaging the undercuts. Resin is added with a plastic instrument. Polymerize the resin, and finish with abrasive disks. Always run the disks from resin to metal at the margins. Disks running from metal to resin discolor the resin with metal particles.

As mentioned previously, some new pre-veneered stainless steel crowns for primary incisors and canines are now commercially available (Kinder Krowns, Mayclin Dental Studios, Minneapolis, MN; Whiter Bite II Crowns, White Bite, Inc., Visalia, CA; NuSmile Primary Crowns, Houston, TX; Cheng Crowns, Peter Cheng Orthodontic Laboratories, Philadelphia, PA). The advantages of these crowns are that an aesthetically pleasing result can be obtained with relatively short operating time, and the steel crown is durable. Additionally, when moisture control is difficult and the resin crowns cannot be placed, these crowns, being less moisture-sensitive, may offer a good alternative. The preparation of the teeth for these crowns is similar to the preparation just described for the nonveneered and the

open-face crown with one important distinction. These preveneered crowns allow for little recontouring or reshaping, and therefore the operator must prepare and adjust the tooth to fit the crown, rather than adjusting the crown to fit the tooth. In general, more tooth reduction, especially on the lingual aspect, is necessary to fit these crowns. When fitting these crowns it is important that a "snap" fit not be achieved. Forcing these crowns onto a prepared tooth under a lot of pressure often leads to microfractures of the veneer and ultimate veneer loss. A snug, sleeve-like fit of the crown over the tooth is recommended.

These crowns have three limitations: (1) crimping is limited primarily to the lingual surfaces, thereby not allowing as close an adaptation, (2) these crowns cost approximately $17–$18.00 apiece, compared with $2.25–$2.50 for plain stainless steel, making an inventory much more costly, and (3) there are no published clinical data available as to the durability of these crowns. Anecdotal information, however, indicates that these crowns can provide aesthetically pleasing results for several years. The most common problem with these crowns is that part of the veneer occasionally chips off. This is usually a result of either trauma or forcing the crown onto the tooth with excessive pressure during cementation. If part of the veneer is lost it can be repaired by the cutting of a small window in the stainless steel, as is done for an open-face crown, and new composite can be added. If the veneer fracture is large, simply replacing the crown may provide a faster, more esthetic result.

PROSTHETIC REPLACEMENT OF PRIMARY ANTERIOR TEETH

Premature loss of maxillary primary incisors as a result of extensive caries, trauma, or congenital absence requires consideration for providing a

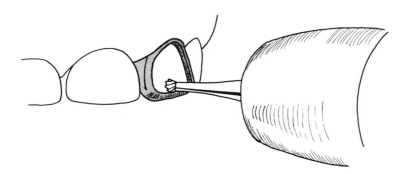

Figure 21–20. Cut the window for the facing in the cemented stainless steel crown and create mechanical undercuts laterally and incisally with an inverted cone bur.

prosthetic tooth replacement for the child (Steffen et al., 1971). In most instances, prosthetic replacement of primary incisors is considered an elective procedure. Space maintenance in this region is not generally necessary. The most frequent reason for placement of a prosthetic appliance is parental concern about esthetics.

Lack of compliance in appliance wear and care by the young child is the greatest limitation of and contraindication for these appliances. If a young child decides that he or she does not like the appliance, the child will find a way to remove it from the mouth and will usually discard it. Education of the parents of this fact is essential before the decision to construct an appliance is made. Another contraindication for prosthetic replacement is the presence of an anterior deep bite.

Prosthetic appliances may be either fixed or removable (Fig. 21–21), and many different designs are used for both. When constructing either type, it is best to allow at least 6 to 8 weeks after the tooth loss before fabrication. This allows for good healing and gingival shrinkage and results in a better fitting, more esthetic appliance.

One fixed appliance design is a Nance-like device, constructed with two bands or, preferably, steel crowns on primary molars that are connected by a palatal wire to which the replacement teeth are attached. These prosthetic appliances can be fabricated by any laboratory, but they are commercially available through Space Maintainers Laboratory of Van Nuys, CA. This appliance is cemented onto the molars and is not easily removed by the child. It requires minimal adjustment. The teeth can be made to sit directly on the ridge of the edentulous space, or acrylic gingiva can be added. Disadvantages of this appliance include (1) possible decalcification around the bands, (2) more difficulty in home cleaning, and (3) bending of the wires with fingers or sticky foods, which may create occlusal interferences and the need for adjustments. Potential loosening of the bands resulting from continual torquing of bands by the movement of the wire during normal chewing may necessitate frequent recementation.

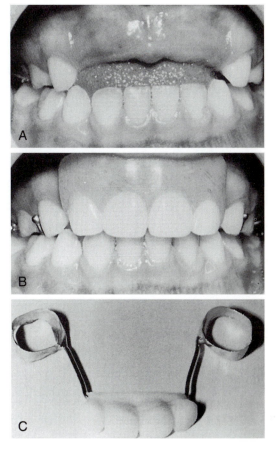

Figure 21–21. Prosthetic replacement of primary anterior teeth. *A,* Edentulous space following extraction of four primary incisors. *B,* Removable prosthetic appliance in place. *C,* Example of a fixed prosthetic appliance replacing four incisors. *Note:* Orthodontic bands are used here; however, stainless steel crowns will often provide better retention and durability for the abutment attachment. (Courtesy of Dr. Gary Nelson, Paradise, CA.)

Atraumatic Restorative Treatment

Michael Kanellis

Atraumatic Restorative Treatment (ART) is a minimally invasive treatment technique for restoring teeth via hand instrumentation for decay removal and fluoride-releasing adhesive materials (glass ionomer) for filling (Frencken et al., 1996) ART has been promoted by the World Health Organization (WHO) as a means of delivering care in underdeveloped countries that do not have electricity or access to sophisticated dental equipment (Phantumvanit et al., 1996; WHO, 1994). Some dentists in developed countries use ART as a means for stabilizing the caries process in young children until they are old enough to cooperate for definitive care or as the definitive treatment of choice for selected procedures.

There are several potential advantages to ART when used with young children. Because hand instrumentation is used, the noise and vibration of dental handpieces is eliminated. Also eliminated is the need for acid etching, water coolant, and the accompanying high-velocity suction. Caries removal using hand instrumentation also often eliminates the need for local anesthesia. Because instrumentation is kept to a minimum, treatment can easily be carried out in the knee-to-knee position. The use of a fluoride-releasing restorative material helps prevent further decay (Figs. 21–22, 21–23, 21–24, and 21–25).

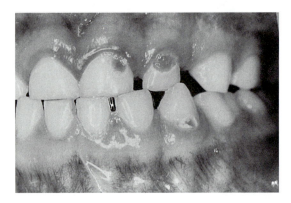

Figure 21–22. Facial caries evident on incisors and cuspid.

Figure 21–23. Spoon excavator positioned for decay removal.

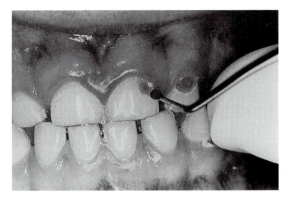

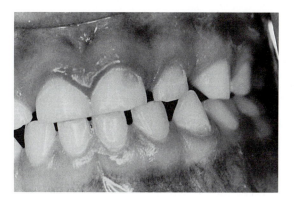

Figure 21–24. Appearance after caries removal with spoon excavator.

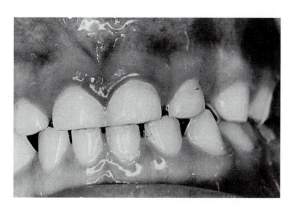

Figure 21–25. Teeth restored with glass ionomer restorative material.

REFERENCES

Frencken JE, Pilot T, Songpaisan Y, Phantumvanit P: Atraumatic restorative treatment (ART): Rationale, technique, and development. J Public Health Dent *56*(3):135-140, 1996.

Phantumvanit P, Songpaisan Y, Pilot T, Frencken JE: Atraumatic restorative treatment (ART): A three-year community field trial in Thailand—survival of one-surface restorations in the permanent dentition. J Public Health Dent *56*(3):141-145, 1996.

WHO: Revolutionary new procedure for treating dental caries. Press release WHO/28, Apr 7, 1994.

The removable appliance is a Hawley-like device that replaces the teeth and utilizes circumferential and ball clasps on the molars. These appliances require the most compliance of any of the prosthetic replacements. They are not indicated in children under 3 years old. Clasps will need adjustment, the frequency of which depends on the child's handling of the appliances. The greatest advantages of these appliances are the ability to remove the appliance for daily cleaning and the fact that adjustments are easily made by the dentist without having to remove and re-cement bands.

REFERENCES

ADA Council on Dental Materials, Instruments, and Equipment: Posterior composite resins. JADA *112*(5):707-709, 1986a.

ADA Council on Dental Materials, Instruments, and Equipment: Posterior composite resins: An update. JADA *113*(6):950, 1986b.

Bhaskar SN, Lilly GE: Intrapulpal temperature during cavity preparation. J Dent Res 44(4):644-647, 1965.

Black GV: A Work on Operative Dentistry, 5th ed, Vol 11. Chicago, Medico-Dental Publishing, 1924.

Black R: Technique for nonmechanical preparation of cavities and prophylaxis. JADA 39:953-965, 1945.

Bouschor CF, Matthews JL: A four-year clinical study of teeth restored after preparation with an air turbine handpiece with air coolant. J Pros Dent 16(2):306-309, 1966.

Christensen GJ: Don't underestimate the class II resin. JADA 123(3):103-104, 1992.

Christensen GJ: Restoration of pediatric posterior teeth. JADA 127(1):106-108, 1996.

Dawson LR, Simon JF, Taylor PP: Use of amalgam and stainless steel restorations for primary molars. J Dent Child 48(6):420-422, 1981.

Donly KJ, Jensen ME, Reinhardt J, Walker JD: Posterior composite polymerization shrinkage in primary teeth: An in vivo comparison of three restorative techniques. Pediatr Dent 9(1):22-25, 1987.

Donly KJ, Wild TW, Jensen ME: Posterior composite Class II restorations: in vitro comparison of preparation designs and restorative techniques. Dent Mater 6:88-93, 1990.

Einwag J, Dunninger P: Stainless steel crown versus multisurface amalgam restorations: An 8 year longitudinal study. Quintess Int 22(5):321-323, 1996.

Goldstein RE, Parkins FM: Air abrasive technology: Its new role in restorative dentistry. JADA 125:551-557, 1994.

Hardison JR, Collier OR, Sprouse CW, et al: Retention of pit and fissure sealants on the primary molars of 3- and 4-year-old children after 1 year. JADA 114(4):613-615, 1987.

Helpin ML: The open-face steel crown restoration in children. J Dent Child 50(1):34-38, 1983.

Houpt M, Fuks A, Eidelman E: The preventive resin (composite/sealant) restoration: Nine year results. Quintess Int 25(3):155-159, 1994.

Humphrey WP: Use of chromic steel in children's dentistry. Dent Surv 26:945-947, 1950.

Lacy AM, Young DA: Modern concepts and materials for the pediatric dentist. Pediatr Dent 18(7):469-475, 1996.

Leinfelder KF: A conservative approach to placing posterior composite resin restorations. JADA 127(6):743-748, 1996.

Leinfelder KF, Sluder TB, Santos JR, Wall JT: Five-year clinical evaluation of anterior and posterior restorations of composite resin. Oper Dent 5:57-65, 1980.

Leinfelder KF, Vann WF: The use of composite resins on primary molars. Pediatr Dent 4(1):27-31, 1982.

Messer LB, Levering NJ: The durability of primary molar restorations: II. Observations and predictions of success of stainless steel crowns. Pediatr Dent 10(2):81-85, 1988.

Myers DR: Factors producing failure of class II silver amalgam restorations in primary molars. J Dent Child 44(3):226-229, 1977.

Nash DA: The nickel-chromium crown for restoring posterior primary teeth. JADA 102(1):44-49, 1981.

Norman RD, Wright JS, Rydberg RJ, Felkner LL: A 5-year study comparing a posterior composite resin and an amalgam. J Prosthet Dent 64(5):523-529, 1990.

Oldenburg TR, Vann WF, Dilley DC: Composite restorations for primary molars: Results after four years. Pediatr Dent 9(2):136-143, 1987.

Paquette DE, Vann WF, Oldenburg TR, Leinfelder K: Modified cavity preparations for composite resins in primary molars. Pediatr Dent 5(4):246-251, 1983.

Pereira JC, Manfio AP, Franco EB, Lopes ES: Clinical evaluation of Dycal under amalgam restorations. Am J Dent 3:67-70, 1990.

Roberts JF, Sherriff M: The fate and survival of amalgam and preformed crown molar restorations placed in a specialist pediatric dental practice. Br Dent J 169(10):237-239, 1990.

Roberts MW, Folio J, Moffa JP, Guckes AD: Clinical evaluation of a composite resin system with a dental bonding agent for restoration of permanent posterior teeth: A 3-year study. J Prosthet Dent 67:301-306, 1992.

Siegal MD, Kumar JV: Workshop on guidelines for sealant use: Recommendations. J Public Health Dent 55:263-273, 1995.

Simonsen RJ: Conservation of tooth structure in restorative dentistry. Quintess Int 16(1):15-24, 1985.

Simonsen RJ: The preventive resin restoration: A minimally invasive, nonmetallic restoration. Compend Cont Educ Dent 8(6):428-435, 1987.

Simonsen RJ, Stallard RE: Sealant-restorations utilizing a dilute filled resin: One year results. Quintess Int 8(6):77-84, 1977.

Spedding RH: Two principles for improving the adaptation of stainless steel crowns to primary molars. Dent Clin North Am 28(1):157-175, 1984.

Steffen JM, Miller JB, Johnson R: An esthetic method of anterior space maintenance. J Dent Child 38(3):154-157, 1971.

Straffon LH, Corpron RE, Dennison JB, et al: A clinical evaluation of polished and unpolished amalgams: 36 month results. Pediatr Dent 6(4):220-225, 1984.

Waggoner WF: Composite restorations of posterior teeth—current status. J Okla Dent Assoc 74(2):39-43, 1984.

Chapter 22

Pulp Therapy for the Primary Dentition

Anna B. Fuks

Chapter Outline

Despite modern advances in the prevention of dental caries and an increased understanding of the importance of maintaining the natural dentition, many teeth are still lost prematurely. This can lead to malocclusion or to esthetic, phonetic, or functional problems that may be transient or permanent (Fuks and Eidelman, 1991; Levine et al., 1988). Maintaining the integrity and health of the oral tissues is the primary objective of pulp treatment. It is desirable to attempt to maintain pulp vitality whenever possible. Pulp autolysis, however, can be stabilized, or the pulp can be entirely eliminated without significantly compromising the function of the tooth.

This chapter briefly reviews the normal histology of the primary pulp and the reaction of the pulp-dentin complex to operative procedures and to dental caries, and it discusses the basis for the different forms of pulpal treatment for the primary dentition.

THE PULP-DENTIN COMPLEX

Histology

The pulp of a primary tooth is histologically similar to that of a permanent tooth. The odontoblasts line the periphery of the pulp space and extend their cytoplasmic processes into the dentinal tubules. These cells have several junctions, which provide a means for intercellular communication and help to maintain the relative position of one cell to another. The cell-free zone is located just below the odontoblastic layer and contains an extensive plexus of unmyelinated nerves and blood capillaries. The core of the dental pulp contains larger blood vessels and nerves, which are surrounded by loose connective tissue (Torneck, 1985). The odontoblasts are highly specialized cells and are responsible for the formation of dentin. Owing to the extension of their cytoplasmic processes into the dentinal tubules, these cells make up the main part of the pulp-dentin complex. When this complex is damaged by disease or attrition or is affected by operative procedures, it reacts in an attempt to defend the pulp.

Reactions to Dental Caries

When the carious process advances from the enamel into the dentin, sclerotic dentin is formed by the apposition of minerals into and between the tubules (intratubular and intertubular dentin), and reparative or tertiary dentin is secreted by other mesenchymal-type cells of the pulp that differentiate into new odontoblasts. The quality and amount of tertiary dentin depend on the depth and rate of progression of the carious lesion. The faster the lesion progresses, the poorer and more irregular is the reparative dentin. In addition, if the noxious irritant is too intense, the cytoplasmic processes of the odontoblasts degenerate and "dead tracts" are formed.

When the carious process advances more rapidly than the elaboration of reparative dentin, the blood vessels of the pulp dilate, and scattered inflammatory cells become evident, particularly subjacent to the area of the involved dentinal tubules (transitional stage). If the carious lesion remains untreated, a frank exposure eventually occurs. The pulp reacts with an infiltration of acute inflammatory cells, and the chronic pulpitis becomes acute. A small abscess may develop under the region of the exposure, and cells of the chronic inflammatory series may be formed further away from the central area of irritation. The remainder of the pulp may be uninflamed (chronic partial pulpitis with acute exacerbation). As the exposure progresses, the pulp may undergo partial necrosis, followed in some instances by total necrosis.

Drainage is apparently the factor determining whether or not partial or total necrosis will occur. If the pulp is open and drainage can occur, the apical tissue may remain uninflamed or chronically inflamed. If drainage is impeded by food packing or a restoration, the entire pulp may become necrotic more rapidly. Figure 22–1 describes the reaction of the pulp to dental caries.

Reactions to Operative Procedures

The factors affecting the dentin-pulp complex during operative procedures (cavity and crown preparations) are mainly the cutting of the dentin per se, the generation of heat, and the desiccation of the tissue. When uninvolved dentin undergoes operation, as in extension for prevention or in crown preparation, tubules that are not protected by reparative dentin are cut. The tissue reaction that occurs is similar to that occurring with caries: intratubular and intertubular mineralization takes place, resulting in sclerotic dentin, followed by the formation of tertiary dentin. The amount and regularity of the tertiary dentin are related to the depth of the cavity preparation: As depth is increased, production of reparative dentin is enhanced but its regularity and quality are compromised. Also, dead tracts may result from damage done to the odontoblastic processes. The effect of cutting the dentin can be observed histologically as a calciotraumatic band, which represents an interruption of the apposition between the secondary and tertiary dentin.

Pulp reactions to operative procedures can be mild or severe, depending on the technique used. When the technique is gentle, the reaction is mild, and minor alterations in the odontoblastic layer can be observed as a result of fluid accumulation. In a severe reaction, the nuclei of the odontoblasts may be aspirated into the dentinal tubules, hemorrhage may be present, and inflammation is extensive, sometimes resulting in cell necrosis. The sequence of pulp reaction to irritation resulting from operative procedures as related to the state of the pulp is summarized in Figure 22–2.

A gentle technique implies using appropriate cooling and minimal pressure. Cutting a cavity without using water cooling might lead to irreversible changes in the pulp owing to the heat generated at the tip of the bur. The application of pressure increases the damage. Prolonged air blasts are also deleterious to the pulp. It has been demonstrated by Langeland (1957) that a blast of air on the dentin for 10 seconds is enough to produce displacement of odontoblastic nuclei. Thus, in order to prevent the generation of heat and damage to the pulp, the following measures should be taken: (1) The cavity should be prepared as shallowly as possible, respecting the principles of cavity preparation, (2) small and sharp burs should be used, (3) appropriate cooling should be employed and minimal pressure exerted, and (4) excessive drying of dentin by air syringe should be avoided.

CLINICAL PULPAL DIAGNOSIS

It is difficult if not impossible to determine *clinically* the *histologic* status of the pulp. With thor-

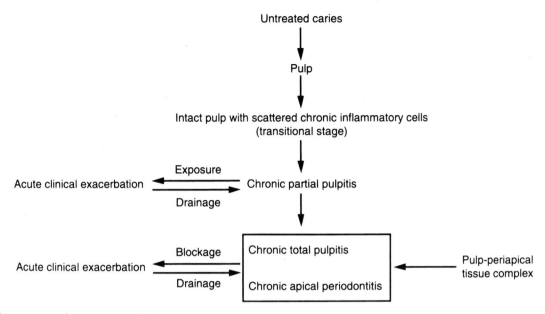

Figure 22–1. Pulp reactions to dental caries. (From Seltzer S, Bender IB: The Dental Pulp, 3rd ed. Philadelphia, JB Lippincott, 1984, p 188.)

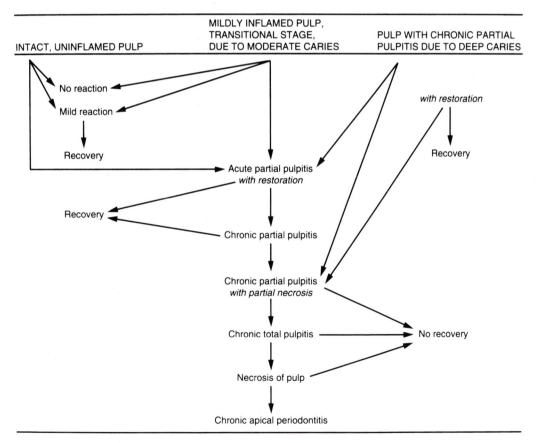

Figure 22–2. Sequence of pulp reaction to irritation from operative procedures. (From Seltzer S, Bender IB: The Dental Pulp, 3rd ed. Philadelphia, JB Lippincott, 1984, p 256.)

ough clinical and radiographic assessment, however, it is possible to determine whether the tooth pulp is treatable. Selection of the appropriate treatment for a tooth is essential to its long-term prognosis. To make the most accurate diagnosis, information must be obtained from several sources, including a careful medical history and notation of the characteristics of the pain, and thorough clinical and radiographic examinations.

History and Characteristics of Pain

The history and characteristics of pain are often important in determining whether the pulp is in a treatable condition. Children may have extensive carious lesions, however, often with draining paruli, with no apparent history of pain or, if dental problems developed early (such as with nursing bottle decay), the child may have no experience of the teeth feeling any other way (Belanger, 1988). Being aware of these limitations, the dentist should distinguish between two main types of dental pain, "provoked" and "spontaneous." Provoked pain is stimulated by thermal, chemical, or mechanical irritants and is reduced or eliminated when the noxious stimulus is removed. This sign frequently indicates dentin sensitivity due to a deep carious lesion or a faulty restoration. The pulp is in a transitional state in most cases (see Fig. 22–1), and the condition is usually reversible.

Spontaneous pain is a throbbing, constant pain that may keep the patient awake at night. This type of pain usually indicates advanced pulpal damage, and the pulp is usually nontreatable. A final diagnosis can only be based on clinical tests in conjunction with radiographic assessment, however. Spontaneous, throbbing pain simulating an irreversible pulp condition can be observed when the dental papilla is inflamed owing to food impaction. This condition may cause bone destruction, and the pulp in these teeth may well be treatable. The symptoms disappear with proper restoration of the tooth and reestablishment of an adequate contact point (Fig. 22–3).

The chief complaint and the history of pain are important factors to be considered when establishing a diagnosis. Additionally, an accurate medical history is imperative. A child with a systemic disease may require an alternative treatment approach than that used for a healthy child.

Clinical Examination

A careful extraoral and intraoral examination can be of extreme importance in detecting the pres-

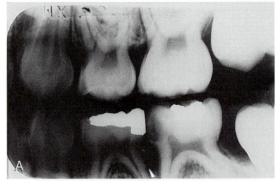
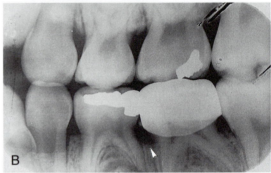

Figure 22–3. *A,* Mandibular second primary molar with extensive mesial caries and alveolar bone resorption (*arrow*) due to food impaction. The history of spontaneous pain associated with tenderness to percussion may suggest pulp involvement. *B,* The same tooth after restoration of the contact point with a stainless steel crown. The symptoms disappeared and bone regeneration is evident (*arrow*). (Courtesy of Enrique Bimstein, CD.)

ence of a pulpally involved tooth. Several signs, such as redness and swelling of the vestibulum or grossly decayed teeth with draining paruli, are definitely indicative of pulpal pathoses. In addition, attention should be paid to missing or fractured restorations or to those with carious marginal breakdown because these may also be indicators of pulp involvement.

Palpation, assessment of tooth mobility, and sensitivity to percussion are helpful diagnostic tools. Fluctuation, felt by palpating a swollen muccobuccal fold, may be the expression of an acute dentoalveolar abscess prior to exteriorization. Bone destruction after a chronic dentoalveolar abscess can also be detected by palpation. Comparing the mobility of a suspicious tooth with its contralateral tooth is of particular importance. If a significant difference is observed, pulpal inflammation might be suspected. Care should be taken not to misinterpret as pathologic the mobility present during the normal time of exfoliation. Sensitivity to percussion may reveal a painful tooth in which inflammation has progressed to involve the periodontal ligament (acute apical periodontitis). Care should be taken in interpreting these tests (see Fig. 22-3). Belanger (1988) suggests that percussion should be done gently—with the tip of a finger and not with the end of a dental mirror—to prevent exposing the child to unnecessary uncomfortable stimuli.

Other classic vitality tests, such as sensitivity to heat or cold or electric pulp testing, are of little value because they seldom provide accurate data in primary teeth. False-positive results may be obtained from stimulation of the gingiva or of the periodontal ligament. In addition, because a child might be apprehensive, use of this type of stimulation by the dentist might lose the child's confidence, causing disruptive behavior.

Radiographic Examination

The clinical examination should be followed by a high-quality bitewing radiograph. Inter-radicular radiolucencies, a common finding in primary teeth with pulpal pathoses, can be better observed in bitewing radiographs. If the apical area cannot be clearly observed in such a film, a periapical view of the affected side should be obtained. The integrity of the lamina dura of the affected tooth should be compared with that of adjacent or contralateral teeth. Radiographs are valuable as aids in visualizing the presence or absence of the following:

1. Deep caries with possible or definite pulp involvement
2. Deep restorations close to a pulp horn
3. Successful or failing pulpotomy or pulpectomy
4. Pulpal changes, such as pulp calcifications (denticles) and pulp obliteration
5. Pathologic root resorption, that may be internal (within the root canal) or external (affecting the root or the surrounding bone). Internal resorption indicates inflammation of a vital pulp, whereas external resorption demonstrates a nonvital pulp with extensive inflammation, including resorption of the adjacent bone.
6. Periapical and inter-radicular radiolucencies of bone. In primary teeth, any radiolucency associated with a nonvital tooth is usually located in the furcation area, not at the apices. This is because of the presence of accessory canals on the pulpal floor area. Thus, a bitewing film is frequently a useful diagnostic aid, particularly in maxillary molars, where the developing premolar obscures the furca in a periapical radiograph.

Belanger (1988) emphasizes that the dentist should be familiar with the normal factors that complicate the interpretation of radiographs in children (i.e., largest bone marrow spaces, superimposition of developing tooth buds, and normal resorption patterns of the teeth).

Operative Diagnosis

There are instances when a final diagnosis can be reached only by direct evaluation of the pulp tissue, and a decision about treatment is made accordingly. For example, if formocresol pulpotomy is planned, the nature of the bleeding from the amputation site should be normal (red color and hemostasis evident in less than 5 minutes with mild cotton pellet pressure). If bleeding persists, a more radical treatment should be undertaken (pulpectomy or extraction), because excessive bleeding is an indication that the inflammation has reached the radicular pulp. Conversely, if a pulp polyp is present and bleeding stops normally after coronal pulp amputation, a formocresol pulpotomy may be performed instead of a more radical procedure.

PULP TREATMENT PROCEDURES

The most important and also the most difficult aspect of pulp therapy is determining the health of the pulp or its stage of inflammation so that an intelligent decision can be made regarding the best form of treatment. Several different types of pulp treatment have been recommended for primary teeth. They can be classified into two categories: *conservative*—those that aim to maintain pulp vitality, and *radical*—consisting of pulpectomy and root filling. When the infection cannot be arrested by any of the methods listed and bony support cannot be regained, the tooth must be extracted.

Conservative Treatment

PROTECTIVE BASE

A protective base or liner is a material placed on the pulpal and axial walls of a cavity preparation to act as a protective barrier between the restorative material and the tooth. Dentin is permeable and allows the movement of materials from the oral cavity to the pulp and vice-versa. For several years it was believed that pulp inflammation was caused by the toxic effects from dental materials

(Stanley, 1990). More recent evidence, however, has demonstrated that pulpal inflammation resulting from dental materials is mild and transient, with adverse reactions resulting from pulpal invasion by bacteria or their toxins (Brannstrom, 1984; Cox et al., 1987). Continued marginal leakage with secondary recurrent caries is probably the most common cause of pulp degeneration under restorations, and this pulpal irritation associated with microleakage is often related to the permeability of the dentin. In deep cavities the dentin covering the pulp is thin, and the tubules are large in diameter and packed close together. This dentin is extremely permeable and should be covered with a material that seals dentin well. Pashley (1990) recommends the use of light-cured calcium hydroxide bases or polycarboxylate cements because this remaining dentin is too thin to permit the use of glass-ionomer cement. Copal varnish has been used to seal the amalgam-tooth interface until corrosion products form to eliminate the gap and to provide a barrier against the passage of irritants from cements (Craig, 1993). The most recent materials to be used as cavity sealers are those that have demonstrated multisubstrate bonding ability to bond the restorative material to the tooth. These include resin cements, glass ionomers, and dentin bonding agents. The benefit of using these materials to bond composite to tooth structure is a well-documented and accepted procedure (Hilton, 1996). Employing them in conjunction with amalgam is more controversial, however. The insoluble adhesive layer may act as a barrier to prevent amalgam corrosion products from ultimately sealing the gap. Thus, the dentin bonding agents may potentially put the patient at a greater risk for marginal leakage and recurrent caries in the long term. In addition, dentin adhesives are more technique-sensitive than varnish and are more expensive and time-consuming (Hilton, 1996). Mahler and colleagues (1996) observed no difference between bonded and unbonded amalgam restorations after 1 year and concluded that the use of bonding agents under traditional amalgam fillings should not be recommended.

INDIRECT PULP TREATMENT

Indirect pulp treatment is recommended for teeth that have deep carious lesions approximating the pulp but *no signs or symptoms of pulp degeneration*. In this procedure, the deepest layer of the remaining carious dentin is covered with a biocompatible material to prevent pulp exposure and additional trauma to the tooth. Two materials are most commonly used in indirect pulp treatment: calcium hydroxide and zinc oxide–eugenol paste. The rationale for indirect pulp treatment is that few viable bacteria remain in the deeper dentin layers, and after the cavity has been sealed *properly* they are inactivated. These facts argue against a two-step procedure, in which the tooth is reentered for the purpose of excavating the previously carious dentin and to confirm the formation of reparative dentin. The procedure risks creating a pulp exposure and further insult to the pulp (Dumsha and Hovland, 1985).

It is difficult to determine whether an area is an infected carious lesion or a bacteria-free demineralized zone. The best clinical marker is the quality of the dentin: soft, mushy dentin should be removed, and hard discolored dentin can be indirectly capped. The ultimate objective of this treatment is to maintain pulp vitality (Eidelman et al., 1965) by (1) arresting the carious process, (2) promoting dentin sclerosis (reducing permeability), (3) stimulating the formation of tertiary dentin, and (4) remineralizing the carious dentin.

Success rates of indirect pulp treatment have been reported to be higher than 90% in primary teeth (Kerkhove et al., 1967), and thus its use is recommended in patients in whom a preoperative diagnosis suggests no signs of pulp degeneration. It has been suggested lately that dentin bonding agents be used for direct and indirect pulp capping (Kanca, 1993). There are some concerns regarding an indirect pulp cap with these materials, however. Nakajima and coworkers (1995) found a significant loss of bond strength to human carious dentin when compared with sound dentin. This finding leads one to question even further the integrity of the bond and subsequent ability to prevent bacterial invasion of a carious substrate.

DIRECT PULP CAPPING

Direct pulp capping is a procedure that is carried out when a healthy pulp has been inadvertently exposed during an operative procedure. The tooth must be asymptomatic, and the exposure site must be pinpoint in diameter and free of oral contaminants. A calcium hydroxide medicament is placed over the exposure site to stimulate dentin formation and thus "heal" the wound and maintain the vitality of the pulp (Levine et al., 1988). Direct pulp capping of a carious pulp exposure in a primary tooth is not recommended. The direct pulp cap is indicated for small mechanical or traumatic exposures when conditions for a favorable response are optimal.

Even in these cases the success rate is not particularly high. Failure of treatment may result in internal resorption (Fig. 22-4) or acute dentoalveolar abscess. Kennedy and Kapala (1985) claim that the high cellular content of the primary pulp tissue may be responsible for the increased failure rate of direct pulp capping in primary teeth. These authors believe that undifferentiated mesenchymal cells may differentiate into odontoclasts, leading to internal resorption, a principal sign of failure of direct pulp capping in primary teeth.

The use of dentin bonding agents for direct pulp capping has been advocated by some investigators (Kanca, 1993; Kashiwada and Takagi, 1991). The rationale is that an effective, permanent seal against bacterial invasion is provided and will allow pulp healing to occur. Animal research has shown good compatibility of mechanically exposed pulps to visible light–activated composite when bacteria are excluded (Cox et al., 1987). A clinical study of 64 cases of direct pulp capping with a bonding agent after carious exposure revealed that 60 of the teeth were vital 1 year later. In the same study, caries-free third molars were intentionally exposed with a bur, pulp capped with a bonding agent, and extracted up to 1 year for histologic evaluation. All cases revealed dentin bridge formation and no inflammatory changes in the pulp (Kashiwada and Takagi, 1991). Similar results were observed by Araujo and associates (1996) in 15 cariously exposed primary teeth, 1 year after capping with a bonding agent and restoration with a composite resin.

Although pulp capping with dentin bonding agents shows promise and offers a distinct future possible treatment modality, the lack of long-term documentation in controlled clinical trials makes its recommendation for clinical practice still premature.

PULPOTOMY

The pulpotomy procedure is based on the rationale that the radicular pulp tissue is healthy or is capable of healing after surgical amputation of the affected or infected coronal pulp (Fuks and Eidelman, 1991). The presence of any signs or symptoms of inflammation extending beyond the coronal pulp is a contraindication for a pulpotomy. Thus, pulpotomy is *contraindicated* when any of the following are present: swelling (of pulpal origin), fistula, pathologic mobility, pathologic external root resorption, internal root resorption, periapical or inter-radicular radiolucency, pulp calcifications, or excessive bleeding from the amputated radicular stumps. Other signs, such as a history of spontaneous or nocturnal pain or tenderness to percussion or palpation, should be interpreted carefully (see Fig. 22-3).

The ideal dressing material for the radicular pulp should (1) be bactericidal, (2) be harmless to the pulp and surrounding structures, (3) promote healing of the radicular pulp, and (4) not interfere with the physiologic process of root resorption. A good deal of controversy surrounds the issue of pulpotomy agents, and, unfortunately, the "ideal" pulp dressing material has not yet been identified. The most commonly used pulp dressing material is formocresol (Buckley's solution: formaldehyde, cresol, glycerol, and water). In a survey, Avram and Pulver (1989) reported that the majority of pediatric dentists in Canada (92.4%) and worldwide (76.8%) use either full-strength or a one-fifth dilution of formocresol as the preferred pulpotomy medicament for vital primary teeth. Issues regarding the selection of pulpotomy medicaments are discussed later in this chapter.

Pulpotomy Technique. After local anesthesia

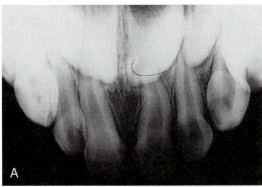
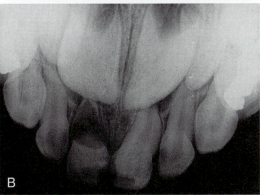

Figure 22–4. *A,* Maxillary primary central incisor treated by direct pulp capping with CaOH$_2$ following pinpoint iatrogenic pulp exposure. *B,* Extensive internal resorption was evident 6 months later.

has been given and the rubber dam placed, all superficial caries should be removed before pulpal exposure to minimize bacterial contamination following exposure. The roof of the pulp chamber should be removed by joining the pulp horns with bur cuts. This procedure is usually accomplished using a No. 330 bur mounted in a water-cooled high-speed turbine. The coronal pulp is then amputated using either a sharp excavator or a slowly revolving round bur. This procedure should be done carefully to prevent further damage to the pulp and perforation of the pulpal floor (Fig. 22-5). Care must be taken to ensure that all the coronal pulp tissue has been removed. Tags of tissue remaining under ledges of dentin may continue to bleed, masking the actual status of the radicular pulp stumps and thus obscuring a correct diagnosis.

After coronal pulp amputation, one or more cotton pellets should be placed over each amputation site, and pressure should be applied for a few minutes. When the cotton pellets are removed, hemostasis should be apparent, although a minor amount of wound bleeding may be evident. Excessive bleeding that persists in spite of cotton pellet pressure and a deep purple color of the tissue may indicate that the inflammation has extended into the radicular pulp. Such signs preclude the tooth from remaining a good candidate for formocresol pulpotomy, and pulpectomy or extraction is indicated. No intrapulpal local anesthesia or other hemostatic agent should be used to minimize hemorrhage because bleeding is a clinical indicator of the radicular pulp status. After hemostasis, a cotton pellet moistened with Buckley's solution (full concentration or one-fifth solution) is placed over the pulp stumps for 5 minutes. When the pellet is removed, the amputation site should appear dark brown (when a full concentration of formocresol is used) or dark

red (when the one-fifth dilution is employed). In both cases, very little or no hemorrhage is present. A base of zinc oxide and eugenol (either plain or reinforced) is placed over the amputation sites and lightly condensed to cover the pulpal floor. A second layer is then condensed to fill the access opening completely. The final restoration, preferably a stainless steel crown, should be placed at the same appointment. If that is not possible, however, the zinc oxide and eugenol base serves as an acceptable interim restoration until the stainless steel crown can be placed.

Clinical and radiographic studies have demonstrated that success rates for formocresol pulpotomies range from 70% to 97% (Berger, 1965; Fuks and Bimstein, 1981; Morawa et al., 1975; Rolling and Thylstrup, 1975). The use of a one-fifth dilution of formocresol has been advocated by several authors (Fuks and Bimstein, 1981; Morawa et al., 1975) because of its reportedly equal effectiveness and potential for less toxicity. This solution is prepared by making a diluent of three parts glycerin and one part water. Four parts of this diluent are then mixed with one part Buckley's solution to make the one-fifth dilution.

Although many studies have reported the clinical success of formocresol pulpotomies, an increasing body of literature has questioned the use of formocresol. Rolling and Thylstrup (1975) demonstrated that its clinical success rate decreased as follow-up time increased. Further, the histologic response of the primary radicular pulp to formocresol appears to be unfavorable. Some investigators claim that, subsequent to formocresol application, fixation occurs in the coronal third of the radicular pulp, chronic inflammation in the middle third, and vital tissue in the apical third (Berger, 1965). Others report that the remaining pulp tissue is partially or totally necrotic (Langeland et al., 1976). In recent decades several reports have questioned the safety and efficacy of formocresol (Block et al., 1978; Fuks et al., 1983; Magnusson, 1978; Myers et al., 1981, 1983), and most authorities now agree that formocresol is at least *potentially* immunogenic and mutagenic. For these reasons, efforts have increased to find a substitute medicament.

Potential Substitutes for Formocresol. Glutaraldehyde (GA) has been proposed as an alternative to formocresol because it is a mild fixative and is potentially less toxic. Because of its cross-linking properties, penetration into the tissue is more limited with less effect on periapical tissues. The short-term success of 2% GA as a pulpotomy agent has been demonstrated in several studies (Davis et al., 1982; Garcia-Godoy, 1986;

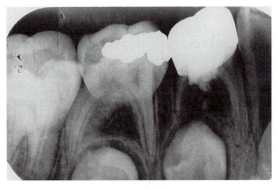

Figure 22-5. Zinc oxide and eugenol (ZOE) paste extruded through a perforated pulpal floor due to improper use of a bur.

Fuks et al., 1986, 1991; Ranly and Lazzari, 1983; Tagger and Tagger, 1984). Longer-term success rates matching those of formocresol, however, have not been reported. Fuks and associates (1990) reported a failure rate of 18% in human primary molars 25 months after pulpotomy when a 2% concentration of GA was used (Fig. 22–6). In the same study sample at 42-month follow-up the authors noted that 45% of the teeth that underwent pulpotomy with GA resorbed faster than their controls (Fuks and Bimstein, 1991).

Some biologic materials have been proposed as pulp dressings on the theory that they would promote physiologic healing of the pulpotomy wound. Freeze-dried bone (Fadavi et al., 1989); autolyzed, antigen-extracted, allogenic dentin matrix; allogenic bone morphogenetic protein (Nakashima, 1989); and enriched collagen solutions (Bimstein and Shoshan, 1981; Fuks et al., 1984) all have led to varying levels of success in early experimental stages. Clinical studies have reported promising results using ferric sulfate, a hemostatic agent, in pulpotomized human primary teeth (Davis and Furtado, 1991; Fei et al., 1991). Fuks and colleagues (1997) reported a success rate of 93% in teeth treated with ferric sulfate (FS) and 84% in those treated with dilute formocresol (DFC). These teeth were followed up for 6 to 35 months. In a preliminary report of the same study, a much lower success rate was described (77.5% for the FS group and 81% for the DFC teeth), with internal resorption evident in five teeth treated with FS and four teeth fixed with DFC (Fuks et al., 1994). This discrepancy can be explained by an excessively severe interpretation of the initial findings. Areas listed initially as internal resorption on the preliminary report remained unchanged after 30 months and

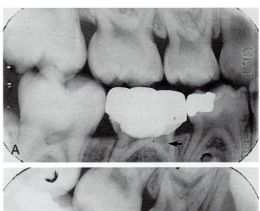

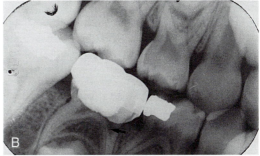

Figure 22–7. *A,* Mandibular second primary molar 6 months after pulpotomy. The radiolucent area in the mesial canal (*arrow*) has been listed as internal resorption. *B,* The area remained unchanged 30 months after treatment.

therefore were reassessed as normal in the last evaluation (Fig. 22–7). Nonpharmacotherapeutic approaches to pulpotomy include the treatment of radicular pulp tissue by electrocautery or laser to eliminate residual infectious processes. Although these techniques are being currently used by a number of practitioners, no long-term controlled clinical studies are available to evaluate their success.

In summary, the search for alternatives to formocresol as a pulp dressing in primary tooth pulpotomies has yet to reveal an agent or technique that has long-term clinical success rates matching those of formocresol. Until such an agent is found, it appears prudent to use formocresol (either in a one-fifth dilution or full strength) in primary tooth pulpotomies.

Radical Treatment

PULPECTOMY AND ROOT FILLING

The pulpectomy procedure is indicated in teeth that show evidence of chronic inflammation or necrosis in the radicular pulp. Conversely, pulpectomy is contraindicated in teeth with gross loss of root structure, advanced internal or external resorption, or periapical infection involving the crypt of the succedaneous tooth (American

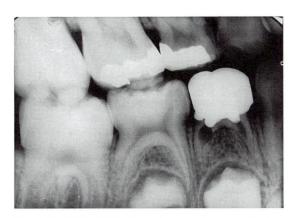

Figure 22–6. Mandibular first primary molar presenting internal root resorption following pulpotomy with 2% buffered glutaraldehyde solution.

Academy of Pediatric Dentistry, 1997). The goal of pulpectomy is to maintain primary teeth that would otherwise be lost. Clinicians disagree, however, about the utility of pulpectomy procedures in primary teeth. Difficulty in the preparation of primary root canals that have a complex and variable morphology and the uncertainty about the effects of instrumentation, medication, and filling materials on developing succedaneous teeth dissuade some clinicians from using the technique. The behavior management problems that sometimes occur in pediatric patients have surely added to the reluctance among some dentists to perform root canal treatments in primary teeth. These problems notwithstanding, the success of pulpectomies in primary teeth has led most pediatric dentists to prefer them to the alternative of extractions and space maintenance.

Certain clinical situations may justify attempting a pulpectomy even when the prognosis may not be ideal. An example of such a case is pulp destruction of a primary second molar that occurs before the first permanent molar erupts. A premature extraction of the primary second molar without placement of a space maintainer usually results in mesial eruption of the first permanent molar with subsequent loss of space for the second premolar (Fig. 22-8). Although a distal shoe space maintainer could be used, maintaining the natural tooth is definitely the treatment of choice. Therefore, a pulpectomy in a primary second molar is preferable, even if that tooth is maintained only until the first permanent molar has adequately erupted and is followed eventually by extraction of the primary second molar and placement of a space maintainer (Fig. 22-9).

Root Filling Materials. Developmental, anatomic, and physiologic differences between primary and permanent teeth call for differences in the criteria for root canal filling materials. The ideal root canal filling material for primary teeth should resorb at a rate similar to that of the primary root, be harmless to the periapical tissues and to the permanent tooth germ, resorb readily if pressed beyond the apex, be antiseptic, fill the root canals easily, adhere to their walls, not shrink, be easily removed if necessary, be radiopaque, and not discolor the tooth (Machida, 1983; Rifkin, 1980). No material currently available meets all these criteria. The filling materials most commonly used for primary pulp canals are zinc oxide–eugenol paste, iodoform paste, and calcium hydroxide.

Zinc Oxide–Eugenol Paste. Zinc oxide-eugenol paste (ZOE) is probably the most commonly used filling material for primary teeth in

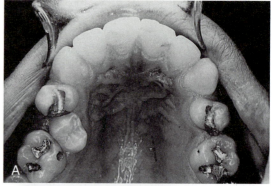

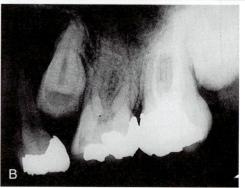

Figure 22–8. *A,* Occlusal view of the permanent dentition following bilateral premature extractions of the maxillary primary second molars. The right second bicuspid erupted ectopically, and the left is impacted. *B,* Radiograph of the area showing the impacted left premolar. (Courtesy of Ilana Brin, DMD.)

the United States. Camp (1984) introduced the endodontic pressure syringe to overcome the problem of underfilling, a relatively common finding when thick mixes of ZOE are employed. Underfilling, however, is frequently clinically acceptable. Primary teeth frequently present with inter-radicular radiolucent areas but without periapical lesions and sometimes even have some vital pulp at the apex (Fig. 22-10). Overfilling, on the other hand, may cause a mild foreign body reaction (Barker and Lockett, 1971). Another disadvantage of ZOE paste is the difference between its rate of resorption and that of the tooth root (Allen, 1979). Although particles of ZOE may remain in the alveolar bone for a long time, it is not certain that this has a clinically significant effect (Fig. 22-11).

Iodoform Paste. Several authors have reported the use of KRI paste (Pharmachemie, Switzerland), which is a mixture of iodoform, camphor, parachlorophenol, and menthol (Barker and Lockett, 1971; Rifkin, 1982). It resorbs rapidly and has no undesirable effects on succedaneous teeth when used as a pulp canal

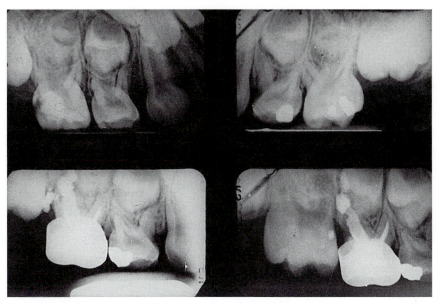

Figure 22–9. Nonvital maxillary second primary molar, treated by pulpectomy with zinc oxide and eugenol (ZOE). *Top left,* Prior to pulpectomy. *Top right,* Contralateral vital tooth. *Bottom left,* Excess of ZOE in palatal and distobuccal canals. *Bottom right,* Primary tooth successfully retained until eruption of first permanent molar.

medicament in abscessed primary teeth. Further, KRI paste that extrudes into periapical tissue is rapidly replaced with normal tissue. Sometimes the material is also resorbed inside the root canal (Fig. 22–12).

A paste developed by Maisto has been used clinically for many years, and good results have been reported with its use (Mass and Zilberman, 1989; Tagger and Sarnat, 1984). This paste has the same components as the KRI paste with the addition of zinc oxide, thymol, and lanolin.

Calcium Hydroxide. This material is generally not used in pulp therapy for primary teeth; however, several clinical and histopathologic investigations of a calcium hydroxide and iodoform mixture (Vitapex, Neo Dental Chemical Products

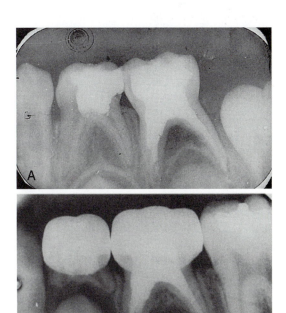

Figure 22–10. *A,* Mandibular second primary molar immediately after completion of root canal treatment with zinc oxide and eugenol (ZOE). Notice the inter-radicular radiolucent area and the underfill of the mesial canals. *B,* The same tooth 5 years later showing healing of the lesion. (Courtesy of Gideon Holan, DMD.)

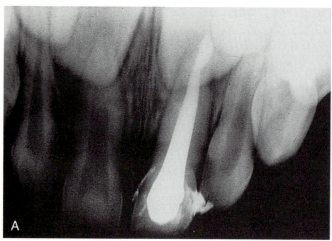

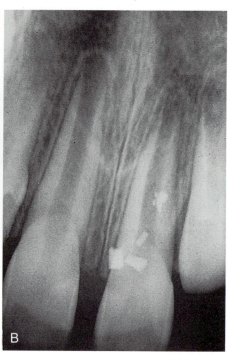

Figure 22–11. *A,* Maxillary primary central incisor with excessive zinc oxide and eugenol (ZOE) immediately after pulpectomy. *B,* Permanent successor of the root-treated primary tooth showing remnants of ZOE in the alveolar bone. (From Fuks AB, Eidelman E: Pulp therapy in the primary dentition. Curr Opin Dent *1*:556–563, 1991.)

Co., Tokyo) have been published in Japan (Fuchino, 1980; Nishino et al., 1980). These authors found that this material is easy to apply, resorbs at a slightly faster rate than that of the roots, has no toxic effects on the permanent successor, and

is radiopaque. For these reasons, Machida (1983) considers the calcium hydroxide–iodoform mixture to be a nearly ideal primary tooth filling material. Another preparation with similar composition is available in the United States under

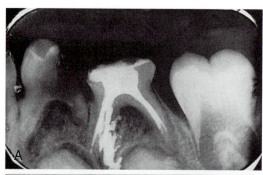

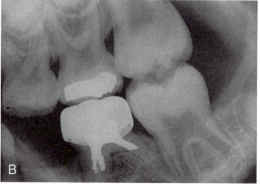

Figure 22–12. *A,* Mandibular first primary molar pulpectomy with KRI paste. Note the excess of material immediately after treatment. *B,* Nine months after treatment, the material has resorbed considerably and the lamina dura appears normal. (Courtesy of Gideon Holan, DMD.)

the trade name Endoflas (Sanlor Laboratories, A.A. 7523 Cali, Colombia S.A.).

Pulpectomy Technique. The pulpectomy procedure should be performed as follows. An access opening should be prepared in a manner similar to that used in a pulpotomy, but the walls may need to be flared more to facilitate access of the canal openings for broaches and files (Camp, 1984). Each canal orifice of the roots should be located, and a properly sized barbed broach should be selected. The broach is used gently to remove as much organic material as possible from each canal. Endodontic files are selected and adjusted to stop 1 or 2 mm short of the radiographic apex of each canal as determined by a radiograph (Fig. 22-13). This is an arbitrary length but is intended to minimize the chance of overinstrumenting apically and causing periapical damage. The removal of organic debris is the main purpose for filing (Belanger, 1988).

The canal should be periodically irrigated to aid in removing debris. A sodium hypochlorite solution may be used because it helps dissolve organic material; however, because of concern about forcing it into the periapical tissues, the solution should be used very carefully and with no excessive irrigation pressure. Sterile saline may be used as an alternative solution. The canal is dried by using appropriately sized paper points.

When a ZOE mixture is used, several filling techniques may be employed (Belanger, 1988). For large canals, as in primary anterior teeth, a thin mixture can be used to coat the walls of the canal, followed by a thick mixture that can be manually condensed into the remainder of the

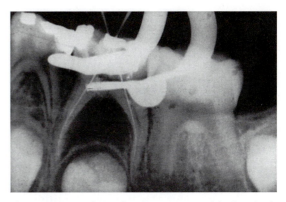

Figure 22-13. Radiographic determination of the length of the canals.

lumen. An endodontic plugger or a small amalgam condenser is useful for compacting the paste at the level of the canal orifice. Care should be taken not to overfill the canal. In primary molars, some of the canals may be quite small and difficult to fill. Commercial pressure syringes have been developed for this purpose. Alternative techniques include using a disposable tuberculin syringe or a local anesthetic syringe, in which the anesthetic Carpule is emptied and the canal is then dried and filled with ZOE paste.

When the root canal is filled with a resorbable paste such as KRI, Maisto, or Endoflas, a lentulo spiral mounted in a low-speed turbine can be used, facilitating the introduction of the material into the canal. When the canal is completely filled, the material is compressed with a cotton pellet. Excessive material is rapidly resorbed (see Fig. 22-12).

Conclusion

Pulp therapy for the primary dentition includes a variety of treatment options, depending on the vitality of the pulp. Conservative treatment is performed when vital pulp remains because recovery is possible once the irritation has been removed. Pulpectomy is indicated in teeth showing evidence of chronic, irreversible inflammation or necrosis in the radicular pulp.

REFERENCES

Allen RK: Endodontic treatment of primary teeth. Aust Dent J *24*:347-351, 1979.

American Academy of Pediatric Dentistry: Guidelines for pulp therapy for primary and young permanent teeth— Reference Manual 1997-1998. Pediatr Dent *19* (Special Issue):43-47, 1997.

Araujo FB, Barata JS, Garcia-Godoy F: Clinical and radiographic evaluation of the use of an adhesive system over primary dental pulps. [Abstract 2101] J Dent Res 75(Special Issue):280, 1996.

Avram DC, Pulver F: Pulpotomy medicaments for vital primary teeth: Surveys to determine use and attitudes in pediatric dental practice and in dental schools throughout the world. J Dent Child *56*:426-434, 1989.

Barker BCW, Lockett BC: Endodontics experiments with resorbable paste. Aust Dent J *16*:364-373, 1971.

Belanger GK: Pulp therapy for the primary dentition. *In* Pinkham JR (ed): Pediatric Dentistry: Infancy Through Adolescence. Philadelphia, WB Saunders, 1988.

Berger JE: Pulp tissue reaction to formocresol and zinc oxide-engenol. J Dent Child *32*:13-28, 1965.

Bimstein E, Shoshan S: Enhanced healing of tooth pulp wounds in the dog by enriched collagen solution as a capping agent. Arch Oral Biol *26*:97-101, 1981.

Block RM, Lewis PD, Sheats JB, et al: Antibody formation to dog pulp tissue altered by formocresol within the root canal. Oral Surg *45*:282-292, 1978.

Brannstrom M: Communication between the oral cavity and the dental pulp associated with restorative treatment. Oper Dent *9*:57-68, 1984.

Camp JH: Pulp therapy for primary and young permanent teeth. Dent Clin North Am *28*:651-668, 1984.

Cox CF, Keall CL, Keall HJ, et al: Biocompatibility of surface-sealed dental materials against exposed pulps. J Prosthet Dent *57*:1-8, 1987.

Craig RG: Restorative Dental Materials, 9th ed. St. Louis, CV Mosby, 1993, p 203.

Davis J, Furtado L: Ferric sulfate a possible new medicament for pulpotomies in the primary dentition: The first year results from a 4 year study in Fortaleza, Brazil. Thirteenth Congress of International Association of Dentistry for Children, Kyoto, Japan, Program and Abstracts, September 27-30, 1991.

Davis MJ, Myers R, Switkes MD: Glutaraldehyde: An alternative to formocresol for vital pulp therapy. J Dent Child *49*:176-180, 1982.

Dumsha T, Hovland E: Considerations and treatment of direct and indirect pulp capping. Dent Clin North Am *29*:251-259, 1985.

Eidelman E, Finn SB, Koulourides T: Remineralization of carious dentin treated with calcium hydroxide. J Dent Child *32*:218-225, 1965.

Fadavi S, Anderson AW, Punwani IC: Freeze-dried bone in pulpotomy procedures in monkey. J Pedodont *13*:108-122, 1989.

Fei AL, Udin RD, Johnson R: A clinical study of ferric sulfate as a pulpotomy agent in primary teeth. Pediatr Dent *13*:327-332, 1991.

Fuchino T: Clinical and histopathological studies of pulpectomy in deciduous teeth. Shikwa Gakubo *80*:971-1017, 1980.

Fuks AB, Bimstein E: Clinical evaluation of diluted formocresol pulpotomies in primary teeth of school children. Pediatr Dent *3*:321-324, 1981.

Fuks AB, Bimstein E, Bruchim A: Radiographic and histologic evaluation of the effect of two concentrations of formocresol on pulpotomized primary and young permanent teeth in monkeys. Pediatr Dent *5*:9-13, 1983.

Fuks AB, Michaeli Y, Sofer-Saks B, et al: Enriched collagen solution as a pulp dressing in pulpotomized teeth in monkeys. Pediatr Dent *6*:243-247, 1984.

Fuks AB, Bimstein E, Michaeli Y: Glutaraldehyde as a pulp dressing after pulpotomy in primary teeth of baboon monkeys. Pediatr Dent *8*:32-36, 1986.

Fuks AB, Bimstein E, Guelmann M, et al: Assessment of a 2% buffered glutaraldehyde solution in pulpotomized primary teeth of school children. J Dent Child *57*:371-375, 1990.

Fuks AB, Cleaton-Jones P, Michaeli Y, et al: Pulp response to collagen and glutaraldehyde in pulpotomized primary teeth of baboons. Pediatr Dent *13*:142-150, 1991.

Fuks AB, Bimstein E: Glutaraldehyde pulpotomies in primary teeth of school children: 42 month results. [Abstract 1654] J Dent Res *70*:473, 1991.

Fuks AB, Eidelman E: Pulp therapy in the primary dentition. Curr Opin Dent *1*:556-563, 1991.

Fuks AB, Holan G, Davis J, Eidelman E: Ferric sulfate versus formocresol in pulpotomized primary molars: preliminary report [Abstract 27]. J Dent Res *73*:885, 1994.

Fuks AB, Holan G, Davis JM, Eidelman E: Ferric sulfate versus diluted formocresol in pulpotomized primary molars: Long term follow-up. Pediatr Dent *19*:327-330, 1997.

Garcia-Godoy F: A 42-month clinical evaluation of glutaraldehyde pulpotomies in primary teeth. J Pedodont *10*:148-155, 1986.

Hilton TJ: Cavity sealers, liners, and bases: Current philosophies and indications for use. Oper Dent *21:*134-146, 1996.

Kanca J III: Replacement of a fractured incisor fragment over pulpal exposure: A case-report. Quintess Int *24:*81-84, 1993.

Kashiwada T, Takagi M: New restoration and direct pulp capping systems using adhesive composite resin. Bul Tokyo Med Dent Univ *38:*45-52, 1991.

Kennedy DB, Kapala JT: The dental pulp: Biological considerations of protection and treatment. *In* Braham RL, Morris E (eds): Textbook of Pediatric Dentistry. Baltimore, Williams & Wilkins, 1985.

Kerkhove BC, Herman SC, Klein AI, et al: A clinical and television densitometric evaluation of indirect pulp capping technique. J Dent Child *34:*164, 1967.

Langeland K: Tissue Changes in the Dental Pulp. Oslo, Oslo University, 1957.

Langeland LK, Dowden W, Langeland K: Formocresol, "mummification," tissue disintegration, microbes, inflammation, resorption and apposition. [Abstract 268] J Dent Res *55*(Special Issue): 1976.

Levine N, Pulver F, Torneck CD: Pulpal therapy in primary and young permanent teeth. *In* Wei SHY (ed): Pediatric Dentistry—Total Patient Care. Philadelphia, Lea & Febiger, 1988.

Machida Y: Root canal therapy in deciduous teeth. Jpn Dent Assoc J *36:*796-802, 1983.

Magnusson BO: Therapeutic pulpotomies in primary molars with the formocresol technique: A clinical and histological follow-up. Acta Odontol Scand *36:*157-165, 1978.

Mahler DB, Engle JH, Simms LE, et al: One year clinical evaluation of bonded amalgam restorations. JADA *127:*345-349, 1996.

Mass E, Zilberman LU: Endodontic treatment of infected primary teeth, using Maisto's paste. J Dent Child *56:*117-120, 1989.

Morawa A, Straffon LH, Han SS, et al: Clinical evaluation of pulpotomies using dilute formocresol. J Dent Child *42:*28-31, 1975.

Myers DR, Pashley DH, Whitford GM, et al: The acute toxicity of high doses of systemically administered formocresol in dogs. Pediatr Dent *3:*37-41, 1981.

Myers DR, Pashley DH, Whitford GM, et al: Tissue changes induced by the absorption of formocresol from pulpotomy sites in dogs. Pediatr Dent *5:*6-8, 1983.

Nakajima M, Sano H, Burrow MF, et al: Bonding to caries affected dentin. [Abstract 194] J Dent Res *74*(Special Issue):36, 1995.

Nakashima M: Dentin induction of implants of autolyzed antigen extracted allogeneic dentin in amputated pulp in dogs. Endodont Dent Traumatol *5:*279-286, 1989.

Nishino M, Inoue K, Ono Y, et al: Clinico-roentgenographical study of iodoform-calcium hydroxide root canal filling material Vitapex in deciduous teeth. Jpn J Pedodont *18:*20-24, 1980.

Pashley DL: Clinical consideration of microleakage. J Endodont *16:*70-77, 1990.

Ranly DM, Lazzari EP: A biochemical study of two bifunctional reagents as alternatives to formocresol. J Dent Res *62:*1054-1057, 1983.

Rifkin A: A simple, effective, safe technique for the root canal treatment of abscessed primary teeth. J Dent Child *47:*435-441, 1980.

Rifkin A: The root canal treatment of abscessed primary teeth—A three to four year follow-up. J Dent Child *49:*428-431, 1982.

Rolling I, Thylstrup A: A three year clinical follow-up study of pulpotomized primary molars treated with the formocresol technique. Scand J Dent Res *83:*47-53, 1975.

Seltzer S, Bender IB: The Dental Pulp, 3rd ed. Philadelphia, JB Lippincott, 1984.

Stanley HR: Pulpal responses to ionomer cements—Biological characteristics. JADA *120:*25-29, 1990.

Tagger E, Tagger M: Pulpal and periapical reactions to glutaraldehyde and paraformaldehyde pulpotomy dressing in monkeys. J Endodont *10:*364-371, 1984.

Tagger E, Sarnat H: Root canal therapy of infected primary teeth. Acta Odontol Pediatr *5:*63-66, 1984.

Torneck CD: Dentin-pulp complex. *In* Ten Cate AR (ed): Oral Histology, Development, Structure and Function, 2nd ed. St. Louis, CV Mosby, 1985.

Chapter	**23**

Patient Management

J. R. Pinkham

Chapter Outline

As has been mentioned several times in this book so far, the usual and customary age of children entering a dentist's office for the first time has been some time around the third birthday. The authors and editors believe that this is *no longer a reasonable entry time.* Strategies for effective prevention of dental disease simply must be implemented much, much earlier in life.

Before dentistry became prevention-oriented, entry at age 3 years made sense from a patient management standpoint. As reviewed in the first section on the dynamics of change (Chapter 12), it is not until around the third birthday that the majority of children have acquired the communication skills and are sufficiently socialized to be able to comply with the demands of a dental appointment. Also, it is not until the age of 3 years that most children have the language and communication skills to learn from the dentist the essential things about what the dentist is doing that allow them to dismiss their fears about a new, unknown, and potentially threatening person and environment.

Obviously, some children as young as 2 years can go to a dentist and learn to be good patients. Conversely, some youngsters as old as 4 years reliably have a difficult time because of their slow development. It is relatively safe, however, to assert that the vast bulk of behavior management techniques practiced, discussed in the literature, and taught in dental schools today are geared primarily toward the preschool-aged child of 3 to 6 years. Most dentists agree that the preschool child clearly requires the most energy and talent for effective management.

THE IMPORTANCE OF CONVICTION, EXPERIENCE, AND GOOD INTENTIONS

Although dentistry for children is doable, not all dentists enjoy working with children. Any dentist who regularly treats preschool children sees some crying, wiggling and kicking, tantrums, and a variety of other avoidance behaviors. Coping with and devoting energy toward intercepting these behaviors exasperates some dentists. Other dentists feel guilty or anxious. Still others feel uncomfortable around the involved parents, and some may dread the next child scheduled on the appointment book.

One aspect of the dental treatment of children (barring burn-out) seems to be predictive of those who can manage children and those who cannot. That aspect is experience. Dental students and young practitioners may be discour-

aged by the anxiety they feel and the insecurity they experience when certain children start to misbehave. With time and dedication to the techniques taught in dental school and outlined in this book, however, a practitioner's skills in child patient management become refined, and with this refinement comes self-confidence in this area of dentistry. The self-confidence of the dentist in his or her management skills is essential to successful interchanges with potentially unruly children.

AN EMBARRASSMENT OF RICHES

In 1977, Dr. David Chambers, a psychologist with extensive interest in dentistry for children and considerable input into the literature on how dentists should manage children, labeled the available ways dentists can manage children as an "embarrassment of riches." Anyone knowledgeable about dentistry for children will concur with Dr. Chambers. So many ways of managing kids have been described in journals and textbooks that few if any dentists can master them all.

There is, however, a basic inventory of skills that remains critical. Some of these management techniques are nice and polite, some have reasonable elegance in psychological terms, and some, on first inspection by a lay person (and perhaps by sophomore dental students, too), may appear rigorous and authoritative.

PATIENT MANAGEMENT BY DOMAIN

There are five basic domains for securing the cooperation of children during the dental experience. These are the physical domain, the pharmacologic domain, the aversive domain, the reward-oriented domain, and the linguistic domain.

For most practitioners the most reasonable domain is the linguistic domain. The importance of this particular domain is discussed later in the chapter. The practitioner should be knowledgeable about certain particulars of the other four domains, however.

Physical Domain

The physical domain ranges from the use of hand restraint by a dental assistant to the use of tools such as the Papoose Board (Olympic Medical Corporation, Seattle, WA) and Pedi-Wrap (Clark Associates, Inc., Worcester, MA). Other restraint systems include tape, sheets with tape, cloth wraps, and belts (Fig. 23-1). The use of mouth props also belongs in the physical domain for child patient management (Fig. 23-2). Obviously, these techniques, when used for the duration of an appointment, are reserved for basically unmanageable children. An alternative to physical restraint usually involves management by drugs or general anesthesia. These techniques can be expensive and are sometimes dangerous.

The physical domain has proven to be useful in treating emergencies on hysterical children and children who cannot be reached in language because of their age. Developmentally disabled children and children who for whatever reason cannot cooperate with the dentist may also need management in this domain. The use of many techniques in the physical domain necessitates explanations to parents, guardians, or caretakers. For instance, the use of a papoose board on a normal child demands informed consent.

Pharmacologic Domain

Pain and anxiety control by way of pharmacologic methods is discussed earlier in this book.

This domain includes modalities as safe and easy to deliver as nitrous oxide/oxygen to the profound management provided by general anesthesia in a hospital setting.

Obviously, any drug that has the capability of decreasing respiration, depressing the gag reflex, or making the child sleepy or causing sleep is potentially dangerous. The smaller the child, the more dramatic the danger. Dentists wishing to work with medications need to have training in such techniques, appropriate monitoring equipment, and a protocol that ensures safety for the child. Again, this domain requires parental understanding about the techniques, risks, and alternatives.

Aversive Domain

A technique can be described as aversive if the use of the technique on a child is objectionable enough that the child will cooperate in order to avoid the technique. Parental spanking is an example of aversive management. Generally speaking, dentists who work with children generally refrain or wish to refrain in bringing any aversion into the dental appointment at all.

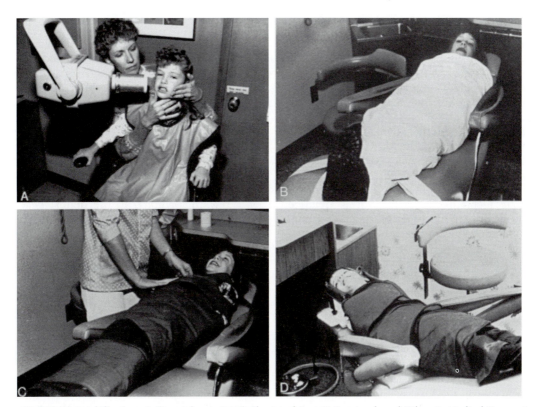

Figure 23–1. Patient stabilization. *A,* Parental restraint. *B,* Sheet and ties. *C,* Papoose board (Olympic Medical Corporation, Seattle, WA). *D,* Papoose board with head stability attachment.

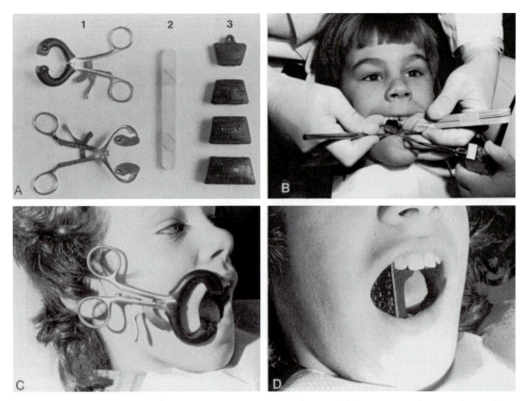

Figure 23–2. Jaw stabilization devices. *A, 1,* Molt mouth gags; *2,* taped tongue blades (sizes can be varied according to size of patient); *3,* McKesson mouth props. *B–D,* Clinical uses of devices.

Some physical techniques can be regarded as aversive if they are used or seem to be used as a punishment. Such practices of these techniques should be avoided: they are unwarranted; they are legally dangerous; they probably will be ineffective.

Hand over the mouth (HOM), sometimes described as hand over the mouth exercise or HOME, is regarded by many to be an aversive technique. It can be practiced as such although, as is discussed later, it can be practiced as a linguistic technique as well. If it is practiced aversively to quiet a crying or screaming child, however, the clinician needs to secure informed consent from the parent or guardian for its use. Use of HOM as well as other techniques is described by guidelines developed by the American Academy of Pediatric Dentistry (1994-95). Any dentist active in the management of children should be aware of these guidelines.

Reward-Oriented Domain

Rewards can be used to secure the cooperation of a child. The reward can be arranged by the dentist, the parent, or the two in concert. The use of rewards by parents may have a negative effect on the appointment. The child may misread the intentions of the parents as their offering a reward because they think the dental appointment will be difficult, frightening, or scary for the child. Certain children who see that they are getting an unusual reward may also conclude that the more anxiety that they develop toward the forthcoming dental appointment, the greater the reward may become. As a rule, I request that parents not promise things like ice cream or toys as a reward for going to the dentist *before the dental appointment.* Afterwards it can come as a surprise and the surprise will have no ramifications on what has already transpired during the dental appointment.

Linguistic Domain: The Linguistic Advantage to Child Patient Management

Linguistic techniques are those communication techniques that involve the conversation of the dentist with the child and the child with the dentist. Therefore, maturity in language is important for the child patient. For the almost complete majority of normally developed and normally socialized children who have no mental or emotional handicaps, the process of coming into maturity in language by way of conversation occurs between 2 and 4 years of age. The vast majority of children are competent in language by their third birthday. Few children are competent to cooperate through language during a complicated dental appointment such as an operative session before 30 months of age, and almost all (normal) children are competent at 42 months of age. Therefore, as a general rule, no child is competent in language before the second birthday and all normal children are competent in language after the fourth birthday.

The linguistic domain demands that the dentist be a communicator. The dentist will be a teacher, a coach, a rewarder, a psychologist, a distracter, and an authority figure when using linguistic techniques.

REQUESTS AND PROMISES

Of all the speech acts that are appropriate to human collaboration and the securing of cooperation, the constitutive speech acts of requests and promises are the most important. Cooperation in the human community happens when two or more individuals take effective actions together. With human beings this can only be done in language. Therefore the basic dental experience of a child is a communication experience of the child with his or her dentist.

To be effective, the dentist must make effective requests of the child and sometimes effective re-requests. For the child to be a good patient, the child must make effective commitments to take responsible actions at the reasonable requests of the dentist. These actions are best described as *promises*. It is when a child declines a request that a management strategy must be initiated. This strategy will ultimately reframe the original request. The essence of this reframing is that it convinces the child that the dentist is serious about the request.

THE DENTIST AS AN ONTOLOGICAL COACH

Ontology means our way of being. The best way of the child being during the dental appointment is quiet, listening for requests, and cooperating with these requests. Obviously, a hysterical screaming child does not have a way of being that works well for the linguistic domain. Therefore, the dentist becomes not just an educator or a requester but an ontological coach in trying to make the child's way of being during the dental

appointment appropriate for linguistic techniques. This can be enhanced with nonverbal techniques as well.

BASICS IN MANAGING CHILDREN IN THE DENTAL EXPERIENCE

Preappointment Experience

The preappointment experience entails bringing the child to the dental office for a tour and orientation. The child is made aware of the fact beforehand that *absolutely nothing* will be done that day. The child meets the receptionist, dental assistant, and dentist. If things go well, certain dental equipment can be shown and explained in "childese," such as "Mr. Wind" and "Mr. Water" for the triplex or "Mr. Buzzer" for the hand piece.

Comments. The preappointment experience provides two offerings that make it powerful for the dentist. First, it removes any unfavorable imaginings as to the realities of the dentist office and its personnel for the child. Today's dental offices are not frightening. The experience in many reception areas, if appropriately furnished and stocked with toys, can be delightful to a child. If the child sees other children who are in the dental experience and having fun, the entire visit is enhanced.

Second, linguistically, the experience sets up a greater likelihood that the requests of the dentist at the first real appointment will be objectively dealt with by appropriate promises of action by the child. People, including children, react more favorably to the requests of familiar persons than we do with strangers.

Preappointment experiences are not used much anymore owing to the time constraints of both the dentist and the parents. This technique is somewhat different from an observation appointment, in which a child watches the dentist treat his or her parent or sibling or someone else. Observation appointments can be useful, but common sense also tells one that they may backfire if children see something that frightens them.

Common sense also dictates that a young child's first appointment should be kept as pleasant and simple as possible. For most children 3 years old or older, an examination and prophylaxis and fluoride treatment can be made a pleasant and even enjoyable experience.

Tell-Show-Do

The tell-show-do method is the backbone of the educational phase of developing an accepting, relaxed child dental patient. The technique is simple and usually works. The technique dictates that before anything is done (except the injection of a local anesthetic or other procedures that defy explanation, such as pulp extirpation), the child is told what will be done and then shown by some sort of simulation exactly what will happen before the procedure is started. For example:

Matt, I'm going to clean your teeth with this special dental toothbrush (prophy angle and rubber cup). You see this soft rubber cup? Well, when I step on this gas pedal this cup turns, and when it is full of toothpaste it can really make your teeth shine. Now, Matt, pinch the cup and you will see how soft it is. Now, let me run it on your fingernail so you can feel how it works. Okay, Matt, please open your mouth for me. Thank you.

Comments. Choice of words is important in the tell-show-do technique. Proper accomplishment requires the dentist to have a substitute vocabulary for his or her tools and procedures that the child can understand. At least four out of five children who are over 3 years old and have a normal social history and emotional status can be guided through a new technique successfully by the use of the tell-show-do method.

Tell-show-do is an educational technique. As the child receives information about an experience, a technique, or piece of equipment, fears of the unknown or the anticipation of pain quickly go away. Again, this technique linguistically enhances the chances that the appropriate request by the dentist will be met by appropriate, effective actions by the child.

Voice Control

Voice control requires the dentist to interject more authority into his or her communication with the child. The tone of voice is important. It must have an "I'm in charge here" ring to it. The facial expression of the dentist must also mirror this attitude of confidence. In fact, a dentist can use "voice control" with facial expressions alone. Voice control can be used with deaf children.

Comments. Voice control is an essential technique for managing preschool children. It is extremely effective at intercepting inappropriate behaviors as they start to happen and is moderately successful at intercepting them after they are full-blown. In other words, voice control is a useful way of reframing a request that has been refused by the child.

As a purely linguistic technique, voice control relies on tonality, cadence, and other aspects of

the quality of the communication of the dentist with the child. I think that voice control is probably a misnomer, however, and should be understood by the practicing dentist to have very nonverbal components. This ramification is discussed further in the nonverbal advantage discussion in this chapter.

Hand-Over-Mouth

The HOM technique calls for the dentist to place his or her hand over the mouth of a hysterically crying child. It is used to intercept tantrums or other fits of rage. It has to be paired with voice control. This technique works reliably with a variety of child personality types (Levitas, 1974). The technique is not intended to scare the child. As said before, it should not be practiced aversively. It is intended to get the child's attention and quiet him or her so that the child can hear what the dentist is saying. Obviously, it reframes the seriousness of a previous request.

Comments. The American Academy of Pediatric Dentistry recognizes HOM as a legitimate technique with certain indications and contraindications. The technique is indicated in the normal child who is old enough to understand the directions of the dentist and to cooperate with the expectations of the appointment but who exhibits "defiant, obstreperous, or hysterical avoidance behaviors to dental treatment." Contraindications include disabled, immature, and medicated children whose understanding of the desires of the dentist are compromised. Prevention of the child from breathing is a second basic contraindication.

The HOM technique has remained somewhat controversial for obvious reasons. Critics have suggested that it may be psychologically aggravating to the child. There is no formal study that verifies this suspicion. The technique remains in many dentists' repertoire of management techniques simply because it works. It works fast and therefore is cost-effective. Patients who qualify for this technique usually would require management with medications, physical restraint, hospitalization, or significant further social and psychological maturation if the technique were not used.

The way that HOM can be regarded as a linguistic technique is when it is not used aversively but rather is practiced as a tap on the lips to remind the child that crying is not appreciated during the dental appointment. Used this way, in which there is no airway restraint intended at all, it becomes a coaching technique and a way of reframing earlier requests to be quiet and cooperative.

Physical Restraint

Physical restraint is its own domain; however, the touching of a child's hands during the injection procedure by a dental assistant, stabilization of a leg that was starting to lift from the chair by a dental assistant, or stabilization of a shoulder by a dentist as a child starts to roll over, when paired with language, becomes part of the entire linguistic management of the child. This is ontological coaching.

Comments. Gentle physical restraint allows for the reframing of a previous request by the dentist.

Praise and Communication

Praise and communication are self-explanatory. All people, including children, react favorably to praise. Furthermore, effective dentistry for children means effective communication of the dentist with the child and vice versa. Both allow for distraction of the anxious child. Language obviously needs to be age-appropriate. Knowing how to talk to children of different ages comes with experience.

Comments. Praise and effective communication combined with tell-show-do form an unbeatable linguistic combination for managing the dental experience for the majority of children age 3 years or older.

Other Methods

There are other management techniques that are readily available to the dentist and are taught in at least some dental schools in North America. Among these are maternal anxiety reduction techniques. (Paternal anxiety reduction has not been studied, but such study probably would lead to similar conclusions.) It has been shown that as a mother's anxiety about her child's dental appointment lessens, so does her child's anxiety. Pairing a frightened child with a "brave" child in the clinic has had some success. Hypnosis and relaxation techniques have some devotees. Play therapy, "time out" to listen to music or "white sound," other distraction techniques, desensitization sessions, gift giving, and observation appointments all have been advocated to some degree at one time or another.

THE NONVERBAL ADVANTAGE TO CHILD PATIENT MANAGEMENT

In 1964, Dr. John Brauer, one of the founders of the specialty of Pediatric Dentistry, noted the following pertaining to the technique called "voice control of the child patient":

> Voice control by the practitioners is an all-important factor in management of the patient. The tone and the emphasis employed in talking with the child produce favorable or unfavorable reactions. While many dentists have recognized the value of voice control and have mastered satisfactory voice techniques, additional research is warranted in this area.

In the same chapter of his textbook, Dr. Brauer went on to offer another conclusion about voice control:

> The voice, with certain qualities under control, has motivated nations in peace as well as war; has captured audiences at all age levels; and it can have a profound influence in the behavior pattern of the individual. It is a powerful instrument employed in too few instances in child behavior problems. The profession must learn more of the positive value of this technique.

The article "Voice Control: An Old Technique Reexamined" (Pinkham, 1985) concluded that facial expression was just as important as the voice (if not more important) during the phenomenon that has been traditionally called "voice control of the child patient." It was noted that facial expression of the dentist conveys to the child that the practitioner is serious and in control. It is the voice and the face that make the dentist powerful in management of the child. A variety of authorities on nonverbal communication from other disciplines were cited to verify this conclusion (Allport, 1961; Baker, 1961; Birdwhistell, 1955; Brandt, 1945; Byrnes, 1950; Darwin, 1904; Goodenough, 1931; Mehrabian, 1968, 1972).

Since that paper, the linguistic phenomena of requests and promises and their importance for the child during the dental experience have been described (Pinkham, 1993, 1995). In fact, these papers portrayed the entire dental experience as being a social interaction based on two constituent speech acts: that of requests made by the dentist and that of promises by the child patient to take effective actions in response to those requests. What this discussion describes is that the request or re-request of the dentist in the domain called "voice control" implies that there is a body posture that may or may not be entirely visible to the child but that takes the dentist to "a place" from which the dentist can speak with authority, command, and self-confidence. This place allows the experience of the nonverbal advantage. This means the clinician is in a posture and body control that empowers his or her coaching of the child patient.

Effectiveness in the nonverbal management of children, even those children who display or develop recalcitrant behavior during their dental appointment, is demonstrated by clinicians who not only make the verbal request to stop such behavior but are able to re-request when needed with more verbal determination, with appropriate facial expression, and from a bodily posture position in which they know that they are competent. The power of re-requesting is the essence of being competent in managing misbehaving children. This ability is both mental (the words) and physical (the face and body). The body is important to both the voice and the face. This body dimension is described, for lack of a better word, as "a place" but it is to be interpreted as total body posture. Feet, hands, and head are in a relationship to the torso, spine, and breathing pattern such that the total posture energizes the clinician and simultaneously (with or without conscious recognition) allows the clinician to adopt a posture and motion from which his or her most powerful articulations and self-expressions can emanate.

The HOM exercise is also favorably enhanced by the nonverbal advantage. In fact, effective voice control either precedes or is concomitant with effective HOM. I argue that effective HOM would be impossible without effective voice control, and effective voice control is probably impossible without the nonverbal advantage.

Where Is "The Place?"

There is no formal research in pediatric dentistry describing the most effective posture in which to practice the nonverbal advantage. It is my observation in watching veteran clinicians intercept the misbehaviors of preschool children that they do so by looking at the child in a downward and forward position of their bodies. Clinicians who notice the deterioration of behavior while in a posture in which they are largely behind the child generally move to a position such that there is frontal facial posture available for the child to see expressions and to have eye contact. The leaning downward and forward dramatizes to the child nonverbally that the original requests of the clinician are important.

This posture also offers the possibility of having a profound positive effect on the confidence of the clinician. This confidence shift is the nonverbal advantage. Leaning away or adjusting to a higher posture could be argued to be contraindicated when looking for the nonverbal advantage while working with a misbehaving child. Importantly, once it is mastered, the clinician will reflexively go to the posture of downward and forward; it does not have to be re-remembered. It is like stepping on the brakes of your car when a red light appears. It lives in your body. It is the fact that it is so reflexive that clinicians who have mastered it are reticent to abandon it. It is also obvious that for practitioners who have never mastered the technique that when they try to practice it consciously that it is not as effective as when it is reflexively practiced.

Nowhere is this philosophy of body affecting confidence so well described in contemporary western literature as it is in the book *Retooling On The Run* by Stuart Heller and David Surrenda (1994). This book addresses the origins of self-confidence as they relate to the body, and is intended for the business world and its executives; however, the issues involved with posture, centered presence, and changing one's experience through motion have direct implications for the dental clinician who works with children as well. Anyone interested in a more thorough description is encouraged to read and study this book.

Figure 23–3, entitled "Your Attitude and Postural Dynamics," is a copyrighted portrayal by Dr. Heller that summarizes how body position affects

Attitude & Postural Dynamics

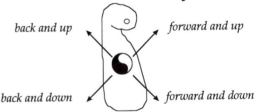

back and up   forward and up

back and down   forward and down

ATTITUDE: **grounded, decisive and powerful**
POSTURE: *forward and down*

ATTITUDE: **supportive, caring and adaptable**
POSTURE: *back and down*

ATTITUDE: **dynamic, inspiring and friendly**
POSTURE: *forward and up*

ATTITUDE: **thoughtful, peaceful and perceptive**
POSTURE: *back and up*

Figure 23–3. Attitude and postural dynamics. (Adapted from art copyrighted by Dr. Stuart Heller.)

attitude. Dr. Heller draws on the research of Dr. Albert Mehrabian, who found that during the communication experience, 7% of one's impact comes from the words that are chosen, 38% come from how those words are said (tone, volume, pacing), and 55% of the impact comes from nonverbal expressions, including such things as movement, posture, gesture, and timing. Dr. Heller also offers that attitude is a function of the interactions between state of mind, feeling, and how one carries oneself. Therefore, an attitude of confidence by a clinician has a great deal to do with the way he or she postures.

From the figure it can be seen that the forward and down position gives a grounded, concise, and powerful attitude. This is what is needed to intercept misbehavior or potential misbehavior of the child patient. It should be noted that this is not the only posture that a clinician needs to work in. In fact, there are times for all four postures. For the domain that has previously been called voice control, however, there seems to be no question that the forward and down posture is the one that is relevant to the clinician who requests and re-requests appropriate behaviors from misbehaving or possibly misbehaving child patients.

This posture is important in the performance of the HOM exercise. In fact, HOM often requires that the practitioner whisper to the child his or her desires for a better behavior and the promise to remove the hand once behavior is restored. This forces the clinician into that downward and forward posture in which, I contend, the nonverbal advantage lies. Being forced into this posture may be one of the reasons *why* those practitioners who effectively use HOM *are* effective. Unknown to them is the fact that the posture they need for the success of the technique is the very posture that is most empowering for them.

An Explanation for Body Affecting Mind

Until recently, Western science has been dominated by the Cartesian notion of the duality of mind and body. This theory has been attacked by a number of disciplines ranging from medicine to philosophy and from biology to linguistics. A recent and popular book, *Descartes' Error* (Damasio, 1994), presents a vivid and convincing argument about the mistakes in this theory.

What is emerging is that clearly there is no duality. Mind belongs to body and body belongs to mind. There is no seam between them. Mental processes such as worry, anxiety, and anger have

profound physiologic effects on the body. Moreover, motion, movement, posture, and breathing have dynamic impacts on attitudes, emotions, and moods. In fact, training the body can sometimes alter mental characteristics and processes faster than information absorbed directly by reading or hearing.

I submit that the power of the requests and re-requests of a competent clinician is enhanced by the clinician's control of the body. This control favorably affects such factors as facial expression and tonality of voice. This is a distinct nonverbal advantage and is a useful predictor that distinguishes those clinicians who have the "knack" of working with children. They have the knack even though their dialogue may be identical to someone who does not have the knack. They may have smaller frames and less muscle mass than their less competent colleagues. They may have a higher voice, be less articulate, or even suffer from a speech impediment and still be more effective than others who have outstanding voice qualities. The nonverbal advantage is a bodily advantage that empowers these clinicians during the communication process of making requests of the child patient.

Categories of Nonverbal Advantage Competency

Clinicians can find themselves to be at various levels of competency in the practice of the nonverbal advantage. I think that no one comes into dentistry having mastered the nonverbal advantage with children even though they may be parents or older siblings or have had educational experiences with children. Simply said, for most American adults today we have little opportunity to interact with children in ways that demand we learn to make bodily adjustments in order to empower our requests and re-requests with the children in our lives. The one exception might be people who have been coaches of children in domains in which fear was an issue that had to be overcome through the coaching. For instance, swimming and diving coaches of young children may have unconsciously experienced a nonverbal advantage as they encouraged children to overcome dreads of water and heights.

BEGINNERS

Dental students come to their dental education as beginners in the domain of the nonverbal advantage. The effectiveness of the curriculum, handouts, textbook assignments, and clinical challenges set the stage for whether a dental student wishes to master the nonverbal advantage or not. Obviously, if the educators do not recognize the nonverbal advantage and do not practice from a nonverbal advantage point of view, the students will probably not even be aware of this phenomenon. If the pediatric dentistry faculty do believe in this, practice it, and serve as role models, however, some students may initially intellectually accept that this does work and, because of curiosity and enthusiasm, may try to develop this talent while in dental school.

It should be noted that this is a difficult technique to teach in that it comes from a level of self-awareness that must be arrived at by each individual in his or her own fashion and time. It is difficult to structure appointments and recruit those kinds of patients in which the nonverbal advantage can be realized. Therefore, it is submitted that, except for those students that have a significant amount of clinical pediatric dentistry, often in extramural clinics in which misbehavior is present, most dental students are not able to develop this advantage until after dental school. It is also submitted that the nonverbal advantage is difficult to learn in the presence of parents in that some degree of experimentation with body, tonality of voice, and facial expression is required while learning. The presence of a parent may arouse enough anxiety in the young clinician so as to thwart experimentation in these dimensions of the nonverbal advantage.

It is also obvious that there are clinicians who, from the very beginning of their dental education, do not want a nonverbal advantage. For the dental student who approaches pediatric dentistry with assessments about children being psychologically delicate or believes that the practice of aspects of the nonverbal advantage such as raising one's voice could either compromise the child's self-esteem or promote anxiety that shows up beyond the dental appointment, mastering the nonverbal advantage will not become a goal. Furthermore, if the student does not believe that the nonverbal advantage is any more effective than other techniques, the nonverbal advantage will not be realized in all likelihood during the course of this dentist's career.

Last, there is evidence of the clinician who once had the nonverbal advantage but lost it. Stories about offices that have routinely opened the operatories up to parents have noted that certain clinicians who practice the nonverbal advantage when not being observed by anyone other than dental staff feel uncomfortable doing such practices in the presence of nondental ob-

servers, particularly parents and guardians. Other clinicians may have sought other solutions: mastery of sedative methods, referral of misbehaving children to other clinicians, willingness to delay treatment, and willingness to work on a crying child stabilized by a papoose board. Clinicians may, through lack of practice, eventually lose the nonverbal advantage even though for years it had lived spontaneously in their bodies and had been reflexively practiced.

EXPERIMENTAL MASTERY

This phase refers to the person who has with conviction tried to find the nonverbal advantage. This clinician has looked for that place in which his or her request or re-request has the strongest design and the greatest impact on the child. Once the person has experienced the positive effects of the nonverbal advantage, he or she will enthusiastically try to practice it more. But until the place that this person has to go is spontaneous and reflexive, the nonverbal advantage may not reliably assist this clinician each and every time a child starts to misbehave. There is a time of trial and error that some clinicians can stay with until they reach mastery. Increasingly for other clinicians, however, the particular climate that we now have to practice dentistry in today, complete with risk management, informed consent issues, litigation, parental presence, and other societal issues that beg dentists not to be as aggressive in the management of children as we were in past decades, can preclude any possibility of obtaining the nonverbal advantage as a reflexive behavior.

MASTERY

Most of the dentists today who reflexively practice with a nonverbal advantage have done so because initially they believed in it. They have experienced it to be powerful. They have had great rewards from it, and they can talk about it in terms that deny the veracity of information implying that there are long-term side effects of these practices. These are mostly older clinicians educated in times where the nonverbal advantage was a technique of choice and when sedative techniques were not necessarily a part of the curriculum of an advanced training program in pediatric dentistry. For younger clinicians who have not seen the nonverbal advantage practiced but who want to, I submit that competent clinicians do exist in virtually all regions of the country and these clinicians could serve as role models for young clinicians looking to develop these skills.

Mastering the Nonverbal Advantage

Figure 23-4 is labeled "Stages of Learning Child Patient Management." This diagram portrays the process of mastering the nonverbal advantage.

The beginning point is making a shift in the language and movement patterns of the clinician around the child patient. Movement encompasses everything the body does, including posture, breathing, action of limbs, walking, concentrating, and emotion. This begins as didactic knowledge gained in the classroom and in homework assignments. Progress here is documented by examinations. The art of working with a child in language complete with appropriate postures is intended to equip the student with techniques and abilities that give his or her actions results. In other words, the purpose of the education is to inform the student about how to manage children. The information by itself, however, does not lead to the nonverbal advantage. Four other steps have to take place.

The second step is labeled a shift in the tone of experience. By this it is meant that the information in teaching language and movement must be accorded credibility by the dental student/ dentist. There must be a verification by the dental student/dentist that a nonverbal advantage is possible.

If a shift is made in the tone of the experience then and only then can there be a shift in presence. This new presence is based on self-confidence in this domain, at least to the extent that the clinician is willing to attempt new behaviors with child patients. It is a change of attitude, a change in the appreciation of the possibilities of personal effectiveness in this domain. The clinician is able to feel this shift. Because of the subtlety of this shift, it may not be visible to the educator/observer.

The shift of presence is what allows for the fourth step: a shift in the set of possible actions that can take place. The clinician now can take effective actions with the child that were impossible before. These new behaviors are visible to the informed observer. It is absolutely verifiable when a dental student/dentist arrives at this level in mastering the nonverbal advantage.

The shift in possible actions allows for a shift in action path, action initiatives, and action results by the clinician. Linguistically this happens by allowing for powerful requests and re-requests that are enhanced by body movement and facial expression. This is the culmination of the nonverbal advantage.

This whole five-step process can happen quickly, and certain dentists can remember learning it on a particular day with a particular patient. The other side of the story is a dentist realizing the shift has happened and that he or she can take more effective actions with child patients in the nonverbal dimension, but the dentist does not know when he or she actually acquired such skill.

Summary: Nonverbal Advantage

The nonverbal advantage has been and still is a powerful management technique of children. Paradoxically, it has probably been called voice control over the years. It belongs in the domain of nonpharmacologic management. It is a linguistic technique because it enhances requests. It

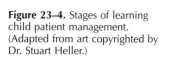

Figure 23–4. Stages of learning child patient management. (Adapted from art copyrighted by Dr. Stuart Heller.)

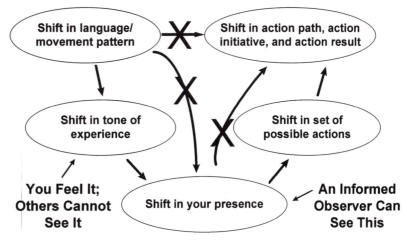

can generally be called a psychological technique. Most importantly, it has to affect the clinician before it has any advantageous effect on the child. The nonverbal advantage affects the voice and its tonality, cadence, and other qualities. It affects facial expression, a powerful part of nonverbal communication. It affects the self-talk of the clinician and therefore the self-confidence about the distinctions the clinician is making about his or her ability to successfully manage the child. There is a distinct and important postural aspect to this. It is my observation that for most clinicians, going to a downward and forward position in front of the child while simultaneously establishing eye contact is the place to which most clinicians go to to find the nonverbal advantage.

(The author wishes to acknowledge his appreciation for the critical review of this part of this chapter by Dr. Stuart Heller, President and Founder of Moving Systems, 513 Santa Fe Avenue, Albany, CA 94706, and for the use of the copyrighted material portrayed in Fig. 23-3.)

PROFILE OF THE GOOD CHILD DENTAL PATIENT

When new acquaintances find out that a dentist treats children, they often offer the conclusion that he or she must be a remarkably patient person. Actually, anything but that conclusion is necessarily true. The reason that people make this false assumption stems in part from a misconception about what it takes to treat children successfully in a dental clinic. These people probably believe that the dentist must sit in his clinic, lovingly holding the hand of every child he or she treats and searching for words and phrases that get the child to cooperate.

Such a perception is generally wrong. The fact remains that the great majority of children over 36 to 40 months of age are astonishingly well behaved and compliant dental patients when handled correctly. In fact, they may be the easiest of all patient types to treat. They don't demand exceptional patience from the dentist. They don't need it.

Performing dentistry for these kids is a pleasant, rewarding professional experience. In many cases, the dentist feels a personal attachment to the child ("He's mine"). It's fun to talk to these children, to ask them questions, to find out what they will wear at Halloween or want for Christmas, to know their favorite television show or food, or to find out how they feel about their new baby brother. Conversing with children is

fun and should be, overall, a relaxing part of a general practitioner's day.

The good child dental patient reacts to "critical moments" of the dental appointment appropriately. This means that he or she reacts *as well as he or she can.* The most frequent critical moments in dentistry for children and how the good child dental patient manages them are described as follows.

CRITICAL MOMENTS IN THE DENTAL APPOINTMENT AND THE GOOD CHILD DENTAL PATIENT

Separation from the Parent

As already discussed, separation from the parent is not always done. Children under 36 to 40 months of age often behave better if the parent accompanies them to the dental operatory. Often the parent of a child younger than 3 years old has an opinion about whether the youngster will be better or worse if he or she is present. After this age, most children do not need their parents to accompany them, but the dentist may prefer to have the parents present during the appointment. The dentist's preference should be known by the parent and child *at least* before the first treatment appointment (e.g., fillings, extractions).

If the parent of a child older than 3 years old does accompany the child to the operatory, he or she should be prepared to leave if the youngster does not behave. This agreement between parent and dentist about leaving should be made *before* the child is seated in the dental chair. It is important for the child to know about the agreement.

The good child dental patient, as a general rule, separates easily from the parent. This is not to say that the separation is easy for the child emotionally, but it does mean that the child has the wherewithal to do it. At his or her best, the child looks eager to get started, shows no observable fear, and talks freely with the dental assistant who escorts him or her from the reception room. At the worst the child acts as a victim so the parent can become the rescuer. The dental appointment is a perfect time for this last scenario to take place. Every dentist who treats children should expect this on some recurring and perhaps even predictable basis.

Getting into the Chair

As simple as it sounds, some kids have difficulty getting into the dental chair. This may stem from natural fears and the perceived vulnerability that goes along with being off one's feet. Some kids need assistance and have to be guided by the hand or even picked up and put into the chair.

The good child dental patient, however, gets right into the chair. It is really pleasant when this happens because it provides the first real opportunity to praise the child for his good behavior and ability to do the things asked of him. ("Wow, John, look at you. I bet your daddy couldn't have gotten into this chair any faster.")

Dentist Seated at Chair

The dentist approaching the chair indicates to the child that treatment is imminent. The well-adjusted child can handle this and responds to his or her name (most dentists have learned the value of nicknames), answer questions, and accept and react to praise. ("What a pretty dress." "Thank you, Mommy got it for me.")

The dentist also represents the most authoritative figure in the dental office, and the good child patient realizes that his or her directives need to be followed. Directives such as "Hands on your tummy and open wide-tall" are obeyed by the child and obeyed quickly.

The Injection

Without question, the injection is the most universally feared procedure in dentistry for children and maybe in dentistry in general. It is, however, not a major obstacle for most children. A large percentage of children do not react at all to the injection. The technique is now so painless that many little kids never even know that they received a "shot" when the dentist gave them "sleepy water." A good-tasting topical anesthetic is usually indicated. It is not indicated in the obviously agitated child who appears to be getting worse.

A small percentage of young children know from siblings, parents, and peers that they will receive an injection. Unfortunately, many youngsters have been given a frightening description of the needle. They expect pain. Fortunately, many of these kids still accept the procedure with only a few tears and with virtually no avoidance behaviors. These kids then learn that the "shot" isn't bad at all, and at later appointments the "pinch" is experienced as just that, a little pinching feeling in the mouth. The dentist must not lie about the needle. If asked whether the injection will hurt, he or she should say, "You will feel a little pinch."

If the child starts to show avoidance behaviors, firm voice control needs to be established. Seldom does delaying the injection result in better behavior. Few dentists have found any benefit in showing the syringe to the child who "wants to see what it looks like." Therefore, clinicians are encouraged not to be hesitant with this procedure. In fact, not using a topical anesthetic may, in certain situations, be wise because of the additional waiting time involved.

A child can cry during the injection and perhaps even need some momentary restraint of arms and body by a dental assistant and still qualify as a very good dental patient. The test is whether the crying and squirming stop when the needle disappears.

Figure 23-5 shows a recommended method for the dental assistant to pass the needle from the tray to the dentist. Obviously, the use of needles around wiggling, thrashing children must be done cautiously.

The Dental Procedure

Nine times out of ten, the dental procedure is restorative treatment if an injection for anesthesia has been given. Fortunately, dentists do not need to extract many teeth in children anymore. For the good child patient, the procedure itself (i.e., the drilling) is easy compared with the injection. Many youngsters fall asleep during the procedure. This may come as a surprise, but most children, even 3-year-olds, can tolerate a fairly long dental appointment without becoming restless. As said before, most kids are great dental patients.

There is still some need for extractions. Here again, most kids do well, but clinical experience still leads many dentists to believe that this can be a scary procedure for little ones. Some authors have assigned Freudian castration implications to this fear. I think that it is the force and torquing applied to the tooth that arouses anxiety. Luckily, most extractions in children are quick and simple.

End of the Appointment

It may seem silly to label the end of the appointment a crisis, but sometimes people spend all their emotional reserves during the heat of battle and then afterward become unglued. A good child dental patient ends his or her appointment

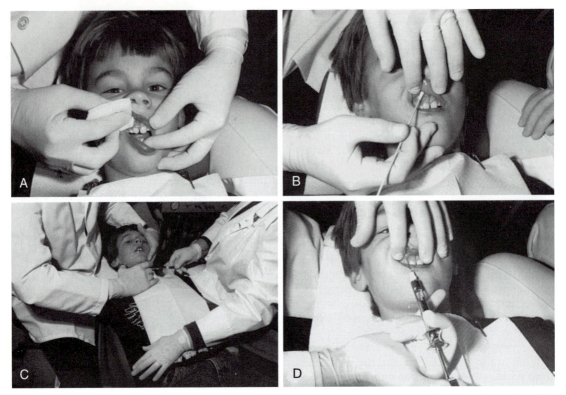

Figure 23–5. *A,* Drying of mucosa prior to using an acceptable-tasting topical anesthetic. *B,* Application of topical anesthetic. This step can be eliminated for very apprehensive children. *C,* Under-the-chin transfer of syringe. Note that the dental assistant is prepared to restrain the child's arms. *D,* Introduction of syringe to oral cavity. Note how the syringe is stabilized by a finger touching the patient's chin.

on a high note. He or she is eager to leave yet is patient enough and human enough to stay around to be congratulated and praised for his or her behavior in the chair.

Return to the Parent

The return of the child to the parent also may not seem like a crisis event. When one understands how some misbehaving child dental patients handle this aspect of their dental appointment, however, this time and its importance become more clear. Some children want their parents to feel guilty about making them go to the dentist and portray themselves as victims. This dramatization can often be intercepted if the dentist or auxiliary is present.

Good child dental patients return to their parents beaming with pride. They know that they have done well and have pleased their parents. They are pleased with themselves. The dentist's compliments to their parents about them are returned by way of smiles and bright eyes. For the dentist, this is a happy occasion.

In summary, most kids turn out to be good, accepting dental patients. There are exceptions, however, and these exceptions need to be understood.

PARENTAL ATTENDANCE IN THE DENTAL OPERATORY

The issue of whether a parent (or parents) should be present in the dental operatory during a child's dental appointment is one that inspires divergent opinions among practitioners of dentistry for children. Parents have varying opinions on this issue also.

Certainly, it can be said that for most of the twentieth century, many dentists as a general rule did not want the parents in attendance during treatment. This was particularly true if the child was over 3 years of age and was of normal social, psychological, and emotional development. A study in 1971 of 120 American Association of Pedodontics diplomates would seem to have verified these facts, at least among specialists. In this study, only five always had the parents back; 18

never did; and 97 did in selected cases. Age of the child was the most often cited reason for allowing parents in attendance. A total of 90 dentists responded to a question about the appropriateness of the parent's attendance compared with the child's age: 71 thought it was appropriate at birth to 1 year; 76 at 1 to 2 years; 35 at 2 to 4 years; and 8 at 4 to 6 years.

The changing times of the 1990s, however, have affected the number of dentists who have reconsidered their policy about admitting parents (Pinkham, 1990). It should be noted that, in a litigious society when risk management is an important feature in running a practice that involves the behavior of children, parental attendance during difficult management circumstances may be a safer approach legally than denying their attendance. Attendance also may foster a more secure feeling in certain parents because they know that, in observing the entire appointment, they can act as an advocate for their child and verify his or her safety (Pinkham, 1991).

It seems reasonable to encourage dentists to think through their own policy regarding parental attendance and to be flexible about the arrangements they have made regarding this presence. It can be argued that there certainly are parents who want to be in attendance and may not remain with the practice or may be anxious about staying in the practice if they are eliminated as a matter of routine procedure because of the philosophy of the dental office. Conversely, there are definitely instances when the presence of the parent may actually heighten the alarm of the child; when being accompanied by the parent allows the child to portray himself or herself as a victim and thereby, it is hoped, recruiting the parent into the role of rescuer; or when the parents frankly are so anxious about dentistry themselves that they heighten the fear responses of the child.

MISBEHAVING CHILD DENTAL PATIENTS

It is now appropriate to explore the types of children who reliably misbehave at the dental office. These are children who just can't cope or, importantly, just *won't* cope with the stimuli and behavioral demands of the dental experience.

The first group are special children who are emotionally compromised. This is not a large group of children, but they do exist. Dentistry as well as many other challenges of life are difficult for these children because of their psychoemo-

tional problems. It is important to realize that the problem may be undiagnosed.

The next largest group are the "shy birds." These are introverted, poorly socialized children who are afraid of the social challenges associated with going to the dentist. The best management technique with these children is to break the barrier of shyness with friendship.

The third group is composed of children who have a hard time with dentistry because they are frightened. (Fear of dentistry is discussed later.) It is my opinion that fear of needles is 90% of the fear of dentistry.

Another group of misbehaving children includes those who do not like authority. These children don't like dental appointments, and their dislike is based on an aversion to compliance with adult directives.

Category I: The Emotionally Compromised Child

A reliable finding in patients with emotional illness is anxiety. When the anxiety of an emotional illness is compounded by the anxiety associated with a dental appointment, a behavioral explosion often occurs. Emotionally compromised children are generally poor dental patients. At best, they are no fun. It is as if there is no child left in a child's body.

The problem with these patients is that often there is no confirmed diagnosis. Parents, even very intelligent, well-informed parents, have no idea that anything is wrong. Because they have grown accustomed to the behaviors of their child, they often overlook the abnormalities of the child's behavior, or they have rationalized an explanation for why their child behaves in certain ways. This situation is extremely unfortunate because most emotional diseases are diagnosable and treatable, and, as is so often the case, the earlier the upset is addressed, the faster and more effective is the therapy.

Emotional illness can also be a problem for children from broken homes and other unfortunate parenting circumstances. The children of poverty probably suffer more from emotionally compromised families than do children from more privileged classes. As a group, abused and neglected children (see Chapter 1) certainly exhibit a high incidence of emotional dysfunction (Pinkham et al., 1988).

The author has had little success in convincing parents that their child's misbehavior during a dental appointment might be due to an unknown emotional problem. It is professional to share any convictions that the dentist may have that are for the child's welfare, however. Of course, if abuse and neglect are suspected, the dentist is legally obligated to report such children to the appropriate authorities.

Category II: The Shy, Introverted Child

Introversion or shyness is a problem for many people, including children, especially very young children. Because the dental experience for children is a fairly intense human encounter that demands rapport and communication between the adult dentist and the child patient, it is obvious that a very shy child will be stressed by the experience. This stress can lead the child to an avoidance behavior such as crying. Usually the crying takes the form of compensatory whimpering. Rarely does the introverted child display aggressive avoidance behavior such as a tantrum. These children can be likened to puppies in some respects. When threatened, they go limp and tremble.

The dental profession has long recognized that shy children have a hard time adjusting to the expectations of a dental appointment. As with all children, the dentist's first objective is to establish rapport, trust, and communication. With shy children, this requires patience because they are unskilled at "feeling people out" and they are categorically mesmerized by the challenge of communicating.

As formidable as the challenge may seem, however, the various techniques of talking to these children on their own level, using praise and the tell-show-do technique, reliably penetrate the oyster shell that these youngsters have secreted around their personalities, and in time, sometimes startlingly fast, they open up. When they open up, they usually become fantastic patients because the dental appointment becomes a social event wherein somebody knows their name, is interested in them, and is willing and ready to talk to them. This opening up does not always happen, but it often does.

Category III: The Frightened Child

A child who is frightened is a formidable challenge to the dentist as well as to teachers, physicians, parents, and everyone else who encounters him or her. In treating such a child, the dentist has a particular problem in that even though the dental encounter is not very long, it is intense and requires, ideally, enormous cooperation from the child. The dentist also contends with the problem of fear to perhaps a greater degree than that encountered by most other adults who react with the child. Such fear ranges from fear of needles to fear of bodily harm to general fear of the unknown. If someone really wanted to make a complete and specific list of all the possible sights, sounds, smells, and expectations that are reasonably unique to the dental experience, it would probably fill up a legal pad. The handheld instruments alone would make an extensive list of possibilities.

The answer to the question of whether a child may misbehave in the dental office because of fear is definitely affirmative. Determining whether a child's misbehavior is motivated by fear or another cause is, as one would expect, a more challenging proposition. Yet, information paired with experience and common sense reliably allows the dentist to determine what is motivating the child.

Some of the established causes of fear that can be used by a parent or clinician to help identify a child who is very fearful of dentistry include the following:

- The child is intellectually unable, even when educated by a parent or dentist, to arrest his or her fears about the dental appointment either because of his or her chronologic age (roughly, 36 to 40 months is the age when most normal children are intellectually able to arrest their fears when given information about what will happen) or because of slow development (perhaps mental retardation).
- The child is overreacting to fears because of other emotional upsets in his or her life. This category includes children who come from homes that are in acute chaos because of an impending divorce or parental separation, children who are abused, and children who are grieving because of the loss of a grandparent or friend. Children who are coping with other health problems are included in this category. These circumstances often yield self-limiting emotional disturbances. The problems resolve in time, but when present they make dentistry, particularly some of the more rigorous appointments such as tooth extraction, difficult for these children to endure.
- The child has been "sold" a set of fears by peers, siblings, or parents. Such fears have been called *acquired fears.*
- The child has had a previous difficult or painful experience at a physician's or dentist's office or at a hospital. These are called *learned fears.*
- The child is emotionally ill.

All of these categories of children, with perhaps the exception of the emotionally ill, are easy to define and identify. Emotional illness, as discussed previously, is something parents often do not address at home, and the real clues to emotional disturbances often do not emerge until these youngsters are enrolled in a formal educational process and are observed by a teacher daily.

One major point is in order here. If the misbehavior occurs because of an intense dread or fear of dentistry, it is important for the parent and the dentist to establish this fact in no uncertain terms. If a child is so frightened that good behavior is impossible, it is the obligation of both of these adults to make sure that everything possible is done to avoid increasing the child's anxieties attendant to dentistry. This may mean postponing dental work, it may mean using drugs, and it may even mean performing dentistry under general anesthesia. Whatever it requires, it is important to take the most appropriate measures regardless of cost, convenience, and efficiency. That is the only humane course to take.

As said before, dreadfully fearful children usually can be screened and identified before dentistry begins. The only gray zone concerns the child who seems to have an emotional illness. When there is a high suspicion of emotional illness (no one can explain why the youngster would be so frightened), it is the most professional and humane course for the dentist to refer the child to a psychiatrist, psychologist, or other counselor. The parent should accept this referral in the spirit in which it is given—that is, the best thing that can be done for this child at this time is to establish whether in fact he or she is emotionally healthy enough to go through a dental appointment without resorting to maladaptive behavior and its sequelae.

Category IV: The Child Who Is Adverse to Authority

The Duke of Windsor, during one of his visits to the United States, noted tongue-in-cheek that one of the things that he liked about America was how well American parents minded their children. Much has been written in the dental literature over the years about children who are difficult because they cannot follow adult directives well (Pinkham, 1983). Some labels applied to these youngsters have been spoiled children, incorrigible or overindulged children, and defiant children. Certainly, even the most casual observer can verify that children exhibit a variety of misbehaviors. One trip to a grocery store, a fast food restaurant, or even a public swimming pool where parents and children congregate will reliably show misbehaving children. If children misbehave in a shopping mall, in the automobiles of their parents, and even in their own homes, why should they not misbehave at the dentist's office?

What is the nature of this misbehavior? Why does it happen? There are children for whom emotional illness, introversion, or fear simply is not the reason for inappropriate behavior at the dental office. The reason is instead that these children have an aversion to authority. On analysis, it is easy to see that a dentist is a strong authoritative figure in his or her own office and therefore a prime candidate for stimulating the worst behavior of such children.

Where did the aversion to authority come from? The works of Dr. Alfred Adler, who was a contemporary of Freud and Jung, and Dr. Rudolph Dreikurs, a student and devotee of Adler, point out that there are four potential misdirected goals in the life of a child (Adler, 1958; Dreikurs, 1964). These goals seep into the personality repertoire of the child, where they subtly satisfy the strong human craving for superiority, believed by Adler to be the main force that drives all human behavior. Noting that one potential way of feeling superior is achieved by manipulating other people, both authors warn parents that their child may adopt a style of behavior with the parents that will carry over to other authority figures whom the child encounters in life, such as the dentist. These misdirected goals and what they mean to the involved children are as follows:

1. *Undue attention:* "In order to satisfy my intense appetite for feeling superior, I will, through manipulative behavior, make sure that my parents pay attention to me any time that I want them to. Because this paying attention to me quickly relieves my insecurities about my being superior, I am likely to want much more attention than is reasonable."
Behavioral characteristics: Annoying, irritating, teasing, disruptive.

2. *Struggle for power:* "In order to satisfy my intense appetite for feeling superior, I am prepared to have a power struggle with my parents about getting attention. This is a challenge and I do intend to win. They will pay attention to me or else."
Behavioral characteristics: Argues and contradicts, does the opposite of instructions, makes people angry, throws temper tantrums.

3. *Retaliation and revenge:* "In order to satisfy my intense appetite for feeling superior, if I do not get what I want, which in a nutshell is attention, I will get even with my parents and I will punish them. I will not let them do this to me without hurting them back."

Behavioral characteristics: Displays violent temper, says things that hurt people, seeks revenge, gets even.

4. *Inadequacy:* "In order to satisfy my intense appetite for feeling superior, I have convinced myself that I am special in the worst sort of way. I am totally unable to grow up, unable to achieve, and in fact I plan to do nothing at all for either myself, my parents, or anyone else on the face of this earth."

Behavioral characteristics: Gives up easily, rarely participates, acts as if he or she is incapable, displays inadequacy.

Space does not permit a detailed discussion of misdirected children. It seems obvious that each of the four misdirected goals becomes more serious from one level to the next. The child who simply wants some attention may very likely find dentistry a nice experience in that it is such a personal one-on-one occasion. The child who engages in a power struggle has a bully's attitude and may not have any compunctions at all about arguing with a dentist or challenging a dentist's authority. The child who engages in retaliation and revenge can frankly be dangerous. This is the type of child who may bite. He or she is not warm and fun and probably will not respond to praise. The child who thinks about himself or herself in a defeated, inadequate way is likely to show a variety of misbehaviors if the dentist asks him or her to cooperate. Overcoming the challenges of the dental appointment is beyond the grasp of this child. When challenges arise, this child tells himself that he is inferior and can't possibly measure up.

I think that misdirected children can often be also described as prefigurative children. The term *prefigurative*, as opposed to postfigurative and configurative, is the description of Margaret Mead. Basically, prefigurative describes a child, raised by prefigurative parents, and prefigurative parents are those that raise their children outside of any consistent cultural tradition. This is a phenomenon that started in the United States after World War II and which Dr. Mead said would happen around the world in time. It has also been noted that the children of prefigurative parents are not well rehearsed in handling the requests of adults. Obviously, with dentistry being such an intense communication experience built on requests and promises, this lack of rehearsal predicts potential problems for the dentist who works with such children.

Another paralleling concern for dentists treating today's child is the phenomenon of learned helplessness. With today's parent being so busy and with often both parents being at work all day long, certain children may find that a strategy of helplessness is one predictable way of getting attention from their parents in their home setting. Because the misdirected behavior of some parents sets the stage on which their child wishes to act as a helpless victim so his or her parents will come to the rescue, the dental experience can easily precipitate this particular phenomenon.

It should also be noted that severely misdirected children present problems in a variety of social circumstances and certainly have troubles in school. Fortunately, most of these children will in time outgrow their misdirection. One may find only remnants or subtleties of their misdirected behavior in adolescence and young adulthood.

Summary: Misbehaving Children

The four categories of misbehaving children have been outlined in what is believed to be the relative frequency with which a practitioner in dentistry encounters them. In other words, there are fewer emotionally disturbed children than there are introverted children, fewer introverted children than frightened children, and fewer frightened children than children who just do not like to comply with authoritative adults. Blends of the four problem groups obviously exist. In fact, a blend is probably the norm.

I think that dental students and clinicians with little experience in dentistry for children and certainly in dealing with the parents of misbehaving children often assign the majority of the reason for misbehavior in the dental office to a fear of dentistry. Conversely, older and more experienced clinicians do not endorse the fear theory as much but assert that inappropriate behavior really has little to do with the dental appointment. They note that these children do not cope well with any sort of stress and that they often simply do not like to work with any adults who make demands on them. Authority, not dentistry, is what these children dread.

The child who has a genuine dreadful fear of dentistry must be handled carefully, and such handling must be, whenever possible, a cooperative effort on the part of the dentist and the parents. Mild to modest fear of dentistry, particularly fear of the needle, is normal. Importantly, for normal children over 3 years of age who have a competent dentist and one who takes the time to educate them with tell-show-do as the primary technique, these fears can be arrested or made manageable.

In summary, the dental experience is a complex social/psychological arena for the three main participants: the dental team, the parents/guardians, and the children. The practice of effective contemporary pediatric dentistry in the linguistic domain demands sophisticated understanding of all the psychosocial themes that can come into play in the course of a child's dental appointment.

THE BOTTOM LINE

It can be offered that the bottom line in employing behavioral management in dentistry for children today is based in part on first managing the parents, their expectations, dreads, uncertainties, and so on. To some extent this is new ground. So is today's keen interest in risk management and informed consent, especially the area of managing the child assertively or pharmacotherapeutically. There is no evidence that the importance of these concepts will diminish in the foreseeable future.

The most important recommendation of this textbook for the dental clinician is to *talk* to the parents of the young children treated in your office, especially if your management style may be an issue. The ability to create a healthy dialogue between you and the parents is the skill needed here. The process of articulating your options and your limits is not only informative to them but good for you. Such communication helps to develop your practice and refine your own convictions about child patient management. It also can be helpful for some parents and their children.

In the final analysis, if everyone, including you, understands your intent, the outcome is more likely to be satisfactory for all involved.

REFERENCES

Adler A: What Life Should Mean to You. New York, Capricorn Books, 1958.

Allport GW: Pattern and growth in personality. New York, Holt, Rinehart and Winston, 1961, p 41.

American Academy of Pediatric Dentistry: Guidelines for Behavior Management. Chicago, American Academy of Pediatric Dentistry. Pediatr Dent *16*(7):49-52, 1994-95.

American Academy of Pediatric Dentistry: Reference manual: Quality assurance criteria for pediatric dentistry: Behavior management. Pediatr Dent *16*(7):84-87, 1994-95.

Baker S: Visual Persuasion. New York, McGraw-Hill, 1961.

Birdwhistell RL: Background to kinesics. Etc., A Review of General Semantics *13*:0-18, 1955.

Brandt HF: The Psychology of Seeing. New York, Philosophical Library, 1945, pp 32, 107.

Brauer JC: Applied psychology in pedodontics. *In* Lindahl RL (ed): Dentistry for Children, 5th ed. New York, McGraw-Hill, 1964, pp 33-68.

Byrnes G: A Complete Guide to Cartooning. New York, Grosset and Dunlap, 1950, p 46.

Chambers DW: Behavior management techniques for pediatric dentists: An embarrassment of riches. J Dent Child *44*(1):30-34, 1977.

Damasio AR: Descartes' Error. New York, GP Putnam, 1994.

Darwin C: The Expression of the Emotions in Man and Animals. London, John Murray, 1904, pp 143, 372-373.

Dreikurs R, Soltz RN: Children, the Challenge. New York, Hawthorn Books, 1964.

Goodenough FL: The expression of the emotions in infancy. Child Dev *2*:96-101, 1931.

Heller S, Surrenda DS: Retooling on the Run. Berkeley, Frog, 1994.

Heller S: The non-verbal advantage from the Art of Coaching Course, a joint presentation of the Education for Life Seminars, Inc. and The Institute for Movement Psychology, 1996.

Levitas TC: HOME—hand over mouth exercise. J Dent Child *41*(3):23-25, 1974.

Mehrabian A: Communication without words. Psychol Today *11*:53, 1968.

Mehrabian A: Nonverbal Communication. New York, Aldine-Atherton, 1972, pp 1-2.

Pinkham JR: Voice control: An old technique reexamined. J Dent Child *52*:199-202, 1985.

Pinkham JR: Classifying and managing child dental patients' misbehaviors: A three-step Adlerian approach. J Dent Child *5*(4):437-441, 1983.

Pinkham JR, Casamassimo P, Levy S: Dentistry and the children of poverty. J Dent Child *55*(1):17-23, 1988.

Pinkham JR: Behavioral themes in dentistry for children: 1968-1990. J Dent Child *57*(1):38-45, 1990.

Pinkham JR: An analysis of the phenomenon of increased parental participation during the child's dental experience. J Dent Child *58*(6):458-463, 1991.

Pinkham JR: The roles of requests and promises in child patient management. J Dent Child *60*:169-174, 1993.

Pinkham JR: Personality development: Managing behavior of the cooperative preschool child. *In* Johnson D, Tinanoff N (eds): Dental Care for the Preschool Child. Philadelphia, WB Saunders, 1995, pp 771-788.

Chapter 24

Periodontal Problems in Children and Adolescents

Ann L. Griffen

Chapter Outline

Children and adolescents are affected by a variety of periodontal diseases and conditions. Gingivitis is common, especially around the time of puberty. Significant loss of periodontal attachment or alveolar bone is more unusual in young patients but can result from systemic disease or occur as isolated dental disease. In addition, gingival anatomic problems, such as lack of attached gingiva, can arise during development and may require early treatment.

GINGIVITIS

Simple gingivitis is characterized by inflammation of the gingival tissues with no loss of attach-ment or bone. It occurs in response to the bacteria that live in biofilms at the gingival margin and in the sulcus. The clinical signs of gingivitis include erythema, bleeding on probing, and edema. In the early primary dentition, gingivitis is uncommon. Younger children have less plaque than adults do and appear to be less reactive to the same amount of plaque. This can be explained both by differences in bacterial composition of plaque and by developmental changes in inflammatory response. Gingivitis occurs in half the population by the age of 4 or 5 years, and it continues to increase with age. The prevalence of gingivitis peaks at close to 100% at puberty, but after puberty it declines slightly and stays

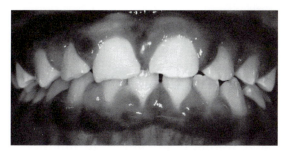

Figure 24–1. Puberty gingivitis in a 13-year-old black male. The dark pigmentation of the gingiva is a normal racial characteristic.

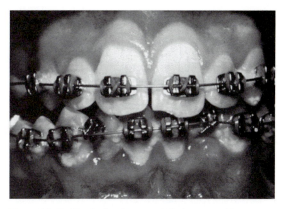

Figure 24–3. Gingival enlargement that occurred in response to long-standing plaque accumulation on the lower incisors secondary to orthodontic appliances.

constant into adulthood (Matsson, 1993). Some children exhibit severe gingivitis at the time of puberty, as is shown in Figure 24-1. Puberty gingivitis is believed to be related to increases in steroid hormones. The gingiva may be enlarged with granulomatous changes similar to those occurring in pregnancy. The peak prevalence of puberty gingivitis is 10 years of age in girls and 13 years of age in boys.

Certain local factors may be important contributors to gingivitis in children. Crowded teeth and orthodontic appliances may make oral hygiene more difficult and predispose to gingivitis. Mouthbreathing may cause chronically dehydrated gingiva in the maxillary labial area and lead to a characteristic localized gingivitis as shown in Figure 24-2. Inflammation, especially erythema, often occurs around erupting primary and permanent teeth.

Gingivitis is reversible and can be treated by improving oral hygiene. Appropriately sized toothbrushes and toothpaste and floss flavored to appeal to children may improve compliance. Young children, especially under 8 to 10 years of age, are not yet capable of performing effective oral hygiene measures and require assistance.

Older children and even adolescents probably need at least some oversight by a parent.

GINGIVAL ENLARGEMENT

Chronic Inflammatory Gingival Enlargement

Longstanding gingivitis in young patients sometimes results in chronic inflammatory gingival enlargement, which may be localized or generalized. It commonly occurs when plaque is allowed to accumulate around orthodontic appliances as shown in Figure 24-3 or in areas chronically dried by mouthbreathing. The interdental papillae and the marginal gingiva become enlarged, and the tissue is usually erythematous and bleeds easily. It may be soft and friable with a smooth, shiny surface. Inflammatory gingival enlargement often slowly resolves when adequate plaque control is instituted, so gingivectomy is rarely required.

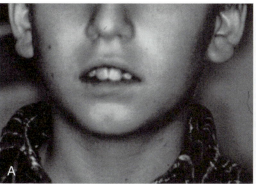
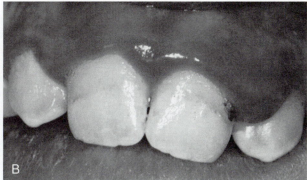

Figure 24–2. *A,* The typical oral posture of mouthbreathing. *B,* The resultant gingivitis of the upper facial gingiva.

Drug-Induced Gingival Overgrowth

Long-term therapy with certain systemic medications can produce an overgrowth of gingival tissue (Fig. 24-4). It can occur after therapy with the anticonvulsant phenytoin (Dilantin), the immunosupressant cyclosporine, or calcium channel blockers. Cyclosporine is used to control host rejection of transplanted organs and to treat autoimmune diseases. The calcium channel blockers such as nifedipine and nitrendipine are cardiac drugs that are sometimes used in children to control hypertension. The overgrowth is painless and differs from chronic inflammatory enlargement in that it is fibrous, firm, and pale pink, often with little tendency to bleed. The enlargement occurs first in the interdental region and may appear lobular. It gradually spreads at the gingival margin. The condition can become extreme, sometimes covering the crowns of the teeth and interfering with eruption or occlusion.

Drug-induced gingival overgrowth occurs slowly and may resolve to some degree when medication is discontinued. There appears to be a genetic component to susceptibility to gingival overgrowth. The severity of the overgrowth is also affected by both the adequacy of oral hygiene and the gingival concentration of the medication. If medication cannot be discontinued or changed, the overgrowth can be surgically removed, but it will recur. The tissue can be removed either by gingivectomy or by a flap with an internal bevel. Surgery is indicated when the appearance of the gingiva is unacceptable to the patient, when the overgrowth interferes with comfortable functioning, or when the overgrowth has produced a periodontal pocket that cannot be maintained in a healthy state. The most severe cases of gingival overgrowth usually occur in mentally retarded patients, in part because of poor oral hygiene. Postoperative discomfort after gingivectomy can be considerable and should be carefully weighed against potential benefits for patients who may not be able to give fully informed consent.

ANATOMIC PROBLEMS

Development and Defects of the Attached Gingiva

When teeth erupt they pierce through an existing band of keratinized gingiva, and the width of this band and its relationship to the teeth change very little during subsequent growth and development. Deflections in the path of eruption, such as those due to crowding or over-retention of primary teeth, may result in a narrowed band of attached gingiva (Andlin-Sobocki and Bodin, 1993). This is particularly common when mandibular incisors erupt labial to the alveolar ridge as shown in Figure 24-5A. If the band of attached gingiva is very narrow, even a small subsequent loss of attachment can result in a mucogingival defect (which occurs when the pocket depth exceeds the width of keratinized gingiva) and recession may occur rapidly as shown in Figure 24-5B. The gingival architecture often makes labially erupted teeth difficult to clean, particularly once recession has occurred, leaving them even more vulnerable to periodontitis and attachment loss. The loss of attachment and recession that occurs with a labially malpositioned tooth is sometimes called *stripping*. Other factors that may contribute to recession are the use of smokeless tobacco and habit-related self-induced injury.

A gingival graft is indicated to stabilize and repair the labial attachment of teeth with significant recession. A free gingival graft using donor tissue from the palate is commonly performed. Orthodontic movement of a labially malpositioned tooth in the direction of the alveolar ridge may produce a small increase in attached gingiva and place the tooth in a periodontally more stable position. Particulary when defects are not severe, it is desirable to postpone grafting until after orthodontic treatment.

Frena

A prominent maxillary frenum, often accompanied by a large midline diastema, is a common finding in children. It is often a cause for concern by parents and health care providers. Unless the

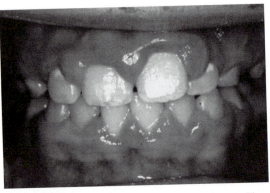

Figure 24–4. Mild gingival enlargement secondary to dilantin therapy.

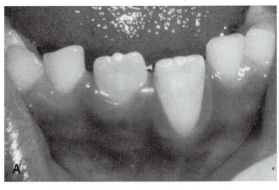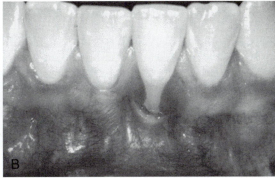

Figure 24–5. *A,* A reduction in the width of keratinized gingiva resulting from labial eruption of the left central incisor. *B,* After orthodontic alignment of the labially positioned left central incisor, a gingival defect was observed. Localized recession occurred as the result of plaque accumulation in an area that was difficult to clean and had inadequate attached gingiva.

frenum attachment exerts traumatic forces on the facial attached gingiva of a permanent tooth—an uncommon situation—immediate treatment is unnecessary. Instead, treatment should be delayed until the permanent incisors and cuspids have erupted to allow natural closure of the diastema. If orthodontic treatment is planned, surgical treatment should generally be postponed until the diastema has been closed. If the appearance is unacceptable after closure, frenectomy is indicated.

A restrictive lingual frenum ("tongue tie") is not uncommon in children (Fig. 24-6). If the attachment limits normal tongue mobility, treatment may be indicated. Children generally accommodate well to the restriction, but if the child cannot protrude the tongue from the mouth or touch the tip of the tongue to the upper alveolar process, a simple frenotomy in

which the attachment is released will make oral functioning, including speech, easier.

PERIODONTITIS

Significant loss of periodontal attachment is common in adults, with what is called "adult-onset" periodontitis affecting the majority of the population. When careful measurements are made, 20% of 14- to 17-year-olds in the United States are found to have attachment loss of at least 2 mm at one or more sites (Bhat, 1991). The number and severity of affected sites increase steadily with age, demonstrating that adult-onset periodontitis often begins in adolescence. Adult-onset periodontitis responds well to oral hygiene measures and can more easily be arrested in its early stages when attachment loss is minimal and deep pockets have not developed.

Smoking is a major risk factor for periodontitis, and smoking is increasing among adolescents, particularly females. Smoking status should be determined as part of a periodontal assessment for young patients and appropriate counseling provided.

Early-Onset Periodontitis

Rare, rapidly progressing forms of periodontitis also affect children and adolescents. Both periodontitis associated with systemic disease and early-onset periodontitis affecting children who are otherwise healthy occur in the pediatric population. Because of their rarity, it has been difficult to study these diseases. For this reason our understanding is often incomplete, and further research is needed on both the etiology and the management of early-onset disease forms.

Figure 24–6. Restrictive lingual frenum in a teenage patient.

Localized Juvenile Periodontitis

Localized juvenile periodontitis (LJP) is characterized by the loss of attachment and bone around the permanent incisors and first permanent molars. The radiographic appearance is distinctive (Fig. 24–7). The attachment loss is rapid, occurring at three times the rate of adult-onset disease. Inflammation in LJP is not as extreme as that occurring in the forms of periodontitis associated with systemic disease such as neutropenia, but both inflammation and plaque accumulation are often greater than that found in the average teenager. The disease is usually detected in early adolescence, but retrospective examination of earlier radiographs has sometimes revealed undetected disease in the primary dentition. This suggests that LJP and prepubertal periodontitis, discussed later, are the same disease entity, differing either in the age of onset or detection. The prevalence of LJP is estimated to be about 1%, and in the United States it most commonly occurs in the African American population. At least some cases appear to be inherited as an autosomal dominant trait, and LJP has been linked to a neutrophil chemotactic defect.

Despite the genetic component, LJP is clearly linked to the presence of high numbers of *Actinobacillus actinomycetemcomitans,* and successful treatment outcomes correlate well with eradication of the bacteria. Treatment consists of local measures in combination with systemic antibiotic therapy and microbiologic monitoring. Systemic tetracylines have been used with some success, but metronidazole alone or in combination with amoxicillin appears to be more effective in arresting disease progression (Saxen and Asikainen, 1993). Some reattachment and resolution of the periodontal defects can occur after antibiotic therapy, but localized surgical intervention is often necessary to treat the residual defects.

Generalized Juvenile Periodontitis

A generalized form of juvenile periodontitis (GJP) sometimes occurs in adolescents and teenagers. In young adults the same disease is called rapidly progressive periodontitis (American Academy of Periodontology, 1996). Unlike LJP, GJP may affect the entire dentition and is not self-limiting. Heavy accumulations of plaque and calculus are found in GJP, and inflammation may be severe. It is not associated with the high levels of *A. actinomycetemcomitans* that occur in LJP but instead seems to have a microbiologic profile more similar to that of adult-onset disease. GJP should be treated aggressively with local therapy plus systemic antibiotics.

Localized Prepubertal Periodontitis

Localized prepubertal periodontitis (LPP) is a form of early-onset periodontitis characterized

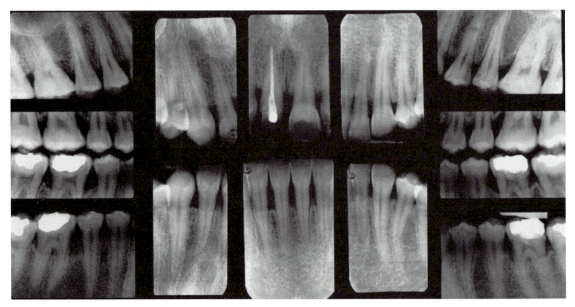

Figure 24–7. Radiographic appearance of localized juvenile periodontitis showing the typical bone loss pattern around first permanent molars and central incisors. Note the root canal treatment of the central incisor. Luxation injuries are common in these patients because of mobility of the incisors.

by localized loss of attachment in the primary dentition. It occurs in children without evidence of systemic disease. The disease is most commonly manifested in the molar area, where localized, usually bilaterally symmetrical loss of attachment occurs (Fig. 24-8). In the United States, LPP occurs most commonly in the African American population. It is usually accompanied by mild to moderate inflammation, and heavier than average plaque deposits may be visible. Calculus may also be present. It is commonly first diagnosed during the late primary dentition or early transitional dentition. LPP may progress to LJP in the permanent dentition and is probably the same disease entity, differing in the age of onset or diagnosis.

LPP is believed to be the result of a bacterial infection combined with specific, but minor, host immunologic deficits. LPP has not been as extensively studied as has LJP, and a causative bacterial species has not been identified. Antibiotic therapy combined with local débridement appears to be effective. Tetracyclines, commonly used to treat LJP, are contraindicated for LPP because of the potential for staining still-developing permanent teeth. Metronidazole is the antibiotic of choice for LPP.

Necrotizing Ulcerative Gingivitis/Periodontitis

Necrotizing ulcerative gingivitis/periodontitis (NUG/P) is characterized by the rapid onset of painful gingivitis with interproximal and marginal necrosis and ulceration. The incidence peaks in the late teens and early twenties in North America and Europe, but in less developed countries it is common in young children. Malnutrition, viral infections, stress, and lack of sleep have been reported as predisposing factors. NUG/P is associated with high levels of spirochetes and *Prevotella intermedia*. Local débridement usually produces rapid resolution of the disease, but antibiotic therapy with penicillin or metronidazole may be indicated when elevated temperature occurs.

SYSTEMIC DISEASES AND CONDITIONS WITH ASSOCIATED PERIODONTAL PROBLEMS

When early loss of periodontal attachment occurs in children, it often is a symptom of systemic disease. Periodontitis may occur in the presence of defects in the immune system that result in a susceptibility to infection, such as leukocyte adhesion deficiency or neutropenia. Early loss of attachment may also occur because of developmental defects in the attachment apparatus as in hypophosphatasia. Periodontal defects and gingival lesions may also result from the invasion of neoplastic cells as in leukemia.

Diabetes

An increased risk and earlier onset of periodontitis occur in both insulin-dependent (IDDM) and non–insulin dependent diabetes mellitus (NIDDM) (De Pommereau et al., 1992), probably because of impaired immune function. As many as 10% to 15% of teenagers with IDDM have significant periodontal disease. Poor metabolic control increases the risk of periodontitis, and untreated periodontitis in turn worsens metabolic control of diabetes. Effective preventive

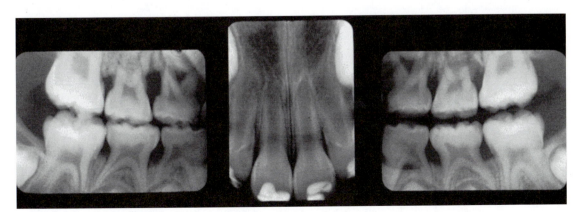

Figure 24–8. Radiographic appearance of prepubertal periodontitis showing the characteristic loss of bone around the primary molars. In this patient the disease has not progressed to include the permanent teeth, as sometimes occurs.

regimens and early diagnosis and treatment of periodontitis are important for the overall health of patients with diabetes.

Down Syndrome

Down syndrome, a genetic form of mental retardation resulting from the presence of three copies of chromosome 21, is accompanied by an increased susceptibility to periodontitis. Most patients develop periodontitis by 30 years of age, and it may first occur in the primary dentition (Reuland-Bosma and van Dijk, 1986). Plaque levels are high in these patients, but the severity of periodontal destruction exceeds that attributable to local factors alone. Various minor immune deficits, particularly in neutrophil function, have been identified in patients with Down syndrome and may be responsible for the increased susceptibility to periodontitis. Severe recession in the mandibular anterior region associated with a high frenum attachment is also common in Down syndrome.

Hypophosphatasia

Hypophosphatasia is a genetic disorder in which the enzyme bone alkaline phosphatase is deficient or defective. Phenotypes of hypophosphatasia can vary from premature loss of deciduous teeth to severe bone abnormalities leading to neonatal death. In general, the earlier the presentation of symptoms, the more severe the disease. In mild forms the early loss of primary teeth may be the first and only clinical sign as shown in

Figure 24-9. The early loss of teeth is the result of defective cementum formation, which in turn results in a weakened attachment of tooth to bone. The teeth are affected in the order of formation, so that those that form the earliest are most likely to be involved and the most severely affected. There currently is no treatment for the disease, but the dental prognosis for the permanent teeth is good. Typically the primary incisors are exfoliated before the age of 4 years, the other primary teeth are affected to varying degrees, and the permanent dentition is normal. Hypophosphatasia can be diagnosed by a finding of low alkaline phosphatase levels in a serum sample.

Leukocyte Adhesion Deficiency

Leukocyte adhesion deficiency (LAD) is a rare, recessive genetic disease. In LAD, surface glycoproteins on leukocytes are defective, resulting in poor migration to infection sites and impaired phagocytic function. This leaves patients susceptible to bacterial infections, including periodontitis. Because of frequent skin abscesses, recurrent otitis media, pnuemonitis, and other bacterial infections of soft tissues, a diagnosis is usually made before dental symptoms appear. Dental symptoms are manifested early in the primary dentition. Bone loss is rapid around nearly all teeth, and inflammation is marked. In the dental literature LAD has sometimes been called generalized prepubertal periodontitis (Watanabe, 1990). Scrupulous oral hygiene measures are necessary to control the periodontitis associated with LAD, but in part because of these patients'

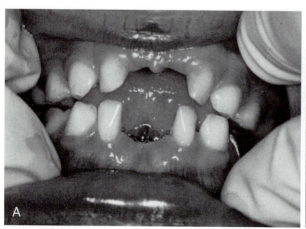
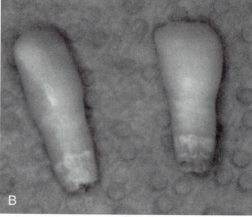

Figure 24–9. *A,* The dentition of a child 4 years of age with early loss of upper and lower central incisors due to hypophosphatasia. *B,* The lower incisors, exfoliated at 13 months of age. Note the incomplete root development at the time the teeth were exfoliated.

chronic problems with illness, adequate compliance may be difficult to achieve.

Neutropenia

Neutropenia is a hematologic disorder characterized by reduced numbers or the disappearance of neutrophils from the blood and bone marrow. In addition to increased susceptibility to recurrent infections such as otitis media and respiratory and skin infections, patients with neutropenia generally suffer from severe gingivitis and pronounced alveolar bone loss. Several different forms of neutropenia, including cyclic neutropenia, have been associated with oral symptoms in children. Neutropenia can be diagnosed by a finding of depressed neutrophils on a differential blood count. Periodontal therapy consists of rigorous local measures to control plaque, but patients are seldom able to maintain the level of oral hygiene necessary to prevent disease.

Papillon-Lefèvre Syndrome

Papillon-Lefèvre syndrome is a rare disease that has as a symptom the onset of severe periodontitis in the primary or transitional dentition. It is a genetic disorder and can easily be identified on clinical examination by the finding of hyperkeratosis of the palms of the hands and soles of the feet. Severe inflammation and rapid bone loss are characteristic of the periodontitis. Therapy consists of aggressive local measures to control plaque. Successful treatment outcomes in children have been reported with antibiotic therapy (Ishikawa et al., 1994).

Histiocytosis

Langerhans' cell histiocytosis (LCH), previously known as histiocytosis X, is a rare disorder of childhood with typical presentation as infiltration of bones, skin, liver, and other organs with hystiocytes. In 10% to 20% of cases, the initial infiltrates occur in the oral cavity, usually in the mandible. Typical findings are gingival enlargement, ulceration, mobility of teeth with alveolar expansion, and discrete, destructive lesions of bone that can be observed on radiographs. Teeth may be left "floating in air" and eventually exfoliated. The lesions of histiocytosis may initially be mistaken for prepubertal periodontitis. LCH may be diagnosed by biopsy. Therapy consists of local measures such as radiation and surgery to remove lesions and systemic chemotherapy for disseminated cases. The prognosis for disseminated early-onset disease is poor, with mortality rates exceeding 60%. Mild, localized LCH, on the other hand, has an excellent prognosis. The lesions of LCH and the local therapy used to remove them may result in the loss or arrested development of teeth.

Leukemia

Leukemia is the most common form of childhood cancer. Acute lymphoblastic leukemia (ALL) is the most common and has the best prognosis. Acute myeloid leukemia (AML) accounts for about 20% of childhood leukemias and has a poorer long-term survival rate. AML, but not usually ALL, may present with gingival enlargement caused by infiltrates of leukemic cells. The lesions are bluish-red and may sometimes invade bone. In addition to the gingival lesions, the patient may have fever, malaise, gingival or other bleeding, and bone or joint pain. AML may be diagnosed by a blood cell count. Anemia, abnormal leukocyte and differential counts, and thrombocytopenia are usually observed.

PERIODONTAL EXAMINATION OF CHILDREN

The periodontal health of children and adolescents should be assessed at each examination. The gingival tissues should be examined for redness, edema, bleeding, or enlargement. Oral hygiene may be assessed via a plaque index. Use of a disclosant provides an excellent oral hygiene instruction tool, and a plaque index provides a method for monitoring and documenting oral hygiene practices. Calculus is not as common in young patients as it is in adults, but it is found in about 10% of children and approximately a third of teenagers. The most common areas in which it occurs are the lingual surfaces of the mandibular incisors followed by the buccal surfaces of the maxillary molars. Patients should always be checked for calculus at periodic examination visits, and deposits should be removed.

Particularly after the eruption of permanent teeth, attachment levels should be determined by periodontal probing, at least of selected sites. Probing of the permanent incisors and first permanent molars provides a diagnostic screening for LJP. Because erupting teeth can be probed all the way to the cemento-enamel junction, transient deep pockets are a normal finding in the transitional dentition and must be distinguished from true attachment loss by locating the cemento-enamel junction (Sjodin and Matsson, 1992).

When radiographs are available, bone levels should be examined. Normal crestal height should be within 1 to 2 mm of the cemento-enamel junction. Once permanent teeth have erupted, the patient should also be examined for deficiencies in the width of attached gingiva and areas of recession noted.

REFERENCES

American Academy of Periodontology: Position Paper: Periodontal diseases of children and adolescents. [Review]. J Periodontol 67:57-62, 1996.

Andlin-Sobocki A, Bodin L: Dimensional alterations of the gingiva related to changes of facial/lingual tooth position in permanent anterior teeth of children. J Clin Periodontol 20:219-224, 1993.

Bhat M: Periodontal health of 14-17-year-old US schoolchildren. J Public Health Dent 51:5-11, 1991.

De Pommereau V, Dargen-Pare C, Robert JJ, Brion M: Periodontal status in insulin-dependent diabetic adolescents. J Clin Periodontol 19:628-632, 1992.

Ishikawa I, Umeda M, Laosrisin N: Clinical, bascteriological, and immunological examinations and the treatment process of two Papillon-Lefèvre syndrome patients. J Periodontol 65:364-371, 1994.

Matsson L: Factors influencing the susceptibility to gingivitis during childhood—a review. Int J Pediatr Dent 3:119-127, 1993.

Reuland-Bosma W, van Dijk LJ: Periodontal disease in Down's syndrome: A review. J Clin Periodontol 13:64-73, 1986.

Saxen L, Asikainen S: Metronidazole in the treatment of localized juvenile periodontitis. J Clin Periodontol 20:166-171, 1993.

Sjodin B, Matsson L: Marginal bone level in the normal primary dentition. J Clin Periodontol 19:672-678, 1992.

Watanabe K: Prepubertal periodontitis: A review of diagnostic criteria, pathogenesis, and differential diagnosis. J Periodontal Res 25:31-48, 1990.

Chapter 25

Space Maintenance in the Primary Dentition

John R. Christensen and Henry W. Fields, Jr.

Chapter Outline

GENERAL CONSIDERATIONS

Management of premature tooth loss in the primary dentition requires careful thought by the clinician because the consequences of proper or improper space management may influence dental development well into adolescence (Fields, 1999). Early loss of primary teeth may compromise the eruption of succedaneous teeth if there is a reduction in the arch length. On the other hand, timely intervention may save space for the eruption of the permanent dentition. The key to space maintenance in the primary dentition is to know which problems to treat (Ngan and Fields, 1995).

Premature tooth loss in this age group is best thought of in terms of anterior (incisors and canines) and posterior (molars) teeth. The causes and treatment of missing teeth differ in these two regions. Anterior tooth loss is due primarily to trauma and secondarily to tooth decay. Injuries to the primary incisors are common because a child of this age is learning to crawl, walk, and

run. Although the prevalence of dental decay appears to be declining, a small number of children still suffer from baby bottle caries and rampant decay. These decay patterns result in tooth loss in both the anterior and posterior regions. The majority of posterior tooth loss is due to dental caries; rarely are primary molars lost to trauma. If no space loss has occurred immediately after tooth loss, space maintenance is appropriate because the permanent successor will not erupt for several years. If space loss has occurred, a comprehensive evaluation is required to determine whether space maintenance, space regaining, or no treatment is indicated. This type of evaluation and decision-making is described in the discussions of mixed dentition, Chapters 30 and 35, because most space-regaining attempts are made at that time.

Missing primary incisors are usually replaced for four reasons: space maintenance, function, speech, and esthetics. Some dentists think that early removal of a primary incisor results in space loss because the adjacent teeth drift into the space formerly occupied by the lost incisor. This does not seem to be true in most clinical situations, however. There may be some re-arrangement of space between the remaining incisors, but there is no net loss of space. Intuitively, this makes sense because there is no apparent movement or drifting of teeth when developmental spacing is present in the primary dentition.

Poor masticatory function has also been proposed as a reason for replacing missing primary incisors. Concerns have been expressed about a child's ability to eat after four maxillary incisors have been removed as a result of nursing bottle decay. Feeding is not a problem, and when given a proper diet, the child continues to grow normally.

Slowed or altered speech development has been cited by some investigators as a justification for replacing missing maxillary incisors. This may be valid if the child has lost a number of teeth very early and is just beginning to develop speech. Many sounds are made with the tongue touching the lingual side of the maxillary incisors, and inappropriate speech compensations may develop if these teeth are missing. However, if the child has already acquired speech skills, the loss of an incisor is not particularly important (Rieckman and ElBadrawy, 1985).

Probably the most valid reason for replacing missing incisors is the esthetic one. Esthetic concerns are voiced by some parents but not by others. If parents do not indicate a desire to replace missing anterior teeth, certainly no treatment is appropriate. If the parents do wish to replace the missing teeth, either a fixed lingual arch or a removable partial denture with attached

primary teeth can serve as a prosthetic replacement (Fig. 25-1). The dentist should present both alternatives and let the parents make an educated decision.

Loss of a primary canine as a result of either trauma or decay is rare. Because it is so rare, there is some debate about whether space loss will occur if the tooth is not replaced. From a conservative point of view, a band and loop space maintainer (see later discussion in this chapter) or a removable partial denture may be placed if the patient is cooperative. Either of these appliances will need to be remade when the permanent lateral incisor erupts because the permanent lateral incisor will require more space than the primary lateral incisor and will interfere with space maintenance. If a space maintainer is not placed in the maxilla, a midline shift to the affected side should be anticipated when the permanent incisors erupt. In the mandible, lingual movement of the incisors and movement of the midline to the affected side will occur. A lingual arch may be appropriate after the permanent incisors erupt to prevent the midline shift.

Therefore, space maintenance during the primary dentition years is aimed primarily at the replacement of primary molars. Loss of interproximal contact as a result of decay, extraction, or ankylosis of an adjacent tooth results in space loss because of mesial and occlusal drift of the tooth distal to the newly created space. There is also evidence that the tooth mesial to the affected molar will drift distally into the space (Owen, 1971). Therefore, loss of space or arch length can occur from both directions (Fig. 25-2).

Space maintenance begins with good restor-

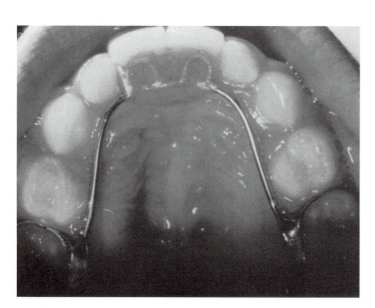

Figure 25–1. A fixed (as shown here) or removable partial denture can be used to replace missing anterior teeth in the primary dentition. In most cases the partial denture is placed for esthetic reasons rather than to prevent space loss in the anterior dental arch.

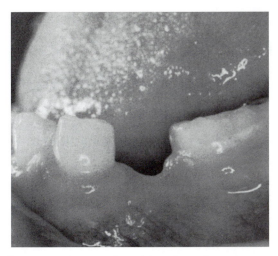

Figure 25–2. Premature loss of the primary first molar results in loss of space from both directions. The primary second molar drifts mesially, and the primary canine drifts distally.

ative dentistry. The dentist should strive for ideal restoration of all interproximal contours. Early restoration of interproximal caries ensures that no space loss occurs. In some instances, however, large carious lesions may make ideal restoration of the tooth impossible and space loss is inevitable. Even if the pulpal tissues have been compromised, pulp therapy should be initiated and the tooth maintained, if at all possible, because the natural tooth is still superior to the best space maintainer available—it is functional, is the correct size, and exfoliates appropriately. In cases of ankylosis, the tooth should be maintained until space loss is imminent; it is then extracted and the space maintained. Ankylosed teeth usually show limited vertical change in the primary dentition years.

Teeth lost during the primary dentition years will cause later-than-normal eruption of the succedaneous teeth. This means that the appliances need to be monitored, adjusted, and possibly replaced over a longer period of time. Abutment teeth for appliances may exfoliate or interfere with adjacent erupting teeth, and decay and decalcification are more likely. These aspects of care need to be considered during treatment planning.

APPLIANCE THERAPY

Four appliances generally are used to maintain space in the primary dentition: the band and loop, the lingual arch, the distal shoe, and the removable appliance.

Band and Loop

The first appliance, the band and loop, is used to maintain the space of a single tooth. This appliance is inexpensive and is easy to fabricate. It requires continuous supervision and care, however, and it does not restore the occlusal function of the missing tooth. In the majority of patients requiring space maintenance in the primary and mixed dentitions, the band and loop appliance is used. The appliance is indicated in the following situations:

1. Unilateral loss of the primary first molar before or after eruption of the permanent first molar (Fig. 25-3)
2. Bilateral loss of a primary molar before the eruption of the permanent incisors (Fig. 25-4)

The initial step in constructing a band and loop appliance is to select and fit a band on the abutment tooth. Band selection is a trial-and-error affair, and bands are fitted until one can be nearly seated on the tooth with finger pressure (Fig. 25-5*A*). A band pusher and band biter are used to achieve the final occlusogingival position (Fig. 25-5*B* and *C*). A properly placed band is seated approximately 1 mm below the mesial and distal marginal ridges (Fig. 25-5*D*). If a band cannot be easily fitted, orthodontic separators should be placed to create space for the band material (Fig. 25-5*E*). This same technique is

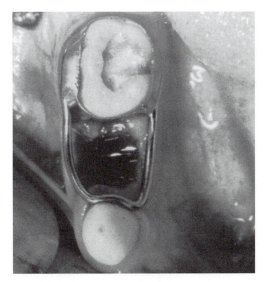

Figure 25–3. The band and loop appliance is used to maintain the space after the premature loss of a single tooth. The band and loop appliance is indicated when there is unilateral loss of a primary first molar before or after the eruption of the permanent first molar. The loop is constructed of 36-mil round wire and is soldered to the band.

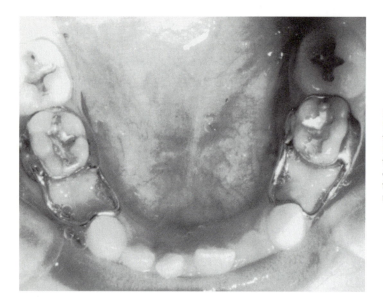

Figure 25–4. If both primary first molars are lost prematurely in the mandibular arch and the permanent incisors have not erupted, bilateral band and loop appliances are used to maintain space. A lingual arch is not indicated in this situation because it may interfere with the subsequent eruption of the permanent mandibular incisors.

used to place orthodontic bands on the posterior teeth when fixed orthodontic therapy is indicated. The next step is to make a quarter-arch impression of the band and edentulous area with either compound or alginate impression material. If alginate impression material is used, the tray should be perforated so that the material can flow through the perforations and prevent the impression from becoming distorted when it is removed. After the impression is made, the band is gently removed with a band remover and is placed and stabilized in the impression in the correct position.

The impression is poured in stone with the band in place. The cast is separated, and a 36-mil wire is formed into a loop and contoured to fit the band and alveolar ridge. The loop should parallel the edentulous ridge 1 mm off the gingival tissue and should rest against the adjacent tooth at the contact point. The faciolingual dimension of the loop should be approximately 8 mm. This dimension should allow the permanent tooth to erupt freely but not impinge on the buccal mucosa or tongue. The loop should not restrict any physiologic tooth movement, such as the increase in intercanine width that occurs during eruption of the permanent lateral incisors. When the band and loop appliance is returned from the laboratory, it should be fitted and adjusted if necessary. Following that, the band should be cemented onto a clean, dry abutment tooth with zinc phosphate or glass ionomer cement. The patient is then recalled every 3 to 4 months to check that the appliance still fits properly, the cement has not washed out, and the abutment teeth are firm. The eruption of the permanent tooth is an easily recognized indication for removal.

Two modifications of the band and loop appliance are not recommended for use in space maintenance therapy. The *bonded band and loop* is a contoured wire similar to the loop portion of the band and loop that is bonded to the abutment tooth with composite resin. There are two reasons why the bonded band and loop is not recommended. First, it is difficult to keep the wire bonded to the tooth because of the shearing force of occlusion. If the bond breaks, there is a potential for space loss and the added danger of aspiration of the wire. Second, the bonded band and loop is nearly impossible to adjust. The other band and loop variation not recommended is the *crown and loop* appliance. The crown and loop technique requires preparation of the abutment tooth for a stainless steel crown and then soldering a space-maintaining wire directly to the crown. Care and maintenance of the band and loop appliance also are easier than that needed for the crown and loop if the appliance is damaged or needs to be modified. If the soldered joint fails and the wire breaks loose, there is no way to repair the crown and loop appliance intraorally. The crown must be cut off, a new crown fitted, and the wire resoldered. It is much easier to restore the abutment tooth with a stainless steel crown and then make a band and loop that fits the crown.

Lingual Arch

The second type of appliance used to maintain posterior space in the primary dentition is the

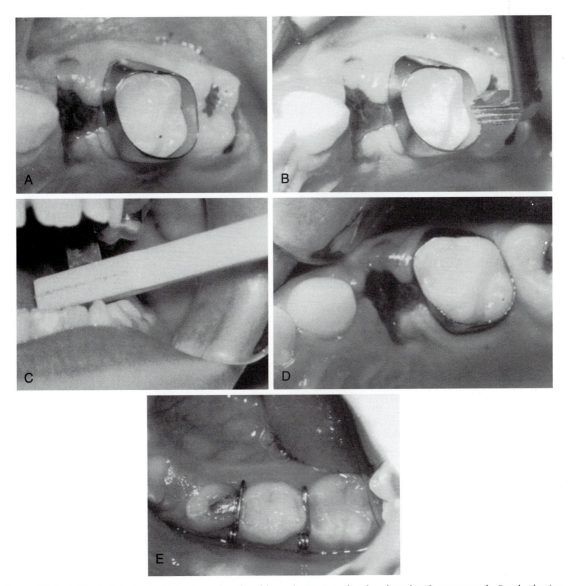

Figure 25–5. *A,* The initial step in fabricating a band and loop device is to fit a band on the abutment tooth. Band selection is a trial-and-error procedure and continues until a band can be nearly seated on the tooth with finger pressure. *B,* A band pusher is used to seat the band to a near-ideal position. The dentist should maintain a good finger rest because soft and hard tissue injury can occur if the pusher slips without proper support. *C,* Final occlusogingival position is achieved with a band biter. In the maxillary arch, the band biter should be placed on the distolingual portion of the band for final positioning. In the mandibular arch, the band biter should be placed on the distofacial portion of the band. *D,* A properly fitted band is seated approximately 1 mm below the mesial and distal marginal ridges. *E,* If a tight interproximal contact prevents the band from seating properly, orthodontic separators are placed to create space for the band material. The separators are removed within 7 to 10 days, and the band is fitted.

lingual arch. The lingual arch is often suggested when teeth are lost in both quadrants of the same arch. Because the permanent incisor tooth buds develop and erupt somewhat lingual to their primary precursors, a conventional mandibular lingual arch is not recommended in the primary dentition: The wire resting adjacent to the primary incisors may interfere with the eruption of the permanent dentition (Fig. 25-6). Instead,

bilateral band and loop appliances are recommended in this situation.

The maxillary lingual arch is feasible in the primary dentition because it can be constructed to rest away from the incisors. Two types of lingual arch designs are used to maintain maxillary space, the Nance and the transpalatal arches. These appliances use a large wire (36 mil) to connect the banded primary teeth on both sides

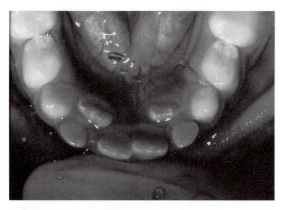

Figure 25–6. Lingual eruption of the permanent mandibular incisors is not uncommon. A mandibular lingual arch is not recommended as a space maintainer in the primary dentition because it may interfere with the eruption of these incisors. Bilateral band and loop appliances are recommended when both primary mandibular first molars are lost prematurely.

of the arch that are distal to the extraction site. The difference between the two appliances amounts to where the wire is placed in the palate. The Nance arch incorporates an acrylic button that rests directly on the palatal rugae. The transpalatal arch (TPA) is made from a wire that traverses the palate directly without touching it (Fig. 25-7). Although the TPA is a cleaner appliance and is easier to construct, many clinicians think that it allows the teeth to move and tip mesially, resulting in space loss.

Distal Shoe

The distal shoe appliance is used to maintain the space of a primary second molar that has been

lost before the eruption of the permanent first molar (Fig. 25-8). An unerupted permanent first molar drifts mesially within the alveolar bone if the primary second molar is lost prematurely. The result of the mesial drift is loss of arch length and possible impaction of the second premolar.

The appliance can be constructed from an impression taken after removal of the primary second molar or from an impression taken before the tooth is extracted. In the former situation, the gingiva needs to be incised when the appliance is placed because of the healing of the extraction site. In the latter situation, the construction cast needs to be modified to simulate loss of the primary second molar, but placement in the extraction site at the time of surgery is easy.

The appliance is constructed very much like the band and loop. The primary first molar is banded and the loop extended to the former distal contact of the primary second molar. A piece of stainless steel is soldered to the distal end of the loop and placed in the extraction site. The stainless steel extension acts as a guide plane for the permanent first molar to erupt into proper position and should be positioned 1 mm below the mesial marginal ridge of the unerupted molar in the alveolar bone. After the permanent molar has erupted, the extension can be cut off or a new band and loop appliance can be constructed. To ensure that the stainless steel extension is in the proper position and in close proximity to the permanent first molar, a periapical radiograph is recommended before the appliance is cemented (Fig. 25-9).

There are many problems associated with the

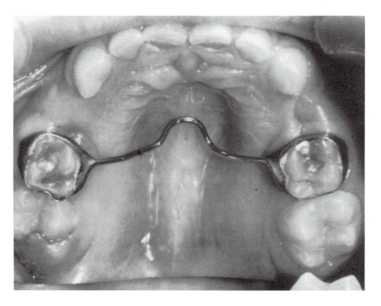

Figure 25–7. The transpalatal arch (TPA) is a fixed lingual arch appliance used to maintain space following bilateral loss of maxillary teeth. The TPA is more hygienic than the Nance appliance because it consists of only the 36-mil palatal wire, but it allows the abutment teeth to tip mesially in some cases, resulting in space loss.

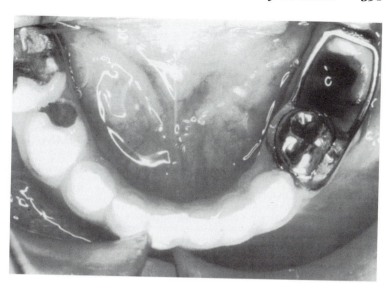

Figure 25–8. The distal shoe appliance is used to maintain the space of a primary second molar that has been lost prematurely before the eruption of the permanent first molar. A stainless steel extension is soldered to the distal end of the band and 36-mil loop; this extension is positioned 1 mm below the mesial marginal ridge of the unerupted permanent first molar. The extension serves to guide the eruption of the permanent first molar.

distal shoe appliance. Because of its cantilever design and the fact it is anchored on the occlusally convergent crown of the primary first molar, the appliance can replace only a single tooth and is somewhat fragile. No occlusal function is restored because of this lack of strength. In addition, histologic examination shows that complete epithelialization does not occur after placement of the appliance (Mayhew et al., 1984). Because the epithelium is not intact, the distal shoe appliance is contraindicated in medically compromised patients and in patients who require subacute bacterial endocarditis coverage.

Removable Appliances

Removable appliances also can be used to maintain space in the primary dentition (Fig. 25–10). The appliance is typically used when more than one tooth has been lost in a quadrant. The removable appliance is often the only alternative because there are no suitable abutment teeth and because the cantilever design of the distal shoe or the band and loop is too weak to withstand occlusal forces over a two-tooth span. Not only can the partial denture replace more than one tooth, it also can replace occlusal function.

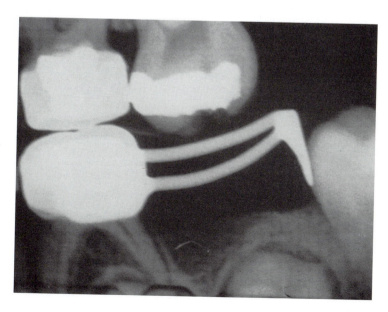

Figure 25–9. A periapical radiograph is recommended prior to cementing the distal shoe appliance to ensure that it is properly positioned in relation to the unerupted permanent first molar.

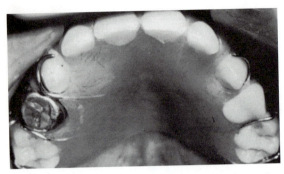

Figure 25–10. A removable partial denture is used to maintain posterior space in the primary dentition when more than one tooth in a quadrant is lost. This appliance is the only suitable space maintainer because the canine is a poor abutment and the cantilever design of the band and loop or distal shoe is too weak to withstand occlusal forces. In the patient portrayed here, both anterior and posterior teeth have been replaced. (From Fields HW, Proffit WR: Orthodontics in general practice. *In* Morris AL, Bohannan HM, Casullo DP [eds]: The Dental Specialties in General Practice. Philadelphia, WB Saunders, 1983, p 299.)

Two drawbacks of the appliance are retention and compliance. Retention is a problem because primary canines do not have large undercuts for clasp engagement. If multiple tooth loss is unilateral, retention problems can be overcome by placing sturdy retention clasps on the opposite side of the arch. If multiple teeth are lost bilaterally, however, retention problems are almost inevitable. Compliance is a problem closely related to retention. Three- to six-year-old children will not tolerate an ill-fitting appliance and will not use it. In fact, some children will not tolerate a retentive appliance. The dentist is then resigned to waiting until the permanent teeth (molars) erupt so that they can be used as abutments for a lingual arch appliance. Partial dentures occasionally need clasp adjustment and acrylic modification to maintain good retention and allow eruption of the underlying or adjacent permanent teeth. Some children are compliant in wearing an appliance but not in cleaning the appliance and the underlying tissue. This can result in decay, tissue irritation, and hyperplasia.

SUMMARY

Space maintenance in the primary dentition should be thought of in terms of anterior and posterior space loss. Space maintenance is not required for missing primary incisors. Primary incisors should be replaced only if esthetic concerns are a factor. Posterior space maintenance is a necessity in this age group and should be undertaken when primary molars are lost prematurely and the space is adequate. The band and loop appliance is used most often; other appliances can be used as different situations dictate. Judicious space maintenance benefits the child patient and may prevent future alignment and crowding problems.

REFERENCES

Fields HW: Treatment of moderate nonskeletal problems in preadolescent children. *In* Proffit WR (ed): Contemporary Orthodontics, 3rd ed. St. Louis, C.V. Mosby, 1999.

Mayhew MJ, Dilley GJ, Dilley DCH, et al: Tissue response to appliances in monkeys. Pediatr Dent 6:148–152, 1984.

Ngan P, Fields HW: Orthodontic diagnosis and treatment planning in the primary dentition. J Dent Child 62:25–33, 1995.

Owen DG: The incidence and nature of space closure following the premature extraction of deciduous teeth: A literature survey. Am J Orthod 59:37–48, 1971.

Rieckman GA, ElBadrawy HE: Effect of premature loss of primary maxillary incisors on speech. Pediatr Dent 7:119–122, 1985.

26

Oral Habits

John R. Christensen, Henry W. Fields, Jr., and Steven M. Adair

Chapter Outline

THUMB AND FINGER HABITS

PACIFIER HABITS

LIP HABITS

TONGUE THRUST AND MOUTH-
BREATHING HABITS

NAIL BITING

BRUXISM

SELF-MUTILATION

The presence of an oral habit in the 3- to 6-year-old child is an important finding during the clinical examination. An oral habit is not usually present in children near the end of this age group. Preferably, a habit that has resulted in movement of the primary incisors or has inhibited eruption will have been eliminated before the permanent incisors erupt. If a habit that causes dental changes is not eliminated before the permanent incisors erupt, they too will be affected. On the other hand, these are not irreversible changes. If the habit is stopped during the mixed dentition years, the adverse dental changes will begin to be reversed naturally. Some appliance therapy may be required, but generally, the teeth will move toward a more neutral position with the absence of the forces of the habit.

If no dental changes have occurred, no treatment can be advocated on the grounds of dental health, but some patients and parents may want to seek treatment because digit or pacifier habits become less socially acceptable as the child becomes older. One study has shown that school age children consider thumb suckers significantly less intelligent, less attractive, and less desirable as friends (Friman et al., 1993). Efforts to discourage the habit may involve as little as a conversation between the dentist and the child, or they may involve more complex appliance therapy. The most important thing to remember about any intervention is that the child must want to discontinue the habit for treatment to be successful.

THUMB AND FINGER HABITS

Thumb and finger habits make up the majority of oral habits. About two thirds are ended by 5 years of age (Helle and Haavikko, 1974). Dentists are often questioned about the kinds of problems these habits may cause if they are prolonged. The malocclusions caused by non-nutritive sucking may be more of an individual response than a highly specified cause-and-effect relationship (Baril and Moyers, 1960). The types of dental changes that a digit habit may cause vary with the intensity, duration, and frequency of the habit as well as the manner in which the digit is positioned in the mouth. Intensity is the amount of force that is applied to the teeth during sucking. Duration is defined as the amount of time spent sucking a digit. Frequency is the number of times the habit is practiced throughout the

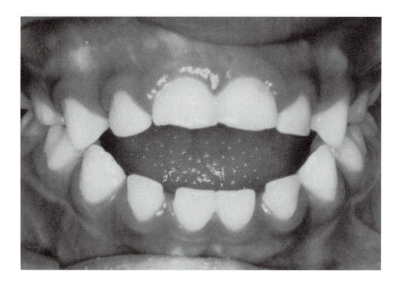

Figure 26–1. This patient's anterior open bite is a direct result of an active thumb-sucking habit. An open bite results when the thumb impedes eruption of the anterior teeth, moves them facially, and allows the posterior teeth to erupt passively. Actual intrusion of the anterior teeth is possible but unlikely.

day. Duration plays the most critical role in tooth movement caused by a digit habit. Clinical and experimental evidence suggests that 4 to 6 hours of force per day are probably the minimum necessary to cause tooth movement. Therefore, a child who sucks intermittently with high intensity may not produce much tooth movement at all, whereas a child who sucks continuously (for more than 6 hours) can cause significant dental change. The most common dental signs of an active habit are reported to be the following:

1. Anterior open bite
2. Facial movement of the upper incisors and lingual movement of the lower incisors
3. Maxillary constriction

Anterior open bite, the lack of vertical overlap of the upper and lower incisors when the teeth are in occlusion, develops because the digit rests directly on the incisors (Fig. 26-1). This prevents complete or continued eruption of the incisors, whereas the posterior teeth are free to erupt. Anterior open bite may also be caused by intrusion of the incisors. Inhibition of eruption is easier to accomplish than true intrusion, however, which would be the result of a habit of great duration.

Faciolingual movement of the incisors depends on how the thumb or finger is placed and how many are placed in the mouth. Some consider this positional variable to be a confounding factor related to intensity, duration, and frequency. Usually, the thumb is placed so that it exerts pressure on the lingual surface of the maxillary incisors and on the labial surface of the mandibular incisors (Fig. 26-2). A child who actively sucks can create enough force to tip the upper incisors facially and the lower incisors lingually. The result is an increased overjet and, by virtue of the tipping, decreased overbite.

Maxillary arch constriction is probably due to the change in equilibrium balance between the oral musculature and the tongue. When the thumb is placed in the mouth, the tongue is forced down and away from the palate. The orbicularis oris and buccinator muscles continue to exert a force on the buccal surfaces of the maxillary dentition, especially when these muscles are contracted during sucking. Because the

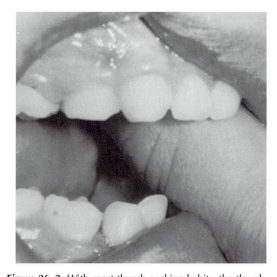

Figure 26–2. With most thumb-sucking habits, the thumb exerts pressure on the lingual surface of the maxillary incisors and on the facial surface of the mandibular incisors. This causes the maxillary incisors to tip facially and the mandibular incisors to tip lingually, resulting in increased overjet.

tongue no longer exerts a counterbalancing force from the lingual surface, the posterior maxillary arch collapses into crossbite.

Data on the amount of skeletal change are not clear. Some believe the maxilla and its alveolar process are moved anteriorly and superiorly (Larsson, 1972). Certainly, if the teeth are moved, some alveolar change is made. Whether this is translated to the skeletal maxilla is not as well known. In one study a significantly higher percentage of distal step molar relationships in 5-year-olds was noted among digit suckers compared with children with no habit (Fukuta et al., 1996).

Timing of treatment must be gauged carefully. If parents or the child do not want to engage in treatment, it should not be attempted. The child should be given an opportunity to stop the habit spontaneously before the permanent teeth erupt. If treatment is selected as an alternative, it is generally undertaken between the ages of 4 and 6 years. Delay until the early school age years allows for spontaneous discontinuation of the habit by many children, often through peer pressure at school. As long as the habit is eliminated prior to full eruption of the permanent incisors, the eruption process will spontaneously reduce the overjet and open bite as the permanent teeth occupy new positions. It is generally agreed that interception of a digit sucking habit does no harm to the child's emotional development, nor does it result in habit substitution. The dentist should, however, evaluate the child for psychological overtones prior to embarking on habit elimination. Such procedures might best be postponed for children who have recently undergone stressful changes in their lives, such as separation or divorce of parents, moving to a new community, or changing schools. Four different approaches to treatment have been advocated, depending on the willingness of the child to stop the habit.

The simplest, yet least widely applicable, approach is counseling with the patient. This involves discussion between the dentist and the patient of the problems created by non-nutritive sucking (NNS). These adult-like discussions focus on the changes that have occurred because of the sucking and their impact on esthetics. Usually an appeal is made to the children on the basis of their maturity and responsibility. Clearly, this approach is best aimed at older children who can conceptually grasp the issue and who may be feeling social pressure to stop the habit. Some children are captured by this approach and successfully eliminate their habit.

The second approach, reminder therapy, is ap-

propriate for those who desire to stop the habit but need some help. The purpose of any of these treatments should be thoroughly explained to the child. An adhesive bandage secured with waterproof tape on the offending finger can serve as a constant reminder not to place the finger in the mouth (Fig. 26-3). The bandage remains in place until the habit is extinguished. Some clinicians have used a mitten or sock to cover the fingers of the hand. This is especially useful during sleeping hours. Another approach is to paint a commercially available bitter substance on the fingers that are sucked. All these methods are aimed at reminding the child not to place the fingers in the mouth. Sometimes this type of therapy is perceived as punishment, however, and may not be as effective as a neutral reminder.

A third treatment for oral habits is a reward system. A contract is drawn up between the child and the parent or between the child and the dentist. The contract simply states that the child will discontinue the habit within a specified period of time and in return will receive a reward. The reward does not need to be extravagant but must be special enough to motivate the child. Praise from the parents and the dentist plays a large role. The more involvement the child takes in the project, the more likely the project is to succeed. Involvement may include placing stick-on stars on a homemade calendar when the child has successfully avoided the habit for an entire day. At the end of the specified time period, the reward is presented with verbal praise for meeting the conditions of the contract (Fig. 26-4). Reward systems and reminder therapy can be combined to improve the likelihood of success.

If the habit continues to persist after reminder and reward therapy and the child truly wants

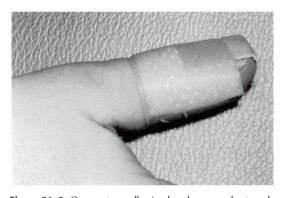

Figure 26–3. One or two adhesive bandages can be taped to a child's finger to serve as a reminder not to place the finger in the mouth. The Band-Aid is worn until the child stops sucking the finger.

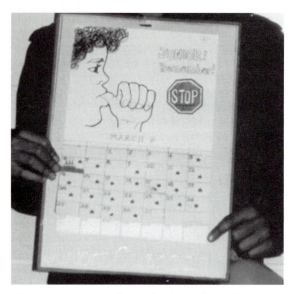

Figure 26–4. A personalized calendar can be used to motivate a child to stop a thumb-sucking habit. Stick-on stars are applied to the calendar on days when the child has successfully avoided the habit. At the end of a month or a specified period of time, a reward and verbal praise can be provided for discontinuing the habit.

to eliminate the habit, adjunctive therapy that includes a method to physically interrupt the habit and remind the patient can be used. This type of treatment usually involves either wrapping the patient's arm in an elastic bandage so it cannot be flexed and the hand inserted in the mouth, or placing an appliance in the mouth that physically discourages the habit by making it difficult to suck a thumb or finger. The dentist should explain to the patient and parent that

the appliance is not a punishment but rather a permanent reminder not to place the finger in the mouth.

The elastic bandage method is usually applied only at night. The bandage is loosely wrapped over the arm extending from below the elbow to above it. The sheer mass of elastic material (not the tightness) prohibits the child from sucking the fingers. Success over several weeks should be rewarded. The total program may take 6 to 8 weeks (anecdotally noted by success in children who have stopped habits while arms were casted for broken bones).

An intraoral appliance approach can also be employed in the adjunct method. The two appliances used most often to discourage the sucking habit are the quad helix and the palatal crib. The quad helix is a fixed appliance commonly used to expand a constricted maxillary arch—a common finding accompanied by posterior crossbite in NNS patients (Fig. 26–5). The helices of the appliance serve to remind the child not to place the finger in the mouth. The quad helix is a versatile appliance because it can correct a posterior crossbite and discourage a finger habit at the same time.

The palatal crib is designed to interrupt a digit habit by interfering with finger placement and sucking satisfaction. The palatal crib is generally used in children in whom no posterior crossbite exists. It may, however, also be used as a retainer after maxillary expansion with a quad helix in a child who has not stopped sucking with the quad helix. For a palatal crib, bands are fitted on the permanent first molars or primary second molars. A heavy lingual arch wire (38 mil) is bent

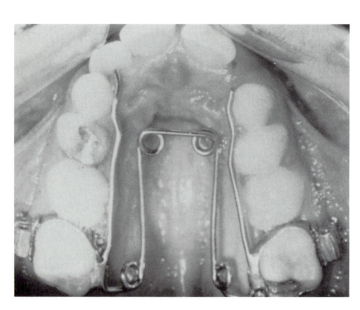

Figure 26–5. The quad helix is a fixed appliance used to expand a constricted maxillary arch. The anterior helices also serve to discourage a sucking habit by reminding the child not to place a finger in the mouth. This appliance is often used in children in whom there is an active sucking habit and a posterior crossbite.

to fit passively in the palate and is soldered to the molar bands. Additional wire is soldered onto this base wire to form a crib or mechanical obstruction for the digit. It is advisable to make a lower cast at the time the appliance is constructed so that the occlusion can be checked for interferences (Fig. 26-6). The parent and child should be informed that certain side effects appear temporarily after the palatal crib is cemented. Eating, speaking, and sleeping patterns may be altered during the first few days after appliance delivery. These difficulties usually subside within 3 days to 2 weeks (Haryett et al., 1970). An imprint of the appliance usually appears on the tongue as an indentation. This imprint disappears soon after the appliance is removed. The major problem with the palatal crib and, to a lesser degree, the quad helix is the difficulty of maintaining good oral hygiene. The appliance traps food and is difficult to clean thoroughly. Oral malodor and tissue inflammation can result.

Adjunctive habit discouragement appliances should be left in the mouth for 6 to 12 months as a retainer. The palatal crib usually stops the child from sucking immediately but requires at least another 6 months of wear to extinguish the habit completely (Haryett et al., 1970). The quad helix also requires a minimum of 6 months of treatment. Three months are needed to correct the crossbite, and 3 months are required to stabilize the movement.

PACIFIER HABITS

Dental changes created by pacifier habits are largely similar to changes created by thumb hab-its, and no clear consensus indicates a therapeutic difference (Fig. 26-7). Anterior open bite and maxillary constriction (with posterior crossbite) occur consistently in children who suck pacifiers. Labial movement of the maxillary incisors may not be as pronounced as that accompanying a digit habit. Manufacturers have developed pacifiers that they claim are more like a mother's nipple and not as deleterious to the dentition as a thumb or conventional pacifier. Research has not substantiated these statements (Adair et al., 1992, 1995; Bishara et al., 1987).

Pacifier habits appear to end earlier than digit habits. Over 90% were reported ended before 5 years of age and 100% by age 8 (Helle and Haavikko, 1974). Pacifier habits theoretically are easier to stop than digit habits because the pacifier can be discontinued gradually or completely withdrawn with discussion and explanation to the child. This type of control is obviously not possible with digit habits, which makes a notable difference in the degree of patient compliance required to eliminate the two types of habits. In a few cases, the child may stop the pacifier habit and then start sucking a digit. Elimination of the subsequent finger habit may become necessary.

LIP HABITS

Habits that involve manipulation of the lips and perioral structures are called lip habits. A number of lip habits exist, and their influence on the dentition is varied. Lip licking and lip pulling habits are relatively benign as far as dental effects are concerned. Red, inflamed, and chapped lips and perioral tissues during cool weather are the

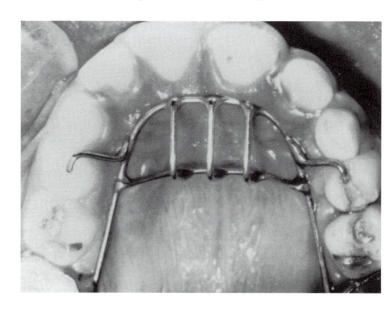

Figure 26–6. A palatal crib is a fixed appliance designed to stop a digit habit by mechanically interfering with digit placement and sucking satisfaction. The parent of the child should expect temporary disturbances in eating, speaking, and sleeping patterns during the first few days after use of the appliance.

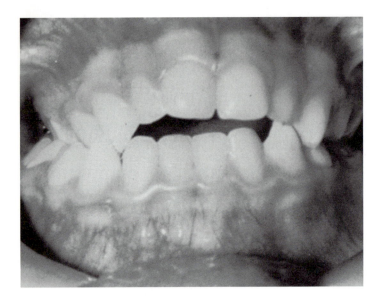

Figure 26–7. A pacifier can create dental changes that are nearly identical to those of a digit habit. The labiolingual movement of the incisors is usually not as pronounced as that associated with a digit habit.

most apparent signs associated with these habits (Fig. 26-8). Little can be done to stop these habits effectively, and treatment is usually palliative and limited to moisturizing the lips, although some have used appliances to interrupt the habits.

Although most lip habits do not cause dental problems, lip sucking and lip biting certainly can maintain an existing malocclusion if the child engages in them with adequate intensity, frequency, and duration. Whether these habits can create a malocclusion is a question that is not easily answered. The most common presentation of lip sucking is the lower lip tucked behind the maxillary incisors (Fig. 26-9). This places a lingually directed force on the mandibular teeth and a facial force on the maxillary teeth. The result is a proclination of the maxillary incisors, a retroclination of the mandibular incisors, and an increased amount of overjet. This problem is most common in the mixed and permanent dentitions. Treatment depends on the skeletal

relationship of the child and on the presence or absence of space in the arch. If the child has a Class I skeletal relationship and an increased overjet that is solely the result of tipped teeth, the clinician can tip the teeth to their original or a more normal position with either a fixed or a removable appliance. If a Class II skeletal relationship exists, however, a more involved growth modification procedure is needed to treat the malocclusion.

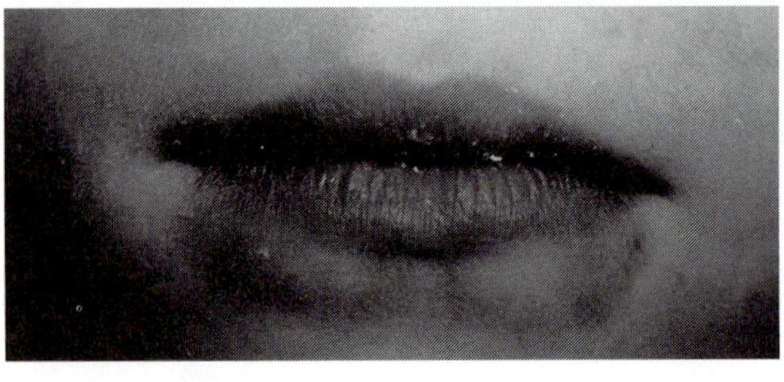

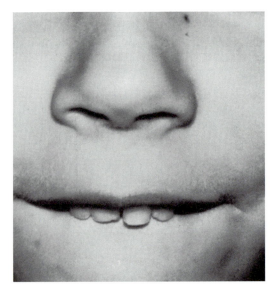

Figure 26–9. The most common habit involving the lips is tucking the lower lip behind the maxillary incisors. The lower lip forces the maxillary teeth facially and the mandibular teeth lingually, resulting in an increased overjet. In addition, the lower lip and other perioral tissues can become chapped and inflamed as a result of constant wetting.

Figure 26–8. Red, inflamed chapped lips and perioral tissues are often indicative of a lip-sucking or licking habit. These problems are more common and severe during the winter months.

TONGUE THRUST AND MOUTH-BREATHING HABITS

Recently, a great deal of attention has been given to tongue thrust and mouth breathing habits as sources of malocclusion. As discussed in Chapter 13, tongue thrust is characteristic of the infantile and transitional swallows, both considered normal for the neonate. Epidemiologic data indicate that the percentage of persons with infantile and transitional swallowing patterns is greater than the percentage of persons with open bite (Kelly et al., 1973). This indicates there is no simple cause-and-effect relationship between tongue thrusting and open bite. Furthermore, data measuring the duration, intensity, and frequency of force associated with tongue thrust suggest that the habit may be able to sustain an open bite but not create one (Proffit and Mason, 1975). Therefore, tongue thrusting should be considered a finding and not a problem to be treated.

Mouth breathing and its association with malocclusion is a complex issue. Research designed to answer questions about this association has not been well controlled. The major problem with this research has been the unreliable identification of mouth breathers. Some persons may appear to be mouth breathers because of their mandibular posture or incompetent lips. It is normal for a 3- to 6-year-old to be slightly lip-incompetent (Fig. 26–10). Other children have been labeled mouth breathers because of a suspected nasal airway obstruction. Two locations have been suggested consistently as sites of obstruction, the nasal turbinates and the nasopharyngeal adenoidal tissues. Clinical judgment is not accurate enough to confirm a diagnosis of nasal airway impairment. The only reliable method of determining the mode of respiratory function is to use a plethysmograph and air flow transducers to determine total nasal and oral air flow. One cross-sectional study used the plethysmograph on normal children and reported that prior to age 8 there were as many oral or predominantly oral breathers as nasal or predominantly nasal breathers. After age 8, the majority of the children were nasal or predominantly nasal breathers (Warren et al., 1990). Despite the difficulties encountered in identifying mouth-breathing persons, there is some indication of a weak relationship between mouth breathing and malocclusion characterized by a long lower face and maxillary constriction. It should be noted that this relationship is very weak, however, and does not imply that turbinectomies or adenoidectomies are required to

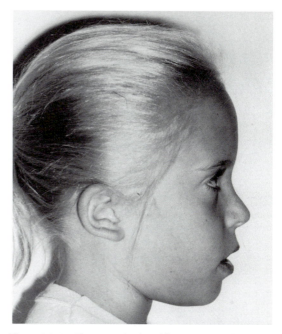

Figure 26–10. The normal relaxed lip posture in the 3- to 6-year-old child is for the lips to be slightly apart or imcompetent. These children are often labeled mouthbreathers because of this posture, but they may in fact be completely nasal breathers.

clear the nasal airway (Bresolin et al., 1984; Wenzel et al., 1985).

NAIL BITING

Nail biting is a rare habit before 3 to 6 years of age. The number of persons who bite their nails is reported to increase until adolescence, but there are very few data on this subject. It has been suggested that the habit is a manifestation of increased stress. There is no evidence that nail biting can cause malocclusion or dental change other than minor enamel fractures; therefore, there is no recommended treatment. Nail biting may damage the fingernail beds, however, and it may be necessary to use appropriate nail care products to protect the nails.

BRUXISM

Bruxism is a grinding of teeth and is usually reported to occur while a child is sleeping. Some children grind their teeth when awake, however. Most children engage in some bruxism that results in moderate wear of the primary canines and molars. Rarely, with the exception of handi-

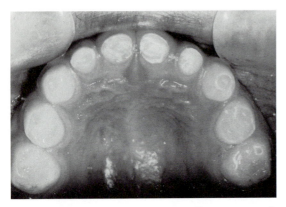

Figure 26–11. This patient's primary maxillary incisors and canines were worn more rapidly than normal owing to a habit of bruxism.

capped persons, does the wear endanger the pulp by proceeding faster than secondary dentin is produced (Fig. 26-11). Masticatory muscle soreness and temporomandibular joint pain have also been attributed to bruxism. The exact cause of significant bruxism is unknown, although most explanations center around local, systemic, and psychological reasons (Kuch et al., 1979). The local theory suggests that bruxism is a reaction to an occlusal interference, high restoration, or some irritating dental condition. Systemic factors implicated in bruxism include intestinal parasites, subclinical nutritional deficiencies, allergies, and endocrine disorders. The psychological theory submits that bruxism is the manifestation of a personality disorder or increased stress. Children with musculoskeletal disorders (cerebral palsy) and severely mentally retarded children commonly grind their teeth. These patients' bruxism is the result of their underlying physical and mental condition and is difficult to manage dentally.

Treatment should begin with simple measures. Occlusal interferences should be identified and equilibrated if necessary. If occlusal interferences are not located or equilibration is not successful, referral to appropriate medical personnel should be considered to rule out any systemic problems. If neither of these two steps is successful, a mouthguard-like appliance can be constructed of soft plastic to protect the teeth and attempt to eliminate the grinding habit. If the habit is thought to be due to psychological factors, which is unlikely, referral to a child development expert is warranted. Rarely is occlusal wear so great that stainless steel crowns are necessary to prevent pulpal exposure or eliminate tooth sensitivity.

SELF-MUTILATION

Self-mutilation, repetitive acts that result in physical damage to the person, is extremely rare in the normal child. The incidence of self-mutilation in the mentally retarded population, however, is between 10% and 20% (DenBesten and McIver, 1984). It has been suggested that self-mutilation is a learned behavior. This may be the case because it is one of the few behaviors that is reliably reinforced—that is, attention is always gained. A frequent manifestation of self-mutilation is biting of the lips, tongue, and oral mucosa. Any child who willfully inflicts pain or damage to himself should be considered psychologically abnormal. Such children should be referred for psychological evaluation and treatment. Self-mutilation has also been associated with biochemical disorders, such as Lesch-Nyhan and de Lange's syndromes. Besides behavior modification, treatment for self mutilation includes use of restraints, protective padding, and sedation. If restraints and protective padding are unsuccessful, extraction of selected teeth may be necessary.

REFERENCES

Adair SM, Milano M, Dushku JC: Evaluation of the effects of orthodontic pacifiers on the primary dentitions of 24- to 59-month-old children: Preliminary study. Pediatr Dent 14:13–18, 1992.

Adair SM, Milano M, Lorenzo I, Russell C: Effects of current and former pacifier use on the dentition of 24- to 59-month old children. Pediatr Dent 17:437–444, 1995.

Baril C, Moyers RE: An electromyographic analysis of the temporalis muscles and certain facial muscles in thumb- and finger-sucking patients. J Dent Res 39:536–553, 1960.

Bishara SE, Nowak AJ, Kohout FJ, et al: Influence of feeding and non-nutritive sucking methods on the development of the dental arches: Longitudinal study of the first 18 months of life. Pediatr Dent 9:13–21, 1987.

Bresolin D, Shapiro CC, Shapiro PA, et al: Facial characteristics of children who breathe through the mouth. Pediatrics 73:622–625, 1984.

DenBesten PK, McIver FT: Oral self-mutilation in a child with congenital toxoplasmosis: A clinical report. Pediatr Dent 6:98–101, 1984.

Friman PC, McPherson KM, Warzak WJ, Evans J: Influence of thumb sucking on peer social acceptance in first-grade children. Pediatrics 91:784–786, 1993.

Fukata O, Braham RL, Yokoi K, Kurosu K: Damage to the primary dentition resulting from thumb and finger (digit) sucking. J Dent Child 63:403–408, 1996.

Haryett RD, Hansen FC, Davidson PO: Chronic thumb-sucking: A second report on treatment and its psychological effects. Am J Orthod 57:164–178, 1970.

Helle A, Haavikko K: Prevalence of earlier sucking habits revealed by anamnestic data and their consequences for occlusion at the age of eleven. Proc Finn Dent Soc 70:191–196, 1974.

Kelly JE, Sanchez M, Van Kirk LE: An assessment of the

occlusion of teeth of children. National Center for Health Statistics, US Public Health Service, DHEW Publication No. HRA 74-1612, 1973.

Kuch EV, Till MJ, Messer LB: Bruxing and non-bruxing children: A comparison of their personality traits. Pediatr Dent *1:*182-187, 1979.

Larsson E: Dummy- and finger-sucking habits with special attention to their significance for facial growth and occlusion: 4. Effect on facial growth and occlusion. Swed Dent J *65:*605-634, 1972.

Proffit WR, Mason RM: Myofunctional therapy for tongue-thrusting: Background and recommendations. JADA *90:*403-411, 1975.

Warren DW, Hairfield WM, Dalston ET: Effect of age on nasal cross-sectional area and respiratory mode in children. Laryngoscope *100:*89-93, 1990.

Wenzel A, Hojensgaard E, Henriksen JM: Craniofacial morphology and head posture in children with asthma and perennial rhinitis. Eur J Orthod 7:83-92, 1985.

Chapter 27

Orthodontic Treatment in the Primary Dentition

John R. Christensen and Henry W. Fields, Jr.

Chapter Outline

The goals of orthodontic care in the primary dentition should be aimed at either intervention in conditions that predispose one to develop a malocclusion in the permanent dentition or monitoring conditions that are better treated later (Ngan and Fields, 1995). Some conditions can be effectively treated, and the result provides a long-term benefit. With other conditions, treatment should be deferred.

The clinician needs to differentiate skeletal problems from dental problems in order to fulfill these goals. Treatment of skeletal malocclusions in this age group is ordinarily deferred until a later age. Three general reasons are offered for delaying treatment. First, the diagnosis of skeletal malocclusion is difficult in this age group. Subtle gradations of skeletal problems and immature soft tissue development make diagnosis of all but the most obvious cases difficult. Second, although the child is growing at this stage, the amount of facial growth remaining when the child enters the mixed dentition years is sufficient to aid in the correction of most skeletal malocclusions. Third, any treatment at this age requires prolonged retention because the initial growth pattern tends to reestablish itself when treatment is discontinued.

On the other hand, several dental problems deserve attention during the primary dentition years. This chapter is devoted largely to these issues.

SKELETAL PROBLEMS

Skeletal problems are addressed only if there is progressive asymmetry as a result of a functional disturbance. The reason for treating these patients early is that treatment at a later time may be more difficult and complex if the child continues to grow asymmetrically and if dental compensation increases. The goal of early treatment is to prevent the asymmetry from becoming worse or to alter growth so that the asymmetry actually improves. The majority of progressive asymmetry cases are treated first with removable functional appliances that are designed to alter growth by manipulating skeletal and soft tissue relationships and allowing differential eruption of teeth. Orthognathic surgery is a second treatment for progressive asymmetry but is reserved for only the most severe cases or those that do not respond to functional appliance therapy. It may be necessary to operate a second time when the child is older because growth often tends to remain asymmetrical even after surgical correction. Because diagnosis and treatment of progressive asymmetry are difficult, it is recommended that these cases be referred to a specialist.

Early treatment of patients with dentofacial anomalies is also advocated. Dentofacial anomalies include a number of environmentally and genetically induced conditions that alter the relationship of the facial structures. Examples of such anomalies include cleft lip and palate, hemifacial microsomia, and mandibulofacial dysostosis (Treacher Collins syndrome). A specialist or specialty team works to minimize the facial disfigurement through early surgical and orthodontic intervention.

DENTAL PROBLEMS

Dental malocclusion in the primary dentition is readily treated by the practitioner who has a knowledge of fixed and removable appliances. The key to successful orthodontic treatment is careful diagnosis and treatment planning, which depend on the database obtained at the initial examination. In this age group, tooth movement should be restricted to tipping teeth into the proper position. Orthodontic appliances designed to move teeth bodily are not indicated.

Before specific treatment problems are discussed, the biology of tooth movement should be reviewed briefly. A force applied to a tooth causes alterations in the periodontal ligament and surrounding alveolar bone. Whether the alterations cause biochemical or electrical changes in these cells is not known exactly. A remodeling process begins that allows the tooth to move, however. This remodeling process may take as little as 3 days or as much as 2 weeks, depending on the amount of force applied to the tooth. After the tooth has moved a certain distance, the force exerted by the orthodontic appliance diminishes to an amount that is below that necessary for tooth movement. During this time, remodeling is completed and the periodontal ligament and alveolar bone cells begin to return to their normal state. This reorganization period is necessary to prevent injury to the tooth and supporting structures. The clinical implication of cellular change, tooth movement, and cellular reorganization is that orthodontic appliances should be reactivated only at 4- to 6-week intervals with a light, continuous force to avoid injury to the periodontium. Therefore, there is some biologic basis behind the recommendation for

monthly visits during orthodontic treatment (Fields, 1999).

After tooth movement is complete, the patient enters the retention phase of treatment. Retention is the period of time that the teeth are held in their new position. Retention is necessary because teeth that have been moved orthodontically tend to move back or relapse into their original position after the appliance has been removed. Relapse may be due to many factors; however, gingival fibers are reported to play a major role. During treatment, gingival fibers tend to be stretched or compressed. They return to their original size unless some reorganization of the fiber network occurs, which generally takes 3 to 4 months (Reitan, 1959). Hence, most clinicians recommend a 3-month retention period after minor tooth movement to allow reorganization.

ARCH LENGTH PROBLEMS

The most common arch length problem in the primary dentition is tooth loss. This is managed as outlined in Chapter 25 with space maintenance if the space is adequate. If space has been lost, which can occur in the posterior sextants because of the tooth loss, space regaining can be instituted. The most notable place to use the appliances is with loss of the primary first molar. If the second primary molar is lost, timely placement of the distal shoe is required and space loss will not be evident if it occurs until eruption of the permanent first molar. Thus, the only realistic space regaining test in the primary dentition is repositioning of the primary second molar prior to permanent first molar eruption. A removable appliance is best used for this purpose. Via multiple clasps and a finger spring, a primary second molar can be repositioned approximately 1 mm per month. Three millimeters of molar movement is a realistic extent of the treatment. This appliance is just like the appliance used to reposition a permanent first molar.

Another primary dentition arch length problem that has implications for the permanent dentition is generalized crowding not due to tooth loss. When a generally crowded primary dentition is encountered, most agree that this is a harbinger of crowding in the permanent dentition. Normally, and in cases when there is adequate space in the permanent dentition, there is spacing between the primary anterior and often posterior teeth.

Some have advocated early expansion of the primary arches with either fixed or removable appliances. This treatment is provided to ensure space for the permanent teeth (McInaney et al., 1980). The expansion provides variable increases in arch width and arch perimeter. Lutz and Poulton (1985) found little long-term benefit in this approach. This early approach to potential crowding remains controversial and unsubstantiated.

INCISOR PROTRUSION AND RETRUSION

In addressing the anteroposterior plane of space, the clinician is mainly concerned with the position of the incisors, particularly the maxillary incisors. The majority of anteroposterior problems involve anterior crossbite, a condition in which the maxillary incisors occlude lingual to the mandibular incisors. A fixed lingual arch or a removable appliance can be used to correct the crossbite. Several things should be kept in mind when moving primary anterior teeth. First, the crowns are extremely short incisogingivally. This means that overly aggressive activation of springs will cause them to not engage the crowns of the teeth but to slip past the lingual surface, for instance, and not engage the tooth. Gentle activation and springs directed gingivally are usually best in these cases. Second, the crowns of some primary first molars converge toward the occlusal surface. This makes banding or clasp retention challenging. Third, there are few or no undercuts on the anterior teeth that will engage a labial bow for retention. For this reason, if a labial bow in the primary dentition is not used for tooth movement, it probably should be discarded. Finally, because the primary teeth will be exfoliated near 6 to 7 years of age, it is probably not wise to consider moving a primary incisor much after 4 years of age.

The lingual arch can be designed in one of two ways. The arch can be activated to tip maxillary teeth into proper position, or it may have auxiliary wires soldered onto it to exert the tipping forces. The lingual arch (36-mil wire) is activated approximately 1 mm per visit because it is such a heavy-gauge wire and exerts such a heavy force. The auxiliary wires can be activated 2 mm, which is the normal amount for a 22-mil wire (Fig. 27-1). Generally, a tooth moves 1 mm per month during treatment. Therefore, if a tooth requires 3 mm of movement to be properly aligned, 3 months of treatment are necessary.

With a removable appliance, wire finger springs are incorporated into the palatal acrylic to move the teeth facially. The appliance is stabi-

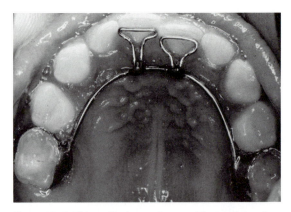

Figure 27–1. This patient's anterior crossbite involving the primary maxillary central incisors is being treated with a T-spring soldered to a lingual arch. The spring is activated 1½ to 2 mm per month until the incisors are tipped out of crossbite.

lized by placing retentive clasps on the posterior teeth. The finger springs are activated 1.5 to 2.0 mm per month. If the patient exhibits a positive overbite and overjet after treatment, retention is probably not necessary because the occlusion generally holds the tipped incisor in its new position. If there is no overbite, the appliance should be maintained until overbite is established to ensure that relapse does not occur.

One further point should be made about anterior crossbite. In some cases of posterior crossbite or occlusal interference, a child positions the jaw forward to achieve maximum intercuspation and an anterior crossbite results. This type of anterior crossbite is due to jaw posturing rather than tooth or jaw malposition. In these cases, treatment is directed toward the posterior crossbite or the occlusal interference and not toward the anterior crossbite.

Excessive overjet in the primary dentition is usually due to a non-nutritive sucking habit or to a skeletal mismatch between the upper and lower jaws. As mentioned previously, because of the tendency for abnormal growth patterns to recur, most skeletal problems should not be treated at this time. Incisor protrusion as a result of a sucking habit can be addressed, however. Treatment is usually directed at eliminating the habit rather than at correcting the incisor protrusion. Incisor protrusion usually corrects itself if the habit is discontinued and if the equilibrium between the tongue, lips, and perioral musculature is reestablished. The quad helix and palatal crib are discussed in Chapter 26 and are the appliances of choice for habit therapy (see Figs. 26-5 and 26-6). Studies designed to determine how long the appliance must remain in place to terminate the habit effectively suggest that 6 months is a minimum time period (Haryett et al., 1970).

POSTERIOR CROSSBITE

Posterior crossbite in the primary dentition is primarily a result of constriction of the maxillary arch. Constriction often results from an active digit or pacifier habit, although there are many cases in which the origin of the crossbite is undetermined. The first step in treating a posterior crossbite is to establish whether there is an associated mandibular shift. If a mandibular shift is present, treatment should be implemented to correct the crossbite. Some authors have implicated a mandibular shift as the cause of asymmetrical growth of the mandible (although few data exist). The asymmetry is thought to occur because the condyles are positioned differently within each fossa. Muscle and soft tissue stretch exert forces on the underlying skeletal and dental structures that may alter normal growth and arch development. If no shift is detected, the mandible should grow symmetrically.

When there is no shift, treatment is usually delayed until the permanent first molars erupt, unless gross crowding is present. In this situation, expansion of the arch should result in more room for the primary and permanent teeth. If the permanent molars erupt into crossbite, treatment can be initiated if no other malocclusion exists. When the permanent molars erupt normally and there is no mandibular shift, treatment may not be indicated for the crossbite of the primary molars until the premolars erupt. Correction of the crossbite in the primary molar region during the mixed dentition does improve the chances that the premolars will not erupt in crossbite (Thilander et al., 1984).

There are three basic approaches to the treatment of posterior crossbite in children: (1) equilibration to eliminate mandibular shift, (2) expansion of the constricted maxillary arch, and (3) repositioning of specific teeth to correct intraarch alignment. In a small number of cases, the mandibular shift is due to interference caused by the primary canines. These cases can be diagnosed by repositioning the mandible and noting the interference. Selective removal of enamel with a diamond bur in both arches eliminates the interference and the lateral shift into crossbite.

In cases of bilateral maxillary constriction, expansion is needed to correct the crossbite and sometimes the lateral shift. This type of case should be treated as soon as it is diagnosed unless it is anticipated that the permanent first molar will erupt within 6 months. In this situation, it is better to allow the permanent molars to erupt and to incorporate these teeth into treatment if necessary. Both fixed and removable appliances can be designed to correct maxillary constriction, although fixed appliances are reliable and require little patient cooperation.

Fixed appliances are variations of a lingual arch bent into the shape of a W. In fact, one of the most popular appliances used to treat crossbites is named the *W arch* (Fig. 27–2). Another popular appliance is the quad helix (see Fig. 26–5). The W arch is constructed of 36-mil wire that rests 1.0 to 1.5 mm off the palate to avoid soft tissue irritation. The W arch is expanded approximately 4 mm wider than its pas-

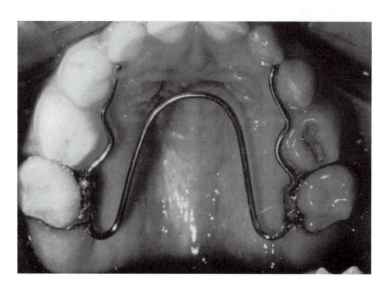

Figure 27–2. The W arch is a fixed appliance used to correct posterior crossbites in the primary dentition. The appliance is activated 3 to 4 mm beyond its passive width or to such an extent that one arm of the W extends over the central grooves of the teeth when the other arm is in the proper position.

sive width or so that one arm of the W is resting over the central grooves of the teeth when the other arm is in the proper position. To move teeth preferentially in the anterior region of the mouth, the appliance is activated by bending the palatal portion of the arm near the solder joint, as demonstrated in Figure 27-3. If more correction is needed in the molar region, the appliance is activated via bending of the anterior palatal portion. The appliance expands the arch approximately 1 mm per side per month.

The patient should return monthly to allow the dentist to check the progress of treatment and to reactivate the W arch if needed. The appliance may be activated intraorally, although the force and direction of activation may be difficult to approximate and unwanted tooth movement can result. Usually it is easier and more accurate to remove, activate, and re-cement the appliance. Expansion should continue until the crossbite is slightly overcorrected and the lingual cusps of the maxillary teeth occlude on the lingual inclines of the buccal cusps of the mandibular teeth. Most crossbites are corrected in 3 months, and the teeth are retained for an additional 3 months.

The quad helix is designed much like the W arch but incorporates more wire into the appliance, making it more flexible. It is constructed of 38-mil wire with two helices in the anterior palate and two helices near the solder joint in the posterior palate. The helices are wound away from the palate and can serve to remind the digit-sucking patient to refrain from the habit. Therefore, this is the preferred appliance for a patient with a finger habit and posterior cross-

bite. Because the quad helix has more wire than the W arch, it has a greater range of action and can be activated farther than the W arch while delivering an equivalent amount of force. Overcorrection and retention are required for the quad helix as well.

Despite activating the W arch or quad helix on one side only, teeth on both sides of the arch react to equivalent amounts of force. In other words, the teeth should all move an equal amount. This is desirable when there is bilateral maxillary constriction. If, however, the crossbite is due to a true unilateral maxillary constriction, it would be more appropriate to move only the teeth at fault. One way to accomplish this with a fixed appliance is to construct an unequal W arch or quad helix that has long and short arms (Fig. 27-4). The short arm touches only the teeth that need to be moved, and the long arm touches as many contralateral teeth as possible. The theory behind the unequal W arch is to pit movement of a large number of teeth against movement of a small number of teeth. The side with the smaller number of teeth tends to move more than the side with the larger number, although there will be expansion on both sides of the arch. An alternative method of unilateral treatment is to place a mandibular lingual arch to stabilize the lower arch and attach cross-elastics to the constricted maxillary teeth. This results in true unilateral movement of the maxillary teeth. This alternative requires more cooperation from the patient and is technically more difficult.

Removable appliances can also be used to correct posterior crossbites but are more difficult to use unless the appliances have good retention.

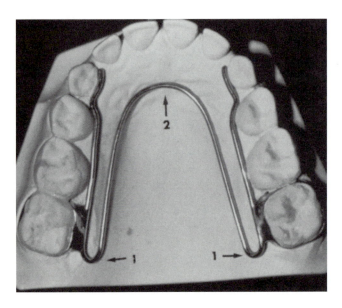

Figure 27-3. The preferred way to move teeth in the anterior region of the mouth is to activate the W arch by bending the arm of the W in the area marked location 1. If more movement is desired in the molar region, the appliance is activated by bending the anterior portion of the W in the area marked location 2.

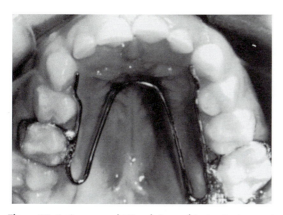

Figure 27–4. An unequal W arch is used to treat a true unilateral crossbite in the primary dentition. The short arm is placed on the constricted side of the arch against the teeth that are to be moved out of the crossbite. The long arm of the arch is placed on the opposite side of the arch, resting against as many teeth as possible to resist tooth movement on that side. In theory, the constricted side of the arch will move more than the opposite side. (From Fields HW, Proffit WR: Orthodontics in general practice. *In* Morris AL, Bohannan HM, Casullo DP [eds]: The Dental Specialists in General Practice. Philadelphia, WB Saunders Co, 1983, p 315.)

The forces used to expand the dental arch are so large that they tend to dislodge removable appliances. Most removable appliances are Hawley split-plate designs that use a variety of clasps to provide retention (Fig. 27–5). If the crossbite is due to a bilateral maxillary constriction, the appliance is split down the middle of the palate. A wire spring or a jackscrew embedded in the acrylic is activated to provide the force necessary for movement. The wire spring is activated approximately 2 mm per month. The jackscrew is turned one time per day; each turn provides 0.25 mm of activation. The wire spring appliance is probably easier for the patient to place and remove than a jackscrew appliance, and compliance may be better as a result. If the crossbite is unilateral or if only one or two teeth are in crossbite, the palatal acrylic can be cut so that the spring exerts force in a manner similar to that of the unequal W arch (Fig. 27-6).

Case Study

M.C., a 6-year-old white male, presented to the dental office for a 6-month dental examination. His mother reported that he still sucked his thumb every night while falling asleep but had stopped sucking during the day. A dental examination revealed a bilateral maxillary constriction in centric relation with a mandibular shift into a left posterior crossbite in centric occlusion. The overjet was 5 mm, and there was a 2-mm open bite in the left central incisor region (Fig. 27–7A).

Reminder therapy and a reward system had been instituted by M.C.'s parents after the last 6-month dental examination. A bandage was placed on his thumb, and M.C. was asked to place stars on a calendar on days when he did not suck. The combination of reminder therapy and reward system was effective enough to help M.C. eliminate the sucking habit during the daytime hours.

A treatment plan was offered to M.C. and his parents to correct the maxillary constriction and stop the bedtime habit. The plan called for a fixed quad helix appliance. The quad helix would be activated monthly to correct the crossbite and then made passive to serve as a retainer. The helices in

Figure 27–5. Removable appliances can be used to correct posterior crossbites in the primary dentition. The split plate appliance is activated by opening the wire spring 2 mm per month. The appliance is more hygienic than the W arch or quad helix because it can be removed to clean the teeth. The appliance requires multiple retention clasps, however, because it tends to dislodge when activated.

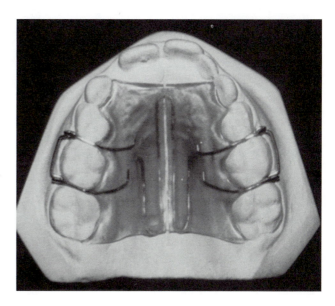

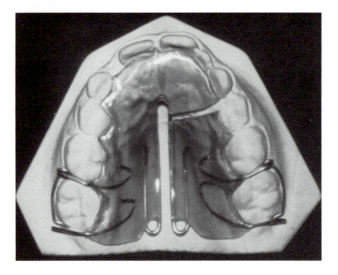

Figure 27–6. The unequal split plate appliance is used to treat true unilateral crossbites. Like the unequal W arch, the appliance is designed to move the constricted teeth preferentially out of crossbite and minimize movement elsewhere. The extent of the crossbite and the number of teeth in crossbite determine where the unequal split is made in the appliance. In this case, the left side is in crossbite.

the appliance would serve as a physical reminder not to suck the thumb.

After three activations over a 3-month period, the crossbite was overcorrected. The appliance was made passive and recemented. The quad helix now served as a retainer. The habit was reported to be extinguished by both M.C. and his parents (Fig. 27–7B). On M.C.'s subsequent 6-month examination, the crossbite correction was found to be stable and the habit had not returned (Fig. 27–7C).

OPEN BITES

Vertical problems in the primary dentition result principally from a finger or pacifier habit. Treatment of an anterior open bite that is due to a sucking habit is discussed in Chapter 26. Deep bite in the primary dentition is generally not treated at this time. The depth of bite usually improves with the eruption of the permanent

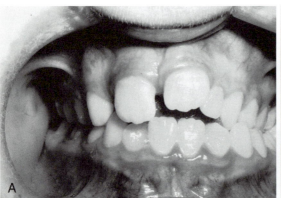

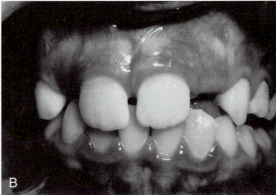

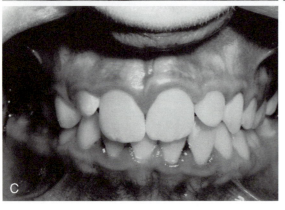

Figure 27–7. *A,* This 6-year-old patient has an anterior open bite, posterior crossbite, and increased overjet as a result of a thumb-sucking habit that is still present. *B,* A quad helix appliance was used to correct the posterior crossbite and extinguish the thumb-sucking habit. Note the overcorrection of the patient's left buccal segment. *C,* At the subsequent recall examination, the posterior crossbite correction is stable, reasonable occlusion has been established, and the habit has not returned.

first molars if the problem is due to dental malocclusion. Skeletal problems, whether anterior open bite or deep bite, are extremely difficult to treat and are appropriately referred to a specialist.

REFERENCES

Fields HW: Treatment of moderate nonskeletal problems in preadolescent children. *In* Proffit WR (ed): Contemporary Orthodontics. St. Louis, CV Mosby, 1999.

Haryett RD, Hansen FC, Davidson PO: Chronic thumbsucking: A second report on treatment and its psychological effects. Am J Orthod *57:*164-178, 1970.

Lutz HD, Poulton D: Stability of dental arch expansion in the deciduous dentiton. Angle Orthod *55:*299-315, 1985.

McInaney JB, Adams RM, Freeman M: A nonextraction approach to crowded dentitions in young children: Early recognition and treatment. JADA *101:*251-257, 1980.

Ngan P, Fields HW: Orthodontic diagnosis and treatment planning in the primary dentition. J Dent Child *62:*25-33, 1995.

Reitan K: Tissue rearrangement during retention of orthodontically rotated teeth. Am J Orthod *29:*105-113, 1959.

Thilander B, Wahlund S, Lennartsson B: The effect of early interceptive treatment in children with posterior crossbite. Eur J Orthod *6:*25-34, 1984.

Chapter 28

Local Anesthesia and Oral Surgery in Children

Stephen Wilson and R. Denny Montgomery

Chapter Outline

Successful management of patients, especially pediatric patients, in terms of allaying their anxiety and discomfort during restorative and surgical procedures is facilitated by the attainment of profound local anesthesia.

Good operator technique in obtaining local anesthesia in pediatric patients is essential and requires mastery of the following areas: (1) child growth and development (physical and mental), (2) behavior management, (3) physiologic pain modulation, and (4) pharmacology of local anesthetics.

Oral surgery procedures in children are similar to and possibly easier than those in adults. There are some important differences as well. This chapter presents an overview of the principles of local anesthesia and oral surgery in children.

LOCAL ANESTHESIA IN CHILDREN

Topical Anesthesia

Topical anesthesia is used to obtund the discomfort associated with the insertion of the needle into the mucosal membrane. The usefulness of topical anesthesia has been debated. For instance, the taste of the anesthetic, the period of time for the patient to anticipate the needle, and the establishment of a conditioned patient response from the needle immediately following the application of topical anesthetic have been considered to be detrimental factors. The operator's effectiveness in interacting with children to distract and increase their suggestibility toward managing their own anxieties may supersede the disadvantages of topical anesthesia, however. Therefore, we recommend the use of a benzocaine topical anesthetic that is good-tasting and that is available in an easy-to-control gel.

A small amount of the topical anesthetic should be applied with a cotton-tipped applicator to the mucosa that has been adequately dried and isolated with a 2 × 2 inch cotton gauze pad (Fig. 28–1). The time required for the topical anesthetic to reach its full effectiveness may vary from 30 seconds to 5 minutes. Although toxic responses to topical anesthesia are rare, excessive amounts should be avoided.

General Considerations for Local Anesthesia

The exact mechanism of action of local anesthetics has not been determined; however, the evidence supports the notion that they block Na$^+$ channels. It is known that a local anesthetic alters the reactivity of neural membranes to propagated action potentials that may be generated in tissues distal to the anesthetic block. Action potentials that enter an area of adequately anesthetized nervous tissue are blocked and fail to transmit information to the central nervous system (Bennett, 1984).

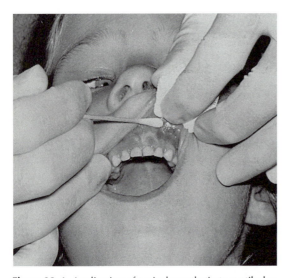

Figure 28–1. Application of topical anesthetic to vestibular tissues for buccal infiltration of incisors. Note a minimal amount of anesthetic on the cotton-tipped applicator. *Technique:* 1. Reflect tissue to expose injection site. 2. Dry soft tissue with 2 × 2 gauze pad. 3. Apply topical gel with cotton-tipped applicator. 4. Maintain applicator on tissue site for minimum of 30 seconds (see manufacturer's recommendations). 5. Remove applicator and proceed with injection.

The efficacy of local anesthesia depends on the concentration of the anesthetic on a segment of the nerve. Beyond a fixed amount of local anesthetic necessary for blockage of neuronal impulses, any excess is wasteful and potentially dangerous. Failure to obtain anesthesia is most likely due either to operator error in depositing the solution sufficiently close to the nerve or to anatomic aberrations (e.g., accessory innervation).

Local infection and inflammation can modify the normal local physiology of tissue by causing the release of neuroactive substances (e.g., histamine, kinins, and prostaglandins) and by lowering the pH. These changes reduce the lipid solubility of the anesthetic and interfere with its ability to penetrate the nervous tissue. Blocking the nerve at a more proximal site distant from the infected area may be a viable alternative. This may include the deposition of local anesthesia in intraligamental or intrapulpal sites. Antibiotic administration may reduce the extent of infection and permit definitive treatment under local anesthesia that would otherwise be impossible.

Local anesthesia may be obtained anatomically by one of three means:

1. *The nerve block,* which is the placement of anesthetic on or near a main nerve trunk. This results in a wide area of tissue anesthesia.

2. *The field block,* which is the placement of anesthetic on secondary branches of a main nerve.

3. *Local infiltration,* which is the deposition of the anesthetic on terminal branches of a nerve. Adequate diffusion of local anesthetic from local infiltration readily occurs in children because their bones are less dense than those of adults.

Local anesthetics used in dentistry are classified as esters or amides. Amides are more frequently used because of their reduced allergenic characteristics and greater potency at lower concentrations. The concentration of the different agents varies, and care must be taken to prevent overdose (Table 28–1). As an example, two full cartridges (Carpules) of 2% lidocaine (Xylocaine) without vasoconstrictor may be easily tolerated by an adult, but the same amount exceeds the maximal allowable dosage (2 mg/lb body weight) for a 20-pound child.

Local anesthetic Carpules (1.8 ml) also contain preservatives, organic salts, and sometimes vasoconstrictors. The preservatives (e.g., methylparaben) may be a source of allergic reactions. The vasoconstrictors (e.g., epinephrine) are used to constrict blood vessels, counteract the vasodila-

TABLE 28–1. Maximum Recommended Doses of Local Anesthetics for Children

Drug	Maximum Dose (mg/kg)	Mg/cartridge*
Lidocaine (2%) w/wo epinephrine	4.4 (300 mg max)	36
Mepivacaine (2%) w/ levonordefrin	4.4 (300 mg max)	36

| Patient Weight (kg/lb)† | Maximum Dosage | |
	mg	*No. of Cartridges*
10/23	44	1.2
15/34.5	66	1.8
20/46	88	2.4
25/57.5	100	2.7
30/69	132	3.6
40/92	176	4.8
50/115	220	6.1
60/138	264	7.3
70/161	300	8.3

Sources: US Pharmacopeial Dispensing Information (USPDI), Drug Information for Health Care Professionals, 1992; Malamed, S: Handbook on Local Anesthesia, 2nd ed. St. Louis, CV Mosby, 1986.
*2% = 20 mg/ml × 1.8 ml/cartridge = 36.
†1 kg = 2.3 lbs.

tory effects of the local anesthetic, and prolong the duration of the anesthetic.

Operator Technique

Communication in a language that the child can understand is important and necessary. The dentist may have to modify his or her wording to accommodate the level of the child's understanding when discussing the injection. For instance, the child may be told that the tooth will be "going to sleep" after a "little pinch" is felt near his tooth. The dentist should not deny that the injection may hurt because this denial may cause the child to lose trust and lack confidence. The dentist should minimize but not reinforce the child's anxieties and fears about the "pinch."

The discomfort of the injection may be lessened by counterirritation, distraction, and a slow rate of administration. Counterirritation is the application of vibratory stimuli (e.g., rapid displacement of loose alveolar tissue) or of moderate pressure (e.g., with a cotton-tipped applicator) to the area adjacent to the site of injection. These stimuli have a physical and psychological basis for modifying noxious input. Distraction can be accomplished by continuing a constant monologue with the child and by maintaining his or her attention away from the syringe. The operator should always aspirate and alter the depth of the needle if necessary prior to slowly injecting the anesthetic. The deposition of a single Carpule should take at least 1 minute. Rapid injections tend to be more painful because of rapid tissue expansion. They also potentiate the

possibility of a toxic reaction if the solution is inadvertently deposited in a blood vessel.

The role of the dental assistant is important during transfer of the syringe and in anticipation of patient movement. During the transfer of the syringe from the assistant to the dentist, the child's eyes tend to follow the dentist's. The eyes of the dentist should be focused on the face of the patient (Fig. 28-2). The hand of the dentist that is to receive the syringe is extended close to the head or body of the child. The body of the syringe is placed between the index and middle finger, with the ring of the plunger being slipped over the dentist's thumb by the assistant. The plastic sheath protecting the needle is then removed by the assistant. The dentist's peripheral vision guides the syringe to the mouth in a slow, smooth movement.

Reflexive movements of the child's head and body should be anticipated (Sanders, 1979, p. 106). The head can be stabilized by holding firmly but gently between the body and arm or hand of the dentist. The assistant passively extends his or her arm across the chest of the child so that potential arm and body movements can be intercepted. The area of soft tissue that is to receive the injection is reflected by the free hand of the dentist. The hand can also be used to block the vision of the child as the syringe approaches the mouth. Once tissue penetration by the needle has occurred, the needle should not be retracted in response to the child's reactions. Otherwise, the child's behavior may deteriorate significantly if he or she anticipates re-injection. Finger rests are strongly advocated.

A short (20-mm) or long (32-mm), 27- or 30-

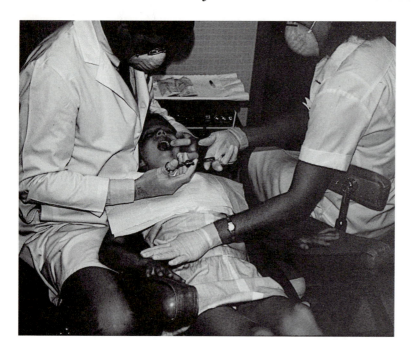

Figure 28–2. Preparing for the injection. Note the hand positions of the dentist and assistant to stabilize the child's head and body during the injection.

gauge needle may be used for most intraoral injections in children, including mandibular blocks. There apparently is little difference in discomfort in comparing 25- versus 30-gauge needles for inferior alveolar injections; thus, the 27-gauge needle would seem less likely to break or bend during injections and is preferred (Brownbill et al., 1987). An extra-short (10-mm), 30-gauge needle is appropriate for maxillary anterior injections.

Maxillary Primary and Permanent Molar Anesthesia

The innervation of maxillary primary and permanent molars arises from the posterior superior alveolar nerve (permanent molars) and middle superior alveolar nerve (mesiobuccal root of the first permanent molar, primary molars, and premolars).

In anesthetizing the maxillary primary molars or permanent premolars, the needle should penetrate the mucobuccal fold and be inserted to a depth that approximates that of the apices of the buccal roots of the teeth (Fig. 28-3). The solution should be deposited adjacent to the bone. The maxillary permanent molars may be anesthetized with a posterior superior alveolar nerve block or by local infiltration.

Maxillary Primary and Permanent Incisor and Canine Anesthesia

The innervation of maxillary primary and permanent incisors and canines is by the anterosuperior alveolar branch of the maxillary nerve. Labial

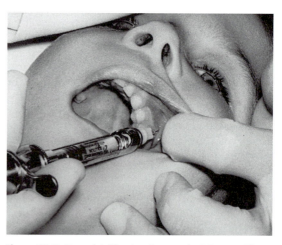

Figure 28–3. Buccal infiltration for anesthetizing maxillary primary molars.
Technique: 1. Reflect tissue to expose injection site. 2. Orient bevel of needle to be parallel to the bone. 3. Insert needle in mucobuccal fold. 4. Proceed to depth that approximates the apices of the buccal roots of the molar(s). 5. The bevel of the needle should be adjacent to the periosteum of the bone. Aspirate. 6. Deposit the bolus of anesthetic slowly. 7. Remove needle and apply pressure with 2 × 2 gauze for 1 minute to obtain hemostasis.

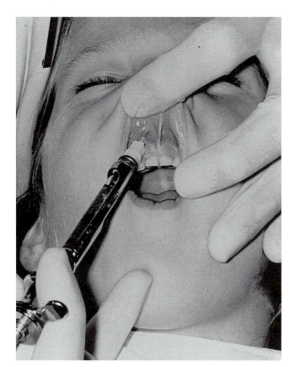

Figure 28–4. Labial infiltration of maxillary incisor area. *Technique for maxillary primary and permanent incisors and canines:* 1. Reflect tissue to expose injection site. 2. Orient bevel of needle to be parallel to the bone. 3. Insert needle in mucobuccal fold. 4. Proceed to depth that approximates the apices of the roots. This depth is less in the primary dentition than in the permanent dentition. 5. The bevel of the needle should be adjacent to the periosteum of the bone. Aspirate. 6. Inject the bolus of anesthetic very slowly. 7. Remove needle and apply pressure to area with 2 × 2 gauze for hemostasis.

infiltration commonly is used to anesthetize the primary anterior teeth. The needle is inserted in the mucobuccal fold to a depth that approximates that of the apices of the buccal roots of the teeth (Fig. 28-4). Rapid deposition of the solution in this area is contraindicated because it produces discomfort during rapid expansion of the tissue. The innervation of the anterior teeth may arise from the opposite side of the midline. Thus, it may be necessary to deposit some solution adjacent to the apex of the contralateral central incisor.

The infraorbital block injection is an excellent technique that may be used in place of local infiltration of the anterior teeth. All ipsilateral anterior maxillary teeth are anesthetized by this block. The needle is inserted anywhere in the mucobuccal fold from the lateral incisor to the first primary molar and is advanced next to bone to a depth that approximates the infraorbital foramen. The foramen is readily palpated as a notch

on the infraorbital rim of the bony orbit. The solution is deposited slowly.

Palatal Tissue Anesthesia

The tissues of the hard palate are innervated by the anterior palatine and nasal palatine nerves. Surgical procedures involving palatal tissues usually require a nasal palatine nerve block (Fig. 28-5) or anterior palatine anesthesia (Fig. 28-6). These nerve blocks are painful, and care should be taken to prepare the child adequately. These injections are not usually required for normal restorative procedures. If it is anticipated that the rubber dam clamp will impinge on the palatal tissue, however, a drop of anesthetic solution should be deposited into the marginal tissue adjacent to the lingual aspect of the tooth. A blanching of the tissue will be observed.

Mandibular Tooth Anesthesia

The inferior alveolar nerve innervates the mandibular primary and permanent teeth. This nerve enters the mandibular foramen on the lingual aspect of the mandible. The position of the foramen changes by remodeling more superiorly from the occlusal plane as the child matures into adulthood. The foramen is at or slightly above the occlusal plane during the period of the primary dentition (Benham, 1976). In adults, it averages 7 mm above the occlusal plane. The foramen is approximately midway between the

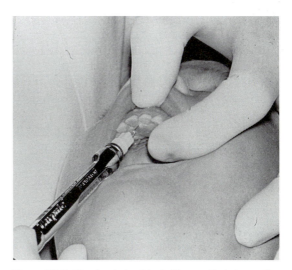

Figure 28–5. Nasal palatine block. The needle is inserted to the left or right side of the papilla. Note the blanching of tissue at the injection site.

anterior and posterior borders of the ramus of the mandible.

For the inferior alveolar nerve block, the child is requested to open his or her mouth as far as possible. Mouth props may aid in maintaining this position for the child. The ball of the thumb is positioned on the coronoid notch of the anterior border of the ramus, and the fingers are placed on the posterior border of the ramus. The needle is inserted between the internal oblique ridge and the pterygomandibular raphe (Fig. 28-7). The barrel of the syringe overlies the two primary mandibular molars on the opposite side of the arch and parallels the occlusal plane. The needle is advanced until it contacts bone, aspiration is completed, and the solution is deposited slowly.

Occasionally, the inferior alveolar nerve block is not successful. A second try may be attempted; however, the needle should be inserted at a level higher than that of the first injection. Care must be taken to prevent an overdose of anesthetic (see Table 28-1).

The long buccal nerve supplies the molar buccal gingivae and may provide accessory innervation to the teeth. It should be anesthetized along

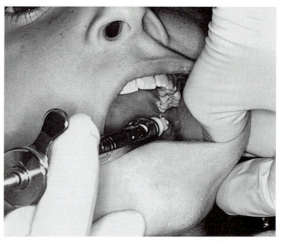

Figure 28–7. Inferior alveolar block.
Technique: 1. With patient's mouth opened as wide as possible place the ball of the thumb on the coronoid notch on the anterior border of the mandible. 2. Position the index and middle fingers on the external posterior border of the mandible. 3. Insert the needle with bevel oriented parallel to the bone and at the level of the occlusal plane between the internal oblique ridge and the pterygomandibular raphe. The barrel of the syringe will be exiting the mouth adjacent to the lip commissure contralateral to the side that is to be anesthetized. 4. Insert the needle to a depth that is adjacent to the bone. Aspirate. 5. Slowly inject the bolus of anesthetic. 6. Remove the needle and apply pressure to area with 2 × 2 gauze for hemostasis.

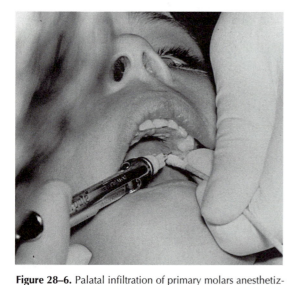

Figure 28–6. Palatal infiltration of primary molars anesthetizing the anterior palatine nerve. The cotton-tipped applicator is being held firmly against the palatal tissue. The needle is inserted in the area between the applicator and tooth. The applicator may provide a masking or distracting effect. *Technique:* 1. Apply pressure with cotton-tipped applicator to site that is to receive the needle. 2. Insert needle with bevel oriented parallel to the bone immediately adjacent to the applicator. 3. Proceed to a depth at which the bevel of the needle is adjacent to the periosteum and aspirate. 4. Inject the bolus of anesthetic very slowly. 5. Remove needle and apply pressure to area with a 2 × 2 gauze for hemostasis.

with the inferior alveolar block. A small quantity of solution is deposited in the mucobuccal fold at a point distal and buccal to the most posterior molar (Fig. 28-8).

Some operators advocate the use of a periodontal ligament injection for anesthetizing singular teeth (Malamed, 1982). An advantage of this method is that soft tissue is not anesthetized, which may prevent inadvertent tissue damage from chewing after dental procedures. There is some evidence, however, that this type of injection may produce areas of hypoplasia or decalcification on succedaneous teeth (Brannstrom et al., 1984).

Complications of Local Anesthesia

The complications of local anesthesia may include local and systemic effects (Malamed, 1986). Local complications may include masticatory trauma (Fig. 28-9), hematomas, infections, nerve damage by the needle, trismus, and, rarely, needle breakage in the soft tissue. These types of complications may be minimized by aspirating, decreasing needle deflection, and warning the parent and child that the soft tissue will be anes-

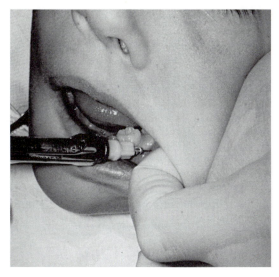

Figure 28–8. Long buccal nerve block.
Technique: 1. Reflect tissue to expose site of injection. 2. Insert needle in the mucobuccal fold at a point distal and buccal to the most posterior molar. The bevel of the needle should be oriented parallel to the bone. 3. Insert needle to a depth that is adjacent to the bone. Aspirate. 4. Slowly inject the bolus of anesthetic. 5. Remove the needle and apply pressure to area with 2 × 2 gauze for hemostasis.

thetized for a period of up to 1 to 2 hours after the restorative procedure.

Systemic complications include allergic reactions and cardiovascular and central nervous system (CNS) dysfunctions. The CNS responses to local anesthetics are complex and depend on plasma concentrations. These responses range from dizziness, blurred vision, and anxiety to tremors, convulsions, CNS depression, and death

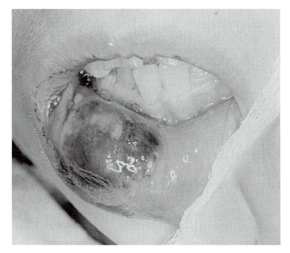

Figure 28–9. Masticatory trauma to lower lip that has been anesthetized with an inferior alveolar block.

(Hersh et al., 1991). The primary effect of local anesthetics on the heart is that of myocardial depression.

Management of overdoses varies, depending on the presenting symptoms and signs. Mild reactions require little more than patient reassurance and, if necessary, termination of the planned treatment. Severe reactions require oxygen supplementation, ventilatory support, and possible hospitalization.

ORAL SURGERY IN CHILDREN

In many ways, oral surgical procedures for children are similar to and possibly easier than those performed for adults. There are some important differences as well. The purpose of this section is to present basic techniques and surgical principles necessary to perform oral surgical procedures safely and competently for the child and adolescent patient. This section discusses the extraction of teeth, minor soft tissue procedures (i.e., biopsies and frenectomies), odontogenic infections, and the recognition and initial care for facial injuries and fractures.

Preoperative Evaluation

The dentist treating the child patient must be careful to evaluate the entire patient and not focus only on the oral cavity. Important considerations in caring for the child patient include the following:

1. Obtaining a good medical history
2. Obtaining appropriate medical and dental consultations
3. Anticipating and preventing emergency situations
4. Being fully prepared to treat emergency situations properly when they occur

In addition to the medical preoperative evaluation, it is important to perform a thorough dental preoperative evaluation, which includes taking appropriate preoperative radiographs. These often include two or more periapical radiographs of the same area in order to determine buccal, lingual, facial, or palatal relationships of impacted teeth. Another preoperative consideration is the future need for space maintenance as a result of the premature loss of primary teeth. Failure to provide immediate space maintenance may allow for the mesial migration of permanent first molars after premature primary molar loss.

Tooth Extractions

ARMAMENTARIUM

Many dentists choose to use the same surgical instruments for their child patients as they routinely use for their adult patients. Most pediatric dentists and oral and maxillofacial surgeons, however, prefer the smaller pediatric extraction forceps, such as the No. 150S and 151S (Fig. 28–10), for the following reasons:

1. Their reduced size more easily allows placement in the smaller oral cavity of the child patient.
2. The smaller pediatric forceps are more easily concealed by the operator's hand.
3. The smaller working ends (beaks) more closely adapt to the anatomy of the primary teeth.

The choice of the proper instrumentation can also depend on special considerations unique to the child and the adolescent. The use of cow horn mandibular forceps is contraindicated for primary teeth, owing to the potential for injury to the developing premolars. Great care must also be given to the routine use of elevators and forceps adjacent to large restorations such as chrome crowns and especially restorations adja-

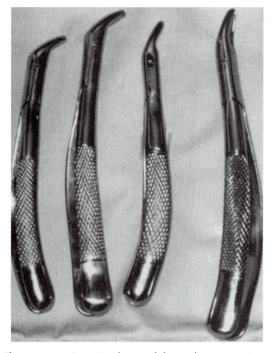

Figure 28–10. Extraction forceps: left to right, No. 151S, No. 151, No. 150S, No. 150.

cent to erupting single-rooted teeth that may easily become dislodged with the slightest force.

GENERAL CONSIDERATIONS

The manual technique used to perform extractions in the child patient is similar to the manual extraction technique used in the adult. The greatest difference is in patient management. It is essential that the dentist take the time to describe the ensuing procedure completely and accurately to the child. The extraction appointment should always begin with proper topical and local anesthesia, with consideration given to oral, intravenous, or nitrous oxide psychosedation on an individual basis (see Chapter 9). A few children require general anesthesia for the surgical procedure to be accomplished. The choice of proper local anesthesia–sedation–general anesthesia technique depends on the psychological constitution of the child and the extent and nature of the surgical procedure. The appropriate local anesthetic technique for each type of tooth is described earlier in this chapter.

A number of aspects of the extraction procedure should be performed with every extraction. The dentist should consult with the child and the parents prior to surgery in order to prepare them for the upcoming procedure. The dentist should provide any preoperative needs, such as prescriptions or any dietary restrictions, that might be necessary as a result of the planned sedative techniques. The entire surgical procedure and the expected postoperative recovery course should also be described. This allows the parents to prepare for any special postoperative arrangements, such as the need for a soft diet or child care support. As noted before, the dentist should perform a thorough review of the patient's medical history, looking especially for medical conditions that might complicate treatment.

There is no other type of dental treatment in which the principles of tell, show, and do are more important than during extractions. The dentist should be sure to obtain profound anesthesia because once the patient has felt pain, it may be difficult to regain the child's confidence to a level in which he or she will behave in a manner that allows completion of the procedure.

Just prior to the actual extraction, the dentist should place the balls of the index finger and thumb in the area of the extraction and demonstrate to the child the types of pressures and movements that he or she will encounter during the extraction. This digital pressure should be firm enough to rock the child's head from side to side in the headrest.

Several factors make it possible for the child patient to aspirate or swallow foreign objects during dental treatment. These factors include (1) the common practice of treating the child patient in a reclining position, (2) poor visibility as a result of the smaller opening into the oral cavity and the proportionately larger tongue of the child, and (3) the increased likelihood of unexpected movements by the child patient. To prevent this from happening, the patient should be positioned in the chair so that the upper jaw is at no more than a 45-degree angle with the floor (Fig. 28–11). If greater than a 45-degree angle is preferred by the operator, consideration should be given to either placing a light gauze pack in the posterior oral cavity (Fig. 28–12) or performing the extraction with the use of a rubber dam.

The dentist should be placed in the position in which he or she can easily control the instrumentation, have good visual access to the surgical site, and control the child's head. The nondominant hand of the dentist in then placed in the patient's mouth. The role of the nondominant hand is to help control the patient's head;

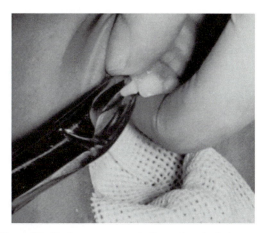

Figure 28–12. A gauze screen in the oral cavity helps prevent aspiration of extracted teeth.

to support the jaw being treated; to help retract the cheek, lips, and tongue from the surgical field; and to palpate the alveolar process and adjacent teeth during the extraction (Fig. 28–13).

Once the proper operator and nondominant hand positions are established, the actual extraction technique may begin. Variations in technique for individual teeth are discussed later in this chapter, but the following general principles apply to all extractions (Kruger, 1984). An instru-

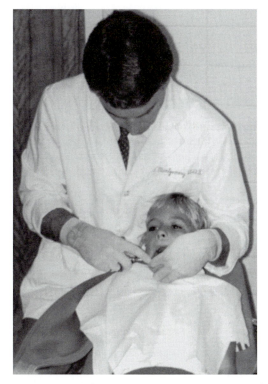

Figure 28–11. To help prevent aspiration of extracted teeth, the child is positioned so that the upper jaw is at a 45-degree angle to the floor.

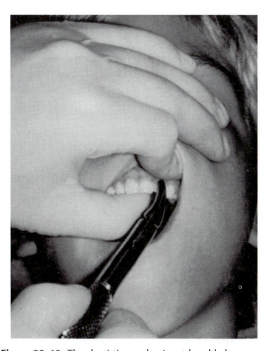

Figure 28–13. The dentist's nondominant hand helps control the child's head, supports the jaw being treated, retracts adjacent soft tissues, and palpates the alveolar process and adjacent teeth during extraction.

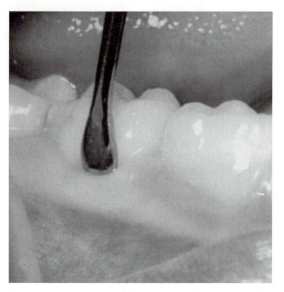

Figure 28–14. A periosteal elevator is used to separate the epithelial attachment of the tooth prior to extraction.

ment such as a dental curette or periosteal elevator is used to separate the epithelial attachment of the tooth to be extracted (Fig. 28–14). Then appropriate elevators may be used to luxate the tooth to be extracted, but great care must be used in order not to damage adjacent or underlying teeth. The appropriate forceps are then placed on the tooth to be extracted, usually seating the lingual or palatal beak first and then rotating the facial beak into proper position. During the entire extraction technique, firm apical pressure should be placed on the forceps. The extraction is then performed via the proper forceps technique.

After the tooth is removed from its socket, the surgical site is evaluated visually and with the use of a curette. The curette should be used as an extension of the dentist's finger to palpate and evaluate the extraction site. No attempt should be made to scrape the extraction site. If a pathologic lesion such as a cyst or periapical granuloma is present at the apex of a permanent tooth socket, it should be gently enucleated. Aggressive manipulation of a curette in a primary tooth socket is contraindicated owing to the potential for damage to the succeeding tooth bud. The operator should palpate both the facial and palatal or buccal and lingual aspects of the surgical site to feel for any bone irregularities or alveolar expansion. Any bone sharpness should be conservatively removed with the use of either a rongeur or a bone file. Digital pressure should be able to return the alveolus to its presurgical configuration if gross expansion has occurred.

The extraction site should now be evaluated for the need for sutures, although they are rarely indicated after extraction of primary teeth. The first postoperative concern is that of obtaining initial hemostasis by way of an intraoral gauze pack. In the anesthetized, deeply sedated, or very young child, a pack that extends out of the oral cavity should be used in order to prevent swallowing of the gauze. Before the patient is dismissed, a written list of postoperative instructions should be given and explained to both the patient and the parents (Table 28–2). The postoperative instruction list should explain how to contact the dentist after hours in case of an emergency.

MAXILLARY MOLAR EXTRACTIONS

Primary maxillary molars differ from their permanent counterparts in that the height of contour is closer to the cementoenamel junction and

---

TABLE 28–2. Postoperative Instruction List for Patients

1. Bite on gauze for 30 minutes. Don't chew on the gauze.
2. Do not use a straw to drink for 24 hours.
3. Brush remaining teeth daily, but don't rinse or use a mouthwash the day of the surgery.
4. Take pain pills and any other medication as directed.
5. If pain increases after 48 hours or if abnormal bleeding continues, call our office.
6. To prevent bleeding, and swelling, keep your head elevated on two or three pillows while you rest and/or sleep.
7. Do not spit. Spitting will cause more bleeding. Excess saliva and a little blood looks like a lot of bleeding.
8. If bleeding starts again, put a gauze, a clean white cloth, or a damp tea bag over the bleeding area and bite on it with firm steady pressure for 1 hour. Do not chew on it.
9. Ice packs can be used immediately after surgery and for the next 24 hours to reduce swelling. Keep ice packs on 10 minutes and off 10 minutes.
10. Black and blue marks are bruises and often occur after surgery. Usually you don't notice them. Sometimes the skin is discolored. Do not worry about this.
11. Drink lots of liquids and eat anything you can swallow.
Call our office about any complications or if you need to change your appointment.
Dr. E. X. Traction. Office No: 555-0123. After hours call 555-3210

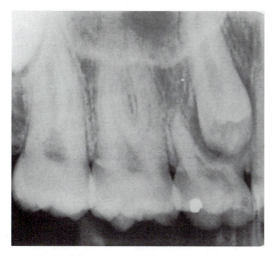

Figure 28–15. Primary molars with roots encircling the developing premolar may need to be sectioned to prevent accidental extraction of the premolar.

their roots tend to be more divergent and smaller in diameter. Because of the root structure and potential weakening of the roots during the eruption of the permanent tooth, root fracture in primary maxillary molars is not uncommon.

Another important consideration is the relationship of the primary molar roots to the succeeding premolar crown. If the roots encircle the crown, the premolar can be inadvertently extracted with the primary molar (Fig. 28-15).

After the epithelial attachment is separated, a 301 straight elevator is used to luxate the tooth (Fig. 28-16). The extraction is completed using a maxillary universal forceps (No. 150S). Palatal movement is initiated first, followed by alternating buccal and palatal motions with slow continuous force applied to the forceps. This allows expansion of the alveolar bone so that the primary molar with its divergent roots can be extracted without fracture.

EXTRACTION OF MAXILLARY ANTERIOR TEETH

The maxillary primary and permanent central incisors, lateral incisors, and canines all have single roots that are usually conical. This makes them much less likely to fracture and allows for more rotational movement during extraction than is possible with multirooted teeth. A No. 1 forceps is useful in the extraction of maxillary anterior teeth (Fig. 28-17).

MANDIBULAR MOLAR EXTRACTIONS

When extracting mandibular molars, the dentist must give special care to the support of the mandible with the nonextraction hand so that

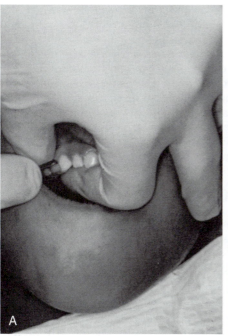
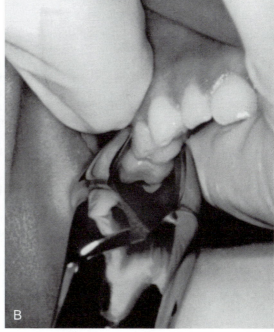

Figure 28–16. *A,* A No. 301 straight elevator is used to luxate the tooth. Extreme care is taken to prevent accidental luxation of adjacent teeth. *B,* The molar is extracted using slow continuous force in alternating buccal and palatal directions.

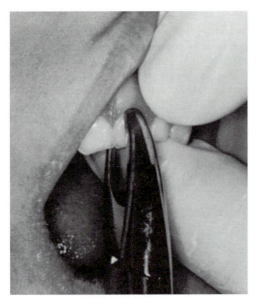

Figure 28–17. Rotational movements and buccolingual motions are used to extract primary incisors.

no injury to the temporomandibular joints is inflicted (Fig. 28–18). After luxation with a No. 301 straight elevator, No. 151S forceps are used to extract the tooth with the same alternating buccal and palatal motions used to extract maxillary primary molars.

EXTRACTION OF MANDIBULAR ANTERIOR TEETH

The mandibular incisors, canines, and premolars are all single-rooted. Because of this fact, one must take great care that the forceps do not place any force on adjacent teeth because they can become easily dislodged. This also enables the dentist to use rotational movements in the extraction process. Then slow, continuous force applied in alternating labial and lingual movements enables these teeth to be removed easily.

MANAGEMENT OF FRACTURED PRIMARY TOOTH ROOTS

Any dentist who extracts deciduous molars occasionally has the opportunity to treat root fractures. Once the root has fractured, the dentist must consider the following factors. Aggressive surgical removal of all root tips may cause damage to the succedaneous teeth. On the other hand, leaving the root may increase the chance for postoperative infection and may increase the theoretical potential of delaying permanent tooth eruption, although most primary root tips will resorb. A common-sense approach is best. If the tooth root is clearly visible and can be removed easily with an elevator or root tip pick, the root should be removed. If several attempts fail or if the root tip is very small or is situated very deep within the alveolus, the root is best left to be resorbed, most probably by the erupting permanent tooth. In some cases, the root tips do not resorb but are situated mesially and distally to the succeeding premolar and do not impede its eruption (Fig. 28–19). The patient and parents should be notified that a root fragment has been retained, and they should be assured that the chance of unfavorable sequelae is remote.

If the preoperative evaluation indicates that a root fracture is likely or that the developing succedaneous tooth may be dislodged during the extraction, an alternative extraction technique should be used. In these cases, the crown should be sectioned with a fissure bur in a buccolingual direction so that the detached portions of the crown and roots can be elevated separately (Sanders, 1979, p 148).

Soft Tissue Surgical Procedures

A number of soft tissue procedures occasionally must be performed for the child patient. Careful presurgical consideration should be given to the following:

1. The expected change in the condition with maturation
2. The optimal time (or age) for the procedure
3. The type of anesthetic or sedation required
4. Postoperative complications or sequelae
5. Expected results

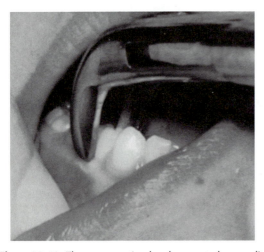

Figure 28–18. The nonextraction hand supports the mandible during extraction of mandibular molars.

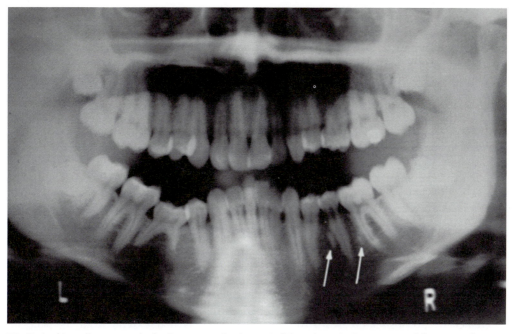

Figure 28–19. In this patient unresorbed primary root tips (*arrows*) did not impede the eruption of the succeeding premolar. Also note that the congenitally missing primary molar roots are not resorbing and the occlusal surface of this tooth is well below the occlusal plane.

BIOPSIES

Biopsy techniques in children are similar to those in adults. A very small lesion is probably best treated with an excisional biopsy, whereas lesions 0.5 cm or larger should probably have an incisional biopsy, especially if there is any doubt regarding the diagnosis of the lesion. Before performing a biopsy on any lesion, the dentist should consider the possibility of a vascular lesion. Any such area should be palpated for intravascular turbulence (thrill), auscultated with a stethoscope for the presence of a bruit, and checked by needle aspiration for the presence of blood within the lesion. Biopsies should not be performed on vascular lesions until a thorough work-up has been completed (Gibilisco, 1985).

Some areas of the oral cavity, such as the mucosa and lips, are easily accessible, whereas other areas, such as the tongue, can be difficult and may require sedation or general anesthesia in order to accomplish the biopsy. The biopsy area should be carefully evaluated for proximity to important anatomic structures, such as the mental nerve or salivary ducts or their orifices. Resorbable sutures are preferred to prevent the necessity of removing sutures in the child patient. The disadvantage of some resorbable sutures is that the knot can be very hard and stiff and irritating to the child. Soaking gut sutures in glycerin prior to their use softens them considerably.

FRENECTOMIES

Maxillary Labial Frenectomies. Recent trends justify significantly fewer maxillary labial frenectomies. These procedures should only be performed after it has been shown that the frenum is a causative factor in maintaining a diastema between the maxillary central incisors. This cannot be determined until after the permanent canines have erupted. Therefore, a maxillary labial frenectomy prior to the age of 11 or 12 is probably not indicated.

Lingual Frenectomies. Evidence from speech pathologists indicates that only the most severe ankyloglossia (tongue-tied) conditions significantly affect speech. Therefore, lingual frenectomies should not be performed until after an evaluation and therapy by a qualified speech therapist.

Dentoalveolar Surgery

More difficult dentoalveolar procedures may involve the use of mucoperiosteal flaps and bone openings of the maxilla or mandible. These are indicated for procedures such as retained roots, bone cysts, impacted teeth (e.g., canines, supernumerary teeth), or intrabony pathologic lesions. Basic technique involves the preparation of an adequate mucoperiosteal flap as well as an adequate bone opening. At the same time, the operator must be cautious to avoid injury to such structures as the mental or inferior alveolar nerves, developing or erupting teeth, and maxillary sinus.

Procedures to uncover impacted maxillary canines are highly successful (Fifield, 1986). Preoperative radiographs are taken to locate the canine within the alveolus accurately. It is often necessary to take two or more periapical radiographs, using the buccal object rule to predict the labiopalatal position of an impacted tooth. The appropriate soft tissue approach (either labial or palatal) is used in a conservative bone uncovering of the crown. Great care is taken not to disturb the root of the impacted canine because it is thought that the chance of ankylosis increases if the cementum is disturbed. If root development has not been complete, the exposed canine may be allowed to erupt passively. If the impacted canine has complete root development or is poorly positioned, an orthodontic bracket may be bonded to the exposed portion of the crown with autopolymerized resin. The exposed canine can now be orthodontically positioned within the maxillary arch.

Facial Injuries

The dentist may be the first health care professional consulted for injuries to the teeth, lips, jaws, or soft tissues of the face. The dentist should be aware of potential problems with each type of injury and treat the patient appropriately or refer him or her to a qualified specialist.

Initial care should be directed toward pain control, hemorrhage control, patient reassurance, wound toiletry if possible, and tetanus prophylaxis. Care should be taken to account for all teeth. Chest or abdominal radiographs may be necessary to find swallowed or aspirated teeth. Traumatic injuries to the teeth are discussed in Chapters 15 and 34.

Facial trauma is rarely life-threatening. A significant number of patients who present with facial trauma may also have acute life-threatening injuries such as chest or abdominal trauma or, more commonly, serious head or neck injury. The dentist must be sure that there are no other serious injuries before treating the facial injuries.

Soft tissue injuries of the face or oral cavity can usually be treated with primary closure. Great care must be taken to be certain that no foreign objects are left hidden within the wound. Gravel or dirt left embedded in soft tissue may leave a permanent tattoo on the face.

Puncture-type wounds often carry glass or debris deep within the wound. When there is doubt about the presence or absence of a foreign body within the soft tissue, a soft tissue radiograph may be helpful in identifying the presence of embedded material (see Fig. 15–7).

Small lacerations of the wet portion of the lips, gingivae, alveolar mucosa, or tongue usually heal very well even if left unsutured. Large lacerations should be closed, regardless of their location. A resorbable suture is most commonly used intraorally, although some practitioners prefer using silk suture material because it has a softer texture. The disadvantage of silk suture is that it requires removal in 5 to 7 days and the patient is still generally tender to manipulation of that area. Lacerations that extend from the face into the oral cavity (through-and-through lacerations) require a layered closure. Principles of a layered closure include a watertight mucosal closure, followed by closure of the muscular, facial, subcutaneous, and skin layers as necessary. Facial lacerations are always reapproximated first at significant anatomic structures, such as the vermilion border, columella of the nose, or eyebrows. Malalignment of these structures produces a noticeable cosmetic defect.

FACIAL FRACTURES

The definitive treatment of facial fractures is best handled by an experienced dental practitioner, such as an oral and maxillofacial surgeon. Often the patient presents to the dentist with an unsuspected fracture.

Patients with maxillary or midface fractures may present with any or all of the following signs or symptoms:

1. Altered occlusion
2. Numbness in the infraorbital nerve distribution
3. Double vision
4. Periorbital ecchymosis (bruising)
5. Facial asymmetry or edema
6. Limited mandibular opening
7. Subcutaneous emphysema (skin cracking upon palpation)
8. Nasal hemorrhage
9. Ecchymosis of the palatal or buccal mucosa
10. Mobility or crepitus upon manipulation of the maxilla

Patients with mandibular fractures may present with any or all of the following signs or symptoms:

1. Mandibular hemorrhage
2. Numbness in the mental or inferior alveolar nerve distribution
3. Altered occlusion
4. Ecchymosis or abrasion of the chin
5. Ecchymosis of the floor of the mouth or buccal mucosa
6. Periauricular pain
7. Mandibular deviation on opening (Fig. 28–20)
8. Mobility or crepitus upon manipulation of the mandible

Initial treatment of facial fractures should be directed toward the immobilization of fractured segments, early antibiotic therapy for open fractures, and pain control (Rowe and Williams, 1985). Definitive treatment should then be performed by a qualified specialist.

Odontogenic Infections

Infections of odontogenic origin are common in the child and adolescent patient. Classic signs and symptoms of infection include redness, pain, swelling, and local and systemic temperature increases. Because of wider marrow spaces in the child, an odontogenic infection can rapidly spread through the bone, possibly resulting in damage to the erupting teeth. Most odontogenic infections in the child are not serious and can be easily treated by pulp therapy or removal of the involved tooth. There are serious complications that uncommonly arise from an odontogenic infection, including cavernous sinus thrombosis, brain abscess, airway obstruction, and mediastinal spread of infection. Signs and symptoms of a more serious infection include an elevated systemic temperature (102–104°F), difficulty in swallowing, difficulty in breathing, nausea, fatigue, and sweating. The child with an odontogenic infection may become dehydrated as a result of his or her refusal to take fluids because of oral pain.

Treatment of odontogenic infections is directed toward providing adequate drainage of the infection. This can be accomplished in minor infections by way of a pulpectomy or extraction. The treatment of more serious odontogenic infections is best accomplished by way of surgical incision and drainage (Sanders, 1979, p. 186). It is often necessary to identify the causative organism or organisms in order to prescribe the most appropriate antibiotic. Because most oral infections are mixed infections (aerobic and anaerobic), penicillin remains the antibiotic of choice for initial therapy.

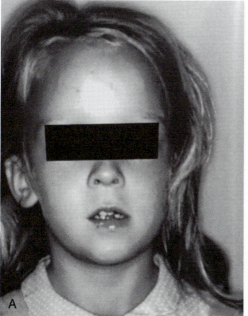 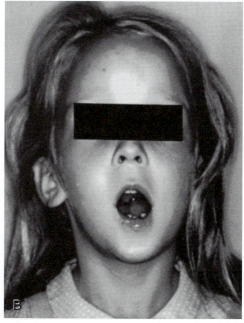

Figure 28–20. *A,* This child suffered a fracture of her left condyle. Note the deviation of the mandible to the left. *B,* The deviation of the mandible toward the side of the condylar fracture is more evident upon opening.

REFERENCES

Benham NR: The cephalometric position of the mandibular foramen with age. J Dent Child *43*:233, 1976.

Bennett CR: Monheim's Local Anesthesia and Pain Control in Dental Practice, 7th ed. St. Louis, CV Mosby, 1984, p 68.

Brannstrom M, Lindskog S, Nordenvall KJ: Enamel hypoplasia in permanent teeth induced by periodontal ligament anesthesia of primary teeth. JADA *109*:735, 1984.

Brownbill JW, Walker PO, Bourcy BD, Keenan KM: Comparison of inferior dental nerve block injections in child patients using 30-gauge and 25-gauge short needles. Anesth Prog *34*:215–219, 1987.

Fifield CA: Surgery and orthodontic treatment for unerupted teeth. JADA *113*:590, 1986.

Gibilisco JA: Oral Radiographic Diagnosis. Philadelphia, WB Saunders, 1985, p 224.

Hersh EV, Helpin ML, Evans OB: Local anesthetic mortality: Report of case. J Dent Child *58*:489–491, 1991.

Kruger G: Textbook of Oral and Maxillofacial Surgery, 6th ed. St. Louis, CV Mosby, 1984, p 52.

Malamed SF: The periodontal ligament (PDL) injection: An alternative to inferior alveolar nerve block. Oral Surg *53*:117, 1982.

Malamed SF: Handbook of Local Anesthesia, 2nd ed. St. Louis, CV Mosby, 1986, p 230.

Rowe N, Williams J: Maxillofacial Injuries. Edinburgh, Churchill Livingstone, 1985, p 538.

Sanders B: Pediatric Oral and Maxillofacial Surgery. St. Louis, CV Mosby, 1979.

USP: Dispensing Information for the Health Care Professional, 17th ed. Rockville, MD, United States Pharmacopeial Convention, 1997.

III

The Transitional Years: Six to Twelve Years

If one examines a group of children younger than 6 years, there tends to be homogeneity in these children regarding such characteristics as height, weight, dental appearance, and facial esthetics. If one could reexamine this group later, when they are over 12 years old, there would be much less overall similarity in these characteristics. Indeed, there would be noticeably tall individuals and short individuals, heavy and slight individuals, dentally unappealing individuals, and facially appealing and facially plain or perhaps even disadvantaged individuals.

The dentist during these years must be concerned with the development of the permanent occlusion, the harmonious relationships of the two jaws, facial posture, and dental appearance. During these years, the child increasingly becomes more conscious of his or her appearance. This consciousness continues to heighten until it is at its most profound point in the adolescent years.

Additionally, parents begin to notice increasingly the appearance of their children from a dental standpoint. In fact, age 6 itself, with the eruption of the two lower permanent central incisors, usually is accompanied by questions by the parents directed to the dentist. A usual question about the two lower permanent central incisors is why they come in rotated and what will happen to these teeth in the future. The maxillary permanent central incisors often appear to parents to be extraordinarily large and very yellow. In the vast majority of cases, these are of normal size and the apparent yellowness is natural compared with the very white enamel of the primary teeth. However, the permanent incisors do look strange to the parent uninformed about the difference in color of the enamel of the permanent dentition and the primary dentition.

From age 6 to 12, the prevention program of the child continues at home, and the parents still need to continue supervision. It is hoped that as the child progresses toward adolescence, it will become less necessary for the parent to supervise the youngster in oral hygiene.

In the dental office, prevention procedures often become more intense during these years. The advent of the first permanent molars in the 6- and 7-year-old and the possibility of buccal pit fissures, lingual pit fissures, and deep grooves on the occlusal surface of these teeth may signal a need for preventive sealants to stop the possibility of pit and fissure caries. Calculus accumulations also loom as more of a problem than in younger years.

With children starting to participate in team sports, ball-throwing sports, and riding bicycles, the chances of facial trauma and trauma to the early permanent dentition increase. This is particularly true for children who for whatever reason present maxillary incisors that are flared forward in their arch and that are likely to absorb the blow from any insult to the face between the nose and the chin.

In summary, everything that the dentist knows how to do for children between 3 and 6 years of age remains important for children between ages 6 and 12 because these youngsters still have primary teeth, particularly the posterior ones, during these years. Some children continue to need space maintenance. Others need interceptive orthodontic treatment. There are children who misbehave and need to be managed, although the incidence of misbehavior is much less than in younger age groups. Obviously, prevention needs remain, and sealants may be indicated. Fluoride supplementation should be encouraged throughout this transitional time. Because of the advent of the permanent dentition, different pulpal therapies and restorative techniques must be mastered to treat the problems presented by this age group effectively. Lastly, the fact that children in this age range can give the dentist more information to aid in decision making about their orthodontic needs is very important, particularly if early treatment is to be attempted.

29

The Dynamics of Change

Chapter Outline

Physical Changes

Body

J. R. Pinkham

The average 6-year-old in the United States is approximately 3 feet, 10 inches tall and weighs about 48 pounds. By the time the child reaches age 12, he or she will be about 5 feet tall and will weigh about 85 pounds. This represents, from age 6 to age 12, an approximately 5% to 6% height increase per year and a weight adjustment of about 10% per year (Watson and Lowrey, 1967).

By age 6, the child's overall body proportions are fairly close to what he or she will be as an adult. The most remarkable proportional change in the body during these years results from the lengthening of the child's limbs.

During the years between the ages of 6 and 12, boys as a group are generally slightly taller than girls until around age 10. From age 10 to around age 15, girls are slightly taller than boys. From a weight standpoint, boys are slightly heavier than girls until around age 11, when girls overtake boys in weight for a brief time. The reasons why boys eventually become taller than girls is dealt with in the discussion of the body's physical changes in the later section on adolescence (Chapter 36).

Other growth and developmental changes that are noteworthy during these years are further increases in blood pressure, continuing decreases in the pulse rate, increased mineralization of the skeleton, and increases in muscular tissue. In addition, the lymphatic tissues reach a peak in development during these years to the point where they exceed the amounts found in adults.

REFERENCE

Watson EN, Lowrey GH: Growth and Development of Children, 5th ed. Chicago, Year Book, 1967.

GROWTH INCREMENTS

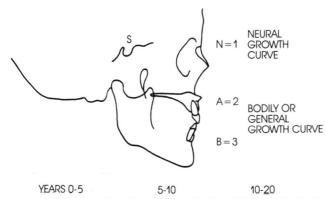

N = 1   NEURAL GROWTH CURVE

A = 2   BODILY OR GENERAL GROWTH CURVE

B = 3

	YEARS 0-5	5-10	10-20
1	85% of Total Growth Completed	96% of Total Growth Completed	Remaining 4% Completed
2	45% of Total Growth Completed	65% of Total Growth Completed	Remaining 35% Completed
3	40% of Total Growth Completed	65% of Total Growth Completed	Remaining 35% Completed

Figure 29–1. Differential growth center rates of craniofacial components. (From Behrents RG: Growth in the Aging Craniofacial Skeleton. Center for Human Growth and Development. Ann Arbor, University of Michigan, 1985.)

Craniofacial Changes

Jerry Walker

The years from ages 6 through 12 represent a continuous progression of the growth in the head and neck noted in the 3- to 6-year-old. In a comparison of the differential growth rates of the craniofacial components from ages 5 to 10 (approximately the age range of interest here), neural and cranial growth are found to be almost entirely complete (Fig. 29–1). During this same age span, the jaws (A = 2 and B = 3 of Fig. 29–1) grow at a rate faster than the cranium. Despite this faster rate, considerable general growth is experienced after age 10.

Using the Bolton Standards for illustrative pur-

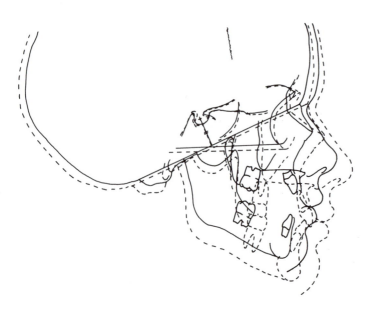

Figure 29–2. This anterior cranial base superimposition of the Bolton Standard for 6- and 12-year-olds (*solid line* and *dashed line*, respectively) demonstrates the magnitude of anteroposterior and vertical skeletal growth during this period as well as the soft tissue change. (Redrawn from Broadbent BH, Sr, Broadbent BH, Jr, Golden WH: Bolton Standards of Developmental Growth. St. Louis, CV Mosby, 1975.)

Figure 29–3. This anterior cranial base superimposition of the Bolton Standard for 6- and 12-year-olds (*solid line* and *dashed line*, respectively) demonstrates the magnitude of transverse and vertical skeletal growth during this period. (Redrawn from Broadbent BH, Sr, Broadbent BH, Jr, Golden WH: Bolton Standards of Developmental Growth. St. Louis, CV Mosby, 1975.)

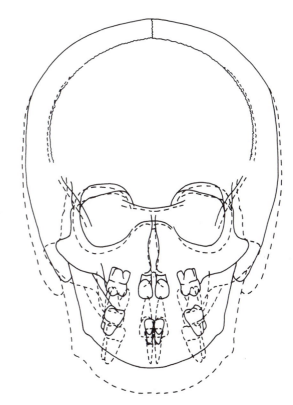

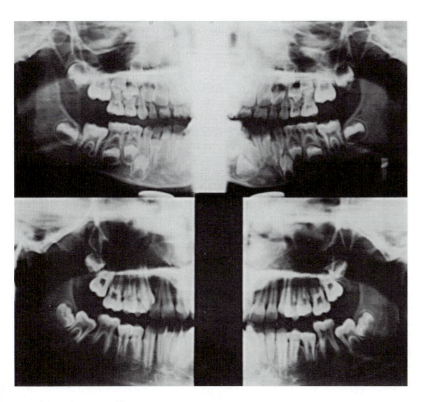

Figure 29–4. These two panoramic radiographs show the transition from the beginning of the permanent dentition to its completion with the exception of the third molars.

poses, nasal projection and increased mandibular prominence are demonstrated (Fig. 29-2). The nasal cartilage and mandibular condyle continue to grow by endochondral bone formation for some time, although the female mandibular growth spurt is most likely completed, and the male's is yet to come. Growth modification can therefore be performed in this age group. Changes in cranial base length caused by endochondral bone formation at the spheno-occipital synchondrosis cease in early adolescence, but some appositional changes continue to occur at the basion and nasion. Vertically, there is a continued lowering of the palatal vault with sutural growth and apposition on the oral side of the palate and resorption on the nasal side as the intramembranous process of bone formation continues.

In the traverse plane, there is continued growth at the maxillary suture and appositional widening of the dentoalveolar ridge with eruption of the permanent teeth (Fig. 29-3). This is especially noticeable with the canines and premolars. Widening of the anterior arch accompanies lateral incisor eruption.

By the end of these transitional years, the complete permanent dentition with the exception of the third molars has erupted (Fig. 29-4). Most of the residual space resulting from either idiopathic spacing or leeway spacing has closed by this time. Further eruption and drift occur in response to continued growth.

REFERENCE

Broadbent BH Sr, Broadbent BH Jr, Golden WH: Bolton Standards of Developmental Growth. St. Louis, CV Mosby, 1975.

Dental Changes

C. A. Full

Early during this period of time, many children experience the eruption of all four first permanent molars and the exfoliation of the mandibular and maxillary primary central and lateral incisors with a subsequent eruption of permanent incisors between the ages of 6 and 7 years (see Table 12-5). The maxillary permanent lateral incisors may erupt later than age 7 in some children.

With the exception of the third molars, all of the permanent teeth usually have erupted by the end of the twelfth year. Except for the third molars, the enamel of all of the permanent teeth is complete by age 8. In the mandibular arch and following the first permanent molars and central incisors, the teeth erupt in immediate succession—that is, centrals, laterals, cuspids, first and second premolars, and second permanent molars from 6 to 7 years through 11 to 13 years of age. The same sequence takes place in the maxillary arch except for the maxillary cuspid, which usually erupts after the bicuspids or premolars and at about the same time or before the eruption of the second permanent molars (Fig. 29-5).

The mandibular central incisor roots are complete by age 9. The roots of the four first permanent molars, the maxillary central incisors, and the mandibular lateral incisors are usually complete by age 10. The roots of the maxillary lateral incisors are complete by age 11.

Because the position of the dental lamina of the permanent teeth is located to the lingual of all of the primary teeth (except for the dental lamina coming off the second primary for the three permanent molars), the anterior teeth develop in their vault or crypt lingual to and near the apex of the primary incisors. When the roots begin to form on the permanent teeth, they start to migrate toward the oral cavity. Generally, they follow a pattern such that they come across the primary root, resorbing it and erupting slightly labial to the location sustained by the primary tooth (Fig. 29-6). Therefore, the permanent teeth are usually always angulated more buccally compared with their primary predecessors (Fig. 29-7). The developing bicuspids develop between the roots of the primary molars and continue to erupt in a slightly mesial position. The permanent molars develop from one dental lamina and, like the bicuspids or premolars, erupt in or at a mesial inclination or angle.

Compared with the primary incisors, the permanent incisors are larger and develop in a more restricted area (Finn, 1973). Their growth, although perpetual, occurs at a much slower rate during their eruption compared with the primary incisors. The inclinations of the eruptive

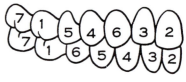

Figure 29–5. Desirable eruption sequence for the permanent teeth. (Reproduced by permission from McDonald RE, Avery DR: Dentistry for the Child and Adolescent, 4th ed. St. Louis, CV Mosby, 1983.)

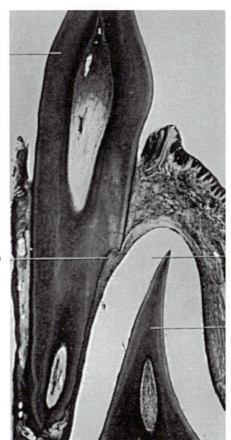

Figure 29–6. Resorption of root of primary incisor owing to pressure of erupting successor. (Reproduced by permission from Bhaskar SN [ed]: Orban's Oral Histology and Embryology, 10th ed. St. Louis, CV Mosby, 1986.)

Deciduous incisor

Root resorption

Enamel of permanent incisor

Dentin

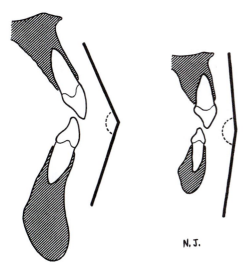

N. J.

Figure 29–7. Angulation of permanent and primary incisors. (Reproduced by permission from Moyers RE: Handbook of Orthodontics, 3rd ed. Copyright © 1973, Year Book Medical Publishers, Inc., Chicago.)

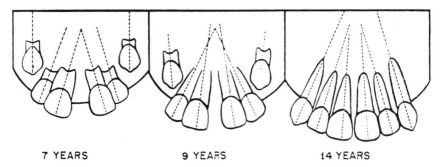

7 YEARS   9 YEARS   14 YEARS

Figure 29–8. The "ugly duckling" stage. (From Finn SB: Clinical Pedodontics, 4th ed. Philadelphia, WB Saunders, 1973; after Broadbent BH: Angle Orthodont *1*:183–208, 1937.)

paths of the permanent incisors account for their flared appearance. Also, it is natural to find diastemas between the incisors, particularly in the maxilla. The permanent canine in the maxillary arch is usually the last permanent tooth to erupt mesial to the first permanent molar. As the permanent canine begins to erupt, its mesial component of force is often adequate to straighten the incisors and close the diastemas. This period of development has been called the "ugly duckling stage" (Fig. 29–8) (Finn, 1973).

REFERENCE

Finn SB: Clinical Pedodontics, 4th ed. Philadelphia, WB Saunders, 1973.

Cognitive Changes
J. R. Pinkham

A book could easily be written describing the incredible cognitive acquisitions, adjustments, and sophisticated changes occurring in a child from age 6 to age 12. Mental capacity alone grows extensively. For example, by age 12 a child can outline on paper or mentally recall the travels of Marco Polo. At age 6 the concept of an ancient man from Italy traveling to China would not be remarkable and probably would be mentally unretainable.

In 1968, White concluded that between the ages of 5 and 7 years a reorganization of the central nervous system may take place that accounts for a dramatically increased ability to remain diligent at a task or attentive to a problem. Unquestionably, the attention span of the child after age 7 is substantially greater than that of the child under 5 years of age.

The school-age years of 6 to 12 are the years when a child becomes literate. Before age 6 few children can do much more than print their names. After age 12 most children have accomplished an appropriate approach to grammar and syntax and have the ability to produce increasingly sophisticated oral and written communications. In some parts of the world it is not uncommon for a child to be fluent in a second language by age 12.

According to Piaget, the ages between 6 and 12 roughly approximate the third major developmental stage of cognition, the phase of concrete operations. Piaget proposed the following four major periods of intellectual development:

1. *Sensorimotor*: birth to 18 months
2. *Preoperational*: 18 months to 7 years
3. *Concrete operations*: 7 to 12 years
4. *Formal operations*: 12 years and onward

So far this book has presented a study of the child through the sensorimotor and pre-operational stages. In the concrete operations stage, Piaget described numerous sophisticated changes in the child's mental abilities. For instance, the 5-year-old may be able to walk "two blocks down, one block right to the second white house" to get to his or her aunt's residence, but the same 5-year-old could not draw this route on a piece of paper. However, by age

7 or 8, the child could portray the route on a self-drawn map. In other words, mental representations of actions become a part of the cognitive abilities of the child during these years. For the dentist who instructs children in the process of tooth decay, it may be helpful in designing his or her preventive presentation to understand the differences in mental representation ability between preschoolers and school-age children. Obviously, two different presentations are needed.

During the years from 6 to 12 (7 to 12, according to Piaget), children acquire the ability to understand the constancies between length, mass, number, and weight despite external differences. Relativity also emerges in the child's evaluation system. To the 4-year-old, the word "dark" means black. The 10-year-old can talk about a "dark" green car. In summary, the child between the ages of 6 to 12 grows up cognitively. By the age of 12 years, his or her mind and mental prowess have matured, and he or she is capable of assimilating real as well as theoretical or abstract information.

REFERENCE

White SH: Changes in Learning Processes in the Late Preschool Years. Presented at a meeting of The American Education Association, Chicago, 1968.

Emotional Changes
J. R. Pinkham

The years from 6 to 12 are years of matriculation toward the acceptance by the child of societal norms of behavior. Crying, tantrums, and other rages will, in normal children, be relinquished as possible modes of expression of frustration. Whereas the preschooler needs and perhaps demands immediate rewards and satisfaction, the child in the transitional years masters the emotional ability to delay gratification. This awareness of delay is reinforced by the child's schooling, and increasingly the child is guided toward the appropriate investment of his or her time into worthwhile activities. Homework, chores at home, caring for pets, newspaper delivery, scouting, team sports, and piano lessons are some of the behaviors expected of this age group, which were almost impossible during the preschool years.

Another emotional refinement that is developed from age 6 to 12 is the ability to utilize life's tasks in ways effective enough to stave off boredom. Previously, the preschooler immersed his mental preoccupation into something until all his energy and attention were spent. Then, at the point of burn-out, he looked for his parents or other attendants to find something else for him to do. Between ages 6 and 12, however, the need for adults to direct the child's attention rapidly recedes, and by age 12 a child usually has a ledger of wants and desires, a sense of the time that should be spent in their pursuit, and an ability to set priorities for which wants and desires should come first or last.

In this age range, body image starts to become an emotional feature of the child's life. Unquestionably, for the majority of children the importance of body image becomes most dramatic during adolescence, but its emergence certainly occurs during these years. Whereas the 6-year-old usually couldn't care less about ketchup on his face or mud on his pants, the 12-year-old may agonize over a blemish or over having clothes that are thought to be not stylish. In summary, body appearance becomes a subject of emotional awareness and emphasis during these years. Unquestionably, this has dental ramifications. The mottled enamel of the 6-year-old may have disturbed only the child's parents. The child was indifferent. By age 12, this condition may account for a lack of smiling, social withdrawal, and a feeling of forlornness by the child. Teasing may make these findings worse.

Although there certainly are exceptions, the majority of children from age 6 to 12 find overall emotional satisfaction only when they are accepted socially by their peers. Lack of acceptance, outright ostracism, and teasing can certainly be very damaging emotionally. During these years, with the help of parents, teachers, role models, and other significant people, it is important for the child to become emotionally resilient. The abilities to handle and recover from humiliation, frustration, loss, and disappointment need at least to start to emerge during these years. If they don't, adolescence presents a real danger.

Social Changes

J. R. Pinkham

The years between ages 6 and 12 are often called middle childhood. These years are clearly more complicated socially than the earlier years because of school, the increasing importance of peers, and the enormous expansion of the child's social environment. These years see the child intensify his or her focus on and pursue some already existing motives, while others are minimized or eliminated completely.

School is certainly extremely important for this age group and represents an extrafamilial world that may reinforce social responses learned at home, portray new ones, and even retrain or deny others. Whether the teacher is encountered earlier in preschool or now for the first time at school, he or she is likely to be the first significant, day-by-day, authoritative adult known outside the child's immediate family. Also, as opposed to baby sitters and relatives, the teacher is encountered by the child in an environment in which the teacher has control. In 1964, Franco concluded that a child's feelings about her or his first teacher correlate closely with the child's feelings about her or his mother.

Perhaps surprisingly, most children anticipate school positively and remain enthusiastic about their experiences there. It has also been noted that children's self-importance, self-control, and ability to be independent (e.g., getting one's own cereal for breakfast) increase quickly during the first few months of school (Stendler and Young, 1951). These findings are less true for children from disadvantaged homes. Also, unfortunately, enthusiasm for school and teachers tends to decline in later years, and this decline appears to be more significant in children from disadvantaged homes than in those from more fortunate social classes. It has been suggested by some investigators that middle- and upper-middle-class parents may be better role models regarding school because their children see them reading, studying, and pursuing other intellectual activities.

Unquestionably, teachers have an important impact on the socialization of a child. Space is far too limited in this text to discuss how different teacher attributes affect pupils, but certainly the characteristics of fairness and consistency, the capacity to maintain order without being overly authoritative, and the ability to praise effectively are appreciated by children and have very positive social effects.

The peer group that a child joins also can be a powerful socializing force. Sometimes the values of the peer group are antithetical to those of the teacher and parents. This presents a conflict for the child in that he or she may risk reprimand from authoritative adults or ridicule or rejection from his or her peers if he or she conforms to one or the other's expectations. It is important for parents to understand these conflicts and how socially strong peer pressure can be for children in this age group. It is also important to note that the child who eagerly accepts a peer value that disappoints her or his parents may in fact be doing so to gain the feelings of acceptance and nurturing that were not provided sufficiently to her or him at home.

One last factor marks the middle childhood years. This is the advent of increasingly stronger, more stable, and more meaningful friendships. Generally, friendships are made with children of the same sex. Friends at this age level as a rule also share similar socioeconomic status, intelligence, maturity, and interests.

REFERENCES

Franco D: The child's perception of "the teacher" as compared to his perception of "the mother." Dissert Abstr *24*:3414–3415, 1964.

Stendler CB, Young N: Impact of first grade entrance upon the socialization of the child: Changes after eight months of school. Child Develop *22*:113–122, 1951.

Epidemiology and Mechanisms of Dental Disease

Steven M. Adair

Dramatic progress has been made in recent decades in the reduction of dental caries in schoolchildren in the United States. Although caries is still perhaps the most common disease of childhood, caries prevalence has declined substantially largely because of the increased availability of fluoride in its different forms. This chapter reviews the epidemiology of caries during the period of the transitional dentition and dietary factors related to caries.

EPIDEMIOLOGY OF CARIES IN THE TRANSITIONAL DENTITION

The most recent, comprehensive data on the caries experience of schoolchildren in the United States were compiled by the Epidemiology and Oral Disease Prevention Program of the National Institute of Dental Research (NIDR) in a nationwide study conducted in 1986–87. Over 39,000 children, ages 5 to 17, were examined. Only visual-tactile criteria were used for caries determinations. No radiographs were taken. Thus, the findings are probably conservative compared with what would have been determined had routine office examination criteria been applied. The 48 contiguous states were divided into seven geographic regions. Each region was further subdivided into urban and rural areas.

Figure 29–9 shows the mean number of decayed, missing, and filled permanent tooth surfaces (DMFS) for children by age and sex. The DMFS for 5-year-olds, who as a group have few erupted permanent teeth, was 0.07. For 8-year-olds, in whom permanent first molars and all permanent incisors generally have erupted, the DMFS was about 10 times higher, 0.71. By age 13, near the end of the transitional dentition, the DMFS was 3.76. These increases reflect the effects of time on an increasing number of permanent tooth surfaces available for decay as children progress through the transitional dentition years (Table 29–1). Females had slightly higher DMFS scores than males.

During the period of the transitional dentition, primary teeth may become carious as well. The 1986–87 survey determined the number of decayed and filled primary tooth surfaces (dfs) for

children ages 5 to 9 years to be 3.91 (Table 29–2). This is a 26% decline in primary tooth decay from the previous large-scale epidemiologic study carried out by the National Institute of Dental Research in 1979–80 (National Caries Program 1981).

In general, the 1986–87 survey found that the DMFS of whites was slightly lower than that of non-whites, and the DMFS of urban children was slightly lower than that of children from rural areas. The explanation for this latter difference is the higher percentage of urban children who were exposed to optimally fluoridated public water supplies.

On a geographic basis, the highest mean DMFS for children ages 5 to 13, 1.80, was found in the Northeast. The region with the lowest DMFS for this age group, 1.11, was the Southwest (Fig. 29–10).

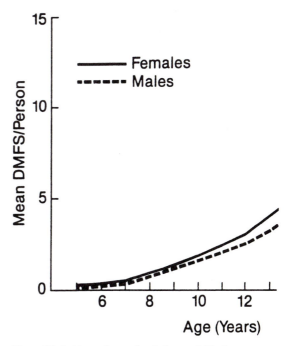

Figure 29–9. Mean decayed, missing, and filled permanent tooth surfaces (DMFS) for children aged 5 to 13 in the United States by age and sex. (Redrawn from National Institute of Dental Research, Epidemiology and Oral Disease Prevention Program: Oral Health of United States Children. The National Survey of Dental Caries in U.S. Schoolchildren, 1986–87. NIH Publication No. 89-2247, 1989.)

TABLE 29–1. DMFS* of Children in the United States Ages 5–13

| Age | DMFS | | | | |
	Whites	Non-whites	Rural	Urban	Total
5	0.06	0.11	0.07	0.07	0.07
6	0.12	0.16	0.15	0.12	0.13
7	0.38	0.46	0.48	0.37	0.41
8	0.72	0.66	0.85	0.65	0.71
9	1.09	1.32	1.25	1.09	1.14
10	1.54	2.14	1.81	1.64	1.69
11	2.31	2.38	2.31	2.34	2.33
12	2.48	3.35	2.82	2.60	2.66
13	3.62	4.23	3.88	3.71	3.76
All ages	1.45	1.70	1.64	1.46	1.52

*Decayed, missing, and filled permanent tooth surfaces.
Data from National Institute of Dental Research, Epidemiology and Oral Disease Prevention Program: Oral Health of United States Children, The National Survey of Dental Caries in U.S. Schoolchildren: 1986–87. NIH Publication No. 89-2247, 1989.

COMPARISONS

The degree to which caries has declined in this country can best be appreciated by comparison with similar surveys. The most complete surveys for comparison are those conducted by the National Center for Health Statistics (NCHS) in 1963–65 and 1971–74, and by the NIDR in 1979–80, as illustrated in Table 29-3. Data for the NCHS studies were collected on subjects ages 6 to 11. Consequently the same age groups have been selected from the NIDR studies as well. The data in Table 29-3 are for decayed, missing, and filled *teeth*, not surfaces, because of the manner in which data were collected in the two earlier NCHS studies. The diagnostic criteria used were practically identical in all studies. As illustrated, the mean DMFT for children in the transitional dentition has declined by 50% since 1963–65 and

by 58% since the 1971–74 NCHS study. These differences would be more striking if comparisons of DMFS could be made.

A similar comparison can be made for the percentage of caries-free 6- to 11-year-old children from each study. As illustrated in Table 29-4, that percentage has increased markedly since the earliest study.

BASIS FOR CARIES REDUCTIONS

Caries results from the interaction of specific microflora with fermentable carbohydrate on a susceptible tooth surface (see Chapter 12). There is no evidence to suggest that *Streptococcus mutans* has become less pathogenic or less prevalent in the population, although it has been proposed that the increased use of antibiotics may have some effect on the oral microflora. Similarly, there seems to be no evidence that per capita consumption of sugars has changed significantly from the 1920s (U.S. Dept. of Agriculture, 1984). Although per capita consumption of sucrose has declined somewhat since the mid-1970s, it has been replaced with fructose and other sugars that are also cariogenic. It is unlikely, therefore, that there has been any discernible change in the disease process itself.

The best explanation for the reduction in caries prevalence is the increased use of fluoride in its various forms, such as community water fluoridation, fluoride-containing dentifrices, and self-administered fluoride supplements. Evidence for this view is supported by the fact that the major caries reductions have occurred on proximal surfaces. These smooth surfaces benefit most from fluoride's protective effects (see Chapter 12).

TABLE 29–2. Caries Experience in the Primary Dentition of Children in the United States, 1979–80 and 1986–87

| Age | Mean dfs* | |
	1979–80	1986–87
5	4.03	3.40
6	4.76	3.73
7	5.52	4.20
8	6.11	4.24
9	5.95	3.89
Total	5.31	3.91

*Decayed and missing tooth surfaces.
Data from National Institute of Dental Research, Epidemiology and Oral Disease Prevention Program: Oral Health of United States Children. The National Survey of Dental Caries in U.S. Schoolchildren: 1986-1987. NIH Publication No. 89-2247, 1989.

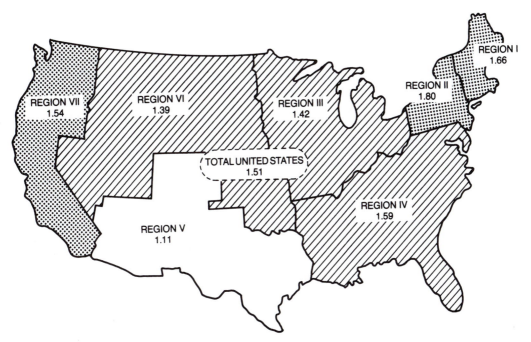

Figure 29–10. Mean decayed, missing, and filled permanent tooth surfaces (DMFS) of 5- to 13-year-old children by geographic region, 1986–1987. (Modified from National Institute of Dental Research, Epidemiology and Oral Disease Prevention Program. Oral Health of United States Children. The National Survey of Dental Caries in U.S. Schoolchildren, 1986–87. NIH Publication No. 89-2247, 1989.)

In the United States, the population exposed to optimally fluoridated water supplies doubled from 40 million to 80 million during the 1960s. Many of the children examined in 1979–80 and in 1986–87 benefitted from lifetime exposure to optimally fluoridated water. Further evidence for this hypothesis can be found by comparing the DMFS scores of children from rural areas and urban areas. A higher proportion of children from cities has been exposed to artificially fluoridated water supplies; however, the increase in the numbers of schoolchildren from fluoride-deficient areas who participate in school fluoride mouthrinse programs and other caries prevention programs has led to reductions in caries in these communities as well.

Other miscellaneous factors may have contributed to the reduction in caries prevalence. These include an increase in the distribution of foods and beverages prepared with fluoridated water to fluoride-deficient areas, known as the "halo effect" (see Chapter 14). A general improvement in education and socioeconomic status may also lead to a more health-conscious population with concomitant changes in dietary patterns. It is also possible that other as yet unclear factors contributing to increased human life span may have some influence on oral health, just as it is possible that improved oral health can contribute to increased longevity.

Dental caries continues to be a common health problem among children. The progress made in

TABLE 29–3. Mean Decayed, Missing, and Filled Teeth of 6- to 11-Year-Old Children in Four National Caries Surveys, 1963–1987

NCHS 1963–65	NCHS 1971–74	NIDR 1979–80	NIDR 1986–87
1.4	1.7	1.1	0.71

Modified from Brunelle JA, Carlos JP: Changes in the prevalence of dental caries in U.S. schoolchildren, 1961–1980. J Dent Res *61*(Special Issue):1346–1351, 1982.

TABLE 29–4. Percentage of Caries-Free 6- to 11-Year-Old Children in Four National Caries Surveys, 1963–1986

NCHS 1963–65	NCHS 1971–74	NIDR 1979–80	NIDR 1986–87
51.1	43.6	56.7	74.3

Modified from Brunelle JA, Carlos JP: Changes in the prevalence of dental caries in U.S. schoolchildren, 1961–1980. J Dent Res *61*(Special Issue):1346–1351, 1982.

recent decades is significant and encouraging, but further substantial reductions in caries prevalence will require redoubled effort. Even if all community water systems were to be optimally fluoridated, only about half of the United States population would benefit. Fortunately, the halo effect has begun to bring about significant decreases in caries prevalence in fluoride-deficient areas, though at the expense of an increase in the prevalence of enamel fluorosis. Increases in the use of self-applied fluoride, whether by fluoride-containing dentifrices or through organized school mouthrinse programs, should continue to be beneficial. Maximizing the use of pit and fissure sealants could greatly reduce the proportion of the caries that is minimally affected by fluoride.

It is interesting to note that although the prevalence of dental caries has been decreasing in the United States, it is increasing in developing nations. The increase is occurring primarily in the more affluent components of the society that are more likely to have adopted a Western-style diet rich in fermentable carbohydrates but who lack the access to quality dental care available in more industrialized nations. The groups that have maintained their more traditional diets have not been affected to the same degree.

DIETARY FACTORS AND DENTAL CARIES

As mentioned in Chapter 12, sugars (sucrose, fructose, glucose, and others) are one of the major etiologic factors in dental caries. Sucrose has been labeled the "arch criminal of dental caries" (Newbrun, 1969), but in fact animal studies have shown other sugars, notably glucose and fructose, to be as cariogenic as sucrose (Koulourides et al., 1976; Stephan, 1966). This poses potential difficulties in making dietary recommendations because many fruits and vegetables contain substantial amounts of naturally occurring sugars (Bibby, 1983).

Sucrose

Speculation has centered on the role of sucrose in caries formation once scientific study of the disease began. One of the first controlled studies to document sucrose as an etiologic factor was the Vipeholm study (Gustafsson et al., 1954). In this study, 436 inmates in a mental institution near Lund, Sweden, were given sugar in various forms to supplement the relatively sugar-free in-

stitutional diets. The sugar was offered as sucrose in solution or in retentive forms, such as sweetened bread and toffee. The sucrose in solution and the bread were introduced with meals, whereas the other forms were given between meals. The study showed that an increase in sucrose intake was associated with an increase in caries activity. Furthermore, this caries activity decreased when the sucrose-rich foods were discontinued. The cariogenic potential of the sucrose was enhanced when it was given between meals and in a more retentive form (caramels and toffees). The time required for the sugar to clear the oral cavity was closely related to the caries activity.

The study also pointed out that caries formation varied among individuals and that caries continued to form in some individuals even after a return to low-sucrose diets. The subjects who received only 30 g of sucrose per day, all at mealtimes, developed an average of 0.27 new carious lesions per year. Those who ingested 330 g of sucrose per day, 300 g of which were in solution, were only slightly worse off, with 0.43 new carious surfaces per year. Subjects in the group that received 24 sticky toffees per day, however, developed 4.02 new lesions per year. This group ingested 300 g of sucrose per day, but 40% of it was eaten between meals. Although there were flaws in the design of this study, the magnitude of the differences in caries development is impressive. The questions regarding the ethics of this type of study ensure that it will probably never be repeated.

Another study corroborating the role of sucrose was conducted with 3- to 14-year-olds who resided at Hopewood House in Bowral, New South Wales, Australia (Sullivan and Goldsworthy, 1958; Sullivan and Harris, 1958). Almost all of these institutionalized children had lived there since infancy and were fed an almost pure vegetarian diet supplemented with milk and an occasional egg yolk. The vegetables were generally served raw, and refined carbohydrate was rigidly restricted. In spite of poor oral hygiene, the caries prevalence in the children was very low. Primary dentition involvement was almost nonexistent, whereas the caries prevalence of the permanent teeth was about one tenth that of the mean score for other Australian children. Almost one third of the children remained caries-free throughout the 5-year study. Children who left Hopewood House at an older age experienced a significant increase in dental caries.

Though there are still some who question the primary role of sucrose and other sugars in the etiology of caries (Walker and Cleaton-Jones,

1989), there is overwhelming evidence to demonstrate its relationship to caries as part of a multifactorial process (Burt and Ismail, 1986).

Relative Cariogenicity of Foods

Further studies into the relationship between diet and dental caries have refined the knowledge given by the Vipeholm and Hopewood House data, but in general the findings of those earlier studies have been confirmed. Much effort in recent years has gone into assessing the relative cariogenicity of a variety of foodstuffs (Bibby and Mundorff, 1975; Bibby et al., 1986). Such comparisons are difficult to make. The variety of methods often leads to differing cariogenicity scores for the same food, and no one method can adequately account for the multiplicity of food and host factors involved in the caries process. Such research, however, has led to the ranking of various foods according the their cariogenic potential, such as the ranking in Table 29–5. This has led to some interesting challenges of preconceived notions. Potato chips produced deeper carious lesions in an artificial oral environment than did cookies, sugared breakfast cereal, or one form of chocolate candy. Similarly, apples were found to dissolve more enamel than did soft drinks, caramel, or sugared breakfast cereal (Bibby, 1977). On the other hand, this system gave different results for two similar types of candy bars, the difference being the presence of almonds in one of the bars. Despite these problems, a cariogenicity ranking system is used in Switzerland to denote "tooth-friendly" foods—those that do not suppress plaque pH below 5.7 for 30 minutes after ingestion.

Other Food Factors

The multiplicity of food factors requires that relative cariogenicity tests be interpreted with caution. These factors include carbohydrate-sucrose concentration, retentiveness, oral clearance rate, detergent quality, texture, the effect of mixing foods, the sequence of ingestion, the frequency of ingestion, and the pH of the food itself. For example, most fruits depress plaque pH by virtue of their own low pH. This occurs even though the low pH of the food inhibits natural fermentation of its sugar content. Low-pH fruits can also demineralize enamel by the direct action of their acids. At the same time, low pH fruits stimulate a flow of saliva that buffers plaque pH drops; other foods, such as vegetables, stimulate salivary flow through the chewing reflex. On balance, however, there is not a strong case for a caries-protective effect from fruits and vegetables (Bibby, 1983).

Another food factor that has received much attention is stickiness or retentiveness. This characteristic has often been equated with the oral clearance of the food, with the underlying assumption being that longer oral clearance times can prolong the period of plaque acid production. Our concepts of food retention on teeth have been challenged in recent years, however, by research that shows a poor correlation between foods judged to be "sticky" and the time required for oral clearance (Kashket et al., 1991). Caramels and candy bars, judged by a lay group to be among the stickiest foods, were found to clear the oral cavity rather quickly; potato chips and white bread, judged as relatively nonsticky foods, were among the last to clear the mouth. Foods high in starch content (breads, cereals, potato chips) were slower to clear the oral cavity, whereas those high in sucrose cleared rapidly from the mouth. It has also been shown that the presence of starch increases the acid production from sucrose (Buehrer and Miller, 1984) and may allow fermentation to take place under otherwise inhibiting concentrations of sugar. On the other hand, high levels of sugar appear to increase the solubility of starchy foods and to hasten the clearance from the oral cavity. Clearly, no one cariogenicity test can account for all these fac-

TABLE 29–5. Comparative Depths of Carious Lesions Produced by Foods in an Artificial Mouth (OroFax)*

Food	Proportionate Depth
Caramel	46.8
Fudge	45.0
Chocolate coconut bar	31.7
Potato chips	30.3
Graham cracker	28.6
White bread	26.7
Chocolate almond bar	26.2
Whole wheat bread	18.3
Plain breakfast cereal	18.2
Sugared breakfast cereal	18.2
Chocolate chip cookie	15.8
Dark chocolate	15.0
Sweet cookie	13.7
Ginger snaps	12.3
Fruit tart	11.2
Milk chocolate	7.5

*Proportionate values calculated from common control used in separate tests.

From Bibby BG: Cariogenicity of foodstuffs. *In* Sweeney EA (ed): The Food That Stays: An Update on Nutrition, Diet, Sugar and Caries. New York, Medcom Inc., 1977, p 53.

tors, except possibly trials in humans. Even in human trials, individual variations exist in plaque composition and amount, salivary buffering capacity, and enamel resistance to dissolution with or without the ability to remineralize.

The frequency with which cariogenic foods are ingested has a strong relationship to the risk of caries development. More frequent contact with sugars at mealtime and frequent between-meal snacks result in prolonged or multiple pH challenges to the teeth and possibly to longer oral clearance times. The net result is an increased likelihood of enamel demineralization that has been demonstrated in animal models (Firestone et al., 1984).

Certain food components and factors may have cariostatic or caries-inhibiting effects. Phosphates, principally sodium metaphosphate, have been shown to reduce caries in animal studies (Nizel and Harris, 1964). The effect is probably local, related to buffering capacity, a reduction of enamel solubility, and other bacterial and biochemical properties. Unfortunately, clinical trials with phosphate supplements in human diets have not proved as effective (Baron, 1977; Lilienthal, 1976). Other animal studies (Featherstone and Mundorff, 1984) have shown that foods high in fat, protein, fluoride, or calcium may protect against caries. Such foods include cheese, yogurt, bologna, chocolate, and peanuts. Fats may pro-

The Cumulative Caries Curves: Clinical Implications of Caries Epidemiology

Burt Edelstein

Universality

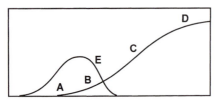

When decay occurrence is plotted against age, two characteristic and universal "S"-shaped curves result—one for primary teeth and one for permanent teeth. Both curves lift slowly from a zero baseline of children too young to experience caries (A), then curve upward as children first experience decay (B). The curves straighten, approaching a fixed slope as decay experience builds with age (C), then round off and flatten as decay experience "tops out" (D). Because these curves are cumulative, they cannot decline unless teeth are lost. As the primary dentition is exfoliated, its curve returns to zero (E).

Implications of Pattern

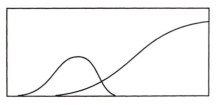

Like a chemical reaction that depends on the presence of all reactants, the curve shows an accelerating start as necessary components (flora, cariogenic diet, and teeth erupting over time) are first combined; a steady state as the reaction progresses through the two developing dentitions; and a decelerating finish as the system becomes saturated and no new teeth present. There is a lag time between tooth eruption and decay occurrence because the caries process takes time to manifest as cavities. This pattern suggests that little new decay will occur after balance between decay attack and resistance is reached. Indeed, caries is overwhelmingly a disease of childhood, with most dental repair for adults addressing re-repair of teeth affected earlier.

Implications of Height

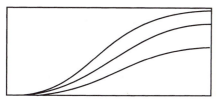

The amount of decay that develops depends on the intensity of caries attack. Groups of children who are particularly efficient at developing cavities—80% of decay occurs in 25% of children—will demonstrate the same shape curve but will reach a higher cumulative caries experience. Because certain teeth are more susceptible to decay than are others, the intensity of caries attack is reflected in specific decay patterns. Generally, occlusal surfaces are most susceptible, followed by interproximal surfaces, then by smooth surfaces. The height of the curve suggests not only how much decay is present but which teeth are most likely to be cavitated.

Implications of Length

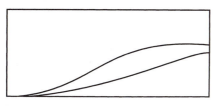

Cavities occur when net decalcification exceeds net recalcification. If decalcification proceeds much more rapidly than recalcification, disease significantly exceeds healing and cavities develop rapidly. If decalcification occurs only marginally faster than recalcification, decay occurs more slowly. When both are in balance, no decay occurs. Fluoride both slows decalcification and speeds recalcification. As fluoride becomes more generally available, the rate of decay slows and the caries curve lengthens. A lengthened curve suggests that the caries process is more attenuated and cavities will not stop occurring until an older age. Indeed, caries rates have slowed dramatically in the United States so that lesions that once occurred in adolescence now occur more commonly in young adulthood.

Implications for Managing Caries

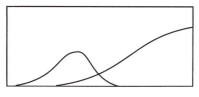

The S shape of these curves is determined by the underlying availability of teeth to the caries process. If a third set of teeth presented in middle age, the pattern would be expected to repeat. Indeed, root surface decay behaves in this way, occurring most rapidly and in greater amounts among persons who had experienced extensive decay earlier in life. To truly change caries experience requires that the underlying caries process be fundamentally altered so that balance between attack and resistance is attained. Failure to manage the underlying caries process relegates the dentist to continually chasing after cavities until new teeth stop presenting themselves in the mouth and the dynamic forces of attack and resistance obtain balance on their own.

tect by coating the teeth and reducing the retention of sugar and even plaque by changing the enamel surface activity. Fats also may have toxic effects on oral bacteria and may decrease sugar solubility. Protein elevates the urea level in saliva and increases the buffering capacity of the saliva.

Protein may also have an enamel-coating effect. Protein and fat in combination may raise plaque pH after exposure to carbohydrate. Tannins and other components of cocoa have been shown to suppress caries activity. The addition of fluoride to dietary sucrose in concentrations as low as 2 ppm has also been found to significantly reduce decay in rats (Mundorff et al., 1986). Similar studies in humans have yet to be undertaken.

It has been proposed that the fibrous quality of some foods, such as celery or apples, may have a detergent effect on the teeth (Caldwell, 1970). Such foods may remove gross debris during mastication, but they are ineffective at plaque removal. By requiring vigorous chewing, these foods may stimulate salivary flow, which, in turn, buffers plaque acid and promotes remineralization of enamel.

Dietary Counseling

Many of these findings have challenged long-accepted notions that have formed the basis of dietary recommendations to reduce the caries activity in children. Is sugared cereal worse than plain breakfast cereal if, in fact, it is cleared from the oral cavity more rapidly? Are potato chips a viable alternative to candy as a snack food?

Stookey (1979) has enumerated the attributes of the ideal snack as follows: (1) It should stimulate salivary flow via its physical forms, (2) it should be minimally retentive, (3) it should be relatively high in protein and low in fat, have minimal fermentable carbohydrate, and have a moderate mineral content (especially calcium, phosphate, and fluoride), and (4) it should have a pH above 5.5 so as not to decrease oral pH, with a large acid buffering capacity and a low sodium content. Certain foods, such as raw vegetables, meet most or all of these requirements. Present day food technology should make it possible to create snacks that are nutritious and noncariogenic, but this will not happen until the food industry finds a reliable cariogenicity test and the incentives to invest in such production.

In the meantime, we are left with the difficult task of attempting to alter the dietary habits of caries-susceptible patients. Although such attempts often fail, the profession has an obligation to make dietary information available to them. Although it is neither feasible nor desirable to eliminate sugar completely from the diet, we can recommend that between-meal snacks be supervised by parents and that, where possible, sugar intake be limited to mealtimes when salivary flow is higher. Lowering the frequency of carbohydrate ingestion may be more important than reducing the total carbohydrate intake.

SUMMARY

Substantial gains in caries reductions have been made for children in the transitional dentition.

The goal of a caries-free generation is achievable for children who have access to care but is not yet within the grasp of many in the lower socioeconomic groups. In addition to the protection afforded by fluoride from various sources, prudent dietary counseling can further reduce an individual child's susceptibility to caries.

REFERENCES

Baron HJ: Modifying the cariogenicity of foods with dicalcium phosphate. *In* Proceedings of Workshop on Cariogenicity of Food, Beverages, Confections, and Chewing Gum. Chicago, American Dental Association, 1977.

Bibby BG: Fruits and vegetables and dental caries. Clin Prev Dent 5:3–11, 1983.

Bibby BG: Cariogenicity of foodstuffs. *In* Sweeney EA (ed): The Food That Stays: An Update on Nutrition, Diet, Sugar and Caries. New York, Medcom Inc., 1977.

Bibby BG, Mundorff SA: Enamel demineralization by snack foods. J Dent Res 54:461–470, 1975.

Bibby BG, Mundorff SA, Zero DT, Almekinder KJ: Oral food clearance and the pH of plaque and saliva. JADA 112:333–337, 1986.

Brunelle JA, Carlos JP: Changes in the prevalence of dental caries in U.S. schoolchildren, 1961–1980. J Dent Res 61(Special Issue):1346–1351, 1982.

Buehrer EA, Miller CH: Sucrose and starch synergism in *Streptococcus sanguis* acid production [Abstract No. 137]. J Dent Res 64(Special Issue):186, 1984.

Burt BA, Ismail AI: Diet, nutrition and food cariogenicity. J Dent Res 65(Special Issue): 1475–1484, 1986.

Caldwell RC: Physical properties of foods and their caries-producing potential. J Dent Res 49:1293–1298, 1970.

Epidemiology and Oral Disease Prevention Program, National Institute of Dental Research: Oral health of United States children: The national survey of dental caries in U.S. school children: 1986–87. NIH publication No. 89-2247, 1989.

Featherstone JDB, Mundorff SA: Identification of the cariogenic elements of foods: Final report for period September 1981–May 1984 prepared for Nation Institute of Dental Research, 1984.

Firestone AR, Schmid R, Mühlemann HR: Effect of the length and number of intervals between meals on caries in rats. Caries Res 18:128–133, 1984.

Gustafsson B, Quensel CE, Lanke L, et al: The Vipeholm dental caries study: The effect of different carbohydrate intake on 436 individuals observed for five years. Acta Odontol Scand 11:232–364, 1954.

Kashket S, van Houte J, Lopez LR, et al: Lack of correlation between food retention on the human dentition and consumer perception of food stickiness. J Dent Res 70:1314–1319, 1991.

Koulourides T, Bodden S, Keller S, et al: Cariogenicity of nine sugars tested with intraoral device in man. Caries Res 10:427–441, 1976.

Lilienthal B: Phosphates and dental caries. *In* Myers H (ed): Monographs in Oral Science. Basel, S Karger, 1976.

Mundorff SA, Glowinsky D, Griffin C: Fluoridated sucrose effect on rat caries [Abstract No. 1017]. J Dent Res 65(Special Issue):282, 1986.

National Caries Program, NIDR: The prevalence of dental caries in United States schoolchildren, 1979–80. NIH publication No. 82-2245, 1981.

National Center for Health Statistics: Decayed, missing and filled teeth among children: United States. Vital and Health Statistics, Series 11, No. 106, DHEW Pub No. (HSM) 72-1003. Washington, DC, US Government Printing Office, 1971.

National Center for Health Statistics: Decayed, missing and filled teeth among persons 1–74 years: United States. Vital and Health Statistics, Series 11, No. 223, DHHS Pub No. (PHS) 81-1673. Washington, DC, US Government Printing Office, 1981.

Newbrun E: Sucrose, the arch criminal of dental caries. J Dent Child *36*:239–248, 1969.

Nizel AE, Harris RS: The effects of phosphate on experimental dental caries: A literature review. J Dent Res *43*:1123–1136, 1964.

Stephan RM: Effect of different types of human foods in dental health of experimental animals. J Dent Res *45*:1551–1561, 1966.

Stookey GK: Developing the perfect snack food. *In* Alfano MC (ed): Changing Perspectives in Nutrition and Caries Research. New York, Medcom, 1979.

Sullivan HR, Goldsworthy NE: Review and correlation of the data presented in papers 1–6 (Hopewood House study). Aust Dent J *3*:395–398, 1958.

Sullivan HR, Harris R: Hopewood House study 2: Observations on oral conditions. Aust Dent J *3*:311–317, 1958.

U.S. Department of Agriculture: Economic Research Service: Sugar and sweetener; Outlook and situation report SSRV9N4. Washington, DC: US Government Printing Office, 1984, pp 3–17.

Walker ARP, Cleaton-Jones PE: Sugar intake and dental caries: Where do we stand? J Dent Child *56*:30–35, 1989.

30

Examination, Diagnosis, and Treatment Planning

Paul S. Casamassimo, John R. Christensen, and Henry W. Fields, Jr.

Chapter Outline

THE HISTORY

THE EXAMINATION

Behavioral Assessment

General Appraisal

Head and Neck Examination

Facial Examination

Intraoral Examination

Radiographic Evaluation

TREATMENT PLANNING FOR NONORTHODONTIC PROBLEMS

Examination of the child in the transitional years presents a diagnostic dilemma of managing oral health at a dynamic stage of development. Although the preschooler's dentition is relatively stable, the child in the transitional years progresses from a full complement of primary teeth through a mixed dentition to a full permanent dentition excluding the third molars. Maintaining the ease and success of this transition constitutes the main challenge for the dentist treating this age group. A large part of this chapter is devoted to orthodontic considerations, but the other elements of significance in dental management of this age group should not be ignored. They are the following:

1. *Preventive considerations related to tooth sealants, nutrition, and fluoride intake*. The eruption of permanent teeth may require a decision to be made about sealant application. Entry into the more heterogeneous, less controlled en-vironment of school places the child at risk for increased carbohydrate exposure. Finally, the child's access to fluoride in school, diet, and other sources makes regular re-evaluation of fluoride exposure a necessity.

2. *Prevention and management of trauma*. The school age child may be active in sports. For a period in the school years, the permanent maxillary incisors are at greater risk for traumatic injury, especially if they protrude.

3. *Development of skills in personal oral hygiene*. The child emerging from the middle school years should acquire the skills and knowledge to conduct effective personal oral hygiene.

4. *Participation in health care decisions*. Classically, dentists are taught to see the school age child as a passive recipient of care. Unfortunately, the result may be poor compliance and a tendency for the child to consider the dentist rather than himself or herself as responsible for his or her own health.

THE HISTORY

Elements of history taking and recording are discussed in Chapter 18. The parent remains the historian of choice, yet the older school age child can provide valid and corroborative information. An important aspect of history taking in this group should be the involvement of the child, whose role initially may be that of listener but can evolve into that of participant. By adolescence, the child can provide accurate, valuable information. Some instances in which this involvement may have profound benefits for both health care provider and patient are (1) when antibiotic premedication for heart disease is required, (2) when there is a history of illness that accompanies a complicated medical history, or (3) when there is a history of a positive reaction to the hepatitis antigen. The payoff for imparting this knowledge to the young patient through a good physician-patient relationship may not be evident until the child seeks care for himself or herself as an adolescent. A health history form should address issues similar to those applicable to the younger child but with different expectations. The differences in patient history for children in this age group in general include the following:

1. *Medical intervention has usually occurred.* Most children have a physician and may have experienced an emergency visit or some invasive procedure. School enrollment has required a physical examination and other treatment in the majority of children.

2. *A health history has evolved.* The coagulation and immunologic systems have been tested and a developmental profile is available. Most childhood-onset disorders manifest themselves at some time during this period, but some have not been noted. Therefore, symptoms remain an important aspect of history taking.

3. *A dental history should be evolving*, and caries experiences and prevention, care delivery, and dental development should be established. Children usually have undergone a dental visit as part of school enrollment.

THE EXAMINATION

As in younger children, the dental examination includes a behavioral assessment; general appraisal; and head and neck, facial, intraoral, and radiographic examinations.

Behavioral Assessment

Another advantage for the dentist is the child's emergence into a period when few children experience behavioral problems that cannot be resolved with a simple tell-show-do method. Even early in this period, most children can be reasoned with to accept dental treatment. The child who resists attempts at careful and compassionate explanations of care may be suffering from a more significant emotional or psychological problem. Significant behavior problems in the presence of normal intelligence signal a serious deviation from normal. The diagnostic process for behavioral problems is clearer in this age group because so few children resist care. The dentist's diagnostic approach should include ruling out major behavioral problems by a history and general appraisal. The next step is to "chair-test" the child, using the dentist's proven techniques of managing children. The technique used may be tell-show-do, positive reinforcement, voice control, or some other method that has worked consistently in the past. Remember, consent should be obtained from the parent if the behavior management technique used is not one that a reasonable parent would expect (Hagan et al., 1984). If behavioral intervention fails, the dentist should consider further evaluation or referral. Some causes of extreme behavior problems in this age group include substance abuse, physical or sexual abuse, family problems, or a minor learning disability.

General Appraisal

The school age population provides a wide range of physical and emotional profiles, yet the general appraisal should be easier from several standpoints. First, the school age child should have developed gross motor skills, and any variations from normal should be obvious. For example, the toddler may be active yet still clumsy. The school age child, even at the early end of this age group, can play with skill. Speech development should also well exceed that of the preschooler, as should the child's emotional and intellectual status. This adaptation is really a manifestation of development of the brain and is one reason why schooling begins at this age.

One advantage available to the dentist who treats children in this age group is the host of health professionals with whom he or she can work if problems are noted. School placement often has identified problem areas, and the appropriate therapy usually has been initiated.

**TABLE 30–1. Selected Development Characteristics
of the 6- to 12-Year-Old Child**
....

Intellectual Development

Demonstrates school readiness early in this period
Should be able to read and write in this period
Becomes capable of logical thought

Psychological Development

Acquires sense of accomplishment for tasks
Learns responsibility for actions
Develops a sense of right and wrong
Looks outside the home for standards or values

Physical Development

Refinement of motor skills occurs as central nervous
  system develops
Spine straightens to improve posture
Sinuses enlarge
Lymphoid system reaches high point of development

Physiologic Development

6-Year-Old	*9-Year-Old*	*12-Year-Old*
Height		
Boys = 121 cm	Boys = 140 cm	Boys = 154 cm
Girls = 119 cm	Girls = 137 cm	Girls = 157 cm

*(Growth rate is approximately 6 cm/year in this
  period)*

Weight (75th percentile)

Boys = 24 kg	Boys = 33 kg	Boys = 44 kg
Girls = 23 kg	Girls = 32 kg	Girls = 45 kg

(Growth rate is approximately 3–3.5 kg/year)

Pulse (average for age)

100/min	90/min	85–90/min

Respiration (50th percentile)

23/min	20/min	18/min

Blood pressure (average for age)

105/60 mm Hg	110/65 mm Hg	115/65 mm Hg

These professionals can assist in clarifying findings made during the dental visit. Table 30–1 lists some characteristics of the school age child that are important in the diagnostic process.

Head and Neck Examination

The head and neck examination should be completed in a manner similar to that outlined in Chapter 18.

Facial Examination

Facial examination of the 6- to 12-year-old child is a systematic examination of the face in three planes of space. It is essentially the same as the facial examination described in Chapter 18, and the reader should review that information if necessary. This section comments on findings that are particularly important for the 6- to 12-year-old.

In examination of the profile one notes the anteroposterior and vertical dimensions of the face and the position of the lips and incisors relative to the face. The ideal soft tissue profile is slightly convex to straight (Fig. 30–1), practically speaking a bit straighter with more mandibular contribution than that of the preschool age group. Most clinicians find that detection of anteroposterior skeletal problems is somewhat easier in this age group, possibly because of reduced soft tissue thickness. In most cases, skeletal relationships can be confirmed by the dental relationships (molar, canine, and overjet). A mild mandibular deficiency in a 4-year-old child may have been difficult to diagnose initially, but it is more apparent at age 8 and even more obvious at age 12. If a skeletal problem exists, the source of the discrepancy is identified by comparing the position of the maxilla and mandible with a vertical reference line (see Chapter 18). This helps to direct treatment if it is indicated to the skeletal component at fault.

In this age group, vertical profile assessment continues to concentrate on the proportionality of the upper, middle, and lower facial thirds. At this point, growth has increased the vertical lin-

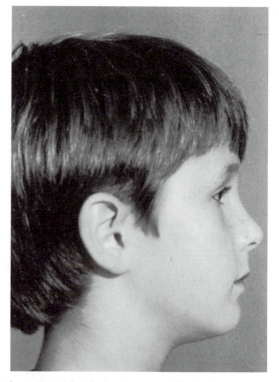

Figure 30–1. The ideal soft tissue profile for the bridge of the nose, the base of the upper lip, and the chin is slightly convex to straight in the anteroposterior dimension in the 6- to 12-year-old child.

ear facial dimensions; however, the proportionality of the well-balanced face remains basically the same. Research has indicated that vertical dysplasia usually is confined to the lower facial third in this age group (Fields et al., 1984). If this is true, the middle and upper thirds can be used as standards to compare with the lower facial third. Incisor and lip position should be examined carefully in this age group. The child is entering the mixed dentition period, and the position of the erupting permanent incisors generally is reflected in the position of the lips. The upper lip is of fairly uniform size and thickness and gives a good indication of the underlying position of the maxillary incisor. The position of the lower lip also depends on the position of the maxillary incisor because the lower lip normally covers 1 to 2 mm of the maxillary incisal edge at rest. Therefore, lip posture is a strong indicator of maxillary dental protrusion. Lip and incisor

position should always be considered in the context of the nose and chin. The lips should be positioned on or slightly behind a line connecting the tip of the nose with the chin (Fig. 30-2). A large nose and chin are more able to accommodate protrusive incisors and lips than are a small nose and chin.

Intraoral Examination

The procedures used for oral examination are similar to those used in the preschool group and include charting of teeth and dental caries. Less emphasis needs to be placed on managing the child's behavior during the examination process because these children are more cooperative. The areas of evaluation that require more emphasis are the periodontal, preventive, and orthodontic aspects.

PERIODONTAL EVALUATION

A thorough examination of this age group involves both periodontal probing and use of a gingival index if inflammation is a problem. If orthodontic treatment is a consideration, it may be delayed or the treatment plan altered if the periodontal tissues are not healthy. Orthodontic treatment initiated during periods of active gingival or periodontal disease may further compromise periodontal health because fixed appliances are difficult to keep clean, and existing inflammatory conditions are exacerbated, resulting in further loss of supporting structures. The periodontal examination should address the following aspects:

1. *Selective probing of anterior teeth and permanent first molars.* A periodontal probe is necessary to evaluate the health of the tissues properly (Fig. 30-3). The probe measures the depth of the sulcus and the amount of free marginal and attached gingiva. Sulcular depths of greater than 3 mm and attached gingiva of less than 1 mm indicate possible periodontal disease, and further evaluation is warranted. The likelihood of bone loss and apical migration of the attachment is low, but some children in this age group experience juvenile periodontitis. Erupting teeth usually have a deep sulcus until the crown is fully erupted. Gingival inflammation in early puberty may also confound pocket-depth measurements.

2. *Evaluation of tissue attachments, especially those of the lower anterior teeth.* Facial clefts as a result of malposition of teeth and inflammation, if identified early, can be success-

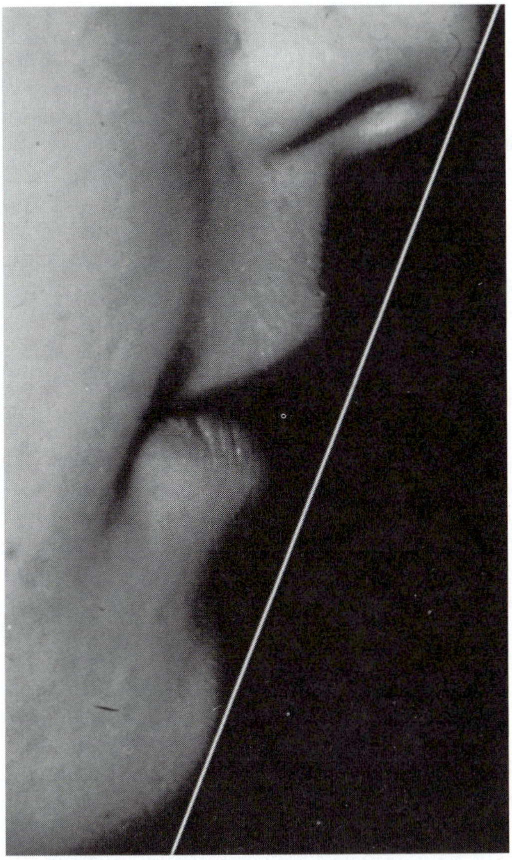

Figure 30-2. In this age group, the lips are positioned on or slightly behind a line connecting the tip of the nose with the soft tissue chin. Lip position must be considered in the context of the nose and chin. A large nose and chin are better able to accommodate protrusive lips than are a small nose and chin.

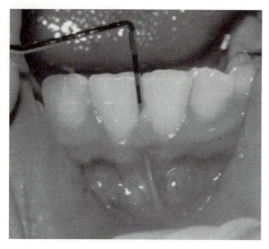

Figure 30–3. During examination of each arch, a periodontal probe is used to evaluate gingival health. Orthodontic treatment that is initiated during periods of active gingival or periodontal disease may further compromise periodontal health.

fully managed with grafting, tooth movement, or a combination of both (Fig. 30-4). The amount of attached gingiva also should be considered in the context of the type of tooth movement being planned. Facial movement of a lower incisor with minimal attached gingiva may cause further loss of attachment, and a gingival grafting procedure should be considered. Lingual movement of the

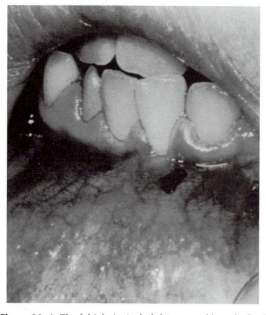

Figure 30–4. The labial gingival cleft is caused by a lack of attached gingival tissue, an abnormally high (coronal) muscle attachment, an anterior crossbite, or a combination of these factors.

same incisor does not involve the risk of loss of attachment and may even contribute to an increase in attached tissue. Last, the position of the frena and their height of attachment on the alveolar ridge should be determined via gentle manipulation of the lips and cheeks. Occasionally, frenal attachments near the crest of the ridge need to be repositioned prior to or after orthodontic treatment because they pull on attached marginal tissue and compromise gingival health or prevent space closure.

3. *Identification of problem areas, such as mandibular and maxillary anterior teeth.* Calculus accumulation, inflammation secondary to anterior crowding, poor cleaning, and eruptive gingivitis are examples of localized problems that require specialized attention.

Numerous gingival indices exist to assess inflammation (Ramfjord, 1967). The gingival index (GI) (Loe and Silness, 1963) can be adapted for pediatric use. The GI uses the following scoring system: 0 = normal gingiva; 1 = mild inflammation: slight change in color, slight edema, no bleeding on probing; 2 = moderate inflammation: redness, edema, and glazing, or bleeding on probing; 3 = severe inflammation: marked redness and edema, tendency toward spontaneous bleeding, ulceration.

In the private practice setting, it may be easier to modify an existing index, using key teeth to provide baseline readings and progress. These readings can be recorded on the examination form adjacent to the data for the teeth being examined. Routine performance of full mouth probing is not warranted.

Oral Hygiene Evaluation. The assessment of clinical needs and patient skills in oral hygiene is a part of the examination process. The history should reveal a pattern of personal care, and the clinical examination should document the effectiveness of care and address problem areas in the oral cavity. A patient's brushing skills and dexterity in flossing can be judged at chairside and are generally directly correlated with classically difficult to clean areas such as plaque accumulation on teeth on the opposite the side on which the brush is held, buccally placed canine teeth, and lingual surfaces. This information should be used to formulate an individual hygiene strategy. If orthodontic treatment is being considered, oral hygiene instructions should be given before orthodontic treatment is started and should be consistently reinforced during the treatment.

OCCLUSAL EVALUATION

The occlusal evaluation is organized around a systematic approach to alignment and the antero-

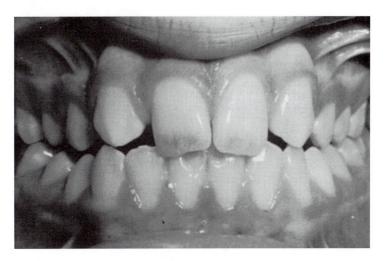

Figure 30–5. This patient is congenitally missing both maxillary lateral incisors. The most common missing teeth in the permanent dentition, besides the third molars, are the maxillary lateral incisor and the mandibular second premolar.

posterior, transverse, and vertical planes of space (Proffit, 1992).

Alignment. The intraoral occlusal examination in the mixed dentition begins with an assessment of arch form and alignment characteristics. An ideal arch should be symmetrical in the anteroposterior and transverse dimensions. Minor asymmetry may exist but is usually confined to the anterior region if there is inadequate space for eruption of the permanent incisors. Significant asymmetry is rare and is usually indicative of skeletal asymmetry or some type of oral habit or crossbite that has displaced the teeth and alveolus. Arch form is described as being either U- or V-shaped. Alignment problems are usually the result of a true arch length deficiency or a transitional arch length deficiency due to the size of the erupting permanent teeth. These are most common in the anterior portions of the arch but can occur anywhere. The type of alignment problem should be noted during the examination. The teeth can be tipped, bodily positioned, or rotated in their aberrant location. These types of positioning errors have definite implications for the type of treatment that can be recommended.

Tooth Number. After the form and symmetry of each arch have been characterized, it is imperative to count the number of permanent and primary teeth. A clinical examination and appropriate radiographs allow the practitioner to determine which teeth are present, developing, or missing. Disturbances in the initiation and proliferation stage of tooth development may lead to an abnormal number of teeth. Teeth that do not form are called congenitally missing teeth (Fig. 30-5). The most common missing teeth in the permanent dentition, with the exception of the maxillary and mandibular third molars, are the

maxillary lateral incisor and the mandibular second premolar (Shafer et al., 1974). In general, the most distal tooth in a class of teeth is most liable to be congenitally missing.

Supernumerary teeth are teeth added to the normal complement of teeth. These teeth are most often found in the maxillary midline region and are called mesiodens (Fig. 30-6). Supernu-

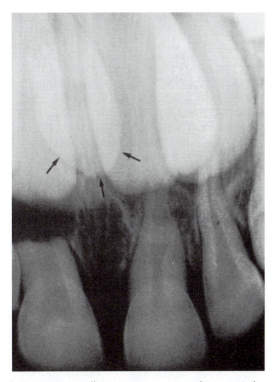

Figure 30–6. A midline supernumerary tooth, or mesiodens, is situated between the unerupted maxillary central incisors. Arrows indicate the position of the mesiodens, which can cause disturbances in eruption and tooth formation.

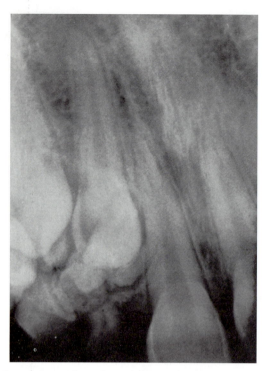

Figure 30–7. In this radiograph, a complete odontoma is impeding the eruption of the maxillary right lateral incisor and canine. The odontoma should be surgically removed before eruption problems arise but late enough to avoid surgical trauma to the adjacent developing teeth. (Courtesy of Dr. Phillip R. Parker.)

merary teeth are also frequently found distal to the maxillary molars and in the mandibular premolar regions (Shafer et al., 1974).

Although not a tooth in the strictest sense, the odontoma is discussed in this section on tooth number. The odontoma is a benign mixed tumor of enamel and dentin that is diagnosed radiographically. Two types of odontomas are identi-

fied. Odontomas that resemble teeth are called compound odontomas; those that are irregular in shape are labeled complex odontomas. Both types may interfere with normal tooth eruption and are usually treated by surgical removal before eruption problems arise but late enough to avoid surgical trauma to adjacent developing teeth (Fig. 30–7). Disturbances in the morphodifferentiation and histodifferentiation stages of tooth development result in alterations of tooth size and shape. Each arch should be examined for generalized large (macrodontia) or small (microdontia) teeth and for localized tooth size discrepancies. Generalized large or small teeth usually can be aligned so that there is a compatible occlusal relationship if the teeth in both arches are equally affected. Localized tooth size problems, however, make it difficult to establish good dental relationships. Again, the most distal tooth in the dental class is the one most often affected. Undersized maxillary lateral incisors and mandibular second premolars are the most common isolated problems in tooth size (Fig. 30–8). Sometimes complex orthodontic and restorative treatment is necessary to achieve a harmonious occlusal relationship and satisfy esthetic requirements when local tooth size problems exist. This type of treatment usually amounts to distributing space between the teeth so that when the teeth are restored to normal size and contour, they fit in a good occlusal relationship that has good anterior esthetics.

Tooth Structure. Teeth with abnormal crown and root structures may create occlusal problems. Careful clinical and radiographic examination is necessary to diagnose these problems. If the abnormality involves the crown (maxillary peg lateral or talon cusp), the crown needs to be recontoured by either adding restorative material to increase crown size or reducing its size by performing selective equilibration to eliminate

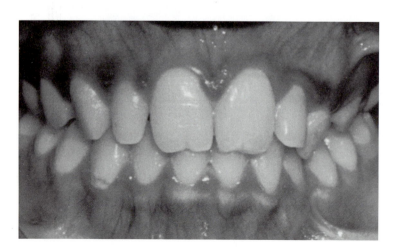

Figure 30–8. This maxillary right lateral incisor is smaller than normal; such a tooth is often called a peg lateral owing to its mesiodistal tapered form. Localized tooth-size problems of this type make it difficult to establish good dental relationships.

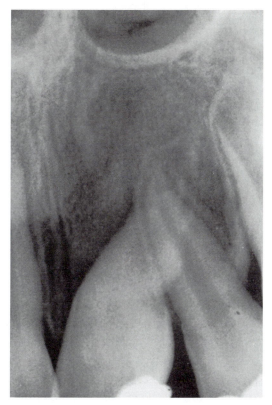

Figure 30–9. Root structure abnormalities, such as this dilacerated maxillary left central incisor, make orthodontic movement of teeth very difficult. A dilaceration of this magnitude makes the root more susceptible to apical resorption and complicates the final positioning of the crown and root.

occlusal interference. Both conditions usually require tooth movement prior to definitive restorative care to obtain an esthetically pleasing and functional result. Root structure abnormalities such as dilaceration may make orthodontic movement of teeth difficult (Fig. 30-9). Often the

portion of the root apical to the irregularity is resorbed or remodeled during tooth movement. Additionally, if a tooth with root abnormalities is scheduled for extraction, it may be prudent to refer the patient to a specialist because the abnormality will certainly complicate the extraction.

Tooth Position. The position of erupted and unerupted permanent teeth in this age group should be noted and compared with the normal sequence and time of eruption. Minor asymmetry in dental eruption is normal, and there is little cause for concern if less than 6 months difference in eruption exists between contralateral sides of the mouth. Four tooth positioning problems are associated with the mixed dentition: ectopic eruption, impaction, primary failure of eruption, and the midline diastema.

Ectopic eruption describes a path of eruption that causes root resorption of a portion or all of the adjacent primary tooth. Ectopic eruption is most often associated with the permanent maxillary first molar and mandibular lateral incisor (Gellin and Haley, 1982; Pulver, 1968). In ectopic eruption, the permanent first molar resorbs a portion of the distal root of the primary second molar (Fig. 30-10). In many cases, the permanent molar spontaneously "jumps" or moves distally and erupts into the correct position. In other cases, the permanent molar lodges under the primary molar crown and no longer erupts. No pain or discomfort is associated with ectopic eruption unless a communication develops between the oral cavity and the pulpal tissue of the primary molar, causing an abscess.

The prevalence of permanent first molar ectopic eruption is reported to be 3% to 4% (Kimmel et al., 1982). Several reasons have been proposed to explain ectopic molar eruption: (1) the maxillary teeth are larger than normal, (2) the

Figure 30–10. In ectopic eruption, the permanent first molar resorbs a portion of the distal root of the primary second molar. In this case, the permanent first molar has lodged under the primary second molar crown. In other cases, the permanent molar spontaneously "jumps" or moves distally and erupts into the normal position.

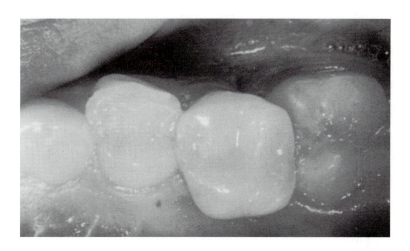

maxilla is smaller than normal, (3) the maxilla is positioned further posteriorly than normal in relation to the cranial base, or (4) the angulation of the erupting maxillary permanent first molar is abnormal (Pulver, 1968). Although ectopic molar eruption may occur in the mandibular arch, it is more common in the maxilla. Ectopic eruption of the permanent lateral incisor is most common in the mandibular arch. The erupting incisor resorbs all or a portion of the primary canine root because the path of eruption is abnormal, there is transitional crowding from the primary to the permanent dentition, or there is a true arch length deficiency (Fig. 30-11). The primary canine either exfoliates prematurely or impedes further eruption of the lateral incisor.

A related phenomenon is *lingual eruption* of the permanent incisors, predominantly the mandibular incisors. The prevalence of lingually erupting mandibular incisors is about 10% (Gellin and Haley, 1982). The cause of ectopic and lingually erupting incisors is not well established. One explanation suggests that ectopic and lingual eruption of the incisors results from an abnormal pattern of resorption. Alternatively, it has been suggested that lingual eruption is a variation of the normal eruption pattern because the lower incisor tooth buds form lingual to the primary incisors and may not migrate facially.

Tooth impaction is diagnosed during the clinical examination or from appropriate radiographs. Impaction of anterior teeth is caused by over-retained primary teeth, supernumerary teeth, severe crowding, or a failure in the eruption mechanism (Fig. 30-12). The permanent tooth usually erupts if the over-retained primary tooth or supernumerary tooth is removed. If the tooth is impacted as a result of crowding, it is necessary to provide space either orthodontically or by extraction to allow eruption. Generally, the last tooth to erupt in an arch or quadrant is impacted

because all of the space is previously spoken for. Treatment is discussed in the next section.

Posterior tooth impaction is normally the result of inadequate arch length. Inadequate arch length is caused by a tooth-jaw size discrepancy or space loss as a result of premature primary tooth loss. If the arch length problem is generalized, either permanent teeth need to be removed or the arch needs to be expanded to allow eruption of all the permanent teeth. Limited, localized crowding due to space loss can be treated by regaining the lost space orthodontically.

Primary failure of eruption is an unusual eruption problem that affects the posterior teeth. It is diagnosed when a tooth fails to erupt despite the presence of adequate space and the absence of overlying hard tissue that prevents eruption. Furthermore, all teeth distal to the affected tooth also fail to erupt. The cause of primary failure of eruption is unknown (Proffit and Vig, 1981).

A small, maxillary *midline diastema* in the early mixed dentition is normal. Typically it is caused by the position of the unerupted lateral incisors or canines (Fig. 30-13). The unerupted teeth are positioned superior and distal to the roots of the central incisors and direct the central incisor roots toward the midline and the crowns toward the distal. As the lateral incisors or canines erupt, the incisors upright themselves slowly, and the midline space begins to close. Treatment to close a diastema is usually delayed until the permanent canines are fully erupted unless the space available for eruption of the lateral incisors is severely limited. If the diastema is larger than 3 mm, the cause may be a mesiodens, a localized tooth size problem, or abnormal incisor positioning. A mesiodens is usually discovered on radiographic examination, and its removal normally allows the diastema to close. A size mismatch between the upper and lower teeth may result in a diastema. Normally, the

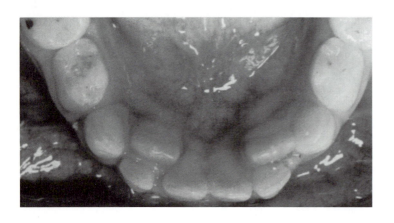

Figure 30–11. Ectopic eruption of the permanent lateral incisors is most common in the mandibular arch. In this example, the mandibular lateral incisors erupted lingual to their ideal position and the primary laterals are still present. In some cases, the lateral incisors erupt into a more normal position but cause premature exfoliation of the primary canine.

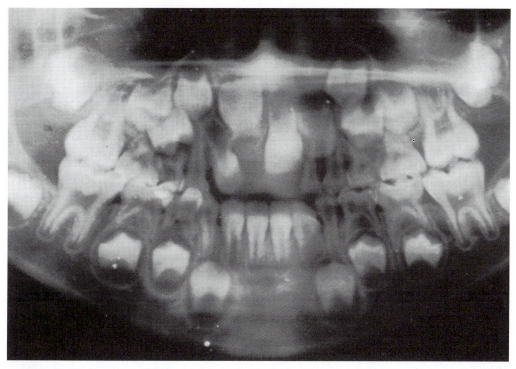

Figure 30–12. In this age group, tooth impaction in the anterior region is usually caused by overretained primary teeth, supernumerary teeth, or severe crowding. In a small number of cases, a failure in the eruption mechanism is responsible for the delayed eruption. In this case, the maxillary right central incisor is completely inverted and is directed toward the nasal cavity.

maxillary incisor crowns are small or excessively tapered, although the mandibular teeth may be too large in relation to the maxillary teeth. If large spaces are present, a combination of tooth movement and anterior restorations is required to correct a size discrepancy. Abnormal incisor positioning and protrusion also may result in a midline diastema. The abnormal positioning may be due to past or present finger habits or to abnormal eruption and is best treated by first eliminating the habit and then retracting the incisors orthodontically and consolidating space.

Anteroposterior Dimension. Permanent molar and canine relationships should be noted

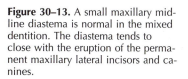

Figure 30–13. A small maxillary midline diastema is normal in the mixed dentition. The diastema tends to close with the eruption of the permanent maxillary lateral incisors and canines.

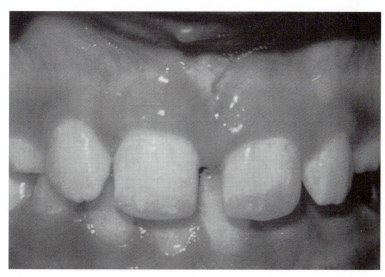

and compared with the anteroposterior skeletal relationships that were determined during the extraoral examination. Permanent molar and canine relationships are illustrated in Figure 30–14. Dental relationships normally reflect the underlying skeletal relationships including asymmetry, although it is feasible to have different dental and skeletal relationships if teeth are missing or have drifted. For example, a person with a Class I skeletal relationship may have a Class II molar relationship on one side if a primary maxillary second molar was lost prematurely and if the permanent maxillary first molar was allowed to drift forward into the space (Fig. 30-15).

If the permanent teeth are properly aligned in the alveolar bone at a normal angulation, overjet is a direct measurement of the relationship between the dental arches. Normal overjet is approximately 2 mm; therefore, the discrepancy between the arches can be calculated by subtracting 2 mm from the measured overjet. Incisor position is not always ideal, however, and estimates of dental arch discrepancies must be adjusted if both upper and lower anterior teeth are not protrusive or retrusive.

Transverse Relationship. Dental midline and posterior crossbite evaluation is conducted in the same manner as described in Chapter 18. Functional deviations of the mandible are identified by noting discrepancies between centric relation and centric occlusion. Posterior crossbites are determined to be either unilateral or bilateral. As the child becomes older, it becomes more critical to identify whether a cross-

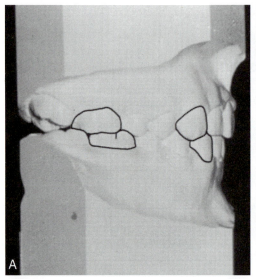

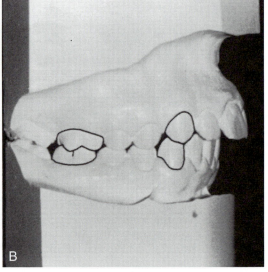

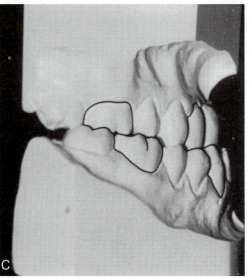

Figure 30–14. *A,* In the permanent dentition, permanent molar and canine relationships are determined and compared with the anteroposterior skeletal relationships. To determine molar relationships, the position of the mesiobuccal cusp of the permanent maxillary first molar is related to the position of the facial groove of the permanent mandibular first molar. If the mesiobuccal cusp occludes in the facial groove, the molar relationship is called Class I. The canine relationship is determined by the relationship of the maxillary canine to the embrasure between the mandibular canine and the first premolar (or primary first molar). If the maxillary canine occludes in the embrasure, the canine relationship is also called Class I. *B,* If the mesiobuccal cusp of the permanent maxillary first molar occludes mesial to the mandibular facial groove, the molar relationship is called Class II. The canine relationship is called Class II if the maxillary canine occludes mesial to the mandibular canine–first premolar embrasure. *C,* If the mesiobuccal cusp of the permanent maxillary first molar occludes distal to the mandibular facial groove, the molar relationship is called Class III. The canine relationship is Class III if the maxillary canine occludes distal to the mandibular canine–first premolar embrasure.

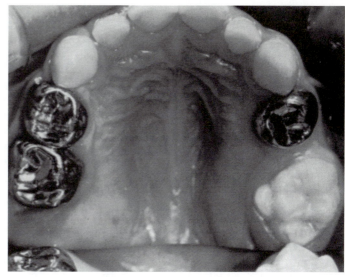

Figure 30–15. Dental relationships usually reflect the underlying skeletal relationships, although different dental and skeletal relationships are possible. In this case, the molar relationship on the left side is different from both the molar relationship on the right side and the skeletal relationship. This situation exists because the primary maxillary left second molar was lost prematurely, and the permanent maxillary left first molar drifted mesially during eruption.

bite is due to skeletal or dental causes. In the early mixed dentition years, treatments for both skeletal and dental crossbites are essentially the same. Treatment of posterior crossbite in the complete permanent dentition, however, varies according to whether the crossbite is skeletal or dental in origin and the estimate of whether the midpalatal suture is bridged or closed.

Vertical Dimension. The vertical dental examination is concerned with overbite and open bite measurements and ankylosis. Normal overbite in this age group is approximately 2 mm. If there is a deviation from normal, the clinician should try to determine if the deviation is due to a dental or a skeletal problem. If the facial examination revealed a vertical skeletal problem, it is sometimes reflected in the dental relationships. Treatment of the malocclusion varies with the source of the problem.

Ankylosis of the primary teeth can present several problems because of the magnitude of vertical dentoalveolar growth. Dental eruption and vertical growth of the alveolus may amount to as much as 10 mm from age 6 to 12. Thus, ankylosis of a primary tooth at an early age may result in large marginal ridge discrepancies, tipping of adjacent teeth, and vertical bone loss. Most of these problems, with the exception of space loss, resolve when the succedaneous tooth erupts. Ankylosed teeth and associated problems are discussed in Chapter 18, and the reader is referred to that chapter for more detail.

SUPPLEMENTAL ORTHODONTIC DIAGNOSTIC TECHNIQUES

Orthodontic treatment in the mixed dentition is more complex than is treatment in the primary dentition. The clinician must consider the difference in size between the primary and permanent dentitions, the amount of space available for the permanent teeth, and the dental and skeletal relationships of the patient. This formidable job requires supplemental information to make accurate orthodontic diagnoses and to develop coherent treatment plans. Diagnostic study casts are an essential part of a thorough evaluation if problems are detected during the examination and definitive analysis or if treatment is required. Findings recorded during the intraoral examination are reviewed and confirmed on the study models. Alignment and tooth position characteristics should receive special attention because appliance design must be appropriate for each rotation and displacement.

After the diagnostic casts are studied, analyses should be performed to determine tooth size relationships and arch length adequacy. The tooth size analysis attempts to compare the size of the teeth in one arch with the size of the teeth in the other. Tooth size must be compatible to ensure that teeth fit together correctly after treatment. The arch length analysis attempts to predict whether there is sufficient space available in the dental arch for the unerupted permanent teeth.

Tooth Size Analysis. The tooth size is calculated using a method developed by Bolton (1958). Bolton selected 55 cases of excellent occlusion and measured the mesiodistal diameter of all teeth on the casts except for the permanent second and third molars. From the measurements, Bolton determined that a certain ratio existed between the size of the upper and lower permanent teeth. A ratio could be determined for either the 6 anterior teeth or all 12 of the measured teeth. Little constructed a table based on the Bolton ratios to simplify tooth size determinations (Proffit, 1992). To use the table, the mesiodistal width of each permanent tooth is measured with a needle-pointed divider or sharp Boley gauge (Fig. 30–16). The widths of the teeth are summed, and the intersection of the mandibular and maxillary totals is located on the table. The intersection gives the tooth size discrepancy in millimeters (Fig. 30–17). Because there is some error in measuring the casts and some error in the analysis itself, tooth size discrepancies of 1.5 mm or less are not considered significant.

Several clinical situations contribute to tooth size discrepancy. Maxillary lateral incisors are commonly smaller than normal, resulting in a mandibular anterior tooth size excess (relatively speaking, the lower teeth are too large even though the problem is in the maxillary arch). The size of the second premolar also varies highly. When significant tooth size discrepancies are discovered, the child is best referred to a specialist because simple tooth movement does not produce an esthetically satisfactory result or good occlusion. Treatment of tooth size discrepancies often requires a combination of tooth movement and restorative dentistry.

Space Analysis. The space analysis is normally completed in the mixed dentition and is used to predict the amount of space available for the unerupted permanent teeth. A number of different methods of space analysis exist; however, all space analyses have two features in common. First, the permanent first molars and the mandibular incisors must be erupted to allow one to perform the analysis. Second, the mandibular incisors (sometimes in addition to other measurements) are used to predict the size of the unerupted canines and premolars. The following four assumptions are made in calculating a space analysis:

1. *All permanent teeth are developing normally.* Although this seems obvious, the analysis is meaningless if teeth are congenitally missing.

2. *There is a correlation between the size of the erupted mandibular incisors and the remaining succedaneous teeth.* The stronger the correlation, the more accurate the prediction of unerupted tooth size.

3. *The prediction tables are valid for a broad population.* The ethnic background of the patients used in most space analysis studies is northwest European. If the patient is not of northwest European descent, the analysis should be interpreted with some caution.

4. *Arch dimensions remain stable throughout growth.* This assumption is made to simplify the procedure, although it is recognized that the intercanine width, intermolar width, and arch length dimensions do change with age and eruption of teeth. Skeletal growth patterns may also

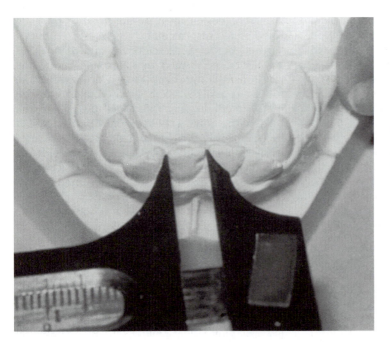

Figure 30–16. To complete the tooth size analysis developed by Bolton, the mesiodistal width of each permanent tooth (except for second and third molars) is measured with a Boley gauge or a needle-pointed divider. The measurements are added together to provide totals for the six anterior teeth and for the overall arch.

BOLTON ANALYSIS

Maxillary Anterior Excess

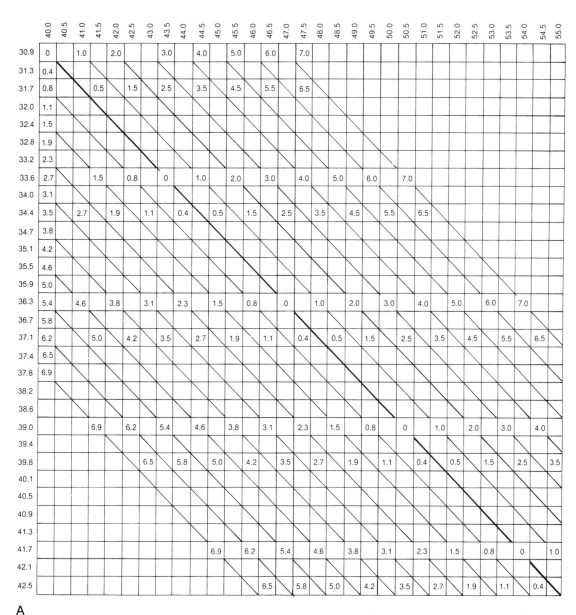

A

Mandibular Anterior Excess

Figure 30–17. To determine whether there is an anterior or overall tooth-size discrepancy, the intersection of the maxillary and mandibular totals is located on the appropriate table. *A,* The width of the mandibular anterior teeth is indicated on the vertical axis, and the width of the maxillary anterior teeth is found on the horizontal axis. The intersection indicates whether a tooth-size discrepancy exists and whether it is a maxillary or mandibular excess, and it indicates the size of the discrepancy in millimeters.

Illustration continued on following page

BOLTON ANALYSIS

Maxillary Overall Excess

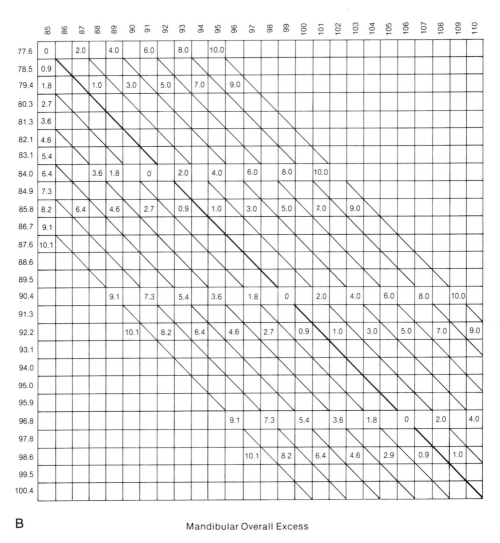

B

Mandibular Overall Excess

Figure 30–17 *Continued. B,* This table provides the same information for overall tooth size relationships. (Courtesy of Dr. Robert Little. Reproduced by permission from Proffit WR, Ackerman JL: Orthodontic diagnosis: The development of a problem list. *In* Proffit WR, et al [eds]: Contemporary Orthodontics. St. Louis, Mosby-Year Book, 1992.)

affect arch dimension stability. Class II mandibular-deficient persons tend to have proclined mandibular incisors to compensate for the deficiency, whereas Class III persons tend to have more upright or retroclined mandibular incisors.

The most accurate space analysis currently available is a modification of the Hixon-Oldfather analysis (Staley et al., 1984). This analysis uses lower incisor widths and the width of the unerupted premolars measured from radiographs to predict permanent tooth size. The Tanaka-Johnston analysis is most clinically useful because it requires no additional radiographs or tables to predict tooth size (Tanaka and Johnston, 1974). The first step in the Tanaka-Johnston analysis is to determine the available arch length. The distance from the mesial of the permanent first molar to the mesial of the contralateral permanent first molar is measured by dividing the arch into several segments (Fig. 30–18A). Each segment is measured over the contact points and incisal edges of the teeth. The segments are added together to provide an approximation of total arch

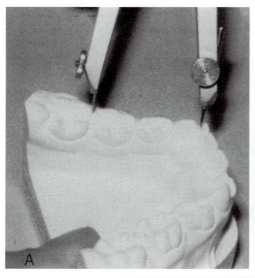
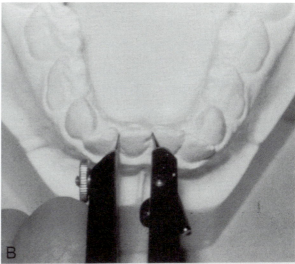

$$\frac{\text{sum of incisors}}{2} + 10.5 \text{ mm} = \begin{array}{l} \text{predicted width of canine} \\ \text{and 2 premolars in one} \\ \text{mandibular quadrant} \end{array}$$

C

$$\begin{array}{c} \text{total arch} \\ \text{length} \end{array} - \begin{array}{c} \text{sum of} \\ \text{incisors} \end{array} - \begin{array}{c} \text{2 (predicted} \\ \text{width)} \end{array} = \begin{array}{c} \text{available} \\ \text{arch length} \end{array}$$

D

Figure 30–18. *A,* The first step in the Tanaka-Johnston space is to determine available arch length. This is accomplished by dividing the arch into several segments and measuring each segment over the contact points and incisal edges of the teeth. *B,* The second step is to measure the width of the four mandibular incisors and add them together. *C,* The mesiodistal width of the unerupted canine and premolars in one quadrant is calculated by using the above formula. In the mandibular arch, 10.5 mm is used to determine the canine-premolar widths. In the maxillary arch, half the sum of the mandibular incisors is still used, but 11.0 mm is substituted for 10.5 mm because the unerupted permanent maxillary teeth are slightly larger. *D,* The final step in the analysis is to subtract the width of the four incisors and the predicted canine-premolar width from the total arch length. The remainder is the available arch length. If the remainder is positive, there is adequate space in the arch. If the remainder is negative, the permanent teeth require more room to erupt than is available in the arch.

length. The second step in the analysis is measurement of the width of the four mandibular incisors (Fig. 30-18*B*). The widths of the four incisors are added together to determine the amount of room necessary for ideal alignment. The mesiodistal width of the unerupted mandibular canine and premolars in one quadrant is predicted by adding 10.5 mm to half the width of the four lower incisors (Fig. 30-18*C*). The final step in the space analysis is to subtract the width of the lower incisors and two times the calculated premolar and canine width (both sides) from the total arch length approximation (Fig. 30-18*D*). If the result is positive, there is more space available in the arch than is needed for the unerupted teeth. If the result is negative, the unerupted teeth require more space than is available to erupt in ideal alignment.

The maxillary space analysis is conducted in the same way. Maxillary arch length is measured, the width of the maxillary incisors is determined, and 11.0 mm is added to half the width of the four lower incisors to predict the size of the unerupted maxillary canine and premolars in one

quadrant. The incisor width and the predicted canine-premolar width are subtracted from the total arch length to determine the amount of space available in the maxillary arch.

After the arch length predictions are made, the clinician should return to the cast and decide whether the results make sense. For example, if the arch appears to be crowded and the analysis predicts 5 mm of excess space, the analysis should be repeated or examined for mistakes. Furthermore, the results should be considered in the context of the patient's soft tissue profile. The space analysis may indicate that the patient is moderately short of space, yet because he or she has very retrusive lips and incisors, the treatment of choice would be to expand the arch by moving the incisors facially to provide better lip support (Fig. 30-19). Conversely, an analysis may predict that there is no crowding, yet extractions are considered necessary because the patient has very protrusive teeth and lips (Fig. 30-20). Dental protrusion and dental crowding are actually manifestations of the same problem. Whether the arch is crowded or the incisors are

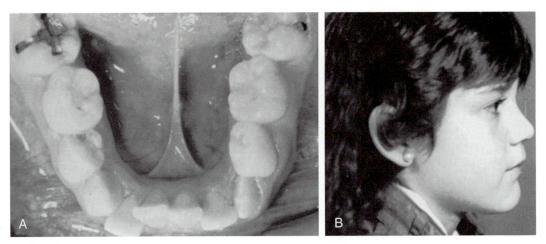

Figure 30–19. The results of the space analysis *(A)* are considered in the context of the patient's soft tissue profile. In this example, the space analysis indicates that the arch length is short. The profile analysis *(B)*, however, indicates that the patient cannot tolerate further loss of lip support. It is more prudent to expand the arch in this case to provide additional space than to extract teeth.

protrusive depends on the interaction between the pressure of the resting tongue and the circumoral musculature.

Two factors must be considered when using the Tanaka-Johnston analysis. It tends to overpredict the width of the unerupted teeth slightly in the study sample. This makes the amount of crowding appear more severe than it actually is. In addition, if the patient is not of northwest European background, it is difficult to know whether the prediction will be over- or understated. An alternative method for determining available space is to measure arch length and incisor width as noted previously and then obtain periapical radiographs of the canines and premolars. The mesiodistal widths of the unerupted teeth are measured on the periapical films and then corrected for magnification by comparing the width of erupted teeth on the films with the actual width of these teeth on the cast. With this technique, an individual space analysis can be performed for every patient. The disadvantages of this technique are that the patient is exposed to more radiation and undistorted radiographs of the canines are difficult to obtain.

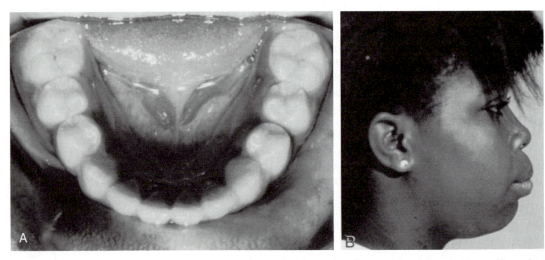

Figure 30–20. In this example, the space analysis *(A)* indicates that there is no shortage of arch length. The profile analysis *(B)*, however, indicates that the patient has extremely protrusive lips and incisors. It is more prudent to extract teeth and retract the incisors and lips in this case. This figure illustrates the fact that dental crowding and dental protrusion are actually manifestations of the same problem.

Analysis of Cephalometric Head Films.
Analysis of lateral cephalometric head films is an additional diagnostic aid used to determine the relationship between the skeletal and dental structures. The cephalometric head film is normally ordered when significant skeletal discrepancies exist and comprehensive orthodontic treatment is being considered. The cephalometric analysis does not replace the facial profile analysis; it provides more specific information about the contribution of each skeletal and dental component to the malocclusion and must be viewed carefully (Fields and Sinclair, 1990). The facial profile analysis should be used by the clinician to gather basic information about the spatial relationships of the teeth and jaws. If the clinician identifies significant anteroposterior or vertical discrepancies, the patient should be evaluated by a specialist. At that time, a lateral cephalometric radiograph may be used to obtain a more precise assessment of the problem.

A large number of cephalometric analyses exist; however, the common goal of all analyses is to determine the size and position of the skeletal structures and the position of the teeth. The first step in the cephalometric analysis is to obtain a diagnostic head film. For the radiograph to be diagnostic, the head must be positioned in a cephalostat in a natural, relaxed posture (Fig. 30-21). In other words, the patient's head should not be tipped up or down or to one side or the other because this alters the perceived relationship of the skeletal structures and makes interpretation of the landmarks more difficult, even to the point of leading one to suspect skeletal asymmetry. A mandibular deficiency may not be apparent if the patient's head is tipped upward. Natural head position is produced by having the patient look at the distant horizon. The teeth should be together and the lips relaxed when the film is exposed.

After the head film is made, the radiograph should be screened for pathologic findings. If none exist, a piece of matte acetate paper is placed over the film, and the anatomic structures are traced and landmarks identified (Fig. 30-22). Linear and angular measurements made from this tracing provide the basis for the analysis. Landmarks on the radiograph can also be directly identified and digitized on a digitizing pad (Fig. 30-23). Computer programs generate linear and angular measurements, and a graphic image of the face constructed from the digitized landmarks provides the basis for the cephalometric analysis (Fig. 30-24).

The analysis, regardless of how the measurements and comparisons were made, should eval-

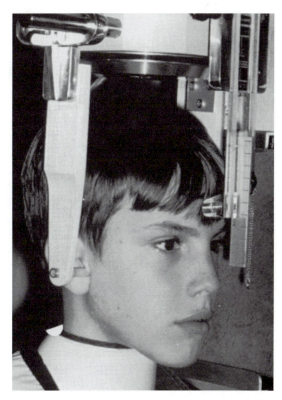

Figure 30–21. The first step in the cephalometric analysis is to obtain a diagnostic head film. After the patient has been appropriately draped with lead aprons, the head is placed in the cephalostat in a natural, relaxed position. Natural head position is produced by having the patient look at the distant horizon.

uate the position of the maxilla and mandible in relation to that of the cranial base and the relationship of the maxilla and mandible to one another. Analysis also should evaluate the position of the teeth in each jaw and the relationship of the upper denture to the lower. Vertical relationships between total, upper, and lower facial heights of the anterior face should be determined. Finally, the analysis should evaluate the soft tissue profile and the position of the lips in relation to the nose and chin. A cephalometric analysis requires two reference lines to orient the position of the teeth and jaws. Historically, the Frankfort horizontal plane has been used as the horizontal reference line because it was thought to be parallel to the true horizontal when the patient was looking at a distant point. The Frankfort horizontal plane connects the upper rim of the external auditory meatus (porion) with the inferior border of the orbital rim (orbitale) (Fig. 30-25). Although the Frankfort horizontal plane is not always parallel to the true horizontal, it is still the most widely used horizontal reference line. The vertical reference line

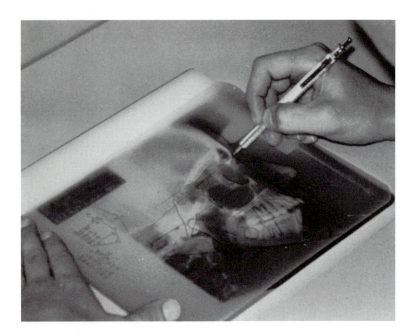

Figure 30–22. After the head film has been screened for pathologic findings, a piece of matte acetate paper is placed over the film, the anatomic structures are traced, and landmarks are identified. Linear and angular measurements can be made manually from this tracing by using a protractor and ruler. These measurements provide the basis for the cephalometric analysis.

can be either a true perpendicular (to the horizon) through the nasion (the bony bridge of the nose) or a line perpendicular to the Frankfort plane through the nasion. The position and size of the maxilla and mandible are evaluated by comparing A point (maxilla) and pogonion (mandible), the most anterior points on these structures, to the vertical reference line. Normal maxillary position and size should place A point 1 to 2 mm behind the vertical line (Fig. 30–26). Pogonion is normally 5 mm behind the vertical with a well-positioned mandible in a preadolescent (McNamara, 1983).

Angular and linear measurements can be used to compare the position of the maxilla with that

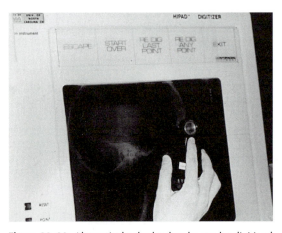

Figure 30–23. Alternatively, the landmarks can be digitized and stored by computer. The measurements are completed electronically.

of the mandible. The angle formed by connecting A and B points with the nasion has traditionally been used to describe the position of the two jaws (Fig. 30–27). In normally related jaws, the angle is between 2 and 5 degrees. Larger positive values suggest a Class II relationship, whereas negative values indicate Class III tendencies. The difference between the size of the lower and upper jaws, as determined from the Harvold measurements, can also be used to relate the jaws (Harvold, 1974).

Vertical facial proportions can be measured in two ways. The most direct method of determining vertical proportions is to measure total, upper, and lower anterior facial heights and to construct facial height ratios or compare linear measurements with age-appropriate norms (Harvold, 1974; Isaacson et al., 1971). Total facial height is normally measured from nasion to menton. The division between the upper and lower facial heights is made at the anterior nasal spine (Fig. 30–28). The upper facial height should compose approximately 45% of the total facial height in a well-proportioned face (Wylie and Johnson, 1952). Vertical facial height can be indirectly determined from the mandibular plane angle (the angle between the mandibular plane and the Frankfort horizontal plane). A long-faced person tends to have a large mandibular plane angle, whereas a short-faced person has a smaller mandibular plane angle (Fig. 30–29). Maxillary and mandibular dental position is evaluated by measuring overjet, overbite, and the axial and bodily position of the incisors. Overjet and overbite

Measurement	Value		Mean	Diff	S.D.	
SNA	82.2	deg	81.2	1.0	3.3	
SNB	77.3	deg	77.3	-0.0	2.7	
ANB	4.9	deg	3.9	1.0	2.1	
Md Unit Length	119.5	mm	114.0	5.5	4.9	*
Mx Unit Length	96.9	mm	92.0	4.9	3.7	*
Unit Difference	22.7		22.0	0.7		
A Pt to N Perp	-4.4	mm	1.1	-5.5	2.7	**
Pg to N Perp	-15.9	mm	-0.3	-15.6	3.8	***
Wits Appraisal	-0.5	mm	-1.1	0.6	2.0	
**************	0.0	mm	0.0	0.0	0.0	
ANS - Menton	66.0	mm	69.6	-3.6	5.0	
SN - GoGn	35.5	deg	33.8	1.7	4.9	
FH to MP	31.7	deg	21.3	10.4	3.9	**
Facial axis	83.9	deg	90.5	-6.6	3.5	*
Nasion - ANS	54.1	mm	54.7	-0.6	3.2	
Total Face Ht	120.1	mm	120.0	0.1	5.0	
⅓ Nasal Height	0.45		0.43	0.02	0.03	
Post Face Ht mm	77.0	mm	77.6	-0.6	5.3	
Ant Face Ht mm	122.2	mm	123.3	-1.1	6.3	
PFH : AFH	0.63		0.62	0.01		
**************	0.0	mm	0.0	0.0	0.0	
U1 to SN	100.3	deg	102.0	-1.7	2.0	
Upper 1 to NA	18.2	deg	22.8	-4.6	5.7	
Upper 1 to NA m	2.0	mm	4.3	-2.3	2.7	
Lower 1 to NB	21.5	deg	26.1	-4.6	6.4	
Lower 1 to NB m	2.9	mm	5.2	-2.3	2.6	
Pogonion to NB	2.5	mm	1.3	1.2	1.6	
**************	0.0	mm	0.0	0.0	0.0	
UL to Steiner	0.1	mm	0.0	0.1	1.0	
LL to Steiner	0.4	mm	0.0	0.4	1.0	
Nasolabial	119.6	deg	102.0	17.6	8.0	**
Nasion' to Sn	50.0	mm	60.0	-10.0	5.0	*
Sn - Stomion s	22.5	mm	22.0	0.5	2.0	
Stomion i - Me'	40.7	mm	44.0	-3.3	4.0	
SLS to Sn Vert	-2.9	mm	-1.7	-1.2	1.0	*
ILS to Sn Vert	-19.2	mm	-8.0	-11.2	2.0	***
**************	0.0	mm	0.0	0.0	0.0	

A

Figure 30–24. Printouts of computer-generated cephalometric analyses often take a form similar to the ones illustrated here. The resulting measurements *(A)* and a graphic image of the face *(B)* are available for analysis. The content usually can be customized by altering the anatomic landmarks and measurements to provide those most useful to the individual clinician.

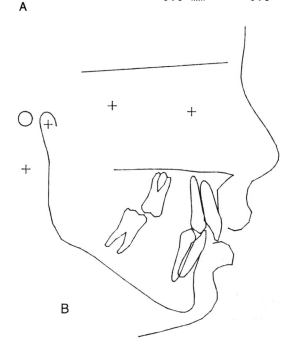

B

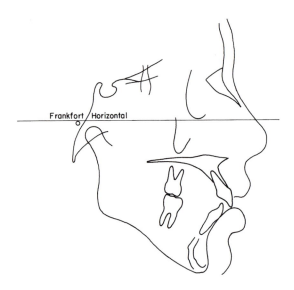

Figure 30–25. Cephalometric analysis requires two reference lines to orient the position of the head and teeth. Historically, the Frankfort horizontal plane has been used as the reference line because it is felt to be parallel to the true horizontal when the patient is looking at the horizon. The Frankfort horizontal plane is constructed by connecting the upper rim of the external auditory meatus (porion) with the inferior border of the orbital rim (orbitale). The vertical reference line is either a true perpendicular to the nasion, the bony bridge of the nose, or a line perpendicular to the Frankfort plane through the nasion.

are simple measurements taken from the facial surfaces and incisal edges of the incisors, respectively (Fig. 30-30). The axial and bodily position of the maxillary incisor is determined relative to the nasion-A point line; the mandibular incisor position is related to the nasion-B point line. Axial inclination is determined from the angle formed by the intersection of the long axis of the incisor with the appropriate nasion-A point or nasion-B point lines. Bodily position is a measure of linear distance from the facial surface of

the incisor to the reference line (Steiner, 1960) (Fig. 30-31).

A number of soft tissue analyses exist to describe the facial profile. The major problem with soft tissue analysis is that the head film is a static representation of a dynamic object. Lip position may be different on the head film depending on whether the patient was in a relaxed posture (as recommended) or was straining to put the lips together when the film was made. This makes clinical assessment of the profile all the more

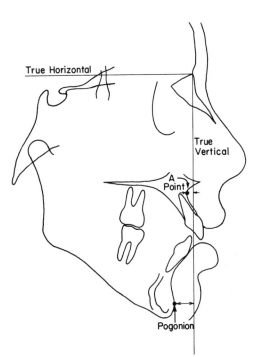

Figure 30–26. The position and size of the maxilla and mandible are evaluated by comparing the A point (maxilla) and pogonion (mandible) with a vertical reference line. In a well-positioned maxilla, A point is located 1 to 2 mm behind the vertical reference line. Pogonion is normally 5 mm behind the vertical line in a properly positioned mandible.

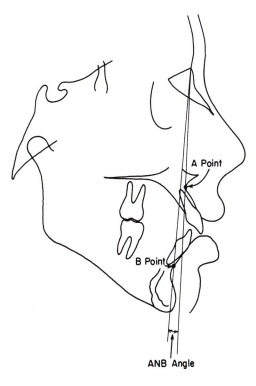

Figure 30–27. The relative positions of the maxilla and mandible are also compared by using an angular measurement. In normally related jaws, the angle formed by connecting A and B points with nasion is between 2 and 5 degrees. Larger positive values suggest a Class II relationship, whereas negative values indicate a Class III tendency.

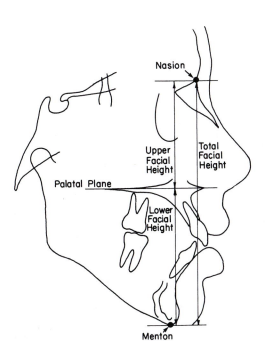

Figure 30–28. Vertical facial proportions are determined by measuring total, upper, and lower facial heights. Total facial height is normally measured from the nasion to the menton. The division between upper and lower facial height is made at the palatal plane (a line connecting the anterior and posterior nasal spines). The measurements are used to construct facial height relations or are compared with age-appropriate norms.

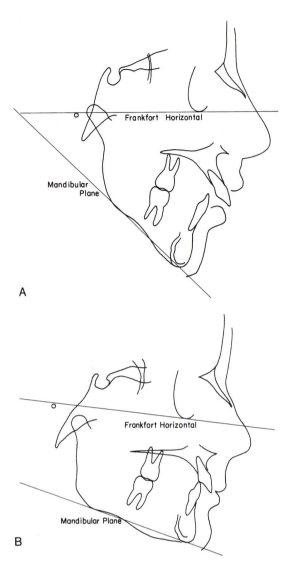

A

Figure 30–29. *A,* Vertical facial height is determined indirectly from the mandibular plane angle (the angle between the mandibular plane and the Frankfort horizontal plane). This angle is usually approximately 24 degrees. A large mandibular plane angle is normally indicative of a long lower facial height. *B,* Conversely, a small mandibular plane angle is indicative of a short lower facial height.

B

important. Nevertheless, lip position is usually compared with the nose and chin. The Ricketts E line, which is convenient to use, is a line connecting the tip of the nose with the anterior contour of the chin (Fig. 30-32). In the permanent dentition, the upper lip is normally 1 mm behind the line and the lower lip is on the line or slightly behind it (Ricketts, 1981).

It is important to realize that the numbers derived as norms serve as references and not as the diagnosis itself. Certain measurements may suggest a discrepancy, and this should be verified by the clinical examination. The clinician also should remember that hard and soft tissue analyses vary according to the ethnic background of the patient. Appropriate analyses and standards should be used. Serial cephalometric radiographs obtained prior to treatment, before and during

treatment, or before and after treatment are often useful for evaluating growth, treatment progress, or treatment result, respectively.

Serial cephalometric head films can be superimposed on each other to illustrate changes in jaw and tooth positions. The observed changes are a combination of tooth movement and growth, and it is difficult to differentiate one from the other. To superimpose head films, one must locate an area within the head that is relatively unchanged over the time period in question—that is, an area that is not affected by growth or treatment from which change can be determined. Traditionally, three superimpositions are made with each pair of serial cephalometric radiographs when growth and treatment changes are being evaluated.

The first superimposition illustrates overall

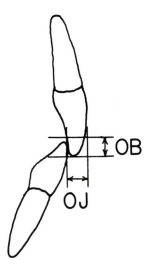

Figure 30–30. The position of the maxillary and mandibular incisors and indirectly the entire dentition is evaluated by measuring the overjet and overbite. Overjet (OJ) is a horizontal measure of the distance between the most anterior points on the facial surfaces of the maxillary and mandibular central incisors. Overbite (OB) is a vertical measure of the overlap between the incisal edges of the maxillary and mandibular incisors.

changes in the face. The comparison is made by superimposing the structures of the anterior cranial base or along the sella-nasion line registering at the sella. The amount and direction of change in the soft tissue profile and position of the jaws are readily apparent (Fig. 30–33*A*). To demonstrate the amount and direction of dental change, structures of the maxilla and mandible are superimposed to eliminate all skeletal change from the evaluation (Fig. 30–33*B, C*). In the maxilla, the maxilla, pterygomaxillary fissure, and zygomatic process are superimposed to find the best fit. In the mandible, the inner surface of the mandibular symphysis, the outline of the mandibular canal, and the unerupted third molar crypts are superimposed.

Radiographic Evaluation

Transition into the mixed dentition requires modification of the basic pediatric survey. Some considerations for radiographs of children in this period are the following:

1. *Identification of missing teeth, supernumerary teeth, and the developmental status of permanent anteriors and premolars require greater periapical coverage on films.* The permanent second premolars are usually evident on radiographs at age 4, but they may not be apparent until age 8.

2. *Potential eruption problems may be diagnosed from the radiographs by study of the unerupted teeth.* Ectopic eruption of permanent first molars has been discussed and is diagnosed from routine bite-wing radiographs. Ectopic eruption of incisors and canine impaction, which are other maxillary eruption problems, are often diagnosed from panoramic radiographs or selected periapical films. Labial or palatal positioning of the canine is determined by using a split-image panoramic film or two periapical radiographs. The image of the canine on the two films shifts as the angulation of the central x-ray beam changes. If the image of the canine moves in the same direction (relative to the other teeth or reference structure) as the central x-ray beam from the first film to the second, the canine is positioned lingual or palatal to the other teeth. If the image moves in the opposite direction to the beam from the first film to the second, the canine is located buccal to the teeth. This technique may also be used to locate supernumerary teeth or other abnormal structures.

3. *Small palate size, especially early in the school age period, prevents or complicates maxillary periapical radiography via a long-cone film-stabilizing apparatus.*

4. *Greater anteroposterior length in the posterior occlusion requires more bite-wing coverage.*

In the early mixed dentition period, a radiograph should be taken to detect supernumerary or missing teeth in the anterior maxilla. All tooth-bearing areas should be surveyed during the early mixed dentition years. This survey could consist of a panoramic radiograph and posterior bite-wing films. The panoramic radiograph offers the advantage of showing the temporomandibular joint (TMJ). Definitive TMJ films are indicated when there are clinical signs of dysfunction or a history of TMJ abnormalities. A traditional intraoral film survey in this age group is composed of appropriate anterior occlusal views and at least one periapical film in each posterior quadrant and posterior bite-wing films (Fig. 30–34). The number of films should be dictated by the size of the tooth-bearing areas, the adequacy of tissue coverage by the size of films tolerated, and the needs of the child. A 12-film survey (four posterior periapical, six anterior periapical, and two posterior bite-wing films) should suffice even for the older school age child if they are performed well.

Radiographic techniques used in children, especially those early in this age group, may include modifications. The anterior area requires

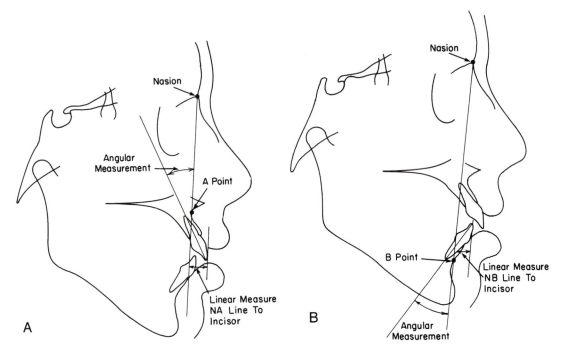

Figure 30–31. *A,* The axial and bodily positions of the maxillary incisor are determined by making angular and linear measurements. Axial position is determined by drawing an angle formed by the intersection of the long axis of the incisor with the nasion–A point line. A large angle (> approximately 22 degrees) suggests that the incisor is axially protrusive; a small angle suggests that the incisor is upright. The bodily position of the incisor is determined by measuring the linear distance between the facial surface of the incisor and the nasion–A point line. On the average, this distance is 4 mm. A large measurement suggests that the incisor is positioned too far anteriorly, whereas a small or negative measurement indicates that the incisor is positioned too far posteriorly in relation to the maxilla. *B,* The position of the mandibular incisor is similarly evaluated, although the nasion–B point line is used as a reference line. For these measurements, the average inclination is 25 degrees and the average linear distance is 4 mm.

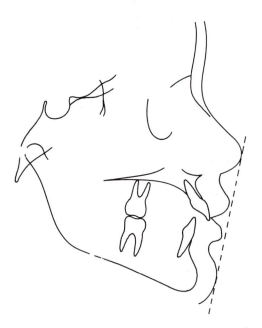

Figure 30–32. The Ricketts E line is a convenient reference line used to assess the position of the lips in relation to the nose and chin. In the permanent dentition, the upper lip is normally 1 mm behind a line connecting the tip of the nose to the anterior contour of the chin. The lower lip is usually on or slightly behind this line.

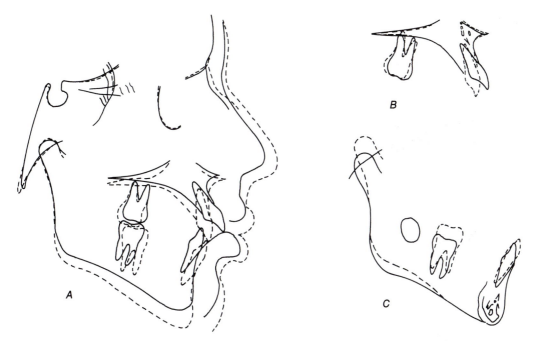

Figure 30–33. *A,* Serial cephalometric head films are superimposed to illustrate changes in jaw and tooth positions during growth and orthodontic treatment. To assess overall change, a stable area within the head that is not influenced by growth or treatment is located. These overall changes in the face are illustrated by superimposing them on structures of the anterior cranial base. In this case, the solid line represents the patient before orthodontic treatment was initiated. The second or dashed line represents the patient after treatment was completed. During treatment, the maxilla moved slightly forward and downward. The horizontal position of the mandible remained virtually unchanged. The mandible did move vertically, however. The position of the lips improved during the treatment period as well. *B,* To illustrate the amount and direction of dental change, structures within the maxilla and mandible are superimposed. In this case, the maxillary superimposition, based on a best fit of palatal morphologic appearance, shows that the incisor and molar were both tipped distally. In addition, there was a change in the vertical position of the incisor. The change in incisor and molar position contributed to an improvement in molar relationships and overjet reduction. *C,* The mandibular superimposition, made by overlaying the inner aspect of the mandibular symphysis, the canal of the inferior alveolar nerve, and the unerupted third molar crypt, shows that both the incisor and molar erupted vertically.

placement of the film positioner deeper in the palate to obtain proper orientation. Two alternatives are to use the prong end of the Snap-A-Ray device (Rinn Corporation, Elgin, IL) with a bisecting angle technique or to use a film with cotton rolls attached (Fig. 30-35). The long-cone technique for posterior teeth is the same as that used in adults with two modifications to help improve the product. Figure 30-36 demonstrates the use of increased vertical angulation to pick up the developing teeth. Figure 30-37 shows the placement of cotton rolls on the bite-block to facilitate positioning in small mouths or when teeth needed for stabilization are absent. A Styrofoam bite-block may be used to obtain anterior films via a bisecting angle technique (Fig. 30-38). The bite-wing technique used in this age group is essentially the same as that used in the preschooler. It may take more skill to open contacts by careful positioning of the beam. Larger films may be preferable because they cover more area in each exposure.

Selection criteria also apply to this age group. Justification of a full-mouth survey of some type is based on the need to identify dental developmental problems and pathology. The number of films made should reflect the adequacy of composite exposure provided by individual views. This translates to making as few films as necessary to reveal tissue areas. In the age range of 6 to 12 years, a variety of combinations of films is possible. No single set of projections is considered best.

TREATMENT PLANNING FOR NONORTHODONTIC PROBLEMS

The planning of care for this age group usually centers around orthodontic considerations, although many patients require additional management. Some elements of treatment planning that may need to be addressed but are only peripher-

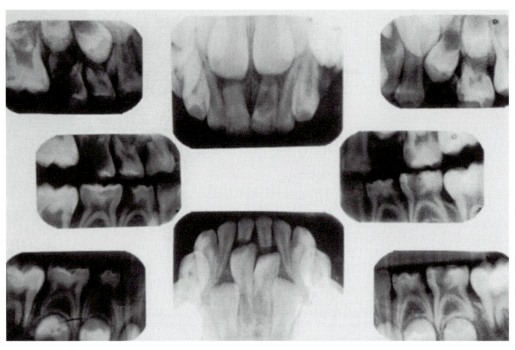

Figure 30–34. An appropriate radiographic examination in this age group consists of anterior occlusal radiographs, at least one periapical film in each posterior quadrant, and posterior bite-wing radiographs. The number of films should be dictated by the size of the tooth-bearing areas, the adequacy of tissue coverage by the size of the films, and the needs of the child.

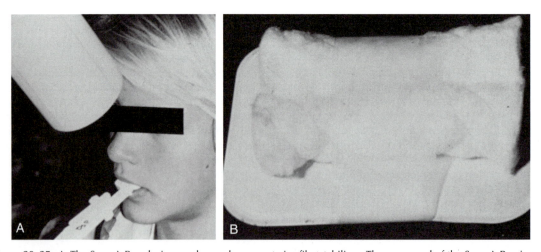

Figure 30–35. *A*, The Snap-A-Ray device can be used as an anterior film stabilizer. The prong end of the Snap-A-Ray is used to hold a film in place by the child. A bisecting angle technique is used. *B*, Alternatively, cotton rolls can be used to stabilize the film. Taping two or three cotton rolls can help fill the space in the palate and stabilize an anterior film. Care must be taken not to bend the film. Bisecting angle technique is used.

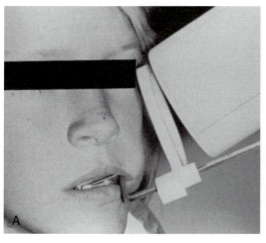 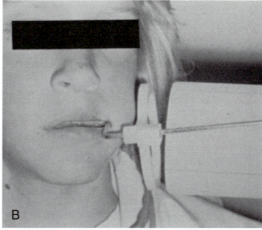

Figure 30–36. *A* and *B,* Increasing the vertical angulation of posterior periapical films will provide more coverage of periapical tissue. This helps the radiographs to include developing premolar roots in this age group.

ally related to orthodontics include the following:

1. *Management of primary caries.* Within this age period, many primary teeth normally exfoliate. A decision to extract a tooth or restore it must be made with its remaining life span in mind as well as the length of time that the child will be without a replacement. Prosthetic replacement for a short time may not be indicated if adequate functional surfaces are available elsewhere and space maintenance is not indicated.

2. *Management of pathosis.* Some forms of oral pathosis, such as supernumerary teeth, odontomas, or missing teeth, are given definitive management in this period owing to the child's better ability to cooperate and the impending effects of the problem.

3. *Prevention of dental disease.* The choice of sealants is also made during this period, as are decisions about how to manage incipient interproximal lesions of permanent teeth. Topical fluoride regimens may be considered if the caries pattern changes for the worse.

4. *Health issues.* Children with disabilities or serious illnesses are in a transitional time. The child with cancer, orofacial clefting, cerebral palsy, or a host of other conditions may need special consideration in regard to such issues as life span, realistic functional requirements, retention of teeth for growth purposes, and the role of the appearance of teeth in social acceptance. Decisions regarding these issues are often complex, and input from parents, the child, and other professionals is helpful in decision making. The dentist's role is to provide information about the need for care, the benefits anticipated, the alter-

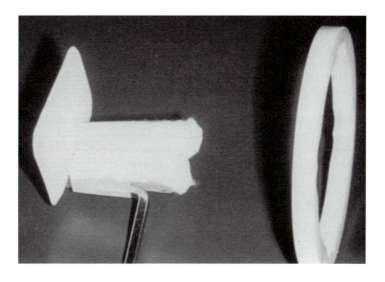

Figure 30–37. Several cotton rolls will help to hold the film holder in place when palate depth is insufficient or teeth are missing. Rolls can be taped both above and below the holder's bite-block.

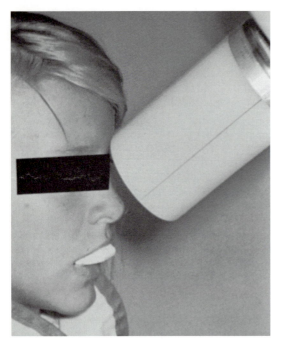

Figure 30–38. A Styrofoam bite-block can be used to aid in film positioning. Most plastic holders can be cut down to fit the child with transitional dentition better.

natives to care (including no treatment), and the burden of maintenance of care. These special patients may tax the dentist's skills in planning care, and they may require careful and frequent observation rather than treatment.

Regardless of the specific situation, dental and periodontal diseases are addressed first and stabilized. Restorative care is rendered next, and more definitive prosthodontic or orthodontic treatment is completed last.

REFERENCES

Bolton WA: Disharmony in tooth size and its relation to the analysis and treatment of malocclusion. Am J Orthod 28:113-130, 1958.

Fields HW, Proffit WR, Nixon WL, et al: Facial pattern differences in long-faced children and adults. Am J Orthod 85:217-223, 1984.

Fields HW, Sinclair PM: Dentofacial growth and development. J Dent Child 57:46-55, 1990.

Gellin ME, Haley JV: Managing cases of overretention of mandibular primary incisors when their permanent successors erupt lingually. ASDC J Dent Child 49:118-122, 1982.

Hagan PP, Hagan JP, Fields HW, et al: The legal status of informed consent for behavior management technique in pediatric dentistry. Pediatr Dent 6:204-208, 1984.

Harvold EP: The Activator in Orthodontics. St. Louis, CV Mosby, 1974.

Isaacson JR, Isaacson RJ, Speidel TM, et al: Extreme variation in vertical facial growth and associated variation in skeletal and dental relations. Am J Orthod 41:219-229, 1971.

Kimmel NA, Gellin ME, Bohannan HA, et al: Ectopic eruption of maxillary first permanent molars in different areas of the United States. ASDC J Dent Child 49:294-299, 1982.

Loe N, Silness J: Periodontal disease in pregnancy: 1. Prevalence and severity. Acta Odont Scand 21:553, 1963.

McNamara JA Jr: A method of cephalometric analysis. In McNamara JA, Ribbens KA, Howe RP (eds): Clinical Alteration of the Growing Face. Monograph 12, Craniofacial Growth Series. Ann Arbor, University of Michigan, Center for Human Growth and Development, 1983, pp 81-105.

Proffit WR: Contemporary Orthodontics, 3rd ed. St. Louis, Mosby-Year Book, 1992.

Proffit WR, Vig KWL: Primary failure of eruption: A possible cause of posterior open-bite. Am J Orthod 80:173-190, 1981.

Pulver F: The etiology and prevalence of ectopic eruption of the maxillary first permanent molar. ASDC J Dent Child 35:138-146, 1968.

Ramfjord SP: The periodontal index. J Periodontol 38:610, 1967.

Ricketts RM: Perspectives in the clinical application of cephalometrics. Angle Orthod 51:115-150, 1981.

Shafer WG, Hine MK, Levy BM: A Textbook of Oral Pathology. Philadelphia, WB Saunders, 1974.

Staley RN, O'Gorman TW, Hoag JF, et al: Prediction of the widths of unerupted canines and premolars. JADA 108:185-190, 1984.

Steiner CC: The use of cephalometrics as an aid to planning and assessing orthodontic treatment. Am J Orthod 46:721-735, 1960.

Tanaka MM, Johnston LE: The prediction of the size of unerupted canines and premolars in a contemporary orthodontic population. JADA 88:798-801, 1974.

Wylie WL, Johnson EL: Rapid evaluation of facial dysplasia in the vertical plane. Angle Orthod 22:165-182, 1952.

31

Prevention of Dental Disease

Arthur Nowak and James Crall

Chapter Outline

FLUORIDE ADMINISTRATION   HOME CARE
Systemic Fluorides   DIET
Topical Fluorides

The patient between 6 and 12 years of age presents an interesting professional challenge for the dentist. At the beginning of this period, the dentist is dealing with a patient who continues to depend on the parents but is now thrust into a new environment for approximately 8 hours a day—the school. By the end of this period, the dentist is dealing with a patient who has gained partial independence from his or her parents and is nearly ready for junior high school and, in the case of the female patient, approaching womanhood.

In addition, all through this period a number of oral-facial changes are taking place. Most of the primary teeth have been replaced with permanent teeth. The alignment and occlusion of the teeth are developing, and the "adult face" is emerging. What "I" look like becomes important, not only to the patient but also to all the people he or she meets each day, especially peers.

Diet and dietary practices are severely challenged by the educational environment and social pressures both during the day and after school hours. Requirements vary from year to year in this period. As the growth pattern of the patient changes from slow progressive physical growth early in the period to substantial physical growth at the end of the period, the requirements of the child need to stay in tune. These dietary requirements depend not only on growth and development but on the level of physical and

mental activity engaged in by the child. Snacking becomes a common practice during this period. With vending machines easily available, convenience stores on many street corners, and the influence of radio and television always pervasive, children are constantly reminded of their hunger needs.

Many changes in manual dexterity take place during this period. Although continuing gross motor development prevails, this is the period when fine motor activity begins to mature. Luckily so, because during this period the child is challenging the parents for independence, especially in areas of personal hygiene, clothes selection, and dietary selection. Conflicts emerge between the parents' desires and the child's wishes. It is a time when parents must have a strong daily influence on all types of activity, including oral care. With eruption of the permanent teeth the fluoride needs begin to shift from systemic administration to topical applications. Periodic review by the dentist is important so that the child receives the optimal protection available.

FLUORIDE ADMINISTRATION

The period from 6 to 12 years is extremely important with regard to fluoride administration for three major reasons: (1) the crowns of many permanent teeth continue to form during this period, (2) the posterior permanent teeth erupt and are at greater risk for developing caries until the process of posteruptive maturation has occurred, and (3) the child becomes increasingly responsible for the maintenance of his or her oral health. The optimal use of all forms of fluoride should be employed to provide protection during this first phase of carious attack on those teeth that will eventually constitute the permanent dentition.

Systemic Fluorides

Studies suggest that a substantial portion of the anticaries protection provided by water fluoridation in humans occurs during the pre-eruptive period (Clarkson, 1991; van Eck et al., 1985). Additional studies in laboratory animals have reported that daily doses of fluoride administered via gastric intubation during the period of tooth formation reduced the incidence of caries in these teeth after their eruption (Hunt and Navia, 1975). Because systemically acquired fluoride may be deposited and redistributed in developing teeth during the mineralization phase as well as during the subsequent period prior to eruption, current recommendations call for systemic fluoride supplements for all children residing in areas where the water is fluoride-deficient until they reach the age of 16. This protocol should help to ensure maximum protection for the posterior teeth, which are more vulnerable to carious attack. The dosage of supplemental fluoride does not change for children past the age of 6.

Topical Fluorides

During the period from 6 to 12 years of age, the child should become increasingly responsible for the maintenance of his or her dentition. Many forms of topical fluoride are appropriate for children in this age group, including fluoride toothpastes, fluoride mouth rinses, and concentrated fluoride preparations for professional and home application.

Accumulating evidence continues to support the effectiveness of frequent application of agents that contain relatively low concentrations of fluoride. The two principal forms of these agents in the United States are fluoride toothpastes and fluoride mouth rinses.

FLUORIDE TOOTHPASTES

The daily use of a fluoride-containing dentifrice should form the foundation of the child's preven-

tive dental activities. Although many toothpastes include fluoride in their formulations, products that have obtained approval by the Council on Dental Therapeutics of the American Dental Association (ADA) should be recommended. Formulations of toothpastes that have not obtained ADA approval may impede the release of fluoride from these products, thereby compromising their effectiveness (Stookey, 1985). Currently approved fluoride toothpastes contain sodium fluoride (NaF) or sodium monofluorophosphate (MFP) as active ingredients. In the United States, the maximum allowable concentration of fluoride in toothpastes that have not received New Drug Approval from the Food and Drug Administration is 1100 parts per million (ppm) (Whall, 1992). Parents should be advised that some over-the-counter products contain higher fluoride concentrations (e.g., 1500 ppm).

FLUORIDE MOUTH RINSES

The use of fluoride mouth rinses has grown considerably as a result of increased use in the home as well as in school-based mouth-rinsing programs. The most popular preparations contain neutral NaF, although stannous fluoride and acidulated phosphate fluoride rinses also are available. Several fluoride mouth rinses, including many 0.05% NaF products, are available on an over-the-counter (nonprescription) basis.

Numerous clinical trials conducted in the 1960s and 1970s reported caries reductions in the 20% and 40% range among children in non-fluoridated areas who rinsed either weekly with a 0.2% NaF rinse or daily with a 0.05% NaF product (Driscoll, 1974; Torrell and Ericsson, 1974). More recent studies, conducted since the overall decline in dental caries in children became evident, have reported that (1) the expected benefits from fluoride rinsing in terms of the actual number of tooth surfaces saved from becoming carious are generally less than previously reported and (2) rinsing appears to have a greater effect in older children ($\geq$10 years of age) (Bell et al., 1984; Poulsen et al., 1984). Nevertheless, the observation that fluoride rinsing provides greater protection to erupting teeth during the time when rinses are being applied provides a rationale for their use in the 6- to 12-year age group.

Rinses are particularly indicated for persons deemed to be at high risk for caries. Included in this category are those who lack the motivation or manual dexterity necessary to carry out effective oral hygiene procedures, patients who wear orthodontic appliances or prostheses that may complicate the process of plaque removal, and patients who have medical conditions that place them at increased risk. Examples of persons in the last group are patients undergoing head and neck radiation therapy, which may compromise their salivary flow, and patients who are required to take frequent doses of liquid or chewable medications that have a high sugar content.

CONCENTRATED AGENTS FOR PROFESSIONAL APPLICATION OR HOME USE

Applications of more concentrated forms of fluoride should be considered for persons who cannot or do not make optimal use of the high-frequency, low-concentration forms of fluoride therapy. Generally, this implies semiannual applications of concentrated fluoride gels or forms in the dental office. Fluoride varnish applications have also been suggested for high-risk patients (see Chapter 14).

Several fluoride gels and solutions, including combinations of acidulated phosphate fluoride and stannous fluoride, are available for home use. Practitioners should be aware that some of these products contain concentrations of fluoride that are similar to those found in fluoride toothpastes or over-the-counter rinses, and in most cases they have not undergone clinical testing. Some of these low-concentration products have also been advocated for professional application, but they are unlikely to be effective when used infrequently (Crall and Bjerga, 1984). Therefore, the advantage of these less-concentrated products over commercially available fluoride toothpastes and mouth rinses is questionable. More concentrated fluoride gels (0.5% APF) have been shown to be effective in reducing the incidence of caries and may be useful in high-risk patients with rampant caries.

HOME CARE

With school activities now emerging as a major influence in the daily schedule of the child, routine personal hygiene must be scheduled. The development of a routine ideally has been reinforced with the routines established during the preschool period. Unfortunately, it is not only the school activity that fills the daily schedule. Music lessons, sports activities, dancing and singing lessons, homework, religious instruction, daily chores, babysitting, and delivering newspapers all begin to influence the daily schedule and the time remaining for personal hygiene.

Although brushing after all meals is ideal, such a schedule is probably unrealistic. A compromise needs to be worked out. An appropriate recommendation would be for a thorough cleaning of the teeth and massaging of the gingiva before bed with additional brushing after breakfast and after the evening meal. Brushing after lunch in school is inappropriate because most children do not remember to bring their toothbrush and they are more interested in physical activity after lunch. Swishing vigorously with water after lunch helps to dislodge any large particles of food remaining and neutralize any acid that may be present.

Parents need to remain active in supervising mouth care during this period. Interference from TV, radio, and computer games cannot be tolerated. A firm stand with appropriate discipline if required is recommended to develop and maintain this important hygiene practice.

Periodic inspection of the mouth by the parent is indeed appropriate. Because fine motor activity is further developing during this period, parental assistance is required to remove all plaque, especially on the buccal surfaces of the posterior maxillary molars and the lingual surfaces of the mandibular posterior molars. Brushes of the appropriate size and contour should be selected to meet the child's needs. With increasing oral dimensions and numbers of teeth, larger brushes should be considered. Soft nylon bristled brushes are recommended over other varieties.

Although mechanical toothbrushes have been available for some time, there has been a dramatic increase in their development and promotion recently. All types, shapes, head size variations, rotations, and vibrations (oscillating and ultrasonic powered) are now available. Some are modified and promoted for children, others only for adults. Some studies show dramatic improvements in plaque removal and gingival health; others report results that are not so impressive (Grossman and Proskin, 1997). The novelty of the device may increase children's compliance with daily brushing. One has to consider the initial cost and brush head replacements when recommending a mechanical brush. Supervision by a caregiver is required for younger children. For patients with special health care needs, especially those with limited motor activity, a discussion as to the benefits is indicated with the caregiver.

With the increased size and independence of the child, the bathroom becomes the ideal location for cleaning. The previously recommended supine position to increase visibility and stability is no longer appropriate. A well-lit bathroom with a wall mirror or hand mirror greatly aids the cleaning process.

Use of disclosing tablets or solutions helps the child and parent to evaluate the thoroughness of the cleaning. At least weekly, the teeth should be disclosed, and with the parent's supervision, the child's mouth should be inspected. Areas of disclosed plaque should be noted with instructions on modification of technique so that it will be removed daily.

With the exfoliation of primary teeth and the eruption of permanent teeth, the mouth may be sore, causing the child to hesitate to do a thorough cleaning. Generally, with the "loosening" of a primary tooth, the gingiva will be tender and even swollen. Careful wiping of this area with the brush should maintain the health of the tissues. As the permanent teeth erupt, the alignment may be irregular, and the gingival tissue may lose its "knife edge" anatomy with the tooth. Instead, a ledge of gingival tissue may emerge that allows plaque to accumulate (Fig. 31-1). Careful manipulation of the brush is necessary until the gingival contour assumes a smooth margin with the tooth. In mouths with a developing discrepancy between arch length and tooth size, the malalignment of the teeth causes retention of food and plaque. Until corrected, additional manipulation of the brush by both child and parent may be necessary.

Toward the end of this period the child may have developed enough fine motor activity to be able to learn the process of flossing. Like any other motor activity, this skill must be learned and practiced frequently. Parents can be helpful in assisting the child. Inappropriate use of the floss by "snapping" it into the interproximal surfaces can injure the gingiva. Once passed through the contact, the floss must be carefully manipulated along one surface of the tooth and then the opposite surface, making sure that it reaches the area just under the gingival crevice. One of the many commercially available floss holders may greatly assist in the process.

Children with developmental disabilities may require partial or total assistance in oral care, depending on their mental and physical capabilities. If a parent must either help with or be totally responsible for mouth care, a mouth prop may be helpful (Fig. 31-2). With good head stability and mouth propping, the cleaning process is enhanced. With severely disabled children, more than one person may be necessary. Stabilization and proper positioning may be necessary, and if so, the bathroom may be an inappropriate location. The bedroom or other living area with available floor space, beds, or couches allows the child to be placed in a supine position and stabilized. In these situations the use of a dentifrice further complicates the process because of the foaming and the need to expectorate.

Last, as the child extends his or her social activities, overnight, weekend, or extended periods away from home occur. As they "pack their bags," toothbrushes, dentifrices, and floss will probably be thought of last, if at all. Again, parents must be responsible for making sure that the appropriate tools are available; whether they will be used is another question.

DIET

Although children are introduced to a new variety of foods during the preschool years, it is during this period, the primary grades, that the

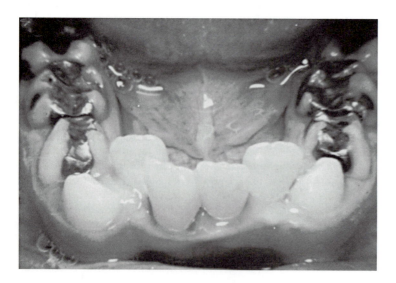

Figure 31–1. Early mixed dentition. Note crowding of teeth and ledge of gingiva.

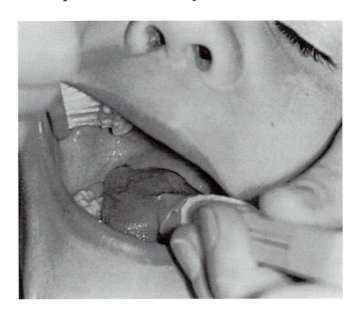

Figure 31–2. A tongue blade mouth prop can be used to facilitate mouth care in a disabled child.

real challenge to well-established dietary habits begins. Again, exposure to a full day in school with frequent treats and school lunches, either from home or purchased at school, and a multitude of after-school activities, usually associated with food, all influence the child's eventual dietary habits. In addition, the child is heavily influenced by the commercial media, especially television. The effect of food choices and purchases has been carefully studied, and although advocacy organizations have attempted to influence the number of commercials related to food shown during the daytime hours, it remains common for the school age child to be exposed to many enticements during a period of TV or radio entertainment. If children accompany parents to the market, a practice not encouraged, the purchases they request are frequently related to television and radio commercials.

Although some dramatic changes have occurred recently in food selection and dietary practices, we know that a large percentage of a family's meals are eaten on the run or in fast food restaurants, seldom with the entire family present, and too often in front of the television set. Per capita consumption of sweeteners is around 150 pounds annually (U.S. Bureau of Census, 1997), although there has been a substantial decrease in the use of ordinary refined table sugar. Annual per capita consumption of soft drinks has increased since the early 1970s from 22.7 gallons to 52.5 gallons in 1996. Forty-four percent of the sweeteners used are refined sugar from sugar cane and beets; 56% are from corn sweeteners. High daily rates of consumption and between-meal intake of sugars remain a risk fac-

tor for children susceptible to proximal caries even though caries development is now declining in the United States (Burt et al., 1988). Nevertheless, caries rates have been dramatically reduced during the last 15 years even as dramatic changes have been taking place in our dietary practices. Can we as dentists make any further impact on the way children eat and what they eat?

For children with a severe caries problem, the dentist must evaluate all etiologic factors, including diet and dietary practices. As reported earlier, the dietary history, whether a 24-hour recall or a 5-day history, is recommended. Once received, the dentist or a designated staff person reviews the history with the parent, paying particular attention to the number of exposures to carbohydrates per day and when they were eaten, whether during meals, after meals, or between meals. Every exposure to a food containing a refined carbohydrate, especially one that adheres to the teeth and dissolves slowly, produces acid in and around the plaque. If a pattern emerges, it should be defined and recommendations for substitute foods or modifications of a dietary practice should be provided. Identifying particular areas of concern and providing specific recommendations will be accepted more readily by both parent and child than sweeping changes of the entire diet. A series of small changes, successfully made over a period of time, eventually leads to a better diet for dental health.

A favorite activity of many school age children is gum chewing. Although frowned on by school officials and parents, it does in fact have an anti-caries effect. Studies have reported an increase in salivary flow and mechanical pumping of saliva to the interproximal sites. This results in a neutralization of interproximal acids. These studies have used both sugarless and sugar-containing gums. All studies agree on the beneficial effects of sugarless gums; but a difference of opinion exists on the effect of sugar-containing gums (Beiswanger et al., 1996; Jensen, 1986; Jensen and Wefel, 1989).

As we learn more about the cariogenic potential of foods, foods "safe for teeth" will be identified and marketed. In the meantime, it is unrealistic to recommend to a parent of a 6- or 7-year-old child to cut out all candy and baked goods. It is better to advise them of possible substitutes—for example, a chocolate candy instead of a caramel—or intake of candy and baked goods only after meals have been eaten and not before or between meals. Children can learn appropriate eating habits, but the habits must be realistic, and the parents must be enthusiastic about the change (Singleton et al., 1992). Regarding meals at school, the parent must work with school authorities to provide wholesome and nutritious meals that also have eye appeal for the child. In addition, parents should work with specific teachers to encourage use of appropriate snacks and party foods for special occasions.

The diets of children with developmental disabilities may be modified for a number of reasons. To increase caloric requirements, supplements are frequently added to routine foods. Unfortunately, these supplements are frequently refined carbohydrates, which increase the risk of acid production. Foods may be altered, minced, pureed, or mashed to assist the child in swallowing and to meet the need for less chewing. Because of these modifications, retention of food in the mouth is enhanced and oral clearance decreased. Because of chewing and swallowing difficulties, fresh fruits and vegetables are withheld from the diet. Substitutes include pastries, canned fruits, puddings, and gelatin desserts, all with a high percentage of refined carbohydrates. The dentist and his or her staff must be aware of these modifications and be realistic in providing dietary recommendations to parents of children with developmental disabilities.

REFERENCES

Beiswanger BB, Elias A, Crawford JL, et al: The effects of sugarless chewing gum use after meals on dental caries. J Dent Res 75:(Special Edition): 1003, 1996.

Bell RM, Klein SP, Bohannan HM, et al: Treatment Effects in the National Preventive Dentistry Demonstration Program. Santa Monica, Rand Corporation, 1984.

Burt BA, Eklund SA, Morgan KJ, et al: The effects of sugar intake and frequency of ingestion on dental caries increment in a three-year longitudinal study. J Dent Res 67:1422–1429, 1988.

Clarkson BH: Fluoride: Biological implications and dietary supplementation. *In* Pinkham JR (ed): Pediatric Dental Care: An Update for the 90's. Evansville, IN, Bristol-Myers Squibb Co, 1991, pp 23–24.

Crall JJ, Bjerga JM: Fluoride uptake and retention following combined applications of APF and stannous fluoride in vitro. Pediatr Dent 6:226–229, 1984.

Driscoll WS: The use of fluoride tablets for the prevention of dental caries. *In* Forrester DJ, Schultz EM Jr (eds): International Workshop on Fluorides and Dental Caries Reductions. Baltimore, University of Maryland, 1974.

Grossman E, Proskin H: A comparison of the efficacy and safety of an electric and manual children's toothbrush. JADA 128:469–474, 1997.

Hunt CE, Navia JM: Pre-eruptive effects of Mo, B, Sr, and F on dental caries in the rat. Arch Oral Biol 20:497–501, 1975.

Jensen ME: Responses of interproximal plaque pH to snack foods and effect of chewing sorbitol-containing gum. JADA 113:262–266, 1986.

Jensen ME, Wefel JS: Human plaque pH responses to meals and the effects of chewing gum. Br Dent J 167:204–208, 1989.

Poulsen S, Kirkegaard E, Bangsbo G, et al: Caries clinical trial of fluoride rinses in a Danish public child dental service. Commun Dent Oral Epidemiol 12:283–287, 1984.

Singleton JC, Achterberg L, Shannon B: Role of food and nutrition in the health perceptions of young children. J Am Diet Assoc 92:67–70, 1992.

Stookey GK: Are all fluoride dentifrices the same? *In* Wei SHY (ed): Clinical Uses of Fluoride. Philadelphia, Lea & Febiger, 1985, pp 105–131.

Torrell P, Ericsson Y: The potential benefits to be derived from fluoride mouth rinses. *In* Forrester DJ, Schultz EM Jr (eds): International Workshop on Fluorides and Dental Caries Reductions. Baltimore, University of Maryland, 1974.

U.S. Bureau of the Census, Statistical Abstract of the United States: 1997 (117th edition), Washington, DC, 1997.

van Eck AAMJ, Groenveld A, Backer Dirks O: Pre- and post-eruptive caries reduction by water fluoridation [Abstract 28]. Caries Res 19:163, 1985.

Whall C: Personal communications. ADA Council on Dental Therapeutics, 1992.

Chapter 32

The Acid-Etch Technique in Caries Prevention: Pit and Fissure Sealants and Preventive Restorations

M. John Hicks and Catherine M. Flaitz

Chapter Outline

Increasingly, the attention of the dental profession has been directed toward prevention of dental caries in pits and fissures. For a number of decades, the prime area of concern has been related to reducing the incidence and prevalence of caries occurring in smooth surfaces. The most recent national surveys during the past several decades on caries incidence and prevalence in pediatric and adolescent groups have shown dramatic reductions in dental caries, especially with respect to smooth surface lesions (National Institute of Dental Research [NIDR], 1989, 1981; National Center for Health Statistics [NCHS], 1974, 1971; Gift and Newman, 1992; Li et al., 1993; Kaste et al., 1996; Brown et al., 1996).

This significant change in the caries status of children and adolescents has been attributed to a number of factors (Hicks et al., 1985; Hicks and Flaitz, 1993). First, this generation of children may have benefited from the optimal use of both systemic and topical fluorides. Second, parents have become increasingly aware of the importance of and need for both preventive and restorative dental care for their young children. Thus, parents bring their children to the dentist at an earlier age when perhaps only preventive measures or minimal restorative procedures are indicated. In addition, the dentist is provided an opportunity to educate both parents and children about the preventive practices available to minimize the caries experience for the child and adolescent. Third, group dental insurance, managed care, and government-funded programs that include expanded preventive and restorative dental care for young children are now common. The availability of such programs has removed some of the financial burden for children's dental care from the family. Fourth, the increase in dental manpower and availability has allowed easy access to state-of-the-art dental care in both urban and rural communities. Finally, the interest of the dental profession in preventive dentistry has increased as the beneficial effects of preventive regimens on dental disease have become evident and both the scientific and the clinical bases of these regimens have been demonstrated.

EPIDEMIOLOGY OF PIT AND FISSURE CARIES

Tooth surfaces with pits and fissures are particularly vulnerable to caries development. With the permanent dentition, caries involving the occlusal surfaces accounts for almost 60% of the total caries experience in children and adolescents according to the 1986–87 NIDR and 1988–91

Third National Health and Nutrition Examination Survey (NHANES III) (Table 32–1). Previously, in the 1974 NCHS survey, occlusal caries represented 49% of total caries. The increased proportion of caries experience attributed to pit and fissure caries is most likely due to the decreasing prevalence of caries with interproximal surfaces. Between the 1974 and 1980 surveys, a 53% reduction in interproximal caries occurred. A further reduction of 50% in interproximal caries occurred between 1980 and 1987 for all children. Surprisingly, interproximal caries declined an additional 25% from 1987 to 1991 (Brown et al., 1996; Kaste et al., 1996). When considering children residing in fluoridated communities, the prevalence of interproximal caries decreased by 75% between 1980 and 1987 and by 88% from 1974 to 1987.

In fluoride-deficient communities, the reduction in interproximal caries was 37% between 1980 and 1987 (see Table 32–1) and may reflect the influence of fluoridated toothpastes, fluoride rinses, school-based water fluoridation programs, and professionally applied topical fluoride. From the information provided by the 1987 NIDR study, interproximal caries were decreased by 60% in fluoridated communities, whereas buccal or lingual and occlusal caries were decreased by only 10% in these fluoridated communities. This discrepancy emphasizes the fact that enamel forming pits and fissures does not receive the same level of caries protection from fluoride as does smooth surface enamel. This finding may also partially explain the fact that occlusal caries are responsible for almost 60% of the total caries experience, although occlusal surfaces account for only 12.5% of the total number of tooth surfaces exposed to cariogenic challenges. The reason for this increased susceptibility is the presence of pits and fissures in these surfaces. When caries occurring in pits and fissures on buccal and lingual surfaces are considered, pit and fissure caries account for over 80% of the total caries experience in all children and adolescents (Bell et al., 1984; Brown et al., 1996; Kaste et al., 1996). In fluoridated communities, over 90% of dental caries occur in occlusal and buccal-lingual surfaces and represent, almost exclusively, pit and fissure caries (NIDR 1989; Brown et al., 1996; Kaste et al., 1996). According to NHANES III (Brown et al., 1996; Kaste et al., 1996), 88% of caries are found in surfaces associated with pit and fissure caries in children and adolescents. From 1987 to 1991, interproximal caries was reduced by 25%, whereas pit and fissure caries decreased by 18%.

In contrast with the permanent dentition, in-

TABLE 32–1. Distribution of Dental Caries in Schoolchildren in the United States by Surface Type

	Occlusal (DMFS)	Buccal/Lingual (DMFS)	Proximal (DMFS)
NCHS 1971-74	49% (3.5)	27% (1.9)	24% (1.7)
NIDR 1979-80	54% (2.6)	29% (1.4)	17% (0.8)
NIDR 1986-87			
All children	58% (1.8)	29% (0.9)	13% (0.4)
Fluoridated	60% (1.7)	31% (0.9)	9% (0.2)
Nonfluoridated	56% (1.9)	30% (1.0)	14% (0.5)
NHANES III 1988-91	56% (1.4)	32% (0.8)	12% (0.3)

Compiled from NCHS 1971, 1974; NIDR 1981, 1989; JADA *127*:335, 1996; J Dent Res *75*(Spec Iss): 631, 652, 1996.

terproximal caries are more common in the primary dentition (Table 32-2). In regional and national surveys (Traubman et al., 1989; Brown et al., 1996; Kaste et al., 1996), caries experience is distributed almost equally among occlusal (35–40%), buccal/lingual (26–29%), and proximal (35%) tooth surfaces. Water fluoridation reduces interproximal caries in primary teeth by 45%. In contrast, occlusal caries in fluoridated communities is decreased by 23%, whereas buccal/lingual caries is reduced by 32%. Pit and fissure caries in occlusal and buccal/lingual surfaces of primary teeth probably accounts for the lessened caries-preventive effect of water fluoridation that occurs in these surfaces when compared with interproximal surfaces.

Pit and fissure caries represent a disease process that has an early onset. Approximately one fifth of children between the ages of 2 and 4 years have experienced caries in the primary dentition. In this age group, caries in occlusal surfaces alone may account for up to 67% of lesions. With the permanent dentition, 65% of first molars in 12-year-old adolescents either have been restored or currently have occlusal caries. In fact, in elementary schoolchildren from a flu-

oridated community, 90% of all lesions in the first permanent molars have been found to be pit and fissure caries (Brown et al., 1996; Kaste et al., 1996; Greenwall et al., 1990; Louie et al., 1990; Traubman et al., 1989; Johnsen et al., 1987; Bohannon et al., 1984; Graves and Burt, 1975; Hennon et al., 1969).

Although previously the incidence of pit and fissure caries in occlusal surfaces was thought to be greatest during the first 4 years after eruption, recent longitudinal studies of caries development in occlusal surfaces of permanent molars (Table 32-3) provide some interesting findings (Vehkalahti et al., 1991; Stahl and Katz, 1992, 1993; Foreman, 1994). The annual incidence of caries development in sound occlusal and interproximal surfaces has been determined over an 8-year period (Vehkalahti et al., 1991). The development of pit and fissure caries in sound occlusal surfaces occurred at a rate of 15% and 10% for ages 8 and 9 years, respectively. From ages 10 through 15 years, pit and fissure caries continued to occur in previously sound first permanent molars at a rate of 4.3% to 6.8% per year. In contrast, interproximal caries occurred at an annual rate of 0.3% to 2.4%. When sound first

TABLE 32–2. Prevalence and Distribution of Caries for Primary Teeth

	Decayed Filled Surfaces, Primary Teeth	Caries-Free	Caries Distribution by Surface		
			Occlusal	*Buccal/Lingual*	*Proximal*
Head Start Program (1990)					
Fluoride-deficient community	7.44	30.4%	35.3%	25.0%	39.5%
Fluoridated community	4.80	36.1%	41.0%	26.3%	32.7%
All children	5.67	34.2%	39.2%	25.9%	34.9%
NHANES III (1988–91)					
2- to 4-year-olds	1.2	83.1%	25.0%	36.5%	36.5%
5- to 9-year-olds	4.1	50.3%	39.0%	24.4%	36.6%
2- to 9-year-olds	3.1	62.1%	35.5%	29.0%	35.5%

Compiled from J Public Health Dent *50*:299, 1990; JADA *127*:335, 1996; J Dent Res *75*(Spec Iss):631, 652, 1996.

TABLE 32–3. Annual Attack Rate of Occlusal and Interproximal Caries Development in Sound Permanent First Molars

Age	Occlusal Surfaces (Caries Incidence)	Interproximal Surfaces (Caries Incidence)
Annual attack rate in 8- to 15-year-olds		
8-year-olds	15.0%	0.3%
9-year-olds	10.1%	1.1%
10-year-olds	5.8%	0.9%
11-year-olds	6.4%	0.9%
12-year-olds	5.2%	2.4%
13-year-olds	5.9%	1.8%
14-year-olds	4.3%	1.3%
15-year-olds	6.8%	2.1%
Average annual attack rate during 8 years		
	5.9%	1.3%
Total percentage with caries after 8 years		
	47%	10%
Prevalence of occlusal caries in molars of young adults		
Coast Guard cadets (Age range 17 to 23 years)		
All molars	11.9%	—
First molars	9.9%	—
Second molars	14.0%	—
Young military recruits (Mean age 20.9 years)		
Permanent molars	25.4%	—

Compiled from J Dent Res *70:*1064, 1991; JADA *125:*182, 1994; J Public Health Dent *53:*212, 1993.

permanent molars were followed in children from age 8 to 15 years, it was found that 47% of occlusal surfaces had developed pit and fissure caries, whereas only 10% of interproximal surfaces had succumbed to caries during this same time period. The mean annual incidence of caries development in previously sound first permanent molars was 5.9% for occlusal surfaces and 1.3% for interproximal surfaces.

A separate clinical study (see Table 32–3) evaluated the development of occlusal caries in college-age young adults ranging in age from 17 to 23 years (Stahl and Katz, 1992, 1993). During the 40-month study period, 32.9% of the young adults developed occlusal caries without radiographic evidence of interproximal lesions in permanent molars and premolars. An additional 9.8% developed occlusal caries with radiographic evidence of interproximal lesions. In this group of persons, it appears that sealant placement during late adolescence or early adulthood would have prevented restoration of the occlusal surfaces in over 75% of cases. The incidence of occlusal caries development without interproximal lesions was found to be 9.9% for first permanent molars 11 to 16 years after eruption, 14.0% for second permanent molars 5 to 10 years after

eruption, and 0.8% for premolars 7 to 12 years after eruption. In another study (see Table 32-3) of young military recruits (mean age 20.9 years, age range 17–25 years), new occlusal caries was identified in 25% of permanent molars (Foreman, 1994). It was also noted that at least one first or second molar needed sealant placement in 47% of the recruits. In almost one third of these young adults, occlusal caries could have been prevented by sealant application. Although the majority of pit and fissure caries was previously thought to occur within 4 years after eruption, these epidemiologic studies emphasize that pit and fissure caries continues to occur throughout late adolescence and well into early adulthood. In fact, it was found that 30% of the 24- to 25-year-old military recruits would benefit from sealant placement. The question of whether to place a sealant over a fissured surface should not be based on how long ago a tooth erupted into the oral cavity but on the clinical impression of whether a sealant is deemed necessary to prevent caries.

MORPHOLOGY OF SURFACES WITH PITS AND FISSURES

The dental profession has known for some time that susceptibility to caries on tooth surfaces containing pits and fissures is related to the form and depth of these pits and fissures. Because of the interest in caries formation in pits and fissures, attempts have been made to provide an elaborate classification system of pits and fissures. For the sake of simplicity, however, two main types of pits and fissures (Fig. 32-1) are usually described: (1) shallow, wide V-shaped fissures that tend to be self-cleansing and somewhat caries-resistant, and (2) deep, narrow I-shaped fissures that are quite constricted and may resemble a bottleneck in that the fissure may have an extremely narrow slitlike opening with a larger base as it extends toward the dentinoenamel junction. These caries-susceptible, I-shaped fissures may also have a number of different branches. The typical fissure usually contains an organic plug composed of reduced enamel epithelium, microorganisms forming dental plaque, and oral debris. Examination of fissures, even with a low level of magnification, reveals the reason for the caries susceptibility of tooth surfaces with pits and fissures. The fissure provides a protected niche for plaque accumulation. The rapidity with which dental caries occur in pits and fissures is most likely related to the fact that the depth of the fissure is close to

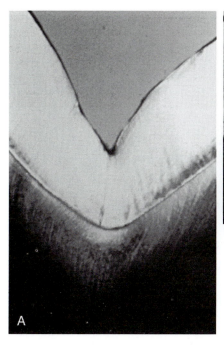

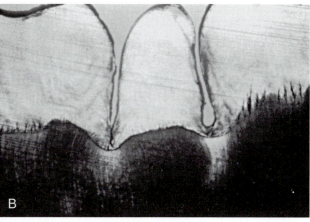

Figure 32–1. Histologic appearance of the main types of pits and fissures in occlusal surfaces (polarized light microscopy; water imbibition). *A*, Shallow, wide V-shaped fissure. *B*, Deep, narrow I-shaped fissure.

the dentinoenamel junction and the underlying dentin, which is highly susceptible to caries (Rohr et al., 1991; Hicks and Flaitz, 1986; Ngano, 1961; Galil and Gwinnett, 1975).

The morphology of occlusal surfaces varies from one tooth to the next and from individual to individual. In general, however, the "typical" premolar (Fig. 32-2*A*) has a prominent primary fissure with usually three or four pits. In the typical molar (Fig. 32-2*B*), as many as 10 separate pits may be present in primary, secondary, and supplemental fissures. In addition, certain surface porosities that would not be noticed clinically become apparent when the surface is examined microscopically.

HISTOPATHOLOGY OF CARIES IN PITS AND FISSURES

At one time, caries formation in fissures was thought to begin at the base of the fissure, involving the deeper aspect of the underlying tooth structure before the walls and cuspal inclines of the fissure became involved by the caries process. This process was expected because the fissure extended into the tooth surface for a considerable depth. Such is not the case, however. Rather, the inclines forming the walls of the fissures are affected first by the caries process. The first histologic evidence of lesion formation occurs at the orifice of the fissure and is usually

represented by two independent bilateral lesions in the enamel composing the opposing cuspal inclines (Fig. 32-3*A*). As the lesion progresses, the depths of the fissure walls become involved, and coalescence of the two independent lesions into a single, contiguous lesion occurs at the base of the fissure. The enamel at the base of the fissure is affected to a greater degree than that of the cuspal inclines, and the lesion spreads laterally along the enamel adjacent to the depth of the fissure and readily toward the dentinoenamel junction (Fig. 32-3*B*). Once the caries process involves the dentin, the progress of the lesion is enhanced because caries susceptibility of dentin is increased compared with enamel. Eventually, cavitation of the fissure occurs owing to loss of mineral and structural support from the adjacent affected enamel and dentin, resulting in a clinically detectable lesion. The unique process of caries formation in pits and fissures is due to the presence of an organic plug in the fissure. This organic plug acts as a buffer against the acid byproducts of plaque and provides a diffusion barrier, which results in a lessened acid attack at the fissural base during the initial phase of caries formation (Hicks and Flaitz, 1986).

Although systemic and topical fluoride use has been shown to be highly effective in prevention of caries on smooth surfaces, enamel surfaces with pits and fissures receive minimal caries protection from either systemic or topical fluoride agents. The reason why fluoride is less effective

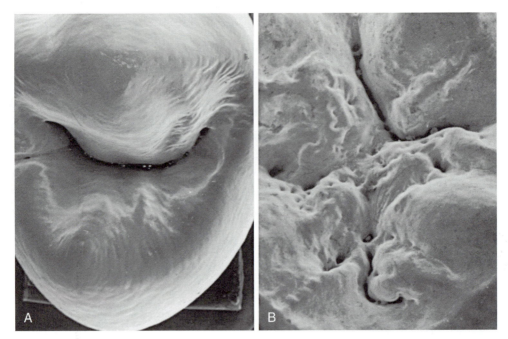

Figure 32–2. Surface morphologic appearance of caries-free premolar *(A)* and permanent molar *(B)* (scanning electron microscopy).

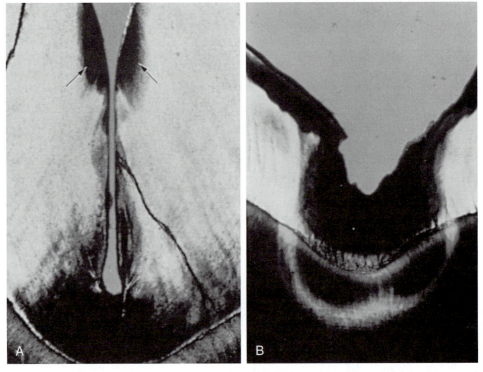

Figure 32–3. Histologic appearance of pit and fissure caries (polarized light microscopy; water imbibition). *A,* Caries formation *(arrows)* begins in the cuspal inclines just above the fissure orifice. The darkened appearance at the base of the fissure is due to the organic material present. *B,* The lesion progresses to the point at which the base of the fissure and underlying dentin become involved. With further progression, cavitation will occur, resulting in a clinically detectable lesion.

in preventing caries in fissured surfaces may be related to the total depth of enamel on smooth surfaces compared with that underlying the fissure (Hicks and Flaitz, 1986; Silverstone, 1984a–c). On smooth surfaces, at least 1 mm of enamel is found superficial to the dentinoenamel junction. In contrast, the base of a fissure or pit may be relatively close to or lie within the dentin. When caries develops in a fissure, the underlying dentin becomes involved rapidly, resulting in a frank, clinically detectable lesion. When caries formation occurs in enamel on a smooth surface, a considerable amount of enamel must become involved before the dentin is involved. It is thought that 3 or 4 years may be required for dentinal involvement to occur. During this time period, remineralization of the smooth surface lesion may occur after exposure to fluoride agents, resulting in the arrest or reversal of the lesion. When pits and fissures are present on smooth surfaces (Fig. 32–4), the pattern of involvement is identical to that seen on occlusal surfaces, and progression of the lesion to a clinically detectable level appears to be related to the lessened thickness of the enamel present and the morphologic form of the pit or fissure.

PREVENTION OF PIT AND FISSURE CARIES: HISTORICAL PERSPECTIVE AND PIT AND FISSURE SEALANT MATERIALS

During the 1920s, two different clinical techniques were introduced in an attempt to reduce the extent and severity of pit and fissure caries in occlusal and smooth surfaces. In 1924, Thaddeus Hyatt advocated prophylactic restorations. This procedure consisted of preparing a conservative Class I cavity that included all pits and fissures at risk for caries development and then placing an amalgam restoration. The rationale for prophylactic restoration of an otherwise caries-free surface was that the procedure prevented further insult to the pulp from caries, decreased loss of tooth structure, and required less time for restoration when the tooth eventually succumbed to caries. A more conservative approach to prevention of pit and fissure caries was presented by Bodecker in 1929. Initially, he advocated cleaning the fissure with an explorer and flowing a thin mix of oxyphosphate cement into the fissure—essentially an attempt to "seal" the fissure. Later, he introduced an alternative method for caries prevention, the prophylactic odontotomy, which involved mechanical eradication of fissures in order to transform deep, retentive fissures into cleansable ones. These two techniques, prophylactic restoration and prophylactic odontotomy, were employed until the use of sealants became prevalent.

The development of pit and fissure sealants was based on the discovery that etching enamel with phosphoric acid increased the retention of resin restorative materials and improved marginal integrity considerably. The initial studies evaluating the effects of acid-etching on enamel were performed by Buonocore in 1955. The first sealant material that involved the acid-etch technique was introduced in the mid-1960s and was a cyanoacrylate substance. Cyanoacrylates were not suitable as sealant materials owing to bacterial degradation of the material in the oral cavity over time. By the late 1960s, a number of different resin materials had been tested, and a viscous resin was found to be resistant to degradation and produced a tenacious bond with etched enamel. This resin was formed by reacting bisphenol A with glycidyl methacrylate, and this class of dimethacrylate resins has become known as BIS-GMA (Bowen, 1982).

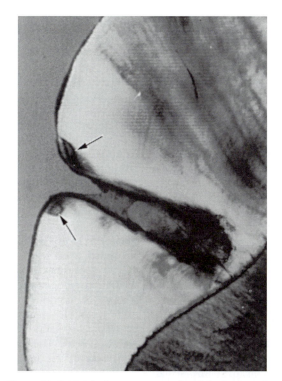

Figure 32–4. Histologic appearance of a pit in the buccal surface of a permanent molar tooth. Caries formation *(arrows)* is evident at the orifice of the fissure. An organic plug is present in the fissure. The base of the pit approaches the dentinoenamel junction (polarized light microscopy; water imbibition).

BIS-GMA is a relatively large epoxy resin-like hybrid monomer in which epoxy groups are replaced by methacrylate groups. BIS-GMA incorporates the rapid polymerization characteristic of methylmethacrylate with the minimal polymerization shrinkage property of epoxy resins. The vast majority of restorative resins are based on the BIS-GMA formulation. They differ from sealants in that restorative resin materials include filler particles such as quartz, glass, and porcelain to improve their strength, whereas the majority of sealants either are unfilled BIS-GMA or have relatively few filler particles added. A few of the sealant products, however, contain up to 50% filler particles in an attempt to improve wear resistance.

BIS-GMA sealants differ in the ways in which the material is polymerized. Two methods of polymerization have been employed. Autopolymerization (chemically cured) systems involve mixing two liquids, a base resin and catalyst resin. The material sets by an exothermic reaction, usually within 1 to 2 minutes. Photoactivated (visible light–cured) polymerization is currently the most popular method used for curing sealants. During the 1970s and early 1980s, ultraviolet light with a wavelength of 365 nm was used to initiate the setting reaction. Because of the inconsistency of the wavelength from the ultraviolet light source and the potential for retinal damage with long-term exposure to ultraviolet light, however, this method of curing sealants was abandoned. In its place, photoactivation of sealant material with a visible light source was introduced.

Photoactivated resins use a diketone initiator such as camphoroquinone and a reducing agent such as a tertiary amine to initiate polymerization. This photoinitiator system is sensitive to light in the blue region of the visible light spectrum, with peak initiator activity centered around 480 nm. Use of visible light sources requires eye protection because of the intensity of the light created. The benefits of light-cured versus chemical-cured sealants are the following: (1) the sealant material sets in 10 to 20 seconds, (2) no mixing of resins is required, eliminating the incorporation of air bubbles that may occur with chemical-cured materials, and (3) the viscosity of the sealant remains constant during infiltration of the etched enamel pores, and the sealant does not set until it is light-activated. The disadvantage of light-cured sealants is the cost of the visible light unit. A number of units may be needed in a dental practice if sealants are placed by auxiliaries.

Laser-curing of visible light–activated sealant and resin materials has been advocated (Hicks et al., 1993; Blankenau et al., 1991; Westerman et al., 1991; Kelsey et al., 1989; Powell et al., 1989). In particular, the argon laser produces a visible blue-green light beam with a monochromatic wavelength similar to that used with visible light sources. The laser light beam also exhibits coherence and may be collimated and focused to a small spot size. The advantages of using a laser for initiating the setting reaction of sealants and restorative resins are (1) a further reduction in the setting time, (2) control over specific radiation energy, wavelength, and area of exposure, and (3) a decrease in the percentage of unpolymerized resin compared with conventional visible light curing. In addition, resin materials exposed to the laser have increased tensile and bond strengths (Kelsey et al., 1989) and lased enamel along the sealant interface and forming the adjacent tooth surface has increased resistance to a cariogenic challenge (Westerman et al., 1991, Hicks et al., 1993). The disadvantages of using a laser for curing resin materials are the cost of the instrument itself and the need for adequate training in laser operation and safety techniques. In the future, the laser may become more common in dental practices and may eventually replace visible light sources for polymerization of resin materials.

Opaque, tinted, and clear sealant materials are commercially available. Opaque and tinted sealants have been advocated because of their ease of detection by the dentist, parents, and child, which allows monitoring of sealant retention. Detection of a clear sealant requires tactile exploration of the sealed surface. A study has shown that the error rate among dentists in identifying the presence or absence of sealants is 1.4% for opaque sealants and 22.8% for clear sealants (Rock et al., 1989). No apparent differences have been reported among opaque, tinted, or clear sealants for retention rates and caries prevention.

In addition to BIS-GMA sealants, conventional glass ionomer materials have also been used as pit and fissure sealants. Glass ionomers bond to both enamel and dentin by physicochemical mechanisms following polyacrylic acid conditioning (Lacy and Young, 1996; McLean, 1994; Forsten, 1994; Burgess et al., 1994; Erickson and Glasspoole, 1994; Hicks et al., 1986). The primary advantage of glass ionomers over conventional BIS-GMA sealants is the ability of glass ionomers to release fluoride. These materials are formed by reacting calcium aluminosilicate with polyacrylic acid in the presence of a fluoride flux. The ionomer powder is created by heating a variable mixture of silica, alumina, calcium fluoride as a flux, cryolite, sodium fluoride, and/or aluminum phosphate to 1100°C to 1500°C. The liquid component is a copolymer of acrylic and itacronic acid or copolymers of maleic and tricarboxylic acids. The liquid component may be freeze-dried and incorporated into the powder. In this situation, a dilute solution of water and tartaric acid as a chelating agent is used to activate the chemical acid-base setting reaction. The resulting material may contain as much as 19% fluoride by weight. This fluoride is readily exchangeable for hydroxyl and chloride ions from the adjacent enamel and dentin. Incorporation of the released fluoride into the adjacent enamel and dentin may enhance caries resistance, remineralize enamel caries and affected dentin, and alter the bacterial composition and metabolic byproducts of plaque (Hicks et al., 1986). The role of glass ionomer "sealants" is currently being defined. Their potential for caries reduction in pits and fissures seems to be high, depending on their long-term retention rate and wear resistance.

Hybrid materials composed of a variable mixture of glass ionomer and composite resin have been advocated as possible pit and fissure sealants because of the improved physical characteristics over glass ionomers, relative ease of placement, adhesive compatibility with various dental substrates, and fluoride-releasing capability (Lacy and Young, 1996; McLean, 1994; Forsten, 1994; Burgess et al., 1994; Erickson and Glasspoole, 1994). Such resin ionomers may be classified into resin-modified ionomers and ionomer-modified resins. The liquid component in both types are acidic monomers (hydroxyethyl methacrylate [HEMA], water, and polyacrylate acid analog with or without pendant methacrylate groups) that may copolymerize with dentin-bonding agents, unfilled bonding resins, or restorative composites and react chemically via an ionomer-type of acid-base reaction with glass fillers (fluoroaluminosilicate glass). The setting reaction is initiated by photoactivation of the resin component through methacrylate groups grafted onto the polyacrylic acid chain and methacrylate groups derived from HEMA. This is followed by an acid-base reaction between the filler and the matrix. Some materials also undergo chemical autocuring via generation of free radical methacrylates that induce polymerization of the resin matrix polymer system and HEMA. Therefore, it is possible that a resin may undergo dual-curing or even tri-curing with chemically cured resin or photoactivated resin, or both types of curing in the presence of a chemical acid-base reaction characteristic of ionomers. These resin-modified ionomers still require a weak acid pretreatment of the tooth structure and visible light curing; however, these materials are considered to be less technique-sensitive than conventional glass ionomers. Ionomer-modified resins are also known as compomers and are composed of a glass filler with an anhydrous acid monomer matrix. The setting reaction between the glass filler and matrix occurs slowly while absorbing water after placement. Etching of dental substrates and placement of bonding primers may be necessary for long-term retention. Although the bond strength of compomers is higher than that for conventional glass ionomers, the occlusal wear resistance is considered to be low.

Selection of a specific sealant product depends on whether the practitioner prefers an opaque, tinted, or clear sealant that is filled or unfilled and whether he or she prefers visible-light curing or autopolymerization of the sealant material. The overall decision should be based on retention rates and caries incidences from longitudinal clinical trials. A number of sealant products (Table 32–4) have met certain biologic, laboratory, and clinical guidelines established by the ADA Council on Scientific Affairs of the American Dental Association (American Dental Association, *http://www.ada.org*, 1997; Freedman, McLaughlin, 1997). Sealant materials may receive a seal of acceptance from this testing agency. Periodically, updates on various dental materials, including sealants, are published by the ADA Council on Scientific Affairs (American Dental Association, *http://www.ada.org*, 1997), and these may serve as guides in selecting a sealant material.

During the mid-1990s, safety concerns were expressed regarding leaching of bisphenol-A (BPA) and bisphenol-A dimethacrylate (BPA-DMA) from sealants, and a possible estrogenic effect (Olea et al., 1996). It is known that incomplete conversion of BPA during the setting reaction may allow this unreacted monomer to be released into the oral environment. BPA and BPA-DMA possess estrogen-like effects on cultures of breast cancer tumor cells, and this was the basis for the safety concerns regarding sealants and composite resins. Sophisticated analysis of seven pit and fissure sealants with high-performance liquid chromatography, ultraviolet spectral analysis, and mass spectrography provided reassuring evidence regarding the safety of these materials (Nathanson et al., 1997). BPA was below the level of detectability (<0.0001 μg BPA/mg of sealant tested) with all seven sealants. BPA-DMA was not detected in five of the seven sealants tested, with the remaining two having mean levels of 0.39 μg and 1.23 μg BPA-DMA/mg of sealant tested. This laboratory investigation used 95%

TABLE 32–4. Pit and Fissure Sealant Materials

Sealant Material	Manufacturer
ADA Seal of Acceptance	
Alpha Fluor Seal II	Confi-Dental Products Co.
Alpha-Dent Chemical Cure	Alpha-Dental Product Co.
Alpha-Dent Light Cure	Alpha-Dental Product Co.
Baritone L3	Confi-Dental Products Co.
Concise Light Cure White Sealant	3M Dental Products Division
Concise White Sealant	3M Dental Products Division
Helioseal F	Ivoclar North America
Helioseal	Ivoclar North America
Prisma Shield	Dentsply LD Caulk Division
Prisma Shield Compule Tips VLC Tinted Pit and Fissure Sealant	Dentsply LD Caulk Division
Prisma Shield VLC Filled Pit and Fissure Sealant	Dentsply LD Caulk Division
Seal-Rite	Pulpdent Corporation
Seal-Rite Low Viscosity	Pulpdent Corporation
Other Sealants	
Bisco Sealant	Bisco Dental Products
Copaliner	Harry J. Bosworth Company
Delton Plus	Dentsply Cavitron/Ash
EcuSeal	Zenith/DMG
Estiseal LC	Heraeus Kulzer Inc.
Fluroseal	Scientific Pharmaceuticals Inc.
FluRestore	DenMat Corporation
Quikseal	Chameleon Dental Products
Team Sealant	Centrix
Teethmate-F	J Morita USA
Total-Seal Pit and Fissure Sealant	American Dental Hygienics
UltraSeal XT Plus Fissure Sealant	Ultradent Products Inc.

ADA Council on Scientific Affairs. Obtained from http://www.ada.org website.
Dental Products Report 1997;16:112–114.

ethanol to extract leachable components, which is a solvent for BPA and BPA-DMA. Studies using water have failed to demonstrate elution of BPA from sealants (Hamid and Hume, 1997). It appears that elution of possible estrogenic chemicals from sealants and composite resins does not require the use of different sealant materials or the restriction of sealant use in children or adults. Further clinical investigations into salivary and serum levels of leachable chemicals from dental materials would be helpful to determine whether these have any biologic effects, either short-term or long-term (Nathanson et al., 1997). To date, no adverse health effects have been attributed to the leachable components in sealants or composite resins (Nathanson et al., 1997).

DIAGNOSIS OF PIT AND FISSURE CARIES

In 1968 at an ADA-sponsored conference on clinical testing of cariostatic agents (Radike, 1972), the criteria for detection and diagnosis of pit and fissure lesions were defined as follows:

Caries is present when the explorer catches or resists removal after insertion into a pit or fissure with moderate to firm pressure and when this is accompanied by one or more of the following signs of caries: (a) softness at the base of the area; (b) opacity or loss of normal translucency adjacent to the pit or fissure as evidence of undermining or demineralization; (c) softened enamel adjacent to the pit or fissure that can be scraped away with the explorer.

Although the incidence and prevalence of pit and fissure caries and the dental technology in dealing with this type of caries have changed dramatically since 1968, the dental profession is still using more or less the same criteria for diagnosis of pit and fissure caries. Diagnosis is based on tactile evaluation with an explorer and visual assessment of the enamel appearance (visual-tactile inspection). Clinical examination varies highly from one practitioner to another owing to the size and shape of the explorer tip, the force applied, and the judgment of the examiner (Houpt et al., 1985b). In general, radiographic evaluation of occlusal surfaces has been found to be of minimal diagnostic value in detecting enamel caries and superficial dentinal caries (McKnight-Hanes et al., 1990; Flaitz et al., 1986).

Attempts to use fiberoptic transillumination to detect caries have been of value for interproximal surfaces but have failed to provide additional information about the caries status of occlusal surfaces (Rock, 1987).

Recently eliminating the explorer in evaluation of pit and fissure caries has been advocated by some for fear of damaging the enamel lining of pits and fissures, resulting in caries development and more rapid progression when enamel caries is present, and because it is thought that probing is unreliable in caries detection (Soderholm, 1995; Workshop on Guidelines for Sealant Use, 1995). Clinical and laboratory studies have indicated that there is no difference in diagnostic accuracy when dentists use either visual-tactile inspection or visual inspection alone. Perhaps this has more to do with the fact that reliability or reproducibility in diagnosis of pit and fissure caries is poor among dentists. In fact, it has been shown that with pit and fissure surfaces, caries is diagnosed correctly in only 42% of cases and only 20% to 48% of lesions histologically involving dentin are detected. It is more likely, however, that dentists will treat carious teeth than restore sound teeth (sensitivity 62%, specificity 84%). Currently, there are a number of techniques to aid the dentist in diagnosis of pit and fissure caries. These include conventional, xeroradiographic, and digital radiography; fiberoptic transillumination; laser fluorescence; caries-detecting dye penetration; ultrasonic imaging; and electrical resistance (Soderholm, 1995; Workshop on Guidelines for Sealant Use, 1995; Angmar-Mansson and ten Bosch, 1993; Peers et al., 1993).

A promising ancillary diagnostic device introduced during the 1980s was the electronic caries detector, which was touted to be superior to the explorer because of its increased sensitivity, specificity, and consistency in pit and fissure caries diagnosis (Ricketts et al., 1996; Ie et al., 1995; Lussi et al., 1995; Verdonschot et al., 1995; Angmar-Mansson and ten Bosch, 1993; Flaitz et al., 1986; White et al., 1981). In laboratory studies comparing the clinical, radiographic, and histologic appearances of occlusal caries, the electronic caries detector was found to correlate well with the extent of histologic involvement of occlusal surfaces by caries. Electronic caries detection was found to have a high sensitivity (0.70 to 1.00) and high specificity (0.71 to 0.96) when compared with histologic extent of pit and fissure caries. In comparison, conventional bitewing radiography had a sensitivity of 0.62 and a specificity of 0.77. Because of the expense of the instrument and the paucity of clinical studies,

however, the electronic caries detector has not been readily accepted as a diagnostic instrument. At this time, diagnosis of pit and fissure caries is based on visual assessment using a mouth mirror and adequate lighting as well as tactile evaluation of the pits and fissures with a sharp explorer. The most important elements in diagnosis of and treatment planning for pit and fissure caries are clinical judgment and experience.

PIT AND FISSURE TREATMENT ALTERNATIVES

With pits and fissures, a number of treatment options may be considered by the dental practitioner: (1) observation only, (2) sealant placement, (3) preventive resin restoration, (4) preventive restorations (glass ionomer-resin preventive restoration, glass ionomer preventive restoration, and sealant-amalgam preventive restoration), and (5) amalgam, glass ionomer, glass ionomer-resin, or posterior composite restoration. The diagnostic criteria and recommended treatments are presented in Table 32-5.

Indications for sealant placement (see Table 32-5; Table 32-6) include the following: (1) deep, retentive pits and fissures, which may cause wedging or catching of an explorer, (2) stained pits and fissures with minimum appearance of decalcification or opacification, (3) pit and fissure caries or restoration of pits and fissures in other primary or permanent teeth, (4) no radiographic or clinical evidence of interproximal caries in need of restoration on teeth to be sealed, (5) use of other preventive treatment, such as systemic or topical fluoride therapy, to inhibit interproximal caries formation, and (6) possibility of adequate isolation from salivary contamination. As noted previously, the development of pit and fissure caries in permanent molars may occur up to 16 years after eruption. Therefore, if a sealant appears to be indicated clinically for a premolar or first or second permanent molar in an older adolescent or adult, a sealant should be placed to avoid caries development. In the past, the philosophy applied to pit and fissures was "drill and fill." With the present state of knowledge and technology in dentistry, the current philosophy should be "seal and heal."

Contraindications for sealant placement (see Tables 32-5 and 32-6) are the following: (1) well-coalesced, self-cleansing pits and fissures, (2) radiographic or clinical evidence of interproximal caries in need of restoration, (3) presence of many interproximal lesions or restorations and no preventive treatment to inhibit interproximal

TABLE 32–5. Protocol for Pit and Fissure Treatment Alternatives

Diagnosis	Treatment
*Caries-free surface: no explorer wedging** No explorer wedging* Well-coalesced, self-cleansing shallow pits and fissures or no identifiable pits and fissures	*No treatment* *Observation* only and *re-evaluation* at 6-month recall examinations
Caries-free surface: No explorer wedging No explorer wedging Stained pits and fissures	*No treatment* *Observation* only and *re-evaluation* at 6-month recall examinations
Caries-free surface: no explorer wedging No explorer wedging Stained or minimal decalcified or opacified appearance of pits and fissures No radiographic or clinical evidence of interproximal caries	*Sealant placement* Adequate isolation from saliva: *place sealant.* Adequate isolation not possible: allow further eruption, and place sealant within 1 to 3 months
*Caries-free surface: explorer wedging** Explorer wedging due to pit and fissure anatomy Stained or decalcified appearance of pits and fissures No radiographic or clinical evidence of interproximal caries	*Sealant placement* Adequate isolation from saliva: *place sealant.* Adequate isolation not possible: *place sealant in accessible fissures* and seal remaining fissures after further eruption (within 1 to 3 months); or *remove overlying tissue and place sealant:* or *allow further eruption,* and place sealant within 1 to 3 months. *Place sealant.*
Incipient caries: minimal involvement Explorer catch† due to incipient or minimal caries involving limited areas of pits and fissures Decalcified appearance of pits and fissures indicative of incipient or minimal caries Involvement of adjacent pit and fissure enamel with possible minimal involvement of underlying enamel and dentin No or minimal undermining of isolated pits and fissures No radiographic or clinical evidence of interproximal caries Possible radiographic evidence of occlusal caries	*Preventive restoration placement* (Restoration of Isolated Pits and Fissures) Preventive resin restoration (sealant alone; sealant and filled resin) Sandwich preventive resin restoration (glass ionomer liner, filled resin and sealant) Glass ionomer preventive restoration (glass ionomer liner, glass ionomer restorative material and sealant) Sealant-amalgam preventive restoration (amalgam in isolated pits and fissures without extension for prevention and sealant) Glass ionomer resin preventive restoration
Carious surface: obvious clinical caries Explorer catch with obvious clinical caries Loss of enamel lining the pits and fissures Demineralized appearance of pits and fissures Generalized involvement of pits and fissures by caries with undermining of enamel Probable radiographic evidence of occlusal caries No radiographic or clinical evidence of interproximal caries	*Restoration* Posterior composite restoration Amalgam restoration Glass ionomer restoration Glass ionomer resin restoration Glass ionomer/posterior composite restoration

*Explorer wedging: Defined as wedging of a sharp explorer in pits or fissures on a clean, dry surface with the following characteristics: (1) pit or fissure is probed vertically, (2) explorer engages a fissure with no clinical or radiographic evidence of caries, (3) action may or may not be reproducible, (4) explorer penetrates into enamel only, and (5) probing by explorer may elicit slight discomfort.

†Explorer catch: Defined as an obvious catch of a sharp explorer in pits and fissures on a clean, dry surface with the following characteristics: (1) pit or fissure is probed vertically, (2) explorer engages a fissure with clinical evidence of incipient enamel or dentinal caries, (3) action is definitely reproducible, (4) explorer engages pit or fissure such that the explorer's weight is supported with minimal stabilization by the operator, (5) explorer penetrates both enamel and dentin, (6) pit or fissure may or may not have radiographic evidence of caries, and (7) explorer possibly elicits slight discomfort or pain on probing.

caries formation, (4) tooth partially erupted and no possibility of adequate isolation from salivary contamination. The presence of an operculum over the distal marginal ridge is associated with loss of sealant material and a reapplication rate of 54% (Dennison et al., 1990). Retreatment has been shown to be necessary in 26% of cases when gingival tissue is at the same height as the distal marginal ridge (Dennison et al., 1990).

Sealant placement should be delayed if adequate isolation and tissue retraction are not possible. If the surface is at immediate risk for caries development, surgical removal of the operculum may be necessary to provide for adequate isolation. These contraindications are relative and should be taken into consideration when pits and fissures are being evaluated for sealant placement. If the clinical impression of whether or not to

TABLE 32–6. Recommendations From Workshop on Guidelines for Sealant Use

Place Sealants

1. Questionable enamel caries in pit and fissures, but caries-free proximal surfaces
2. Enamel caries in pit and fissures, but caries-free proximal surfaces
3. Enamel caries and proximal caries not involving pit and fissures
4. Caries-free pit and fissures
   a) Pit and fissure surface morphology at risk for caries
   b) Patient's current and prior caries pattern (pit and fissure caries [≥1 lesion per year] or caries-free pattern in primary and/or permanent dentition)
   c) Eruption status of teeth adequate for sealant placement
   d) Patient's/parent's perception and desire for sealant placement
5. Medical history with factors associated with increased caries incidence or xerostomic medications
6. Routine dental care with active preventive dentistry program
7. Community-based sealant program
   a) Identify population at moderate and high risk for caries
   b) Individual caries-risk assessment
   c) Sealant placement in pits and fissures of at-risk teeth using above criteria

Do Not Place Sealants

1. Dentinal caries (consider preventive restoration, conventional restoration)
2. Proximal caries or restoration involves pit and fissures
3. Teeth cannot be isolated adequately (delay sealant until isolation possible)
4. Life expectancy of primary tooth is limited
5. Patient's risk pattern (caries-free or extensive caries pattern in primary and/or permanent dentition)
6. Pit and fissure morphology not at risk for caries (monitor for change in caries risk)
7. Sporadic dental care and lack of preventive dentistry practices (instigate routine dental care and preventive practice)

J Public Health Dent 55:259, 55:263, 55:274, 55:292, 55:302, 1995.

---

seal an occlusal surface is questionable, however, it is more appropriate to err toward sealant placement than toward observation of the surface and development of caries over time.

In 1994, a consensus workshop was held to establish general guidelines for sealant use in individual patients as well as for community-based sealant programs. A summary of the recommendations from this workshop is presented in Table 32–6 (Rozier, 1995; Brown, 1995; Corbin, 1995; Solderholm, 1995; Siegal, 1995).

A well-accepted clinical procedure used for restoring isolated pits and fissures and simultaneously preventing caries in the remaining unaffected pits and fissures is known as the preventive resin restoration and involves the acid-etch technique. This technique was introduced by Simonsen in 1978 as an alternative to sealing questionable pits and fissures or restoring the entire surface with an amalgam restoration. The technique involves widening the pits and fissures and removing the enamel or dentin affected by caries. Depending on the extent of this removal, either an unfilled or a filled resin is used to restore the resulting cavity. A sealant material is placed over the remaining intact pits and fissures as well as over the restored pits and fissures.

Three types of preventive restorations were described initially (Simonsen, 1978a,b). The Type I preventive resin restoration requires minimum preparation of pits and fissures prior to placing a sealant. The Type II preventive restoration is defined by minimal preparation of pits and fissures but with a small area or areas of caries that involve dentin. Filled composite resin is placed in the areas of dentin exposure after application of an appropriate base. The remaining pits and fissures are covered with a pit and fissure sealant. The Type III preventive resin has more extensive dentinal involvement and requires restoration of the preparation with a posterior composite material after application of either an unfilled bonding resin or a dentinal bonding agent. An appropriate base should be placed over the dentin. The adjacent pits and fissures are protected by a sealant material. It must be emphasized that only isolated pits and fissures with caries of clinical significance are prepared and intact pits and fissures without clinical evidence of caries are not included in the preparations. Also, removal of additional tooth structure to aid retention is not necessary.

In recent years, additional types of preventive restorations have been introduced to deal with more extensive caries in isolated pits and fissures that require restoration of the prepared cavities with dental materials of greater strength. These techniques include (1) the glass ionomer-resin preventive restoration, (2) the glass ionomer preventive restoration, and (3) the sealant-amalgam preventive restoration. These preventive restorations adhere to the principle of conservation of tooth structure.

With the glass ionomer-resin and the glass ionomer preventive restorations, no attempt is made to remove additional tooth structure for retention. Instead, these restorations rely on mechanical and physicochemical bonding of the materials to the tooth structure. In the glass ionomer-resin preventive restoration, a glass ionomer restorative material is placed in the deeper aspect of the prepared cavity, filling the lower third to half of the cavity. Posterior composite resin material fills the remaining superficial portion of the cavity preparation, and sealant material is placed over the restoration as well as over the remaining intact pits and fissures. In the glass ionomer preventive restoration, the dentinal cavity floor is covered with a glass ionomer lining material, and the remaining cavity is filled with a conventional glass ionomer, a glass ionomer-silver (cermet) restorative material, or a glass-ionomer modified resin. Again, the preventive restoration and remaining intact pits and fissures are coated with a sealant material. Finally, the sealant-amalgam preventive restoration attempts to conserve the maximum amount of tooth structure. The ultraconservative preparation of carious pits and fissures, however, requires the dentist to pay some attention to retention form to allow placement of the amalgam material. Depending on the practitioner's preference, a glass ionomer lining material may be placed over the dentinal cavity floor. Amalgam restores most of the cavity preparation. Sealant material is placed over the ultraconservative amalgam restoration and the remaining intact pits and fissures. Clearly, these innovative techniques all share a common goal—namely, conservation of tooth structure with removal of only carious enamel and dentin.

More recently, the World Health Organization (WHO) endorsed a minimal intervention technique for management of dental caries in developing countries lacking dental personnel, equipment, and facilities (Horowitz, 1996; Holmgren, 1996; Frencken et al., 1994, 1996; Holmgren and Pilot, 1996; Ismail, 1996; Phantumvanit et al., 1996). It is estimated that over 90% of dentinal caries in Africa go without treatment because restorative care is not available to the majority of Africans. Carious teeth are left untreated and eventually extracted because of pain, pulpal involvement, and jaw infections. In less economically developed countries, the predominant oral care procedure is extraction. Many of the citizens of these countries suffer from pit and fissure caries that over time becomes extensive and results in pulpal involvement and eventual tooth loss. A minimal-intervention technique called atraumatic restorative treatment (ART) has been touted by WHO for controlling dental caries in disadvantaged countries. ART involves the following:

1. Isolation of the tooth with cotton rolls
2. Cleansing the tooth surface with water-moistened cotton pellets, followed by drying with cotton pellets
3. Widening the cavitated tooth surface with a dental hatchet by rotating the instrument backwards and forwards
4. Removing frank caries using a circular scraping motion with an excavator
5. Removing undermined, unsupported enamel with a dental hatchet and washing with lukewarm water
6. Placing calcium hydroxide paste over limited areas of very deep cavities
7. Cleansing the tooth surface with a wet cotton pellet
8. Applying dentin conditioner to the cavity and tooth surface followed by cotton pellet washing and drying
9. Inserting glass ionomer and slightly overfilling
10. Applying pressure to the entire occlusal surface using a vaseline-coated, gloved finger
11. Removing excess material if necessary
12. Instructing the patient not to eat for at least 1 hour

The major advantages of the ART technique are that no anesthesia is required, no mechanical or electrical devices are needed, and the restorations may be applied by dental personnel or others trained in the procedure. This technique has undergone several years of clinical trials with impressive results. WHO has established an electronic network (Holmgren, 1996) for information regarding ART (*majordomo@who.ch*, subscribe art-odont *[your email address]*).

The final treatment alternative is restoration of the entire occlusal surface with removal of all pits and fissures that are at risk for caries development in the future. This treatment is reserved for surfaces that have generalized involvement of all pits and fissures and appear to be undermined clinically. These surfaces most likely have radiographic evidence of dentinal involvement without interproximal lesions. The choice of restorative material includes posterior composite resins, hybrid resins-ionomers, amalgam, and glass ionomer-silver (cermet). As with preventive restorations, a variety of clinical techniques incorporating the beneficial effects of different restorative materials are employed in restoring surfaces with pit and fissure caries.

RETENTION AND CARIES PREVENTION WITH SEALANTS, PREVENTIVE RESTORATIONS, AND ATRAUMATIC RESTORATIVE TREATMENT: CLINICAL TRIALS

Pit and Fissure Sealants

Numerous clinical trials, ranging in length from 6 months to 15 years, have been carried out to assess retention rates, caries incidence, and the effectiveness of sealants in preventing pit and fissure caries (Fig. 32–5*A*). In the majority of clinical studies, a single application of sealant is provided, followed by periodic evaluations to determine the retention rate and caries incidence. A review (Weintraub, 1989) of clinical sealant trials carried out over two decades has been published (Table 32–7). The complete retention rate varied from 92% after 1 year to 28% after 15 years. Caries incidence increased from 4% after 1 year to 14% after 3 years. Seven years after sealant placement, caries incidence had increased to 31%. The 10-year results from two separate trials were encouraging, with a complete retention rate of 53% and a caries incidence of 22% (Romcke et al., 1990; Simonsen, 1987). Even 15 years after initial sealant application, the caries incidence was found to be 31% and the complete retention rate was 28% (Simonsen, 1991). The effectiveness of sealants in preventing caries ranged from 83% after 1 year to 53% after 15 years.

The caries protection provided to pits and fissures by a single application of sealant material is therefore remarkable, especially considering the limited wear resistance of this resin material. In addition, even though sealant material may be judged clinically to be partially or completely lost, it may be present within the depths of pits and fissures and may protect against caries development.

Reapplication of sealants to pits and fissures that have lost their sealant cover provides a greater degree of caries reduction than that reported by most single-application sealant trials. Clinical studies allowing reapplication of sealant material after sealant loss have shown that retention rates ranging from 88% to 96% may be achieved at each annual evaluation (Straffon and Dennison, 1988; Charbeneau, 1982). Over periods of up to 7 years, it was found that 56% of sealed tooth surfaces required no retreatments, 28% required one reapplication, 8% required two reapplications, and only 8% required three reapplications. The anticipated annual reapplication rate is approximately 8%, with the highest rate of reapplication occurring 6 months after initial sealant application. The 5- to 7-year-old age group required the greatest number of sealant reapplications (Dennison et al., 1990). No doubt this high rate was due to the difficulty of isolating partially erupted first permanent molars from sal-

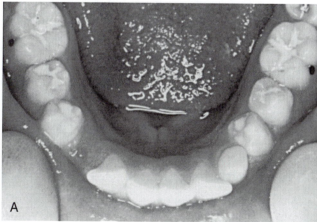
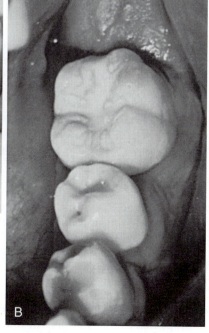

Figure 32–5. Clinical appearance of fissure sealants and a preventive resin restoration. *A*, These sealants have been retained for 6 years with the permanent first molars and for 2 years with the premolar teeth and are protecting these teeth from occlusal caries formation. *B*, After 5 years, this preventive resin restoration is still present and is responsible for the occlusal surface of the first molar remaining caries-free.

TABLE 32–7. Retention and Effectiveness of Pit and Fissure Sealants in First Permanent Molar Teeth

Length of Time Since Application	Complete Retention (Median)	Caries Rate (Median)	Effectiveness of Sealants (Median)
1 year	92%	4%	83%
2 years	85%	7%	81%
3 years	71%	14%	69%
5 years	67%	26%	55%
7 years	66%	31%	55%
10 years*	53%	22%	68%
15 years†	28%	31%	53%

*Represents results from two separate 10-year sealant studies. JADA *115:*31, 1987; J Can Dent Assoc *56:*235, 1990.
†Represents a single 15-year sealant study. JADA *122:*34, 1991. Compiled from J Public Health Dent *49:*317, 1989.

ivary contamination. When an operculum covered the distal marginal ridge, 54% of the sealed teeth required retreatment. Slightly less than one quarter required retreatment if the gingival tissue was at the same height as the distal marginal ridge. If the gingiva was below the distal marginal ridge, no retreatments were required. Of great interest was the fact that this type of sealant reapplication protocol was found to be 100% effective in preventing caries within pits and fissures. In a dental practice that maintains an active recall system for sealant evaluation and that reapplies sealant as necessary, a relatively high degree of caries prevention may be anticipated.

The effectiveness of sealants placed by dental students in a pediatric dentistry clinic (Walker et al., 1996a) has been assessed and provides some interesting findings. A total of 7838 permanent molars underwent sealant placement and were followed for up to 7.9 years. Complete or partial retention not requiring sealant application occurred in 78.6% of molars. Reapplication of sealant was necessary in 13.2%. A preventive resin or one-surface composite was placed in 6.4%. Caries requiring a one-surface or two-surface amalgam occurred in 1.0% and 0.8% of cases, respectively. Two thirds of sealant reapplications occurred in children under 8 years of age. This probably reflects the eruption status of the teeth at the time of sealant placement.

Although fewer sealant studies have been completed with primary teeth, caries incidence and retention rates are similar to those for permanent teeth (Vrbic, 1997; Hardison et al., 1987; Simonsen, 1981). Retention rates have been reported to be 95% and 93% after 1 and 3 years, respectively. During these time periods, none of the sealed primary molar surfaces was affected by caries. A clinical study compared retention rates in primary and permanent molars 12 months after placement of a fluoride-releasing sealant (Vrbic, 1997). Complete retention was 98% for primary teeth and 97% for permanent teeth; partial retention was 2% for primary teeth and 3% for permanent teeth. None of the fluoride-releasing sealants was lost during this limited 12-month period.

Several clinical studies (Table 32–8) have investigated the use of conventional glass ionomers, glass ionomer-silver cermets, and resin-modified glass ionomers as pit and fissure sealants (Winkler et al., 1996; Aranda and Garcia-Godoy, 1995; Komatsu et al., 1994; Forss et al., 1994; Mills and Ball, 1993; Ovrebo and Raadal, 1990; Torppa-Saarinen and Seppa, 1990; Mejare and Mjor, 1990; McKenna and Grundy, 1987). Conventional glass ionomers used as pit and fissure sealants have a relatively low complete and partial retention rate when compared with resin-based pit and fissure sealants. Although conventional glass ionomers were assessed as completely lost in almost 50% of sealed teeth, only 5% were affected by caries after 2 years.

Two factors may account for the caries protection afforded by glass ionomers. First, glass ionomer materials release a significant amount of fluoride. The released fluoride may become incorporated into the adjacent enamel forming the pits and fissures, providing increased caries resistance. Second, replica impression studies of surfaces that have experienced complete loss of their glass ionomer sealants have shown glass ionomer material within the depths of the pits and fissures in 93% of cases. This retained glass ionomer sealant may still provide an effective barrier against caries development. Both glass ionomer-silver cermet and resin-modified glass ionomer sealants have improved retention rates when compared with conventional materials. Over a 2-year period, almost 95% of glass ionomer silver sealants were retained, whereas all

TABLE 32–8. Glass Ionomers as Pit and Fissure Sealants: Retention and Caries Preventive Effects

Single-Application Glass Ionomer Materials as Pit and Fissure Sealants

	6 mos	*12 mos*	*24 mos*	*36 mos*
Glass ionomer		*12 mos*	*24 mos*	
Complete retention		20%	26%	
Partial loss		70%	26%	
Complete loss		10%	48%	
Caries development		0%	5%	
Glass ionomer-silver cermet	*6 mos*	*12 mos*	*24 mos*	
Complete retention	93%	81%	83%	
Partial loss	3%	13%	12%	
Complete loss	4%	6%	6%	
Caries development	0%	0%	0%	
Resin modified glass ionomer	*6 mos*	*12 mos*		
Complete retention	78%	51%		
Partial loss	22%	49%		
Caries development	0%	5%		

Reapplication of Glass Ionomer Material as Pit and Fissure Sealants

	6 mos	*12 mos*	*24 mos*	*36 mos*
Complete retention	37%	41%	51%	53%
Partial loss	46%	28%	20%	17%
Complete loss	17%	31%	29%	30%
Caries reduction (compared with age-matched controls)	—	76%	70%	67%
No reapplications required	—	50%	17%	10%

Compiled from JADA *125:*543, 1994, *127:*1508, 1996; J Clin Pediatr Dent *19:*273, 1995; Community Dent Oral Epidemiol *22:*21, 1994; Oper Dent *18:*148, 1993.

resin-modified glass ionomer sealants were retained over a 1-year period. Caries developed in 5% of teeth sealed with a resin-modified glass ionomer. In contrast, no caries developed in the pits and fissures protected by glass ionomer-silver cermets.

With a reapplication protocol for conventional glass ionomer sealants, caries may be reduced considerably. When age- and gender-matched controls were used for comparison, pit and fissure caries was reduced by 76% after 1 year and by 67% after 3 years. As with conventional resin pit and fissure sealants, the highest percentage of reapplications occurred within 1 year of glass ionomer placement. By year 3 of the clinical trial, only 10% of sealed teeth required reapplication of the glass ionomer sealant. It is anticipated that if a reapplication protocol is used and resin-modified or glass ionomer-silver sealants are placed instead of conventional glass ionomer materials, the replacement rate would probably decrease while providing a high degree of caries protection.

Preventive Resin Restorations

Since the introduction of preventive resin restorations (see Fig. 32-5*B*) in 1978, the retention rate of preventive resins and caries incidence have been studied in both longitudinal and cross-

sectional studies (Table 32-9). The results of a representative longitudinal trial indicated complete retention rates similar to those recorded for pit and fissure sealants (Houpt et al., 1984, 1985a, 1986, 1988, 1994). The caries incidence, however, was considerably reduced compared with pit and fissure sealants during the first 6.5 years of the study. Only 11% of surfaces with preventive resins were affected by caries 78 months after placement. In comparison, caries incidence for surfaces with sealants was 31% after 84 months. Nine years after placement, almost 80% of the preventive resins were either completely or partially retained. The caries incidence was 24% by year 9 and was similar to that for sealants that had been in place for 10 years. These findings are remarkable when one realizes that the clinical protocol allowed only for placement of the preventive resin material and monitoring for retention and caries development over the 9-year period. If periodic repair of the preventive resin material had occurred, one can imagine that the caries incidence would have been reduced considerably with a concomitant increase in retention rate.

A cross-sectional study evaluated preventive resin restorations placed by dental students over a period of 3 to 65 months (Walker et al., 1990). A relatively high retention rate was noted, with slightly more than 1% of restorations being completely lost. Considering the fact that the preven-

TABLE 32–9. Preventive Resin Restorations (PRR): Retention Rates and Caries Incidence/Prevalence

	Retention			Caries
Length of Time Since PRR Placement	*Complete*	*Partial*	*Lost*	*Incidence/Prevalence*
Longitudinal PRR Study				
3 years	84.5%	14.7%	0.8%	3.6%
4 years	77.2%	18.8%	4.0%	6.9%
5 years	72.1%	21.2%	6.7%	6.7%
6.5 years	65.4%	19.2%	15.4%	10.6%
9 years	54.4%	25.3%	20.3%	24.0%
Cross-Sectional PRR Studies				
1.3 years (mean) (range = 0.3–5.5 years)	81.7%	11.9%	1.2%	5.2%

Compiled from J Dent Child *57:*257, 1990, *51:*270, 1984; JADA *110:*352, 1985; J Prosth Dent *55:*164, 1986; Pediatr Dent *10:*304, 1988; Quint Int *25:*155, 1995.

tive resins had been in place for a mean period of 15 months, the caries incidence was at least comparable to that for pit and fissure sealants. In the longitudinal trial, it appears that preventive resin restorations may provide a retention rate and caries protective effect similar to those associated with pit and fissure sealants.

The assessment of preventive resins placed by dental students in a pediatric dentistry clinic provides further support for the utility of this technique in simultaneous caries restoration and prevention (Walker et al., 1996b). Over 5000 preventive resin restorations were followed for up to 6.5 years. No additional treatment was required in 83.2%, whereas 6.2% required replacement of the pit and fissure sealant component and another 1.5% were retreated with a preventive resin restoration. Slightly less than 7% required a one-surface restoration, with most of these being composite resin restorations (81%). Two or more surface restorations were placed in 3.6% of the teeth. The most common reason for treatment intervention was either the loss of sealant material or failure to place sealant into the distal pits of maxillary molars and buccal pits of mandibular molars. Interproximal caries occurred in 3.6% of all teeth with preventive resins, whereas caries developed around preventive resin restorations in 8% of cases. Of the 10.6% of teeth restored, one third possessed intact preventive resin restorations but were affected by interproximal caries.

The preventive resin restoration is an acceptable alternative to restoration of an entire occlusal surface when only isolated pits and fissures with caries are present. Currently, clinical trials involving glass ionomer preventive restorations are in progress but of limited duration. Because of the ability of glass ionomer materials to release fluoride, combined with the caries-preventive ef-

fects of the sealant material, results similar to those reported for preventive resin restorations are anticipated.

Preventive Restorations

Relatively few clinical studies have evaluated ultraconservative restoration of isolated pit and fissure caries followed by sealant placement over the restored areas and remaining intact pits and fissures (Mertz-Fairhurst et al., 1987, 1991, 1992, 1995, 1998). The 10-year results from a clinical trial of sealant-amalgam and sealant-composite restorations on paired molars and premolars have now been reported (Table 32–10). Isolated pits and fissures with clinical and radiographic evidence of superficial dentinal caries were prepared for either ultraconservative composite or amalgam restorations. With the sealant-composite restorations, no attempt was made to remove undermined demineralized enamel or affected dentin. With the sealant-amalgam restorations, an ultraconservative preparation was performed with complete removal of caries and attention to retention form. During the 10-year study period, complete and partial retention of the sealant material was comparable in both the sealant-composite and sealant-amalgam restorations. Complete and partial retention rates ranged from 88% to 97% in the sealant-amalgam restorations and from 76% to 95% in the sealant-composite restorations. Complete loss of sealant material occurred more often in the sealant-composite restorations with 10% of restorations lost 6 years after initial placement and a dramatic increase in lost restorations by year 10. Cumulative failures after 10 years amounted to 22% of sealant-composite restorations and only 6% of sealant-amalgam restorations. Despite the higher number of failures

TABLE 32–10. Sealant-Amalgam and Sealant-Composite Preventive Restorations: Comparison of Sealant Retention, Caries Development, and Restoration Failure

Length of Time Since Placement	Sealant Retention			Caries Incidence	Restoration Failure (Cumulative)
	Complete	*Partial*	*Lost*		
Sealant-Amalgam Preventive Restorations					
1 year	68%	28%	4%	0%	2%
2 years	52%	45%	3%	0%	2%
3 years	46%	51%	3%	2%	3%
4 years	48%	47%	5%	0%	3%
5 years	43%	54%	3%	0%	3%
6 years	41%	53%	6%	0%	6%
9 years	23%	71%	6%	0%	6%
10 years	27%	61%	12%	0%	6%
Sealant-Composite Preventive Restorations					
1 year	74%	21%	5%	0%	1%
2 years	57%	34%	9%	1%	1%
3 years	59%	32%	9%	0%	8%
4 years	55%	47%	8%	0%	8%
5 years	50%	40%	10%	0%	9%
6 years	55%	35%	10%	0%	12%
9 years	28%	48%	24%	1%	16%
10 years	20%	69%	11%	0%	22%

Compiled from JADA *115*:689, 1987; Am J Dent *4*:43, 1991, *5*:5, 1992; Quint Int *23*:827, 1992; J Dent Child *62*:97, 1995; JADA *129*:55, 1998.

in the composite group, caries occurred in only 1% of cases after 2 years. By year 10, an additional 1% had been affected by caries during the remaining period of the study in the composite group. The results from this longitudinal paired trial demonstrate convincingly the ability of sealant-composite and sealant-amalgam preventive restorations to provide a caries-protective effect for pits and fissures while conserving tooth structure. In addition, the isolation of dentinal caries from the oral environment by the sealant-composite materials allowed arrest of these lesions, with no radiographic evidence of advancement in any case noted during the entire study period.

Atraumatic Restorative Treatment

Field trials of ART (Table 32-11) have been performed in developing countries, such as Thailand and Zimbabwe, using the minimal intervention technique for caries control (Phantumvanit et al., 1996; Frencken et al., 1994). In Thailand, extensive data are available regarding this WHO-endorsed tooth-saving technique. When compared with one-surface amalgams, ARTs are not retained to the same extent. Considering the lack of technology, personnel, and physical facilities and equipment necessary to place amalgam restorations in these underdeveloped rural country settings, ART is the only viable option except for

extraction when caries becomes extensive. ARTs placed in children, in occlusal surfaces, and by dentists have a slightly reduced retention rate than when ARTs are placed in adults, in nonocclusal surfaces, and by dental nurses. Primary teeth and restoration of two or more tooth surfaces had much higher loss rates than one-surface restorations and permanent teeth restored with ARTs. During the 3-year clinical field trial in Thailand, 71% of ARTs were retained for up to 3 years. The Zimbabwe clinical trials also included placement and assessment of glass ionomer sealants. Over a 2-year period, less than 4% of sealed teeth were affected by caries despite the fact that the retention rate was less than 60%. Both primary and permanent teeth with glass ionomer sealants had similar retention rates after 1 year. These findings from economically less developed countries with limited resources and dental manpower are encouraging and emphasize the importance of using relatively simple, low-technology procedures to improve the dental health and overall quality of life for less advantaged persons. Even in developed countries, a technique such as ART incorporating the use of modern dental equipment may provide a rapid means for controlling rampant caries, offering a means for fluoride delivery via fluoridated glass ionomer materials, and alleviating dental pain in the moderately to severely caries-affected child. This interim ART technique may then be followed by appropriate restorative and timely care.

TABLE 32–11. Atraumatic Restorative Treatment and Glass Ionomer Sealants in Caries Management in Developing Countries: Retention Rates

Thailand	1 Year	2 Years	3 Years
Alloy restoration (one-surface restorations)	98%	94%	85%
Atraumatic restorative treatment (one-surface restorations)	93%	83%	71%
Children	92%	80%	67%
Adults	93%	86%	77%
Occlusal	91%	80%	62%
Non-occlusal	95%	88%	85%
Dentist placed	92%	79%	66%
Dental nurse placed	93%	85%	73%
Primary teeth			
One surface	79%		
≥Two surfaces	55%		
Permanent teeth			
One surface	93%		
≥Two surfaces	67%		

Zimbabwe		2 years	
Atraumatic restorative treatment (one-surface restorations)		89%	

Glass ionomer sealants	1 year	2 years	
Primary teeth	73%	—	
Permanent teeth	78%	58.3%	
Caries present	—	3.8%	

Compiled from J Public Health Dent 56(Spec Issue):135, 141, 1996; Int Dent J 44:460, 1994.

Longevity of Amalgam Restorations in Children

The longevity of sealants and preventive restorations compares favorably with the longevity of conventional amalgam restorations placed in children (Walls et al., 1985). The median survival for amalgam restorations placed in first permanent molars ranged from 26 months for 6-year-olds to 8 years and 11 months for 12-year-olds. The overall median survival for amalgams placed in first molars of 5- to 15-year-old children was 71 months. The age of the child at the time of placement is a major factor in restoration longevity. The 5-year survival rate for occlusal amalgams is 30% in 5- to 7-year-olds, 43% in 7- to 9-year-olds, and 62% in 9- to 15-year-olds. Sealants and amalgam restorations appear to follow a similar course with respect to retention in children and adolescents. The major difference is that sealant placement is associated with a conservative, preventive technique, whereas amalgam placement represents a restorative procedure in which loss of tooth structure is significant. In fact, it has been shown that preventive resin restoration results in considerable conservation of tooth structure, with the restored portion occupying only 5% of the occlusal surface compared with 25% of the occlusal surface removed in order to place an amalgam restoration (Wellbury et al., 1990). Perhaps even more importantly, when replacement of a defective amalgam is necessary, the area of the cavity preparation is further increased by 38%, resulting in an even greater loss of tooth structure (Elderton, 1976).

COMBINED EFFECT OF SEALANT AND FLUORIDE RINSING PROGRAMS

The combination of sealant and fluoride rinsing programs significantly reduces the incidence and prevalence of pit and fissure and smooth surface caries in schoolchildren from fluoride-deficient communities. A longitudinal study compared the effect of fluoride rinsing alone with sealant placement combined with fluoride rinsing in caries-free second- and third-grade schoolchildren (Ripa et al., 1986, 1987). After a 2-year period, 78% of the children in the fluoride rinse group were caries-free. In comparison, 96% of children receiving the benefits of both fluoride rinsing and sealant placement were caries-free. The caries incidence in children in the fluoride rinse group was 13 times that noted in children in the combined fluoride-sealant group.

Perhaps even more impressive is the effect of combined fluoride rinsing and sealant therapy in children living on the previously fluoride-deficient island of Guam (Sterritt et al., 1990, 1994). After a baseline survey of caries prevalence in schoolchildren in Guam (Table 32–12), a school-based fluoride rinsing program was initiated in

TABLE 32–12. Effect of Fluoride and Sealant Programs on Caries Prevalence in Fluoride-Deficient Communities

	Occlusal	Buccal/Lingual	Proximal	Total
Guam Preventive Dentistry Program				
Prior to fluoride rinse DMFS*	3.27	2.48	1.31	7.06
Fluoride rinse DMFS (% reduction in caries compared with baseline levels)	3.04	1.72	0.51	5.27 (25%)
Sealant and fluoride rinse DMFS (% reduction in caries compared with baseline levels)	1.38	1.09	0.46	2.93 (59%)
Water fluoridation, sealant, and fluoride rinse DMFS (% reduction in caries compared with baseline levels)	0.92	0.72	0.28	1.92 (73%)
Nelson County School Preventive Dentistry Program				
7- to 11-year-olds				
School fluoride program DMFS	0.88	0.56	0.06	1.50
Fluoride and sealant DMFS (% reduction in caries compared with baseline levels)	0.19 (78%)	0.26 (54%)	0.04 (33%)	0.49 (67%)
14- to 17-year-olds				
School fluoride program DMFS	3.71	1.78	0.73	6.22
Fluoride and sealant DMFS (% reduction in caries compared with baseline levels)	2.43 (35%)	1.32 (26%)	0.33 (55%)	4.07 (35%)

*DMFS = decayed, missing, filled surfaces, permanent teeth.
Compiled from Community Dent Oral Epidemiol *18*:288, 1990, *23*:30, 1995; J Public Health Dent *54*:153, 1994.

1976. Assessment of caries prevalence in 1984 indicated that fluoride rinsing had resulted in a 25% reduction in the mean incidence of decayed, missing, and filled tooth surfaces (DMFS). The effects were most prominent in the proximal (61% reduction) and buccal-lingual surfaces (31% reduction). As would be expected, fluoride rinsing had the least effect on the occlusal surfaces (7% reduction). In 1984 a sealant application program was initiated while the fluoride rinsing program was maintained. In 1986, 2 years after the sealant program had begun, caries prevalence on surfaces with pits and fissures decreased dramatically. During this 2-year period, a more than 50% reduction in caries occurred on the occlusal surfaces, and a 36% reduction occurred on the buccal-lingual surfaces. The proximal surfaces showed the least degree of change, with a slightly less than 10% decrease in caries prevalence. With the addition of sealant placement to the existing fluoride rinsing program, caries prevalence was reduced by 44%. In Guam, the total reduction in caries prevalence from 1976 until 1986 was slightly less than 60%, translating into more than four tooth surfaces per child being saved from caries involvement.

In 1986, community water fluoridation (0.5 to 1.0 ppm) reaching over 90% of the island's population was successfully implemented. This allowed an evaluation in 1989 of the effect of adding water fluoridation to the ongoing fluoride rinse and sealant programs. Three years after water fluoridation, the use of three preventive regimens in concert provided an overall reduction of over 70% in the DMFS for all surfaces when compared with the 1976 baseline prior

to fluoride rinsing. The introduction of water fluoridation resulted in an additional DMFS reduction of 35% over that for the combined fluoride rinsing and sealant program. Proximal surfaces experienced a 40% DMFS reduction, while occlusal surfaces had undergone a 33% decrease in DMFS. Over the 13-year period since the initial introduction of fluoride rinsing, 5.1 tooth surfaces per child were saved from dental caries. Perhaps more impressive is the fact that children from Guam in 1989 had a mean DMFS of 1.92, whereas children from the United States in 1991 had a mean DMFS of 2.50. This further emphasizes that with optimization and integration of various caries-preventive regimens, including sealants, further reductions in caries experience may be achieved.

Within the United States, a longitudinal study was performed to assess a preventive program in a fluoride-deficient community that initially instituted a weekly school-based fluoride rinsing regimen and later introduced school-based sealant application (Selwitz et al., 1995; Horowitz et al., 1986). After an 11-year fluoride rinsing program, the overall prevalence of dental caries was lowered by 65%. Four years after implementing the sealant program (see Table 32–12), the DMFS had decreased by two thirds in 7- to 11-year-olds and by one third in 14- to 17-year-olds. The younger age group experienced a 78% reduction in occlusal caries, while the older age group experienced a 35% reduction in occlusal caries. Buccal-lingual caries, which is considered to predominantly involve pits and fissures, decreased by 54% in the younger age group and by 26% in the older age group. The percentage of proximal caries reduction was lower in 7- to 11-year-olds and greatest in 14- to 17-year-olds. This probably reflects the fact that 14- to 17-year-olds are in a period when proximal surfaces may be more susceptible to caries development and the caries-preventive effect of the fluoride rinsing program on smooth surfaces is becoming realized.

CLINICAL TECHNIQUE: SEALANT APPLICATION AND PREVENTIVE RESIN RESTORATION PLACEMENT

Sealant Application

Step 1: Isolate Tooth Surface From Salivary Contamination. The tooth should be isolated from salivary contamination, ideally by using rubber dam isolation (Fig. 32–6). Cotton roll isolation with adequate suctioning to remove saliva from the operating field is also acceptable and is the preferred method of isolation for many practitioners.

Step 2: Cleanse Tooth Surface. Prophylaxis of the tooth surface to be sealed should be carried out via a pumice slurry applied with a rubber cup or pointed bristle brush in a prophy angle. An alternative method is to clean the surface with an air-polishing device using an air-powder abrasive (sodium bicarbonate slurry) system (Goldstein and Parkins, 1995). Some practitioners merely use toothbrush prophylaxis with toothpaste or pumice followed by copious water rinsing to prepare the pits and fissures (Waggoner and Siegal, 1996). Rinse the tooth surface thoroughly to remove the prophylactic paste or slurry and oral debris. Trace the pits and fissures with a sharp, fine-pointed explorer to remove any cleansing material lodged within the pits and fissures. If a sodium bicarbonate slurry has been used, it is necessary to neutralize the retained slurry with phosphoric acid for 5 to 10 seconds. Some practitioners recommend cleaning the surface with 3% hydrogen peroxide after using a prophylactic paste to remove additional debris from the fissure. Once the tooth surface has been thoroughly cleansed, rinse and air dry the surface.

Step 3: Acid-Etch Tooth Surface. Apply the etching agent to the tooth surface with a fine brush, a cotton pledget, or a minisponge using the manufacturer's recommended exposure time. Exposure time varies from 20 seconds for permanent teeth to 30 seconds for primary teeth (IADR Sealant Symposium, 1991) with additional etching time for fluorosed teeth. Gently rub the etchant applicator over the tooth surface, includ-

ing 2 to 3 mm of the cuspal inclines and reaching into any buccal and lingual pits and grooves that are present. Periodically add fresh etching agent to the tooth surface. Be careful to avoid spillage of the etchant onto the interproximal surfaces. Interproximal etching may lead to gingival irritation or sealing of adjacent interproximal surfaces together. The sealant may be either a gel or a liquid agent. The advantage of the gel material is increased control over the areas to be etched and a decreased likelihood of spillage onto the interproximal surfaces.

Step 4: Rinse and Dry Etched Tooth Surface. Rinse the etched tooth surface with an air-water spray for 30 seconds (IADR Sealant Symposium, 1991). This removes the etching agent and reaction products from the etched enamel surface. Dry the tooth surface for at least 15 seconds (IADR Sealant Symposium, 1991) with uncontaminated compressed air. If cotton roll isolation has been used, replace the cotton rolls at this time, making certain that salivary contamination of the etched enamel does not occur. The dried, etched enamel should have a frosted-white appearance. If the enamel does not have this appearance, repeat the etching step. If salivary contamination does occur at this stage, re-isolate the tooth, rinse the entire tooth surface, dry thoroughly, and repeat the etching process. Avoid contact with the dry, etched enamel surface.

Step 5: Apply Sealant to Etched Tooth Surface. Apply the sealant material to the etched tooth surface and allow the material to flow into the pits and fissures. With mandibular teeth, apply the sealant at the distal aspect and allow it to flow mesially. With maxillary teeth, apply the sealant at the mesial aspect and allow it to flow distally. Allowing the sealant material to flow into the etched pits and fissures should avoid incorporating air into the material and creating voids. Add additional material as necessary to seal all pits and fissures. Using a fine brush, minisponge, or applicator provided by the manufacturer, carry a thin layer of sealant up the cuspal inclines to seal secondary and supplemental fissures, and to allow the sealant material to flow into buccal or lingual pits and grooves. With autopolymerizing sealants, working time varies from 1 to 2 minutes. With photoactivated sealants, the setting reaction is initiated by exposing the sealant to visible light and usually requires 10 to 20 seconds for complete setting. The manufacturer's recommended curing time should be considered a minimal exposure period and the addition of 5 to 10 seconds of curing time to that recommended may allow for maximal polymerization. With light-cured sealants, penetration

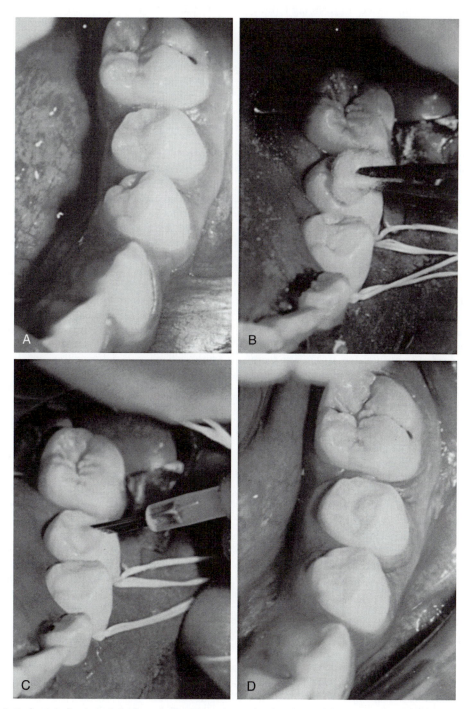

Figure 32–6. Sealant application. *A,* Sealant application to the occlusal surfaces of these premolar teeth is necessary because of the presence of deep retentive fissures. *B,* Following rubber dam isolation and pumice prophylaxis, phosphoric acid is applied to the teeth for 20 seconds via a cotton pledget. The etched surface is then rinsed thoroughly and dried. *C,* An opaque sealant is applied with a fine brush. Polymerization of the sealant is completed with a visible light unit for 10 to 20 seconds. With chemical-cured sealants, setting time varies from 1 to 2 minutes after mixing of the materials. *D,* Following removal of the rubber dam, the occlusion should be evaluated to determine if adjustment is necessary.

of the resin into the etched enamel may be increased by up to 300%, based on resin tag length, if curing is delayed for 10 seconds (Chosak and Eidelman, 1988). This delay in curing may be possible if isolation from salivary contamination is adequate.

Step 6: Explore the Sealed Tooth Surface. Explore the entire tooth surface for pits and fissures that may not have been sealed and for voids in the material. If deficiencies are present, apply additional sealant material. Usually a sticky layer of apparently unreacted sealant is present on the tooth surface. This is an air-inhibited layer of sealant that has not undergone polymerization. Remove the rubber dam or cotton rolls.

Step 7: Evaluate the Occlusion of Sealed Tooth Surface. Evaluate the occlusion of the sealed tooth surface to determine whether excessive sealant material is present and needs to be removed. A small discrepancy in occlusal interference with an unfilled sealant is easily tolerated by the child because the sealant will abrade away, allowing proper interdigitation. With filled sealant materials and in adult and adolescent age groups, occlusal adjustment should be completed to avoid discomfort due to excess material. Evaluate the interproximal regions for inadvertent sealant placement by performing tactile examination with an explorer and passing dental floss between the contact regions.

Step 8: Periodically Reevaluate and Reapply Sealant as Necessary. During routine recall examination, it is necessary to reevaluate the sealed tooth surface for loss of material, exposure of voids in the material, and caries development. The need for reapplication of sealant material is usually highest during the first 6 months after placement. Should reapplication be necessary, the steps involved in reapplying sealant material to an existing sealant are identical to those used for initial placement.

Placement of Preventive Resin Restoration

A preventive resin restoration (Fig. 32–7) requires the same steps as those used for sealant placement except that caries are removed from isolated pits and fissures.

Step 1: Isolate Tooth Surface From Salivary Contamination. Isolate tooth surfaces as described previously.

Step 2: Remove Caries From Isolated Pits and Fissures. Remove caries from isolated pits and fissures using an inverted cone, round or pear-shaped bur in a high-speed handpiece. The size of the bur and the resulting cavity preparation will be dictated by the amount of caries present. Remove caries while making no attempt to incorporate retention into the preparation.

Step 3: Cleanse Tooth Surface. Perform prophylaxis as previously described, followed by rinsing and drying.

Step 4: Place Cavity Base or Lining Material. If dentin is exposed, place a calcium hydroxide or glass ionomer base prior to acid-etching.

Step 5: Acid-Etch Tooth Surface. Etch, rinse, and dry tooth surface as previously described.

Step 6: Place Resin and Sealant Material. Place a thin layer of resin bonding agent or dentinal bonding agent in the cavity preparation, followed by a diluted composite material for a Type 2 cavity or posterior composite material for a Type 3 cavity. If the restorative material is chemically cured, allow time for complete setting reaction to occur. Expose light-cured material to the visible light source to initiate the setting reaction. If adequate isolation is present, allow resin to penetrate into etched tooth structure for 10 seconds before initiating light curing. Apply sealant material over the restored area and the adjacent intact etched pits and fissures. Carry the sealant material up the cuspal inclines for 2 to 3 mm and into the buccal-lingual grooves and pits. Initiate the sealant setting reaction. With a Type 1 preventive resin restoration, sealant material is applied only to the tooth surface, including the prepared enamel.

Step 7: Explore the Sealed and Restored Tooth Surface. Explore the sealed and restored surface as previously described. If necessary, apply additional sealant material. Remove rubber dam or cotton roll isolation.

Step 8: Evaluate the Occlusion of Sealed and Restored Tooth Surface. Evaluate the occlusion of the sealed and restored tooth surface to determine whether excessive material is present and adjust as necessary. Evaluate the interproximal regions for inadvertent resin placement by tactile examination with an explorer and passage of dental floss between the contact regions.

Step 9: Periodically Reevaluate the Restoration Repair and Reapply Sealant as Necessary. During routine recall examinations, it is necessary to reevaluate the sealed and restored tooth surface for loss of material and development of caries. Repair of the restored regions and reapplication of sealant material may be necessary periodically.

Although both techniques involved in sealant application and preventive resin restoration placement appear to be simple, a high failure

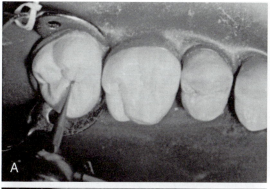

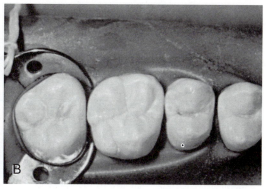

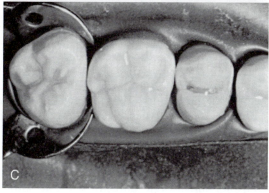

Figure 32–7. Preventive resin restoration placement. *A,* After isolation with a rubber dam, pits and fissures with caries of clinical significance are removed with a round bur in a high-speed handpiece. *B,* After minimal cavity preparation, a pumice prophylaxis is carried out. If dentin is exposed, a cavity base should be placed prior to etching the occlusal surface. *C,* Type A preventive resin restorations have been completed. The occlusion should be evaluated to determine if adjustment is necessary.

rate may occur if the practitioner does not pay strict attention to the steps in the acid-etch technique. Of particular importance to the success of the acid-etch procedure is avoidance of salivary contamination of the enamel surface once the surface has been etched.

The remaining types of preventive restorations follow in general the same steps outlined for the preventive resin restoration. The major difference lies in the selection and substitution of different restorative materials. Each of the materials requires certain modifications in the restoration steps. (The reader is referred to Chapters 20 and 21 for details on glass ionomer, posterior composite, and amalgam restorative materials.)

SCIENTIFIC BASIS FOR THE ACID-ETCH TECHNIQUE

The initial studies of acid-etching of surface enamel involved a solution of 85% phosphoric acid. Since the 1950s, a considerable number of laboratory and clinical studies have been performed to determine the appropriate acid type, acid concentration, and etching time that would yield optimal bonding characteristics with minimal loss of surface enamel. Phosphoric acid in the range of 35% to 40% with an application time

of 15 to 60 seconds for permanent and primary teeth has been shown to produce adequate resin bonding while minimizing the loss of surface enamel (Tandon et al., 1989; Eidelman et al., 1988; Redford et al., 1986; Silverstone, 1984a–c). No significant differences in sealant retention rates or caries incidence have been found with variations in the etching time for either primary or permanent teeth. The currently recommended etching times are 20 seconds for permanent teeth and 30 seconds for primary teeth (IADR Sealant Symposium, 1991). The etching time should be extended for fluorosed teeth.

Acid-etching of surface enamel has been shown to produce a certain degree of porosity (Silverstone, 1984a–c). In fact, sound enamel etched with phosphoric acid is affected at three levels microscopically (Fig. 32–8). First, a narrow zone of enamel is removed by etching. In this manner, plaque and surface and subsurface organic pellicles are effectively dissolved. Fully reacted, inert mineral crystals in the surface enamel are also removed, resulting in a more reactive surface, an increase in surface area, and a reduced surface tension that allows resin to wet the etched enamel more readily. This etched zone is approximately 10 μm in depth. The second zone is the qualitative porous zone, which is 20 μm in depth. Because of the relatively large

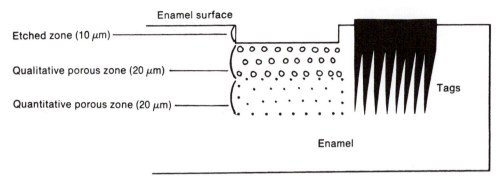

Figure 32–8. Histologic zones created in sound enamel by the acid-etch technique. Resin penetrates into the porosities in etched sound enamel, forming retentive resin tags.

porosities created by the etching process, this zone may be distinguished qualitatively from adjacent sound enamel via polarized light microscopy. The final zone is the quantitative porous zone; as its name implies, it has relatively small porosities created by the etching process that may be identified only by quantitative methods involving polarized light microscopy. This zone extends into the enamel for an additional 20 μm. After acid-etching and creation of these various zones, sealant material is applied to the etched enamel, and the resin material penetrates into the porosities created. This provides a mechanical bond between the etched enamel and the resin material that may extend 40 μm or more into the underlying tooth structure.

Three characteristic etching patterns occur after exposure of sound enamel to phosphoric acid (Fig. 32–9). The Type 1 etching pattern has lost the prism cores, but the prism peripheries remain. In the Type 2 etching pattern, the prism peripheries are lost, and the prism cores appear to be relatively intact. Some regions of etched enamel show a generalized surface roughening and porosity with no exposure of prism cores or peripheries. This surface morphology is characteristic of the Type 3 etching pattern. No specific etching pattern is preferentially created during the etching procedure, and the three types of etching pattern are often found adjacent to one another. The type of etching pattern has not been found to be related to increased or decreased sealant retention rates or caries incidence (Silverstone, 1984a–c).

ENAMEL-RESIN INTERFACE

After sealant application to an etched occlusal surface, the pits and fissures are occluded with resin material (Fig. 32–10A, B). The surface mor-

phology then changes from one in which plaque and oral debris can accumulate easily (see Fig. 32–2) to a self-cleansing surface with no readily apparent pits or fissures (see Fig. 32–10A, B). The interface between enamel and resin is intimate and shows no detectable microspaces between the resin and the adjacent etched enamel (see Fig. 32–10B, C).

Sealant materials do not simply bond to the enamel surface but actually penetrate into the microporosities created in the surface enamel during the etching procedure (see Fig. 32–10C, D). Infiltration of the etched enamel results in formation of resin tags, which provide the mechanical means for sealant retention. Typically, resin tags penetrate etched enamel to a depth of 25 to 50 μm, with some tags terminating at depths of up to 100 μm (Silverstone, 1984a–c). As noted previously, resin tag length may be increased by allowing visible light–cured resin to penetrate the etched enamel for 10 seconds or more prior to initiating the setting reaction (Chosak and Eidelman, 1988).

Resin tags serve a number of functions. They provide a mechanical means for retention of the sealant. The resin tags surround the enamel crystals and may provide resistance to demineralization by acid byproducts from plaque. BIS-GMA sealant materials are resistant to acid dissolution and provide protection against caries formation along the enamel-resin interface (Fig. 32–11). Finally, the enamel-resin interface creates a protective barrier against bacterial colonization of the sealed fissure and does not allow passage of nutriments into the fissure (Hicks and Silverstone, 1982a,b).

Although the acid-etch technique produces an intimate, interdigitating interface between the etched enamel and the resin, microspaces are present between the cavosurface enamel and amalgam and glass ionomer materials used in

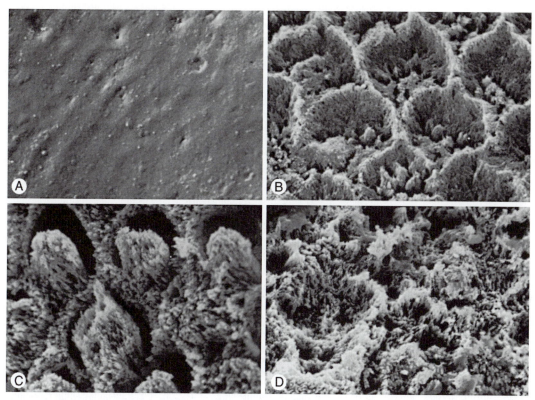

Figure 32–9. Effects of the acid-etch technique on surface morphology (scanning electron microscopy). *A,* The surface of sound enamel is relatively smooth, with occasional depressions representing terminations of enamel prisms. *B,* Type 1 etching pattern, with loss of prism cores after etching. *C,* Type 2 etching pattern, with loss of prism peripheries after etching. *D,* Type 3 etching pattern, with surface porosities but without a distinct prism morphologic appearance.

restoration (Hicks, 1984a,b; Hicks et al., 1986). These microspaces may allow passage of acidic bacterial byproducts from plaque along the restoration-enamel interface and may result in secondary caries formation in the cavosurface enamel. With amalgam restorations, there is a release of metallic ions, which may be bacteriostatic or bactericidal, into the microspace. This may reduce bacterial colonization of the amalgam-enamel interface. In addition, certain amalgam materials produce corrosion-like products that may effectively seal the microspace over time. With glass ionomers, fluoride released into the microspace may become incorporated into the cavosurface enamel, providing increased caries resistance. In addition, the acidic nature of glass ionomers enhances the antimicrobial effects of fluoride on plaque. Clinical studies have shown that secondary caries is responsible for replacement of amalgams in over 70% of cases (Mjor, 1985; Mjor and Leinfelder, 1985). In limited clinical studies of glass ionomers used as sealants, massive clinical loss of material from pits and fissures occurs; however, only 1% of previously

sealed surfaces were affected by caries (Ovrebo and Raadal, 1990; Mejare and Mjor, 1990).

These clinical findings are consistent with laboratory studies (Hicks et al., 1992, 1990, 1986; Hicks, 1984a,b; Hicks and Silverstone, 1982a,b) on artificial secondary caries formation around restorative materials (see Fig. 32–11). Typically, secondary caries-like lesions form along the amalgam-enamel interface in all cases. This reflects the ready access of acidic byproducts to the microspace between the amalgam and the cavosurface enamel. In contrast, artificial secondary lesions are found in up to 17% of cases when sealants or composite resins have been placed via the acid-etch technique. With glass ionomer materials, up to 7.5% of specimens develop artificial secondary caries. The difference in prevalence of secondary lesions between amalgams and sealants reflects the intimate interface created by the acid-etch technique during placement of the resin material. The differences noted between sealant and glass ionomer materials, however, are related to the fluoride released from glass ionomers. This release results in incorpora-

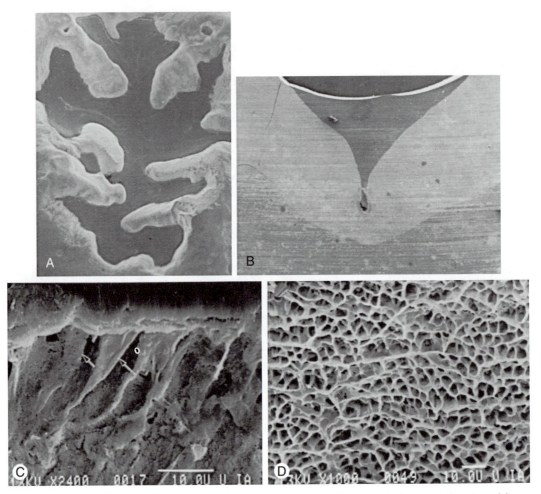

Figure 32–10. The enamel-resin interface (scanning electron microscopy). *A,* After sealant placement, the pits and fissures on this occlusal surface are protected from cariogenic challenges by the acid-resistant sealant. *B,* The interface between the enamel forming the fissure and the sealant appears to be an intimate one, with no apparent space between the etched enamel and sealant. *C,* After partial demineralization of enamel that has been sealed, resin tags *(arrows)* may be seen in the etched enamel. *D,* Complete demineralization of enamel that has been sealed allows one to visualize the appearance of the acid-resistant resin tags.

tion of fluoride into the cavosurface enamel, thereby enhancing the resistance of the enamel to caries. The effect of glass ionomers on caries formation also is visible in the surface enamel adjacent to the restoration. In fact, primary surface lesion depths are reduced by 40% to 50% when the surface enamel is in close proximity to a glass ionomer restoration or a fluoride-releasing sealant (Hicks et al., 1992, 1990). The importance of protecting the cavosurface enamel and the enamel–dental material interface from secondary caries formation cannot be overemphasized.

FLUORIDE-RELEASING SEALANTS

Initial attempts to incorporate fluoride into BIS-GMA sealants were disappointing. Typically, a relatively large amount of fluoride was released during the first 24 hours after sealant placement; however, fluoride levels returned to baseline within a 1-week period. The great majority of the fluoride incorporated into the sealant was trapped within inert sealant material and was unavailable for release. Loosely bound fluoride that was present on the surface of the sealant was responsible for the initial burst of fluoride released into the oral environment (Roberts et al., 1984).

Instead of incorporating fluoride into an inert sealant material, ion-exchanging resins were developed (Tanaka et al., 1987; Rawls and Zimmerman, 1983). These resins have a relatively high fluoride content and exchange fluorine ions from the sealant material for hydroxyl and chloride ions in the oral environment. In laboratory stud-

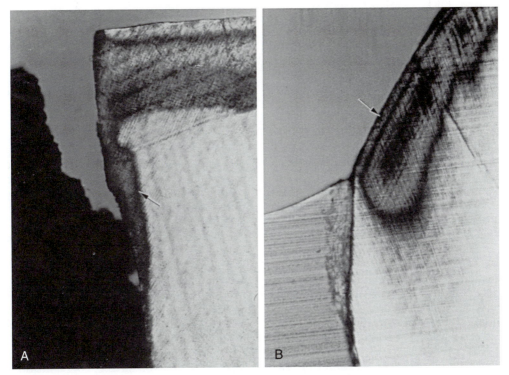

Figure 32–11. Caries-like lesion formation adjacent to amalgam and sealant materials (polarized light microscopy; water imbibition). *A,* Secondary caries formation *(arrow)* may be seen along the cavity wall of this amalgam restoration, indicating that microleakage between the restoration and cavity wall has occurred. Fracturing of the restoration occurred during preparation of the section for microscopic examination. *B,* The primary surface lesion *(arrow)* terminates at the point where bonding occurs between the etched enamel and sealant material. No secondary cavity wall lesion exists. Resin tags provide resistance against a cariogenic challenge at the enamel-resin interface.

ies, fluoride levels of 5 to 10 ppm/day are released for periods of up to 2 years. Inhibition of caries formation and remineralization of enamel caries have been shown to occur in vitro and in vivo. A significant level of fluoride is taken up by the sealed enamel. Both superficial and deep enamel layers incorporate the released fluoride, with fluoride levels of 3500 ppm and 1700 ppm reported for enamel biopsy depths of 10 μm and 60 μm, respectively. In comparison, fluoride levels in contralateral control teeth were 650 ppm and 200 ppm for enamel biopsy depths of 10 and 60 μm, respectively. The potential benefits of these fluoride-exchanging resins in prevention and remineralization of both smooth surface and pit and fissure caries appear to be considerable.

A fluoride-releasing sealant material composed of a modified urethane-BIS-GMA resin has become available for clinical use (Cooley et al., 1990; Hicks et al., 1992, 1990; Jensen et al., 1990). Preliminary laboratory and clinical studies have shown that a burst of fluoride release occurs during the first week after sealant placement, and a relatively constant release of low levels of fluoride follows for at least 12 months. In the first year of clinical trials, retention rates have been similar to those reported for conventional sealants, and caries incidence has been reduced with no caries development. The caries-protective effect of this fluoride-releasing sealant has also been assessed with an artificial caries system. A reduction of approximately 60% of secondary caries formation occurs with use of the fluoride-releasing sealant compared with conventional sealant material. In addition, primary caries formation in surface enamel adjacent to the fluoride-releasing sealant shows a 35% reduction in lesion depth, indicating an enhanced degree of caries resistance. The fluoride released from the sealant material apparently becomes incorporated into the adjacent enamel and provides an increased level of caries resistance.

SALIVARY CONTAMINATION OF ETCHED ENAMEL

Perhaps the most frequent reason for sealant failure is a lack of proper isolation of etched enamel from contamination with saliva (Fig. 32–12). In the initial sealant studies, the effect of salivary contamination on the success of the acid-etch technique was not known. A high level of sealant loss and caries development most likely occurred because saliva had contaminated the etched enamel and prevented resin penetration into the porosities of the etched enamel.

Protection of the etched enamel from salivary contamination is considered the key to success with the acid-etch technique. A tenacious surface coating forms rapidly over etched enamel surfaces exposed to saliva (see Fig. 32–12). These coatings form within a few seconds of salivary contamination and cannot be removed entirely by rinsing with an air-water spray unless the etched enamel has been exposed to saliva for 1 second or less. This means that if salivary contamination occurs, the tooth surface should be reisolated from saliva and then rinsed and dried thoroughly; repetition of the etching step in its entirety follows prior to placement of the resin (Silverstone et al., 1985; Waggoner and Siegel, 1996).

In general, two methods of isolation from salivary contamination are used—the rubber dam and cotton roll isolation. Approximately two thirds of practitioners prefer to use cotton roll isolation during placement of sealants, and the remainder prefer rubber dam isolation. Retention rates for sealants placed using the rubber dam or cotton roll have been compared. In one study in which a single application protocol was used, retention rates were 96% for rubber dam isolation and 88% for cotton roll isolation 2 years after placement of the sealant (Eidelman et al., 1983). A separate 3-year study in which a sealant reapplication protocol was used showed no dif-

ference in retention rates between the two isolation methods (Straffon et al., 1985). When sealant reapplication was used, the average retention rate at each 6-month recall period was 95% for cotton roll isolation compared with 94% for rubber dam isolation. If the need for sealant reapplication had been classified as sealant loss, the retention rates would have been 65% for cotton roll isolation and 62% for rubber dam isolation after 3 years. Using the reapplication protocol, 68% of sealed surfaces required no reapplication, 25% required one reapplication, 5% required two reapplications, and 1% required three reapplications. During the 3-year study period, no carious lesions developed.

A potential source of contamination of etched enamel is the air-water syringe. It is possible for oil or water to contaminate the air line. If contamination occurs, a thin film of oil or water may be deposited on the etched surface, which would interfere with resin penetration into the etched enamel. Periodically, the air line should be evaluated for contamination by blowing air onto a mirror surface. If oil or water droplets form on the mirror surface, contamination of the air line has occurred, and filtration to remove these contaminants will be necessary.

SEALING OVER CARIES

Because caries may be present histologically for a considerable time before being detected clinically and radiographically, it is possible that sealant placed over a clinically caries-free surface may result in sealing over enamel caries and cariogenic organisms within pits and fissures. This has caused a great deal of concern among

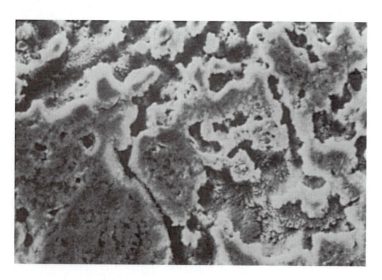

Figure 32–12. Etched enamel that was exposed to saliva for only 10 seconds. A tenacious surface coating, which would interfere with resin bonding, is present, even though the surface was rinsed thoroughly after salivary contamination (scanning electron microscopy).

practitioners and has resulted in limited use of sealants since they were introduced. It should be reassuring to the practitioner to know that the acid-etching procedure itself eliminates 75% of the viable microorganisms from pits and fissures. Clinical studies in which sealants were placed over intact pits and fissures with radiographic evidence of dentinal lesions showed that after a 2-week period, only 4.5% of microorganisms were viable. Two years after sealant placement, viable microorganisms had been reduced by 99.9%. Of the remaining viable microorganisms, less than 3% were of an acidogenic variety associated with caries formation. Sealant placement effectively creates an impermeable barrier that isolates the remaining viable organisms from their source of nutriments and prevents colonization of the sealed fissure by other oral microorganisms (Mertz-Fairhurst et al., 1979a,b, 1986, 1987, 1992, 1993; Jensen and Handelman, 1980; Handelman et al., 1976).

Of clinical significance is the radiographic appearance of sealed surfaces with caries. Following sealant placement, the dentinal lesions are arrested, and some studies report reversal of these lesions in up to 89% of cases. Longitudinal studies have shown that although dentinal lesions in matched control teeth progressed an average depth of 640 μm, dentinal lesions present beneath the contralateral sealed teeth were arrested and advanced no further. This finding is convincing because each pair of control and sealed molars was exposed to the same intraoral cariogenic environment. On removal of the sealant and bacterial sampling of the underlying dentin, the superficial affected dentin was noted to be dry, leathery, and somewhat powdery. The more deeply situated dentin had become sclerotic with a glassine appearance, which was indicative of reparative dentin formation (Mertz-Fairhurst et al., 1979a,b, 1986, 1987, 1992, 1995; Handelman et al., 1986).

Retention rates of sealants placed over carious and sound tooth surfaces have been found to be similar. After 2 years, complete retention was 64% and 65% for sealed carious and sound molars, respectively. Partial retention of sealant material was present in 35% of carious molars and 34% of sound molars (Handelman et al., 1987). Similar results were obtained for sealant-composite preventive restorations in which dentinal caries remained sealed beneath the resin material (Mertz-Fairhurst et al., 1991, 1992). At the end of this 6-year clinical trial, complete or partial retention was present in 90% of cases with caries occurring in only 1% of cases. These findings are not surprising because previous laboratory studies showed identical etching patterns for both sound enamel and enamel caries (Hicks and Silverstone, 1984a,b). It has also been shown that if the sealant appears to be lost clinically from an etched surface, resin tags remain embedded within the enamel and provide protection against a cariogenic challenge (Hicks and Silverstone, 1982a,b). The placement of an unfilled resin over caries-like lesions has been shown to protect against caries progression (Garcia-Godoy et al., 1997).

These results obtained from sealing over caries involving enamel and dentin emphasize the fact that if sealants are applied properly and are monitored periodically, caries arrest beneath a sealant can be expected. If clinically undetectable dentinal involvement has occurred, sealing over the lesion may allow odontoblasts to effect biologic repair of the affected dentin.

SEALANT USE

Since the introduction of commercially available sealant products in the early 1970s, dental practitioners have been somewhat hesitant to incorporate sealants into their practices. The initial ADA sealant use survey in 1974 found that only 38% of general dentists were placing sealants (Gift et al., 1975). The reasons given for the poor acceptance of sealants were concern about the effectiveness of sealants in preventing caries, the possibility of sealing over caries, and the longevity of sealants. A follow-up survey by the ADA in 1982 showed a modest increase in the proportion of practitioners placing sealants (Gift and Frew, 1986). Almost 60% of general dentists had accepted sealants as a preventive procedure and provided this service for their pediatric patients. Because of the overwhelming laboratory and clinical results attesting to the caries-preventive capabilities and retention rates of sealants, one would have expected an even higher level of acceptance. This lack of acceptance, however, can be explained in part by the fact that 41% of surveyed dentists believed that amalgam restorations were effective in preventing pit and fissure caries in children, whereas only 10% believed that sealants were effective in preventing caries. The reasons given for limiting sealant use included concerns about sealant longevity, sealing over caries, lack of reimbursement by third-party providers, and a preference for restoration of pits and fissures.

During the late 1980s and 1990s, it has become apparent that sealants have been incorporated into the preventive regimens of almost all general and pediatric dentists. Both regional and national surveys (Table 32-13) have indicated that between 80% and 95% of general dentists use sealants to some extent in their practices (Siegal et al., 1996; Gonzalez et al., 1991; Hicks et al., 1990; Bowman and Fitzgerald, 1990; Romberg et al., 1988; Cohen et al., 1988; Faine and Dennen, 1986). This rapid adoption of sealants since the previous ADA survey is consistent with the finding that slightly over 50% of dentists have been using sealants for 3 years or less (Faine and Dennen, 1986).

Using a self-assessment method for determining sealant use (see Table 32-13), a regional survey found that 83% of general dentists and 96% of pediatric dentists used sealants (Hicks et al., 1990). Although 73% of pediatric dentists indicated that they used sealants routinely, only 40% of general dentists claimed to be routine users of sealants. By grouping dentists into sealant use categories based on the number of sealants placed per week, it can be seen that most general dentists (53%) are in the low-use category and the majority of pediatric dentists (65%) are in the moderate- and high-use categories. These figures may reflect the relatively low pro-

portion of children in general dentistry practices, resulting in less frequent applications of sealants during a specific time period. Still, pediatric dentists placed sealants in slightly less than 40% of their patients, whereas less than 20% of children in general dentistry practices have received sealants (Cohen et al., 1988; Romberg et al., 1988). Almost 50% of general dentists reported placing sealants in less than 10% of their child patients. In contrast, 50% of pediatric dentists indicated that they placed sealants in more than 40% of their patients. Delegation of sealant placement is similar for pediatric and general dentists, with slightly over half delegating the responsibility for sealant placement to hygienists or assistants (Foreman, 1993; Farghaly et al., 1993). Pediatric dentists tend to delegate this responsibility more frequently to dental assistants, whereas general dentists delegate more frequently to dental hygienists. This probably reflects the fact that relatively few pediatric dentistry practices employ hygienists.

Incorporation of sealants into general practice is associated with the dentist's age and number of years in practice (Faine and Dennen, 1986; Call et al., 1988; Siegal et al., 1995). In fact, one

TABLE 32–13. Comparison of Sealant Use by Pediatric and General Dentists

	Pediatric Dentists	General Dentists
Self-assessment category		
Routinely Use Sealants	73%	40%
Occasionally Use Sealants	16%	33%
Seldom Use Sealants	7%	10%
Do Not Use Sealants	4%	17%
Sealant use category		
High Use (>20 sealants/wk)	38%	8%
Moderate Use (11–20 sealants/wk)	27%	12%
Low Use (1–10 sealants/wk)	31%	53%
Non Use (0 sealants/wk)	4%	27%
Percentage of children in private practice receiving sealants		
0%	6%	31%
1–9%	11%	13%
10–19%	14%	18%
20–39%	21%	19%
40–59%	18%	11%
60–79%	17%	5%
80–89%	8%	2%
90–100%	7%	2%
Average percentage of children in private practice receiving sealants	39%	19%
Delegation of sealant placement	61%	53%
Sealant placed by:		
Dentist	50%	40%
Dental hygienist	9%	51%
Dental assistant	18%	9%
Dental assistant or hygienist	23%	—

Compiled from J Pedodont *14*:97, 1990; J Public Health Dent *48*:26, 1988, *48*:138, 1988, *53*:246, 1993; J Dent Child *55*:257, 1988, *60*:193, 1993.

survey found that 97% of dentists under 30 years of age provided sealants for their child patients. Among dentists in practice for 10 years or less, 90% used sealants, whereas among dentists with 30 or more years of practice, approximately two thirds used sealants. In the latter group, slightly less than 50% used sealants either routinely or occasionally, whereas 78% of dentists with 10 years or less of practice experience claimed to use sealants routinely or occasionally.

Although incorporation of sealants into general practice has become more or less a standard of care, the proportion of children receiving the benefits of sealants is unexpectedly low (Table 32-14). In both regional and national surveys carried out between 1985 and 1991, the proportion of children who had undergone sealant placement ranged from 6% to 21% (Selwitz et al., 1996; Palmer, 1992a; Lang et al., 1988; Simonsen, 1989a, b). A 1989 U.S. Public Health Service survey noted a trend toward an increased prevalence of sealants, with 17% of 8-year-olds and 13% of 14-year-olds having received sealants (Palmer, 1992a).

The most recent NHANES III survey of sealant prevalence (see Table 32-14) indicates a continuing increase in sealant application by dentists. Sealants are found in 18.5% of all children and adolescents. Slightly over one quarter of 14-year-olds have undergone sealant placement, whereas slightly over 20% of 8-year-olds have sealants. The highest sealant application rates are associated with white, non-Hispanic race. Overall, both Hispanics and blacks have sealants applied infrequently. Slightly over 5% of 18- to 24-year-old young adults have sealants. In contrast, persons over 25 years of age rarely have sealants.

An exemplary, aggressive campaign for sealant placement in Ohio (see Table 32-14) has been waged in conjunction with state and local dental societies, a sealant product manufacturer, and federal agencies (Palmer, 1992b). Sealant prevalence in second-grade children in one Ohio community increased from 7% to 24% between 1986 and 1992. Among third-grade students evaluated in 1992, sealants were found to be present in 35%. Perhaps even more surprising was a program initiated by the Indian Health Service to provide sealants to at least 75% of 9-year-old Native American children by 1990 to complement the preventive effects of water fluoridation (Palmer, 1992c). In 1990, the Indian Health Service announced that 74% of 9-year-olds had received sealants. Also in 1990, the director of the U.S. Public Health Service established oral health goals for the next decade (Palmer, 1992a). One of the 16 goals for the year 2000 is to achieve

TABLE 32-14. Prevalence of Sealants in Children in the United States

	Children With Sealants
Michigan Sealant Prevalence Study 1985–86	
All age groups	6.4%
NIDR Sealant Prevalence Study 1985–87	
All regions of United States	7.6%
USPHS Sealant Prevalence Study 1987	
8-year-olds	11%
14-year-olds	8%
USPHS Sealant Prevalence Study 1989	
8-year-olds	17%
14-year-olds	13%
NHANES III 1988–91	
8-year-olds	20.9%
White	26.6%
Hispanic	9.9%
Black	8.6%
14-year-olds	28.2%
White	35.7%
Hispanic	10.9%
Black	4.7%
5- to 17-year-olds	18.5%
Males	17.1%
Females	19.9%
White	21.7%
Black	7.0%
Hispanic	6.9%
18- to 24-year-olds	5.5%
25- to 34-year-olds	1.6%
>35-year-olds	0.6%
Ohio Bureau of Dental Health Sealant Project 1986–1992	
1986 second-grade schoolchildren (Columbus, Ohio results only)	7%
1992 second-grade schoolchildren	24%
1992 third-grade schoolchildren	35%
US Indian Health Services Sealant Project 1990	
9-year-olds	74%
USPHS Oral Health Goal for the Year 2000	50%

Compiled from J Public Health Dent *48*:133, 1988; Quint Int *20*:785, 1989; ADA News *23*:1, 4, 1992a–c; J Dent Res *75*(Spec Iss):652, 1996.

sealant protection of the pits and fissures of permanent molar teeth in at least 50% of schoolchildren in the United States between the ages of 5 and 17 years. Recent trends tend to indicate that a dramatic increase in protection of children with sealants will be realized by the year 2000; however, it is unlikely that 50% of schoolchildren in the United States will have sealants in place by the year 2000.

With children who had sealants, the number of permanent teeth with sealants and tooth type (Table 32-15) were analyzed in the NHANES III survey (Selwitz et al., 1996). In the 5- to 11-year-

TABLE 32–15. Sealant Placement: Number of Teeth Sealed and Tooth Type Sealed

Number of Permanent Teeth Sealed

	5- to 11-Year-Olds	12- to 17-Year-Olds
1 tooth	8.0%	12.7%
2 teeth	18.3%	8.8%
3 teeth	18.6%	21.3%
4 teeth	50.5%	8.8%
≥5 teeth	4.6%	—
5 teeth	—	8.9%
6 teeth	—	7.1%
7 teeth	—	5.2%
8 teeth	—	14.1%
9 to 12 teeth	—	3.8%
13 to 16 teeth	—	5.9%

Permanent Tooth Type Sealed

	5- to 11-Year-Olds	12- to 17-Year-Olds
Maxillary		
First molar	15.6%	10.5%
Second molar	5.5%	8.0%
First premolar	0.8%	2.5%
Second premolar	0.6%	2.6%
Mandibular		
First molar	15.3%	11.7%
Second molar	5.6%	9.5%
First premolar	0.6%	2.4%
Second premolar	1.7%	2.7%

From J Dent Res 75(Spec Iss):652, 1996.

old age group, four teeth had been sealed in 50% of children; in the 12- to 17-year-old age group, eight teeth had been sealed in 14%, three teeth in 21%, and one tooth in 13%. The number of permanent teeth sealed varied greatly, with as many as 16 teeth sealed in 12- to 17-year olds. The most frequently sealed tooth types were maxillary and mandibular first molars (10.5–15.6%) followed by maxillary and mandibular second molars (5.5–9.5%). Less than 3% of premolars had been sealed in 12- to 17-year-olds.

Even though remarkable increases are occurring in the number of children with sealants, there still appears to be a significant discrepancy between the percentage of dentists using sealants in their practices and the proportion of children receiving sealants. Perhaps the most frequent reason cited for limiting sealant use may be helpful in understanding why more children are not receiving the caries-protective benefit of sealants (Table 32–16). Although concerns about sealing over caries, sealant retention, and cost-effectiveness were cited, lack of reimbursement for sealant placement was the most frequent cause of limiting sealant use (Siegal et al., 1996; Hicks et al., 1990). In fact, dentists report that

only 11% of their patients' insurance policies cover sealant placement (Romberg et al., 1988; Cohen et al., 1988). In addition, lack of insurance coverage influenced the level of sealant use by slightly over 50% of dentists. In one regional survey, approximately 15% of dentists did not place sealants in their patients because insurance plans did not provide reimbursement for this procedure (Faine and Dennen, 1986). Without insurance coverage, parents are required to accept financial responsibility for sealant placement or decline this preventive procedure. Without sealant placement, susceptible tooth surfaces will most likely develop caries and require placement of a permanent restoration that will be covered by the patient's insurance program. The lack of insurance coverage for sealants and the reimbursement for restorative procedures may partially explain the lower-than-expected prevalence of sealants in children. When one examines the reasons for limiting sealant use by sealant nonusers and sealant users, however, the major concerns expressed by the nonusers are based on lack of confidence in sealant ability to prevent caries and be retained. With sealant nonusers, the least frequent reasons cited for limiting sealant use are related to insurance coverage issues. In contrast, sealant users appear to limit sealant use in their practices when the parents are unwilling to pay for sealant placement, insurance does not reimburse for sealants, or the patients/parents do not understand the value of sealants in preventing caries.

Surveys of insurance companies that do not provide sealant coverage have been carried out to determine the reasons for lack of reimbursement (Glasrud, 1985; Glasrud et al., 1987). The most frequently cited reasons for nonreimbursement (Table 32–17), in descending order, were (1) low cost-effectiveness of sealants, (2) guidelines for sealant placement not defined, (3) more clinical research deemed necessary, and (4) potential for inappropriate use and fees. It is obvious that these reasons for nonreimbursement are not well founded. Because the same third-party providers reimburse the patient for restoration placement, it seems logical to assume that sealant placement may provide additional savings for the insurance companies based on the cost to place and maintain sealants compared with that to place amalgam restorations. Of the insurance companies that do provide sealant coverage, approximately two thirds define certain clinical conditions for reimbursement. Some of these conditions are age limitations; restriction of sealant placement to permanent teeth, with some specifying first and second molars only; and car-

TABLE 32–16. Reasons for Limiting Use of Pit and Fissure Sealants by General Practitioners

	Ranking (1 = most frequent)
Lack of insurance reimbursement	1
Concern with sealing over caries	2
Concern with sealant retention	3
Cost-effectiveness of sealants low	4
Sealant Nonusers	
Concern regarding sealing in decay	1
Occlusal fillings preferred	2
Sealants do not last long	3
Patients not requesting sealants	4
Additional research necessary	4
Better materials needed	4
Insurance coverage lacking	4
Sealant Users	
Patients unwilling to pay for sealants	1
Insurance companies do not reimburse	2
Patients do not understand value of sealants	3

Compiled from J Pedodont *14*:97, 1990; J Public Health Dent *56*:12, 1996.

ies-free status of teeth to be sealed. One insurance company requires that only opaque sealants be used (Faine and Dennen, 1986).

In recent years, significant gains have been realized in sealant coverage by Medicaid programs. In 1985, less than 10% of Medicaid programs provided sealant reimbursement (Glasrud et al., 1987). A 1991 ADA survey found that 58% of Medicaid programs covered sealant protection (Palmer, 1992a). In 1992 it was reported that 92% of Medicaid programs provided reimbursement for sealant placement (Palmer, 1992a), and by October 1994, all 50 states included sealants in their Medicaid programs (Siegal, 1995). With the oral health goal for the year 2000 of sealant protection provided to 50% of schoolchildren, it is hoped that inclusion of sealants in comprehensive dental insurance plans will become common among third-party and managed-care providers.

PARENTAL AND PHYSICIAN KNOWLEDGE AND ATTITUDES TOWARD SEALANTS

Education of parents and physicians regarding the importance of caries prevention is of considerable importance in improving the dental health of infants and young children. With the majority of dentists claiming to use sealants in their practices, expansion of the knowledge base and attitudes of parents and physicians may be required to further the acceptance of this preventive technique. Certain parental factors (Table 32–18) are associated with acceptance of sealants for their children (Ismail and Gagnon, 1995; Gonzalez et al., 1995; Bowman and Zinner, 1994; Holloway and Clarkson, 1994; Mafeni and Messer, 1994; Selwitz et al., 1992). Some of the parental factors

TABLE 32–17. Reasons for Limited Coverage of Sealants by Third-Party Payment Plans

Reason	Ranking (1 = Most Frequent)
Cost-effectiveness of sealants low	1
Guidelines for sealant placement not defined	2
More clinical research necessary	3
Potential for inappropriate use and fees	4
Most insurers do not provide sealant coverage in policies	5
Sealants are temporary treatment	6
Policy premiums would increase	7
Employers exclude sealant coverage from dental plans	7

Compiled from J Dent Child *57*:81, 1987.

TABLE 32–18. Parental and Physician Knowledge and Attitude Toward Sealants

Parental Factors Associated With Acceptance of Sealant Placement

Education beyond high school, especially college-educated
Caucasian race
Female parent decision-maker
Prior knowledge of sealants
Recommendation by dentist or dental staff
Regular dental care for children
Dental insurance coverage
Middle and upper socioeconomic group

Parental Rating of Preventive and Restorative Dental Care

	Important	*Not Important*	*Not Sure*
Professional cleaning	76%	10%	13%
Filling decayed teeth	88%	3%	10%
Decrease sugar intake	88%	7%	5%
Sealant placement	45%	6%	49%
Sealants prevent decay	53%	2%	46%
Fluoride and sealants may prevent most caries	53%	3%	44%
Sealants important for permanent teeth	43%	5%	52%
Sealants protect for >1 yr	31%	3%	66%

Physician's Knowledge Base Regarding Sealants

69%	Not very familiar with sealants
64%	Unsure which type of teeth to recommend for sealants
35%	Sealants protect against caries
32%	Benefit of combining sealants and fluoride
3%	Acceptable to place sealant over incipient caries

Compiled from Aust Dent J *39*:172, 1994; J Dent Hyg *68*:279, 1994; J Dent Child *62*:335, 1995; J Dent Res *74*:1583, 1995; J Public Health Dent *52*:137, 1992.

associated with sealant acceptance as a preventive measure include (1) education beyond high school, (2) female parent decision-maker, (3) recommendation by dentist or dental staff, and (4) regular dental care for children. Although a number of parents are familiar with sealants from friends or the popular press, recommendation by the dentist and his or her staff is most important. Dental coverage for sealants is more commonly associated with sealant placement. The parental knowledge of preventive and restorative dental care may also give the dentist a sense of the parent's knowledge base and the need for education in caries prevention. Although most parents understand the importance of professional prophylaxis, restoring carious teeth, and decreasing sucrose intake, a large percentage (44–66%) are not certain of the effect of sealants on caries prevention. Many times pediatric and general dentists depend on the knowledge base and attitude of pediatricians and family practice physicians for referral of infants and young children in need of preventive and restorative care. Over two thirds of physicians are not familiar with sealants (see Table 32-18) and are unsure which type of teeth benefit from sealant placement. Only one third of physicians realize that sealants alone or in combination with fluoride protect

against caries formation. It is obvious that the dental profession needs to develop educational material directed toward parents and physicians regarding the role of sealants in a complete prevention program. With an improved knowledge base and attitudes toward sealants, requests by parents and physicians for evaluation of children for sealant placement may increase the prevalence of sealants in our pediatric and adolescent population.

COST-EFFECTIVENESS OF SEALANTS

Although it has become apparent that sealants provide a significant degree of caries protection for pits and fissures, the use of sealants has been limited in the past owing to questions about their cost-effectiveness. In a regional survey of sealant use during 1987, the mean professional fee for sealant placement per tooth surface was $9.05 (Faine and Isman, 1989). In comparison, a national survey completed in 1988 found that mean costs for sealant placement were $13.50 and for amalgam placement they were $26.50 (Cohen et al., 1988). The average cost per child for sealant application and reapplication was determined to be $28.78 per year (Faine and Isman, 1989).

These fees are based on those reported by private practitioners. An extensive study of dental insurance claims for sealants and one-surface posterior restorations placed in 1.35 million children across the United States over a 39-month period provided a means to calculate the cost ratio of sealant versus a one-surface restoration placement (Kuthy, 1992; Kuthy and Clive, 1992). Of interest was the difference between the range of fees for sealant placement from $11.63 to $38.91 and those for one-surface restoration from $28.48 to $76.69. The mean cost of a sealant was $17.80 contrasted with $41.00 for a one-surface restoration. By applying a sealant to an at-risk surface, a cost reduction of 57% could be realized. Appropriate placement of a sealant would provide a significant initial savings for governmental health care agencies, third-party payers, and parents. Some additional maintenance expenses may be incurred secondary to sealant loss and caries development over time. It has been suggested that the cost of placing sealants may be reduced by as much as 80% if sealants are placed by dental auxiliaries either in the dental office or in a school-based public dentistry facility (Mitchell and Murray, 1989).

The total expense incurred with sealant placement must be compared with the cost of restoration of the teeth should sealants not be placed and caries eventually develop. Over a 10-year period, it was found that the cost of restoring unsealed surfaces was 1.64 times the cost of a single application of sealant (Simonsen, 1987). Using a sealant maintenance program that includes the cost of initial sealant placement, sealant reapplication, and restoration placement when sealants fail, the total expenditure for this type of program would be 25% less than that for restoration of unsealed surfaces when caries developed. Perhaps more important is the fact that even with a single application of sealant material, 4.7 and 4.1 tooth surfaces per child are "saved" from caries over 10-year and 15-year periods, respectively (Simonsen, 1987, 1991). When comparing the cost of a preventive program including sealants with the expense of restoration placement, one must also consider the intangible value of maintaining caries-free tooth surfaces and promoting a low incidence of dental caries in our child and adolescent population.

SUMMARY

At the present time, pit and fissure caries accounts for approximately 90% of the total caries experience in childhood and adolescence. The development of pit and fissure caries occurs not only in 6- to 14-year-old children but also in adolescents and young adults. With the introduction of sealants, a clinical procedure for prevention of caries in pits and fissures became available. Laboratory studies and clinical trials have provided overwhelming evidence supporting the ability of this resin material to resist caries development. With innovative applications of the acid-etch technique, tooth surfaces with isolated involvement of pits and fissures may also benefit from the conservation of tooth structure afforded by preventive restorations. It also appears that both fluoride-releasing sealant and glass ionomer materials act as fluoride reservoirs for adjacent enamel and dentin, provide enhanced caries resistance for sound enamel, and perhaps remineralize enamel and dentinal caries.

During the latter part of the 1980s and into the 1990s, increased acceptance of sealants as a preventive regimen has occurred, with 80% to 95% of dentists placing sealants in their practices. Sealants apparently will be adopted as a standard of care for prevention of pit and fissure caries. Although the percentage of children receiving sealants is increasing, certain factors still limit sealant use. The primary concern limiting sealant use is lack of third-party reimbursement for this procedure. To make significant gains in caries reduction in the child, adolescent, and adult populations in the near future, it is necessary for the dental profession to educate and inform the general public, parents, physicians, underwriters of dental care plans, and funding agencies about the cost-effectiveness and caries-preventive benefits of sealants and preventive restorations. With widespread use of the acid-etch technique, it may be possible to provide the majority of children, adolescents, and adults with a caries-free dentition.

REFERENCES

American Dental Association, Council on Scientific Affairs, *http://www.ada.org*, 1997.

Angmar-Mansson B, ten Bosch JJ: Advances in methods for diagnosing coronal caries—A review. Adv Dent Res 7:70, 1993.

Aranda M, Garcia-Godoy F: Clinical evaluation of the retention and wear of a light-cured pit and fissure glass ionomer sealant. J Clin Pediatr Dent *19*:273, 1995.

Bell RM, Klein SP, Bohannon HM, et al: Treatment Effects in the National Preventive Dentistry Demonstration Program. Publication No. R-3072-RWS, Santa Monica, CA, The Rand Corporation, 1984.

Blankenau RJ, Kelsey WP, Powell GL, et al: Degree of composite resin polymerization with visible light and argon laser. Am J Dent *4*:40, 1991.

Bodecker CF: The eradication of enamel fissures. Dent Items Interest *51*:859, 1929.

Bohannon HM, Disney JA, Graves RC, et al: Indications for sealant use in a community-based preventive dentistry program. J Dent Educ *48*:45, 1984.

Bowen RL: Composite and sealant resins—past, present and future. Pediatr Dent *4*:10, 1982.

Bowman PA, Zinner KL: Utah's parent, teacher and physician sealant awareness surveys. J Dent Hyg *68*:279, 1994.

Bowman PA, Fitzgerald CM: Utah dentists sealant usage survey. ASDC J Dent Child *57*:134, 1990.

Brown LJ: The impact of recent changes in the epidemiology of dental caries on guidelines for the use of dental sealants. J Public Health Dent *55*:274, 1995.

Brown LJ, Kaste LM, Selwitz RH, Furman LJ: Dental caries and sealant usage in US children, 1988–91: Selected findings from the third national health and nutrition examination survey. JADA *127*:335, 1996.

Buonocore MG: Simple method of increasing the adhesion of acrylic filling materials to enamel surfaces. J Dent Res *34*:849, 1955.

Burgess J, Norling B, Summitt J: Resin ionomer restorative materials: The new generation. J Esthet Dent *6*:207, 1994.

Call RL, Mann J, Hicks J: Attitudes of general practitioners towards fissure sealant use. Clin Prev Dent *10*:9, 1988.

Charbeneau GT: Pit and fissure sealants. J Dent *32*:315, 1982.

Chosak A, Eidelman E: Effect of time from application until exposure to light on the tag length of a visible light-polymerized sealant. Dent Mater *4*:302, 1988.

Cohen L, LaBelle A, Romberg E: The use of pit and fissure sealants in private practice: A national survey. J Public Health Dent *48*:26, 1988.

Cooley RL, McCourt JW, Huddleston AM, et al: Evaluation of a fluoride-containing sealant by SEM, microleakage and fluoride release. Pediatr Dent *12*:38, 1990.

Corbin SB, Clark NL, McClendon BJ, et al: Patterns of sealant delivery under variable third party requirements. J Public Health Dent *50*:311, 1990.

Dennison JB, Straffon LH, More FG: Evaluating tooth eruption on sealant efficacy. JADA *121*:610, 1990.

Eidelman E, Fuks A, Chosak A: The retention of fissure sealants: Rubber dam or cotton roll isolation in private practice. J Dent Child *50*:259, 1983.

Eidelman E, Shapira J, Houpt M: The retention of fissure sealants using twenty-second etching time: Three-year follow-up. J Dent Child *55*:119, 1988.

Elderton RJ: The cause of failure of restorations: A literature review. J Dent *4*:257, 1976.

Erickson RL, Glasspoole EA: Bonding to tooth structure: A comparison of glass-ionomer and composite-resin systems. J Esthet Dent *6*:227, 1994.

Faine RC, Dennen T: A survey of private dental practitioners' utilization of dental sealants in Washington state. J Dent Child *53*:337, 1986.

Faine RC, Isman R: The use of dental sealants in the Washington state medical assistance program: A second-year report. J Dent Child *56*:450, 1989.

Farghaly MM, Lang WP, Woolfolk MW, et al: Factors associated with fissure sealant delegation: Dentists characteristics and office staffing patterns. J Public Health Dent *53*:246, 1993.

Flaitz CM, Hicks MJ, Silverstone LM: Radiographic, histologic, and electronic comparison of occlusal caries: An in vitro study. Pediatr Dent *8*:24, 1986.

Foreman FJ: Sealant prevalence and indication in a young military population. JADA *125*:182, 1994.

Foreman FJ: Effects of delegation, state practice acts, and practice management techniques upon sealant utilization: A national survey of pediatric dentists. J Dent Child *60*:193, 1993.

Forss H, Saarnium, Seppa L: Comparison of glass-ionomer and resin-based fissure sealants: A 2-year clinical trial. Community Dent Oral Epiderm *22*:21, 1994.

Forsten L: Fluoride release of glass ionomers. J Esthet Dent *6*:216, 1994.

Freedman G, McLauglin G: Sealants buyer guide. Dental Products Report *16*:112, 1997.

Frencken JE, Pilot T, Songpaisan Y, Phantumvanit P: Atraumatic restorative treatment (ART): Rationale, technique and development. J Public Health Dent *56*:135, 1996.

Frencken JE, Songpaisan Y, Phantumvanit P, Pilot T: An atraumatic restorative treatment (ART) technique: Evaluation after one year. Int Dent J *44*:460, 1994.

Galil KA, Gwinnett AJ: Three-dimensional replicas of pits and fissures in human teeth: A scanning electron microscopic study. Arch Oral Biol *20*:493, 1975.

Garcia-Godoy F, Summitt JB, Donly KJ: Caries progression of white spot lesions sealed with an unfilled resin. J Clin Pediatr Dent *21*:141, 1997.

Gift HC, Frew RA: Sealants: Changing patterns. JADA *112*:391, 1986.

Gift HC, Frew RA, Hefferren J: Attitudes toward and use of pit and fissure sealants. J Dent Child *42*:460, 1975.

Gift HC, Newman JF: Oral health activities of US children: Results of a national health interview survey. JADA *123*:96, 1992.

Glasrud PH: Insuring preventive dental care: Are sealants included? Am J Public Health *75*:285, 1985.

Glasrud PH, Frazier PJ, Horowitz AM: Insurance reimbursement for sealants in 1986: Report of a survey. J Dent Child *54*:81, 1987.

Goldstein RE, Parkins FM: Using air-abrasive technology to diagnose and restore pit and fissure caries. JADA *126*:761, 1995.

Gonzalez CD, Frazier PJ, Messer LB: Sealant use by general practitioners: A Minnesota survey. J Dent Child *58*:38, 1991.

Gonzalez CD, Frazier PJ, LeMay W, et al: Sealant status and factors associated with sealant presence among children in Milwaukee, WI. J Dent Child *62*:335, 1995.

Graves RC, Burt BA: The pattern of the carious attack in children as a consideration in the use of fissure sealants. J Prev Dent *2*:28, 1975.

Greenwall AL, Johnsen D, DiSantis TA, et al: Longitudinal evaluation of caries pattern from the primary to the mixed dentition. Pediatr Dent *12*:278, 1990.

Hamid A, Hume WR: Release of estrogenic component bisphenol-A not detected from fissure sealants *in vitro*. J Dent Res *76*:321, 1997.

Handelman SL, Leverett DH, Espeland M, et al: Clinical radiographic evaluation of sealed carious and sound tooth surfaces. JADA *113*:751, 1986.

Handelman SL, Leverett DH, Espeland M, et al: Retention of sealants over carious and sound tooth surfaces. Community Dent Oral Epidemiol *15*:1, 1987.

Handelman SL, Washburn F, Wopperer P: Two-year report on the sealant effect on bacteria in dental caries. J Dent Res *93*:967, 1976.

Hardison JR, Collier OR, Sprouse CW, et al: Retention of pit and fissure sealant on primary molars of 3- and 4-year-old children after 1 year. JADA *114*:613, 1987.

Hennon DK, Stookey GK, Muhler JC: Prevalence and distribution of dental caries in preschool children. JADA *79*:1405, 1969.

Hicks MJ, Flaitz CM, Westerman GH, et al: Caries-like lesion initiation and progression around laser-cured sealants. Am J Dent *6*:176, 1993.

Hicks MJ, Flaitz CM: Caries-like lesion formation around fluoride-releasing sealant and glass ionomer. Am J Dent *5*:329, 1992.

Hicks MJ: Preventive resin restorations: Etching patterns, resin tag morphology and the enamel-resin interface. J Dent Child *51*:116, 1984a.

Hicks MJ: Caries-like lesion formation around occlusal alloy and preventive resin restorations. Pediatr Dent *6*:17, 1984b.

Hicks MJ, Flaitz CM: The epidemiology of dental caries in pediatric and adolescent population: A review of past and current trends. J Clin Pediatr Dent *18*:43, 1993.

Hicks MJ, Flaitz CM: Caries-like lesion formation in occlusal fissures: An in vitro study. Quint Int *17*:405, 1986.

Hicks MJ, Flaitz CM, Call RL: Comparison of pit and fissure sealant utilization by pediatric and general dentists in Colorado. J Pedodont *14*:97, 1990.

Hicks MJ, Flaitz CM, Silverstone LM: The current status of dental caries in the pediatric population. J Pedodont *10*:57, 1985.

Hicks MJ, Flaitz CM, Silverstone LM: Secondary caries formation in vitro around glass ionomer restorations. Quint Int *17*:527, 1986.

Hicks MJ, Silverstone LM: Fissure sealants and dental enamel: A histological study of microleakage in vitro. Caries Res *16*:353, 1982a.

Hicks MJ, Silverstone LM: The effect of sealant application and sealant loss on caries-like lesion formation in vitro. Pediatr Dent *4*:111, 1982b.

Hicks MJ, Silverstone LM: Acid-etching of caries-like lesions of enamel: A scanning electron microscopic study. Caries Res *18*:326, 1984a.

Hicks MJ, Silverstone LM: Acid-etching of caries-like lesions of enamel: A polarized light microscopic study. Caries Res *18*:315, 1984b.

Holloway PJ, Clarkson JE: Cost:benefit of prevention in practice. Int Dent J *44*:317, 1994.

Holmgren CJ: ART-ODONT: An electronic network for information concerning minimal intervention techniques for caries. J Public Health Dent *56*:166, 1996.

Holmgren CJ, Pilot T: Preliminary research agenda for minimal intervention techniques for caries. J Public Health Dent *56*:164, 1996.

Horowitz AM: Introduction to the symposium on minimal intervention techniques for caries. J Public Health Dent *56*:133, 1996.

Horowitz HS, Meyers RJ, Heifetz SB, et al: Combined fluoride, school-based program in a fluoride-deficient area: Results of an 11-year study. JADA *112*:621, 1986.

Houpt M, Eidelman E, Shey Z, et al: Occlusal restoration using fissure sealant instead of "extension for prevention." J Dent Child *51*:270, 1984.

Houpt M, Eidelman E, Shey Z, et al: Occlusal composite restorations: 4-year results. JADA *110*:351, 1985a.

Houpt M, Eidelman E, Shey Z, et al: The composite/sealant restoration: Five-year results. J Prosth Dent *55*:164, 1986.

Houpt M, Fuks A, Eidelman E: Measuring the stickiness of pits and fissures in enamel. Clin Prev Dent 7:28, 1985b.

Houpt M, Fuks A, Eidelmann E: The preventive resin (composite resin/sealant) restoration: Nine-year results. Quint Int *28*:155, 1994.

Houpt M, Fuks A, Eidelman E, et al: Composite/sealant restoration: 6-year results. Pediatr Dent *10*:394, 1988.

Hyatt TP: Occlusal fissures: Their frequency and danger. How shall they be treated? Dent Items Interest *46*:493, 1924.

IADR Sealant Symposium. J Dent Res *70(Special Issue)*:266, 1991.

Ie YL, Verdonschot EH, Schaeken MJM, van't Hof MA: Electrical conductance of fissure enamel in recently erupted molar teeth as related to caries status. Caries Res *29*:94, 1995.

Ismail AI: Rector paper: Minimal intervention techniques for dental caries. J Public Health Dent *56*:155, 1996.

Ismail AI, Gagnon P: A longitudinal evaluation of fissure sealants applied in dental practices. J Dent Res *74*:1583, 1995.

Jensen OE, Billings RJ, Featherstone JD: Clinical evaluation of Fluroshield pit and fissure sealant. Clin Prev Dent *12*:24, 1990.

Jensen OE, Handelman SL: Effect of an autopolymerizing sealant on viability of microflora in occlusal dental caries. Scand J Dent Res *88*:382, 1980.

Johnsen DC, Schechner TG, Gerstenmaier JH: Proportional changes in caries patterns from early to late primary dentition. J Public Health Dent *47*:5, 1987.

Kaste LM, Selwitz RH, Oldakowski RJ, et al: Coronal caries in the primary and permanent dentition of children and adolescents 1–17 years of age: United States, 1988–1991. J Dent Res *75(Special Issue)*:631, 1996.

Kelsey WP, Blankenau RJ, Powell GL, et al: Enhancement of physical properties of resin restorative materials by laser polymerization. Lasers Surg Med *9*:623, 1989.

Komatsu H, Shimokobe H, Kawakamis, Yoshimura M: Caries-preventive effect of glass ionomer sealant reapplication: Study presents three-year results. J Am Dent Assoc *125*:543, 1994.

Kuthy RA: Charges for sealants and one-surface, posterior permanent restorations: Three years of insurance claims data. Pediatr Dent *14*:405, 1992.

Kuthy RA, Clive JM: Comparison of number and mean charge between dental sealants and one-surface restorations. J Public Health Dent *52*:227, 1992.

Lacy AM, Young DA: Modern concepts and materials for the pediatric dentist. J Pediatr Dent *18*:469, 1996.

Lang WP, Weintraub JA, Choi C, et al: Fissure sealant knowledge and characteristics of parents as a function of their child's sealant status. J Public Health Dent *48*:133, 1988.

Li S-H, Kingman A, Forthofer R, Swango P: Comparison of tooth surface-specific dental caries attack patterns in US schoolchildren from two national surveys. J Dent Res *72*:1398, 1993.

Louie R, Brunelle JA, Maggiore ED, et al: Caries prevalence in Head Start children, 1986–87. J Public Health Dent *50*:299, 1990.

Lussi A, Firestone A, Schoenberg V, et al: *In vivo* diagnosis of fissure caries using a new electrical resistance monitor. Caries Res *29*:81, 1995.

Mafeni JO, Messer LB: Parental knowledge and attitudes towards pit and fissure sealants. Aust Dent J *39*:172, 1994.

McKenna EF, Grundy GE: Glass ionomer cement fissure sealants applied by operative dental auxiliaries: Retention rate after one year. Aust Dent J *32*:200, 1987.

McKnight-Hanes C, Myers DR, Salama FS, et al: Comparing treatment options for occlusal surfaces utilizing an invasive index. Pediatr Dent *12*:241, 1990.

McLean JW: Evolution of glass ionomer cements: A personal view. J Esthet Dent *6*:195, 1994.

Mejare I, Mjor IA: Glass ionomer and resin-based fissure sealants: A clinical study. Scand J Dent Res *98*:345, 1990.

Mertz-Fairhurst EJ, Curtis JW, Ergle JW, et al: Ultraconservative and cariostatic sealed restorations: Results at year 10. JADA *129*:55, 1998.

Mertz-Fairhurst EJ, Adair SM, Sams DR, et al: Cariostatic and ultraconservative sealed restorations: Nine-year results among children and adults. J Dent Child *63*:97, 1995.

Mertz-Fairhurst EJ, Call-Smith KM, Schuster GS, et al: Clinical performance of sealed composite restorations placed over caries compared with sealed and unsealed amalgam restorations. JADA *115*:689, 1987.

Mertz-Fairhurst EJ, Richards EE, Williams JE, et al: Sealed restorations: 5-year results. Am J Dent *5*:5, 1992.

Mertz-Fairhurst EJ, Schuster GS, Fairhurst CW: Arresting caries by sealant: Results of a clinical study. JADA *112*:194, 1986.

Mertz-Fairhurst EJ, Schuster GS, Williams JE, et al: Clinical progress of sealed and unsealed caries. Part I: Depth changes and bacterial counts. J Prosth Dent 45:521, 1979a.

Mertz-Fairhurst EJ, Schuster GS, Williams JE, et al: Clinical progress of sealed and unsealed caries. Part II: Standardized radiographs and clinical observations. J Prosth Dent 42:633, 1979b.

Mertz-Fairhurst EJ, Smith CD, Williams JE, et al: Cariostatic and ultraconservative sealed restorations: Six-year results. Quint Int 23:827, 1993.

Mertz-Fairhurst EJ, Williams JE, Pierce KL, et al: Sealed restorations: 4-year results. Am J Dent 4:43, 1991.

Mills RW, Ball IA: A clinical trial to evaluate the retention of a silver-cement-ionomer used as a fissure sealant. Oper Dent 18:148, 1993.

Mitchell L, Murray JJ: Fissure sealants: A critique of their cost-effectiveness. Commun Dent Oral Epidemiol 17:19, 1989.

Mjor IA: Frequency of secondary caries at various anatomic locations. Oper Dent 10:88, 1985.

Mjor IA, Leinfelder KJ: Operative dentistry. In Mjor IA (ed): Dental Materials: Biological Properties and Clinical Evaluations. Boca Raton, FL, CRC Press, 1985, p 93.

Nathanson D, Lertpitayakun P, Lamkin MS, et al: In vitro elution of leachable components from dental sealants. JADA 128:1517, 1997.

National Center for Health Statistics: Decayed, Missing and Filled Teeth Among Children: United States. Vital and Health Statistics, Series 11, No. 106. DHEW Publication No. (HSM) 72-1003. Washington, D.C., U.S. Government Printing Office, 1971.

National Center for Health Statistics: Decayed, Missing and Filled Teeth Among Youths 12–17 Years: United States. Vital and Health Statistics, Series 11, No. 144. DHEW Publication No. (HRA) 75-1626. Washington, D.C., U.S. Government Printing Office, 1974.

National Institute of Dental Research, National Caries Program: The Prevalence of Dental Caries in United States Children, 1979–1980. NIH Pub. No. 82-2245. Bethesda, MD, National Institutes of Health, 1981.

National Institute of Dental Research, National Caries Program: Epidemiology and Oral Disease Prevention Program: Oral Health of United States School Children: The National Survey of Dental Caries in U.S. School Children: 1986–1987. NIH Publ. No. 89-2247, Bethesda, MD, National Institutes of Health, 1989.

Ngano T: Relationship between form of pits and fissures and the primary lesion of caries. Dent Abstr 6:426, 1961.

Olea N, Pulgar R, Perez P, et al: Estrogenicity of resin-based composites and sealants used in dentistry. Environ Health Perspect 104:298, 1996.

Ovrebo RC, Raadal M: Microleakage in fissures sealed with resin or glass ionomer cement. Scand J Dent Res 98:66, 1990.

Palmer C: How many will have sealants in 2000? ADA News 23:1, 1992a.

Palmer C: Ohio effort shows rise in sealants. ADA News 23:4, 1992b.

Palmer C: Sealant use for Indians nears 75%. ADA News 23:4, 1992c.

Peers A, Hill FJ, Mitropoulos CM, Holloway PJ: Validity and reproducibility of clinical examination, fibre-optic transillumination, and bite-wing radiology for the diagnosis of small approximal carious lesions: An in vitro study. Caries Res 27:307, 1993.

Phantumvanit P, Songpaisan U, Pilot R, Frencken JE: Atraumatic restorative treatment (ART): A three-year community field trial in Thailand—Survival of one-surface restorations in the permanent dentition. J Public Health Dent 56:141, 1996.

Powell GL, Kelsey WP, Blankenau RJ, et al: The use of an argon laser for polymerization of composite resin. J Esthet Dent 1:34, 1989.

Radike AW: Criteria for diagnosis of dental caries. In Proceedings of the Conference on the Clinical Testing of Cariostatic Agents, October 14-16, 1968. Chicago, American Dental Association, 1972, pp 87–88.

Rawls HR, Zimmerman BF: Fluoride-exchanging resins for caries protection. Caries Res 17:32, 1983.

Redford DA, Clarkson BH, Jensen ME: The effect of different etching times on sealant bond strength, etch depth and pattern in primary teeth. Pediatr Dent 8:11, 1986.

Ricketts DNJ, Kidd EAM, Liepins PJ, Wilson RF: Histological validation of electrical resistance measurements in the diagnosis of occlusal caries. Caries Res 30:148, 1996.

Ripa LW, Leske GS, Forte F: The combined use of pit and fissure sealants and fluoride mouthrinsing in second and third grade children: One-year clinical results. Pediatr Dent 8:158, 1986.

Ripa LW, Leske GS, Forte F: The combined use of pit and fissure sealants and fluoride mouthrinsing in second and third grade children: Final clinical results after two years. Pediatr Dent 9:118, 1987.

Roberts MW, Shern RJ, Kennedy JB: Evaluation of an auto-polymerizing fissure sealant as a vehicle for slow release of fluoride. Pediatr Dent 6:145, 1984.

Rock WP: The diagnosis of early carious lesions—A review. J Pediatr Dent 3:1, 1987.

Rock WP, Potts AJC, Marchment MD, et al: The visibility of clear and opaque fissure sealants. Br Dent J 167:395, 1989.

Rohr M, Makinson OF, Burrow MF: Pit and fissures: Morphology. J Dent Child 58:97, 1991.

Romberg E, Cohen LA, LaBelle AD: A national survey of sealant usage by pediatric dentists. J Dent Child 55:257, 1988.

Romcke RG, Lewis DW, Maze BD, et al: Retention and maintenance of fissure sealants over 10 years. Can Dent J 56:235, 1990.

Rozier RG: Reaction paper: The impact of recent changes in the epidemiology of dental caries on guidelines for the use of dental sealants: Epidemiologic perspectives. J Public Health Dent 55:292, 1995.

Selwitz RH, Colley BJ, Rozier RG: Factors associated with parental acceptance of dental sealants. J Public Health Dent 52:137, 1992.

Selwitz RH, Nowjack-Raymer R, Driscoll WS, et al: Evaluation after 4 years of the combined use of fluoride and dental sealants. Community Dent Oral Epidemiol 23:30, 1995.

Selwitz RH, Winn DM, Kingman A, et al: The prevalence of dental sealants in the US population: Findings from NHANES III, 1988-1991. J Dent Res 75(Special Issue):652, 1996.

Siegal M: Promotion and use of pit and fissure sealants: An introduction to the special issue. J Public Health Dent 55:259, 1995.

Siegal MD, Garcia IA, Kandray DP, et al: The use of dental sealants by Ohio dentists. J Public Health Dent 56:12, 1996.

Silverstone LM: The current status of fissure sealants and priorities for future research: Part I. Comp Cont Educ 5:204, 1984a.

Silverstone LM: The current status of fissure sealants and priorities for future research: Part II. Comp Cont Educ 5:299, 1984b.

Silverstone LM: State of the art on sealant research and priorities for further research. J Dent Educ 48:107, 1984c.

Silverstone LM, Hicks MJ, Featherstone MJ: Oral fluid contamination of etched enamel surfaces: An SEM study. JADA 110:329, 1985.

Simonsen RJ: Preventive resin restorations (I). Quint Int 1:69, 1978a.

Simonsen RJ: Preventive resin restorations (II). Quint Int *2*:95, 1978b.

Simonsen RJ: The clinical effectiveness of a colored pit and fissure sealant at 36 months. JADA *102*:323, 1981.

Simonsen RJ: Retention and effectiveness of a single application of white sealant after 10 years. JADA *115*:31, 1987.

Simonsen RJ: Cost-effectiveness of pit and fissure sealants at 10 years. Quint Int *20*:75, 1989a.

Simonsen RJ: Why not prevention? Quint Int *20*:785, 1989b.

Simonsen RJ: Retention and effectiveness of dental sealants after 15 years. JADA *122*:34, 1991.

Soderholm K-JM: Reactor paper: The impact of recent changes in the epidemiology of dental caries on guidelines for the use of dental sealants: Clinical perspectives. J Public Health Dent *55*:302, 1995.

Stahl JW, Katz RV: Occlusal dental caries incidence in college students: Implications for sealants. J Dent Res *71*(AADR Abst):250, 1992.

Stahl JW, Katz RV: Occlusal dental caries incidence and implications for sealant program in a US college student population. J Public Health Dent *53*:212, 1993.

Sterritt GR, Frew RA, Rozier RG: Evaluation of Guamamian dental caries prevention programs after 13 years. J Public Health Dent *54*:153, 1994.

Sterritt GR, Frew RA, Rozier RG, et al: Evaluation of a school-based fluoride mouthrinsing and clinic-based sealant program on a non-fluoridated island. Community Dent Oral Epidemiol *18*:288, 1990.

Straffon LH, Dennison JB: Clinical evaluation comparing sealant and amalgam after 7 years: Final report. JADA *117*:751, 1988.

Straffon LH, Dennison JB, More FG: Three-year evaluation of sealant: Effect of isolation on efficacy. JADA *110*:714, 1985.

Tanaka M, Ono H, Kadoma Y, et al: Incorporation into human enamel of fluoride slowly released from a sealant in vivo. J Dent Res *66*:1591, 1987.

Tandon S, Kumari R, Udupa S: The effect of etch-time on the bond strength of a sealant and on the etch pattern in primary and permanent enamel: An evaluation. J Dent Child *56*:186, 1989.

Torppa-Saarinen E, Seppa L: Short-term retention of glass-ionomer sealants. Proc Finn Dent Soc *86*:83, 1990.

Traubman A, Silberman SL, Meydrech EF: Dental caries assessment of Mississippi Head Start Program children. J Public Health Dent *49*:167, 1989.

Vehkalahti MM, Solavaara L, Rytomaa I: An eight-year follow-up of the occlusal surfaces of first permanent molars. J Dent Res *70*:1064, 1991.

Verdonschot EH, Rondel P, Huysmans MC: Validity of electrical conductance measurements in evaluating the marginal integrity of sealant restorations. Caries Res *29*:100, 1995.

Vrbic V: Sealing of primary and permanent teeth with Helioseal F [Abstract No. 1421]. J Dent Res *76(Special Issue)*:191, 1997.

Waggoner WF, Siegal M: Pit and fissure sealant application: Updating the technique. JADA *127*:351, 1996.

Walker JD, Floyd K, Jakobsen J: The effectiveness of sealants in pediatric patients. J Dent Child *63*:268, 1996a.

Walker, JD, Floyd K, Jakobsen J, Pinkham JR: The effectiveness of preventive resin restorations in pediatric patients. J Dent Child *63*:338, 1996b.

Walker JD, Jensen ME, Pinkham JR: A clinical review of preventive resin restorations. J Dent Child *57*:257, 1990.

Walls AWG, Wallwork MA, Holland IS, et al: The longevity of occlusal amalgam restorations in first permanent molars of child patients. Br Dent J *158*:133, 1985.

Weintraub JA: The effectiveness of pit and fissure sealants. J Public Health Dent *49*:317, 1989.

Wellbury RR, Walls AWG, Murray JJ, et al: The management of occlusal caries in permanent molars: A 5-year clinical trial comparing minimal composite with an amalgam restoration. Br Dent J *169*:361, 1990.

Westerman G, Hicks MJ, Flaitz CM, et al: Argon laser-cured sealant and caries-like lesion formation. J Dent Res *70*:493, 1991.

White GE, Tsamtsouris A, Williams DL: A longitudinal study of electronic caries detection of occlusal caries. J Pedodont *5*:91, 1981.

Winkler MM, Deschepper EJ, Dean JA, et al: Using a resin-modified glass ionomer as an occlusal sealant: A one-year clinical study. J Am Dent Assoc *127*:1508, 1996.

Workshop on Guidelines for Sealant Use: Recommendations. J Public Health Dent *55*:263, 1995.

33

Pulp Therapy for Young Permanent Teeth

Gary K. Belanger

Chapter Outline

PULPAL ASSESSMENT
Patient History
Clinical Examination
Clinical Diagnostic Procedures
Radiographic Examination
Direct Pulpal Evaluation

PULP TREATMENT PROCEDURES
Caries Control
Indirect Pulp Cap
Direct Pulp Cap
Formocresol Pulpotomy
Apexogenesis (Calcium Hydroxide or Vital Pulpotomy)
Apexification (Frank Procedure or Root-End Closure)

Mature teeth are those that have experienced complete apical development, whereas young permanent teeth are those recently erupted teeth in which apical root closure has not been completed. Pulp protection and therapy for young permanent teeth require consideration of many of the same objectives and techniques that are necessary for both deciduous teeth and mature permanent teeth. A major additional concern for the young permanent tooth with a diseased or traumatized pulp, however, may be the need either to promote normal apical completion or to stimulate an atypical apical closure. These outcomes are sought in order to ensure that an adequate crown-to-root ratio is established and to allow, if necessary, a definitive root canal procedure to be successfully completed at a later date. Because normal physiologic root closure of permanent teeth may take 2 to 3 years after the tooth's eruption, young permanent teeth are a developmental stage in children from 6 years of age until the mid-teens.

Numerous factors can affect the pulpal health of teeth, but the two major conditions detrimental to young permanent teeth are deep caries and traumatic injuries. Deep caries is much more likely to affect the posterior teeth, especially the permanent first molars. Trauma is much more likely to affect the anterior teeth, especially the maxillary incisors.

PULPAL ASSESSMENT

Assessment of the pulp status of young permanent teeth is divided into the same five categories as are used for deciduous teeth: (1) patient history, (2) clinical examination, (3) clinical diagnostic procedures, (4) radiographic examination, and (5) direct pulpal evaluation.

Patient History

A child may report complaints of spontaneous dental pain or pain and sensitivity that is precipitated from external sources such as air, heat, cold, food, or pressure. Spontaneous pain occurs without provocation and is indicative of significant damage to the pulp that is usually irreversible. Precipitated (or stimulated) pain that does not persist after removal of the stimulus is often a more favorable finding, indicating dentinal sensitivity (Seltzer and Bender, 1984).

A complaint of pressure sensitivity may indicate a serious situation, such as total pulpal necrosis, extending to the periodontal ligament and causing extrusion of the tooth from its socket. It may also indicate a fairly innocuous situation, however, such as a previously placed restoration or a sealant that is in hyperocclusion. A foreign body (such as a popcorn kernel) that has wedged into the sulcus can also account for sensitivity to pressure. Historical information must be compared with other findings in order to properly investigate a child's complaints about pressure pain.

Any historical findings regarding dental caries should include an assessment of the length of time during which the lesion may have been developing; how long it has been bothersome; whether there is any facial or intraoral redness, swelling, or drainage; and whether there has been any previous treatment or recommendation. Anything that the child is able to do that reduces or eliminates pain should also be noted. Many children complain of "toothaches" during the eruption of permanent first molars around age 6. In such instances, the dentist should be careful to rule out whether the child is really only reacting to a pericoronitis or to biting on an operculum.

In the assessment of a traumatic injury to a young permanent tooth, time is a critical element for the dentist to consider. The longer a pulp has been exposed, the greater the opportunity has been for bacterial infection and degenerative pulpal changes. Thus, conservative techniques (such as direct pulp cap) are possible with a very recently fractured incisor (less than 1 hour), but as the elapsed time increases, progressively more aggressive therapy is required.

Clinical Examination

Young permanent teeth with pulpal involvement that is due to a carious lesion will likely be obvious during clinical inspection. Some deep lesions, however, progress through poorly coalesced pits, fissures, or hypoplastic enamel and display minimal enamel destruction clinically. Sensitivity to explorer probing, review of radio-graphs, and clinical excavation can confirm a suspicion that the lesion is more advanced than it appears (Fig. 33-1).

Traumatized teeth may show evidence of injury in many ways. Fractures may involve enamel, dentin, cementum, or pulp of dental crowns or roots. Displacement injuries affect the periodontal structures and may range from minor loosening to complete avulsions. In all situations, the pulp is affected to some degree (see Chapter 34 for a discussion of treatment of traumatized teeth). With some injuries, the effect on the pulp may be neither apparent nor diagnosable initially and actually may take months or years to become manifest. With severe injuries, however, the pulp is almost always deleteriously affected and requires immediate or subsequent treatment.

Clinical Diagnostic Procedures

Heat, cold, and an electrical pulse are classic tests for pulpal sensitivity, vitality, and viability. In young permanent teeth, these measurements can provide some clues to the histopathologic status of the pulp in a carious or traumatized tooth in comparison with noninvolved teeth. Interpretation of testing data must be cautious, however, because an open apex provides a significantly enlarged vascular supply but an incompletely developed nervous innervation when compared with mature permanent teeth (Bernick, 1964). In traumatized teeth especially, the reactions to pulp tests should not be interpreted literally because the pulp can be in a state of shock for many days or weeks and may register negatively to tests and then return later to normal status. Nevertheless, testing should be performed because test results serve as good baseline data for subsequent comparisons and for evaluation of changes over time.

Tests of mobility and percussion sensitivity should also be performed for comparison with antimeres or unaffected teeth. Increased mobility in carious teeth is indicative of periodontal ligament involvement. Traumatized teeth often suffer slight to extreme increases in mobility, which indicates damage to the supporting structures and possibly an altered pulp status.

Radiographic Examination

A diagnostically accurate periapical radiograph is essential for correct pulpal evaluation of a deeply carious or traumatized young permanent tooth.

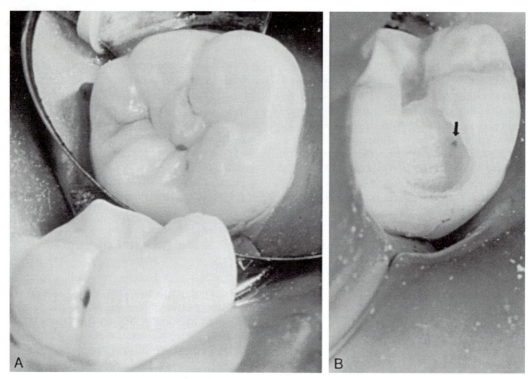

Figure 33–1. *A,* Clinical view of permanent first molar with poorly coalesced occlusal fissures and buccal pit but without gross decay. *B,* Same tooth at time of treatment, showing a carious pulp exposure *(arrow).*

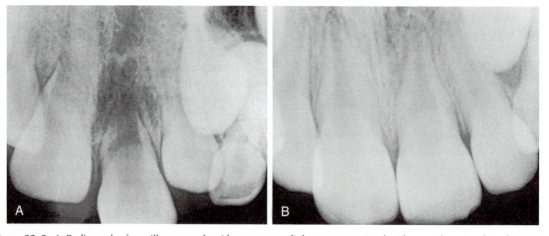

Figure 33–2. *A,* Radiograph of maxillary centrals with apparent radiolucency associated with recently erupted tooth No. 9. There was no history of trauma, pain, or excess mobility, however, and the tooth was within normal limits for all pulp tests; thus, no treatment was begun. *B,* Radiograph of same maxillary centrals 12 months later, showing symmetrical apical development of No. 8 and No. 9 and no evidence of periapical pathosis.

The interpretation may be difficult, however, because of a normally large and open apex; the dentist must be careful to never make treatment decisions based on radiographic information alone (Fig. 33-2). It is also helpful to have a view of the antimere available for the sake of comparison. Several additional factors worthy of consideration are as follows:

1. More than one view of the area of interest, each taken at a different angle, is helpful for locating subtle changes (e.g., root fractures).

2. Pathologic changes should not be confused with normal anatomy (e.g., mandibular canal, mental foramen, incisive fossa, nasopalatine canal).

3. Internal resorption is possible in permanent teeth but does not occur as often as in primary teeth. Pathologic external root resorption is frequently a later sequela of severe disruption of the periodontal ligament (e.g., avulsions).

4. Treatment-induced calcification (i.e., bridging or apical closure) may be too thin to visualize radiographically. Clinical probing, although potentially dangerous, may be necessary to confirm development of calcification.

Direct Pulpal Evaluation

As for primary teeth and mature secondary teeth, important information may become apparent at the time of actual clinical treatment. Careful visual inspection, tactile evaluation during instrumentation, and even detection of foul odors given off by a pulp provide important clues about lesion depth and pulpal status. The texture of carious dentin must be judged as well as its proximity to the pulp. The quality (color) and quantity of bleeding from a direct exposure of pulp tissue (unintended, planned, or traumatic) must be assessed. The dentist develops clinical experience and judgment of how these direct findings may confirm or alter planned treatment.

PULP TREATMENT PROCEDURES

Young permanent teeth are considered good candidates for many pulp-healing procedures because of their increased apical perfusion, which is thought to enhance the pulp's ability to react to various insults successfully (Massler, 1972). As for primary and mature permanent teeth, protection of exposed dentin during any mechanical preparation or restorative phase of treatment is mandatory. Calcium hydroxide preparations should be placed routinely over dentin in any area that is appreciably deeper than the dentinoenamel junction because of mechanical preparation, caries excavation, or a coronal fracture involving dentin. This is intended to protect dentinal tubules, odontoblasts, and pulp by sealing the dentin and protecting the pulp through sclerosis of dentinal tubules.

More recent reports (Cox and Suzuki, 1994), however, have challenged this conventional form of pulp protection and instead recommend using newer adhesive systems because calcium hydroxide preparations have no inherent ability to affect pulp and produce a favorable biologic response. Acid treatment of dentin is recommended to modify the smear layer, allowing for hybridization using compatible adhesive systems that seal the dentin, over which a final restoration can be immediately placed. North American dental schools are teaching less the use of calcium hydroxide for bases or liners, and glass ionomers and dentin bonding agents are becoming increasingly popular (Weiner et al., 1996).

Caries Control

A child may present with uncontrolled multiple carious teeth, one or more of which may have frank pulp involvement or deep dentinal caries encroaching on the pulp. Rather than trying to complete all pulp and restorative procedures sequentially, the dentist may recommend that the initial treatment visit be used to try to arrest all deep active carious lesions and halt their advancement toward pulpal involvement. In such a case, under rubber dam isolation, the gross caries are removed followed by calcium hydroxide placement (or glass ionomer or a dentin bonding agent) and an interim restoration with a reinforced zinc oxide and eugenol product such as I.R.M. (LD Caulk Co., Milford, DE). The goal is to arrest the progression in a caries-active mouth and promote a favorable pulpal response. Definitive restorations and further pulp treatment, if necessary, are completed at subsequent visits.

Indirect Pulp Cap

Given the situation of a deep carious lesion in an asymptomatic young permanent tooth in which a pulpal exposure would most likely occur if total removal of carious dentin were attempted (Fig. 33-3A), in the indirect pulp cap procedure a very thin layer of carious dentin is left in place

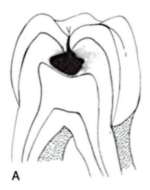 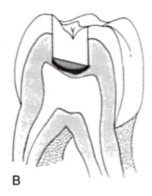 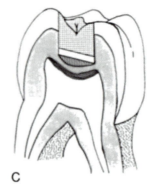

A   B   C

Figure 33–3. Indirect pulp cap. *A,* Carious lesion *(black area)* progressing through enamel and dentin toward pulp; if all carious and decalcified dentin were removed, a pulpal exposure would likely occur. *B,* A small layer of soft dentin is left over pulp, over which a calcium hydroxide preparation *(vertical lines)* is placed directly, followed by reinforced zinc oxide and eugenol interim restoration *(white area). C,* Reparative dentin that has formed *(horizontal lines in pulp chamber roof),* sclerosis of the dentin that was left, calcium hydroxide, base (or previous interim restoration if it was not totally removed at second instrumentation), and final amalgam restoration *(stippled area).*

directly over the pulp. A calcium hydroxide preparation is placed over the soft carious dentin, followed by a reinforced zinc oxide and eugenol interim restoration in order to seal the cavity (Fig. 33-3*B*). The goal is to promote pulpal healing by removing the majority of infective bacteria and by sealing the lesion, which stimulates sclerosis of dentin and reparative dentin formation (King et al., 1965). As the procedure was originally practiced, after a minimum of 6 weeks the zinc oxide and eugenol, calcium hydroxide, and remaining carious dentin were removed. It was hoped that this second instrumentation of the tooth would confirm the intended goals and would be followed by placement of a permanent restoration (Fig. 33-3*C*). For the experienced clinician using good case selection, however, it may be preferable to avoid the second instrumentation (and the potential risk of pulpal exposure). If the dentist is confident in the case selection and has good technical expertise for the procedure, a final (rather than interim) restoration may be placed and the procedure performed in one step. Periodic follow-up of the tooth's history along with appropriate pulp vitality testing and radiographic assessment is necessary. Indirect pulp capping is an excellent and conservative treatment option for some deep carious lesions in permanent teeth (especially if it avoids complete root canal treatment).

It should be emphasized that the indirect pulp cap procedure is intended to *avoid* a direct carious exposure. Therefore, cautious caries removal is required prior to calcium hydroxide placement. Unfortunately, some dentists use the term *indirect pulp cap* whenever calcium hydroxide

is placed over dentin. The term should be reserved for the procedure as described previously.

Direct Pulp Cap

Actual clinical exposure of the pulp of a young permanent tooth may sometimes render it a candidate for a direct pulp capping procedure (Camp, 1983). Several situations in which this would be indicated include the following:

1. A small mechanical exposure caused by overpreparation has occurred with a rubber dam in place.
2. A small carious exposure in a tooth that has not been associated with any spontaneous pain, redness, swelling, or fever shows no radiographic signs of pulp degeneration or changes in the periapical areas and presents controllable bleeding at the exposure site (see Fig. 33-1).
3. A traumatic injury has caused a coronal fracture involving the pulp, the exposure is no larger than 2 mm in diameter, and the injury has occurred within the past few hours. If time since the injury is longer than that or if the exposure is larger in size than 2 mm, apexogenesis may be indicated or the dentist may choose to remove several millimeters of infected surface pulp and place calcium hydroxide at a slightly more apical level where healthy pulp tissue is encountered (see Chapter 34 for a description of the shallow calcium hydroxide pulpotomy treatment of traumatized teeth).

In any of these situations, the child and parents need to be informed that problems may develop later (with or without symptoms) and that periodic monitoring is necessary. Monitoring should occur every few weeks initially and then less frequently if no signs, symptoms, or radiographic problems develop. After a direct pulp cap of a carious exposure, an interim restoration is indicated (usually a reinforced zinc oxide and eugenol preparation), followed by a final restoration once success appears to be ensured. A mechanical exposure and direct pulp cap is usually restored by whatever final restoration had originally been planned. For trauma cases, a composite or glass ionomer interim palliative restoration (or "bandage") can be placed over the direct pulp cap and enamel. A final composite restoration is seldom indicated at the same appointment during which the direct pulp cap is placed for two reasons:

1. The additional manipulation necessary to complete a final restoration may be additive to any pulpal and periodontal damages already sustained from the traumatic injury.

2. A final restoration that is esthetically pleasing in a child who is not in pain may discourage the parents from returning for important follow-up monitoring visits.

Formocresol Pulpotomy

The formocresol pulpotomy procedure has enjoyed high clinical success in primary teeth. Dentists have attempted to extrapolate its use in permanent teeth. Results have been equivocal, and the routine use of this procedure cannot be recommended. Given the situation in which (1) deep caries involves an especially critical tooth (e.g., permanent first molar), causing extensive pulpal involvement, (2) the parents have ruled out conventional endodontic treatment, and (3) the dentist wishes to avoid extraction if at all possible, formocresol pulpotomy may be attempted (Trask, 1972). Although there may be clinical success for several years afterward, deterioration usually occurs in time. The procedure should be considered and tried only as a last alternative in attempting to temporarily forestall an eventual need for conventional and definitive endodontic treatment.

Apexogenesis (Calcium Hydroxide or Vital Pulpotomy)

If a young permanent tooth has a sufficiently large or long-standing pulp exposure such that

its coronal (but not radicular) pulp is infected, inflamed, or judged unlikely to retain its viability, the coronal portion of the pulp can be removed and the remaining radicular pulp treated with calcium hydroxide (Fig. 33-4, *left middle*). The goal is to maintain the radicular pulp's viability to allow apexogenesis or apical closure (Dannenberg, 1974). Calcium hydroxide placed directly on the radicular pulp stump stimulates a calcific response immediately adjacent to it, which later becomes visible on a radiograph as a radiopaque "bridge" over the amputation site (Fig. 33-4, *left bottom*). If degenerative and irreversible coronal pulp changes have not progressed into the radicular pulp, successful root closure can progress to completion (Figs. 33-5 and 33-6). The procedure can be thought of as analogous to a direct pulp cap except that it is performed at a more apical level.

For apexogenesis candidates, a radiograph should be taken to confirm that no pathologic

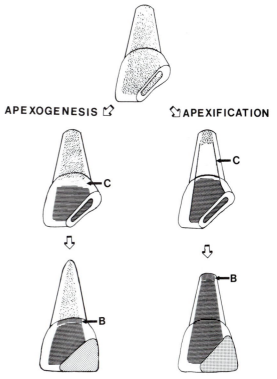

Figure 33–4. Top diagram indicates that pulp exposure of immature permanent incisor can be treated by apexogenesis *(left arrows)* if radicular pulp is vital or by apexification *(right arrows)* if radicular pulp is necrotic. For both procedures, C indicates the level where calcium hydroxide is placed at initiation of the procedure; B indicates the location of a bridge formation with time. *Horizontal lines* represent the interim restoration and final base; *stippled area* represents final composite restoration.

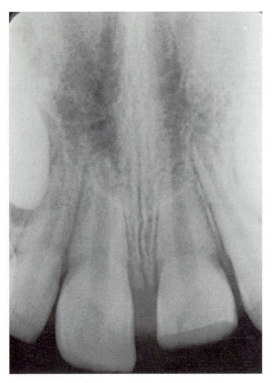

Figure 33–5. Apexogenesis was started on tooth No. 9 several days after a dentinoenamel fracture with pulp exposure; note open apex.

Apexogenesis is a useful treatment for saving young permanent teeth with exposed vital but infected coronal pulps. (If the apex is closed, conventional endodontic procedures can be performed.) Periodic clinical and radiographic observation is mandatory.

Recent research, however, indicates that complete amputation of the coronal pulp may not be necessary. A "shallow pulpotomy" of several millimeters with a large round diamond bur followed by placement of calcium hydroxide is an increasingly popular treatment option, even if considerable time has elapsed since a traumatic injury with pulp exposure (Heide and Kerekes, 1986). This technique has also been employed successfully with deep carious lesions and exposed pulps (Mejàre and Cvek, 1993).

Apexification (Frank Procedure or Root-End Closure)

If a young permanent tooth has a pulp with extensive degeneration or necrosis throughout (usually with clinical and radiographic signs of a periapical reaction), the pulp should be totally

periapical changes are present. Even though hemorrhage will occur at the amputation site, it should not be profuse or have an abnormal color. Slight pressure for several minutes with a sterile cotton pellet should significantly reduce bleeding. The calcium hydroxide can be either U.S.P. powder or a proprietary calcium hydroxide pulp-capping preparation such as Pulpdent (Pulpdent Corporation of America, Brookline, MA). It is placed directly on the pulp amputation site and then covered with a base and interim restoration. Although a final restoration may be placed, it is preferable to wait until success is evident so that the time and expense of a permanent restoration are warranted.

The child and parent should be informed that there is a risk that the procedure may not be successful and that more aggressive treatment (i.e., apexification) will be necessary later. Also, conventional gutta percha endodontic treatment after the apical closure has occurred is recommended even in the absence of a problem owing to a concern that complete canal obliteration through continued calcification will progress after apexogenesis and make endodontic procedures impossible later (Fuks et al., 1982).

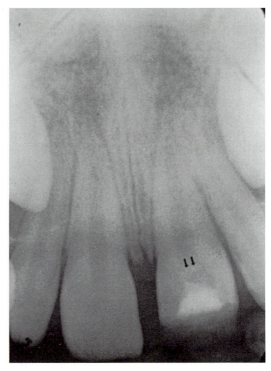

Figure 33–6. Apexogenesis (radiograph taken 6 months after Fig. 33–5) showing bridge formation *(arrows)* and apical maturation.

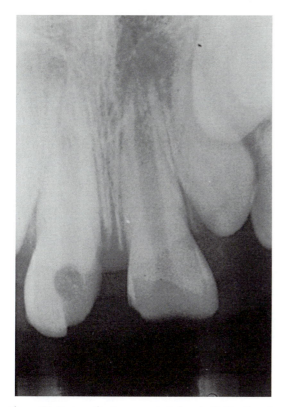

Figure 33–7. Apexification was started on both No. 8 and No. 9 after pulp exposures with necrosis.

is placed at the apical end of the radicular canal; a proprietary calcium hydroxide preparation (Pulpdent) or a mixture of U.S.P. calcium hydroxide mixed with sterile saline or local anesthetic can be carried to the apical portion of the root, covered with a sterile cotton pellet, and sealed with an interim restoration. The calcium hydroxide gradually washes out; therefore, it must be replaced every several months until apical closure occurs. In 6 months to 1 year (possibly longer), an apical barrier will develop, against which a conventional gutta percha endodontic procedure can be completed. Although a complete apical closure is occasionally visible radiographically, it may actually be a porous osteodentin or cementoid bridge (Goldman, 1974). Careful clinical probing within the root should be performed to confirm closure and the readiness of the tooth for a definitive endodontic filling.

Apexification is analogous to two other conditions in mature permanent teeth for which the

débrided and the canal treated with calcium hydroxide (Figs. 33-4, *right*, 33-7, and 33-8). Were a conventional endodontic procedure attempted, it would be compromised as a result of incomplete root formation, a blunderbuss canal (which would be difficult if not impossible to seal apically), and a decreased crown-to-root ratio. Apexification is used to promote root elongation or a calcific root closure across the enlarged apex of the tooth (Frank, 1966). Even though the pulp has been necrotic and is removed, Hertwig's epithelial root sheath is thought to persist and be capable of generating the response (Michanowicz and Michanowicz, 1967). A conventional endodontic procedure is performed after apexification is complete (Fig. 33-9).

In apexification, the entire pulp contents are removed to the level of the radiographic apex via endodontic broaches and files. Care must be taken not to file against the incompletely formed thin and tapered internal walls of the root. Liberal irrigation with a sodium hypochlorite solution or a nonirritating solution (e.g., sterile saline or local anesthetic solution) helps to remove all organic and necrotic tissue. Calcium hydroxide

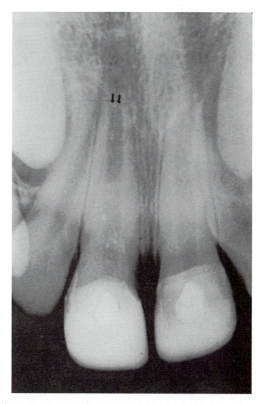

Figure 33–8. Apexification (radiograph taken 14 months after Fig. 33–7) showing radiographically apical bridging of tooth No. 8 *(arrows)* but not of No. 9. Later, both teeth were obturated with gutta percha when clinical probing confirmed apical closure; note interim composite restorations.

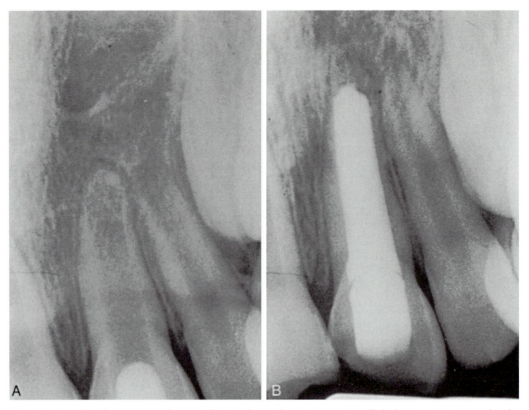

Figure 33–9. *A,* Apical bridge apparent after apexification (but without increase in wall thickness). *B,* Gutta percha obturation of canal.

entire root canal contents are removed and replaced with calcium hydroxide. This procedure is performed in cases of developing internal or pathologic external root resorption after a traumatic injury in an attempt to halt progressive root destruction (Andreasen, 1981).

REFERENCES

Andreasen JO: Traumatic Injuries of the Teeth, 2nd ed. Philadelphia, WB Saunders, 1981.

Bernick S: Differences in nerve distribution between erupted and non-erupted human teeth. J Dent Res *43*:406–411, 1964.

Camp JH: Pedodontic-endodontic treatment. *In* Cohen S, Burns RC (eds): Pathways of the Pulp, 3rd ed. St. Louis, CV Mosby, 1983.

Cox CF, Suzuki S: Re-evaluating pulp protection: Calcium hydroxide liners vs. cohesive hybridization. JADA *125*:823–831, 1994.

Dannenberg JL: Pedodontic endodontics. JADA *18*:367–377, 1974.

Frank AL: Therapy for the divergent pulpless tooth by continued apical formation. JADA *72*:87–93, 1966.

Fuks AB, Bielak S, Chosak A: Clinic and radiographic assessment of direct pulp capping and pulpotomy in young permanent teeth. Pediatr Dent *4*:240–244, 1982.

Goldman M: Root-end closure techniques, including apexification. Dent Clin North Am *18*:297–308, 1974.

Heide S, Kerekes K: Delayed partial pulpotomy in permanent incisors of monkeys. Int Endo J *19*:78–89, 1986.

King JB, Crawford JJ, Lindahl RL: Indirect pulp capping: A bacteriologic study of deep carious dentine in human teeth. Oral Surg *20*:663–671, 1965.

Massler M: Therapy conducive to healing of the human pulp. Oral Surg *34*:122–130, 1972.

Mejàre I, Cvek M: Partial pulpotomy in young permanent teeth with carious lesions. Endod Dent Traumatol *9*:238–242, 1993.

Michanowicz JP, Michanowicz AE: A conservative approach and procedure to fill an incompletely formed root using calcium hydroxide as an adjunct. J Dent Child *34*:42–47, 1967.

Seltzer S, Bender IB: The Dental Pulp: Biologic Considerations in Dental Procedures, 3rd ed. Philadelphia, JB Lippincott, 1984.

Trask PA: Formocresol pulpotomy on (young) permanent teeth. JADA *85*:1316–1323, 1972.

Weiner RS, Weiner LK, Kugel G: Teaching the use of bases and liners: A survey of North American Dental Schools. JADA *127*:1640–1645, 1996.

34

Managing Traumatic Injuries in the Young Permanent Dentition

Dennis J. McTigue

Chapter Outline

Injuries to the primary dentition are discussed in Chapter 15. Also covered are the following fundamental areas relevant to managing trauma in children of any age:

1. Classification of traumatic injuries to teeth
2. Medical and dental history
3. Clinical and radiographic examinations
4. Common reactions of teeth to trauma

This chapter deals with injuries to the young permanent dentition, but the reader is strongly advised to review the fundamental areas just noted in Chapter 15. Frequent references are made to them.

ETIOLOGY AND EPIDEMIOLOGY OF TRAUMA IN THE YOUNG PERMANENT DENTITION

Falls during play account for most dental injuries to young permanent teeth. Children engaging in contact sports are at greatest risk for dental injury, though the use of mouth guards greatly reduces their frequency (see Chapter 40). In the teenage years, automobile accidents cause a significant number of dental injuries when occupants not wearing seat belts hit the steering wheel or dashboard. As noted in Chapter 15, children with seizure disorders also injure their permanent teeth more frequently. In contrast with the primary dentition, permanent teeth suffer crown fractures more frequently than luxation injuries. The smaller crown-to-root ratio and denser alveolar bone in the permanent dentition contribute to this phenomenon. Maxillary central incisors are again most commonly injured, and protruding incisors are at greatest risk (Jarvinen, 1978) (Fig. 34-1).

CLASSIFICATION OF INJURIES TO YOUNG PERMANENT TEETH

Classification of tooth fractures and luxation injuries is discussed in Chapter 15. Refer to Figure 15-1.

HISTORY

The essential elements of the medical and dental history are discussed in Chapter 15. The use of a trauma assessment form to help organize the gathering of historical and clinical data is emphasized (see Fig. 15-5). The reader is reminded to determine the status of the child's tetanus prophylaxis and to consult the child's physician if there is any question about its adequacy.

Another issue worthy of review relates to the potential for injury to the central nervous system. Older children are likely to suffer harder blows at play, and thus the dentist should find out if the child lost consciousness or became disoriented or nauseated after the injury. Positive findings indicate immediate medical consultation. As noted in Chapter 15, significant head injuries can

lead to symptoms many hours after the initial trauma and parents should be cautioned to watch for the signs just noted for 24 hours and to wake the child every 2 to 3 hours through the night (Tecklenburg and Wright, 1991).

CLINICAL EXAMINATION

Refer to Chapter 15 for a thorough discussion of the clinical examination. An important difference between the primary and permanent dentition exists in respect to vitality testing. Whereas it is not routinely performed in the primary dentition, vitality testing can be a useful diagnostic aid in the permanent dentition. The dentist should be aware that pulp testing may not elicit reliable responses from erupting permanent teeth and from those with open apices. Further, recently traumatized teeth may not respond to any vitality test for several months. Positive findings after a traumatic injury are thus more valuable for assessing pulp vitality than are negative responses.

Electrical vitality testing is preferable to heat and cold testing because the former technique utilizes a stimulus that can be gradually increased and precisely recorded. Temperature tests are less exact and tend to elicit "all or none" responses. Although carbon dioxide snow does elicit more reliable results, the thermal shock of the low temperature applied can cause infraction lines in the enamel (Andreasen and Andreasen, 1994). Laser Doppler flowmetry has potentially great clinical value because this technique directly measures blood flow and does not rely on sensory nerve response (Vongsavan and Matthews, 1993). The technique is also painless and

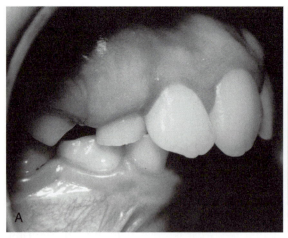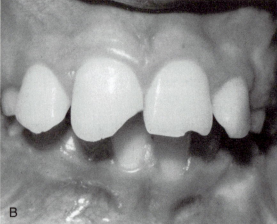

Figure 34–1. *A*, Lateral view, showing large horizontal overjet. *B*, Same patient with fractured central incisors. (From McTigue DJ: Management of orofacial trauma in children. Pediatr Ann *14*:125, 1985.)

is reliable in teeth with immature apices (Mesaros and Trope, 1997). Modifications in this instrument's design, however, and a significant reduction in its cost are necessary before it can achieve general use.

Principles of radiographic diagnosis for permanent teeth do not differ from those for primary teeth. A frequent error made by dentists in diagnosing traumatic injuries is taking an insufficient number of radiographs. Additional views taken from slightly different angles both vertically and horizontally can significantly improve the accuracy of diagnosis (Andreasen and Andreasen, 1985).

It is important to note the urgency of follow-up radiographs after injury. Reviewing radiographs at 1 month after injury detects signs of pulpal necrosis and inflammatory resorption. At 2 months, replacement resorption can be detected.

PATHOLOGIC SEQUELAE OF TRAUMATIZED TEETH

Refer to Chapter 15 for a discussion of the pathologic sequelae of traumatized teeth.

TREATMENT OF TRAUMATIC INJURIES TO THE PERMANENT DENTITION

The dentist treating a traumatic injury follows essentially the same principles of gathering historical information and completing a clinical examination, regardless of the child's age. Further, the pathologic sequelae of injuries to teeth are similar for both primary and permanent teeth. There are many significant differences, however, in the way that injuries to permanent teeth are treated. As in the primary dentition, a complete diagnostic work-up (described in Chapter 15) should precede all treatment. Even though a blow may cause little if any obvious injury to a permanent tooth, it may lead to pulp necrosis as a result of disruption of the neurovascular bundle at the apex of the tooth. Post-treatment evaluation is indicated for all traumatic injuries.

Enamel Fractures

In some cases, minor enamel fractures can be smoothed with fine disks. Larger fractures should be restored using an acid-etch/composite resin technique (see Chapter 39).

Enamel and Dentin Fractures

The primary issue in managing fractures that expose dentin is to prevent bacterial irritants from reaching the pulp. Standard care in the past called for covering exposed dentin with calcium hydroxide or glass ionomer cement to seal out oral flora. More recent research indicates that exposed dentin sealed with a bonding agent enables the unexposed pulp to form reparative dentin. Some clinicians are thus advocating simultaneous acid etching of dentin and enamel followed by dentin and enamel bonding without placement of calcium hydroxide or glass ionomer (White et al., 1992). In the absence of long-term clinical data documenting the success of this technique, however, I recommend covering the deepest portion of dentin fractures with glass ionomer cement, followed by a dentin bonding agent (see Chapters 20 and 39). The tooth can then be restored with an acid-etch/composite resin technique (Fig. 34-2). If there is not enough time to restore the tooth completely, an interim covering of resin material (a resin "patch") can temporize the tooth until a final restoration can be placed. Some dentists routinely place such a partial restoration to ensure an appropriate post-treatment evaluation when the patient returns for the final restoration. This is a reasonable strategy provided that care is taken to ensure an adequate seal.

Fractures Involving the Pulp

Crown fractures that expose the pulp are particularly challenging to treat (Fig. 34-3). The pertinent clinical findings that dictate treatment include the following:

1. Vitality of the exposed pulp
2. Time elapsed since the exposure
3. Degree of root maturation of the fractured tooth
4. Restorability of the fractured crown

The objective of treatment in managing these injuries is to preserve a vital pulp in the entire tooth (see Chapter 33). This allows for physiologic closure of the root apex in immature teeth. It is important to note that root end closure does not signal completion of root maturation. Progressive deposition of dentin normally continues in roots through adolescence, making them stronger and more resistant to future traumatic insult. Maintaining a vital pulp in the tooth crown allows the clinician to monitor the tooth's vitality periodically.

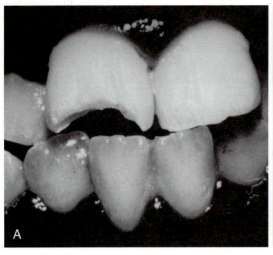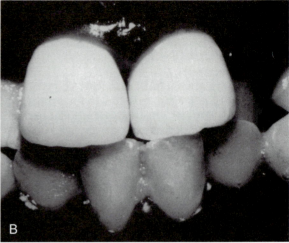

Figure 34–2. A fractured incisor *(A)* can quickly be restored using an acid-etch/composite resin technique *(B)*.

It is not always possible to maintain vital tissue throughout the tooth. Three treatment alternatives are available, based on the clinical findings just noted:

1. Direct pulp cap
2. Pulpotomy
3. Pulpectomy

DIRECT PULP CAP

The direct pulp cap is only indicated in small exposures that can be treated within a few hours of the injury. The chances for pulp healing decrease if the tissue is inflamed, has formed a clot, or is contaminated with foreign materials. The objective, then, is to preserve vital pulp tissue

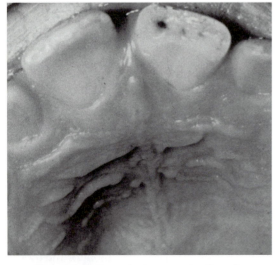

Figure 34–3. Crown fracture exposing the pulp.

that is free of inflammation and physiologically walled off by the calcific barrier.

A rubber dam is applied, and the tooth is gently cleaned with water. Commercially available calcium hydroxide paste is applied directly to the pulp tissue and to surrounding dentin. It is essential that a restoration be placed that is capable of thoroughly sealing the exposure to prevent further contamination by oral bacteria. As in the treatment of dentin fractures, it is acceptable to use an acid-etch/composite resin system for an initial restoration. The calcific bridge stimulated by calcium hydroxide should be evident radiographically in 2 to 3 months.

In fractures exposing pulps of immature permanent teeth with incomplete root development, a direct cap is no longer the treatment of choice. Failure in these cases leads to total pulpal necrosis and a fragile, immature root with thin dentinal walls. Thus, the preferred treatment in pulp exposures of immature permanent teeth is the pulpotomy.

PULPOTOMY

The objectives of the pulpotomy technique are to remove only the inflamed pulp tissue and to leave healthy tissue to enhance physiologic maturation of the root. As previously noted, this technique is favored for immature permanent teeth with exposed pulps. It is also indicated in large exposures or for pulps exposed for longer than several hours. Owing to its higher success rate, many clinicians have totally abandoned the direct pulp cap in favor of this technique.

It is difficult to determine clinically how far the inflamed pulp extends. The tooth shown in

Figure 34-4 had been fractured for 4 days with a pulp exposure approximately 3 mm in diameter. The dentist elected to remove all tissue in the pulp chamber, with obvious success. Figure 34-4B demonstrates complete maturation of the root, including apical closure and dentinal wall thickening as well as a calcific barrier at the amputation site. Maintaining some pulp tissue in the crown, however, allows the dentist to monitor the vitality of the tooth and is thus preferable when possible.

In 1978, Cvek noted that in most cases of pulps exposed for more than a few hours, the initial biologic response is pulpal hyperplasia. Inflammation in these cases rarely extends beyond 2 mm. In his study involving 60 teeth with pulps exposed from 1 hour to 90 days, Cvek removed only 2 mm of the pulp and the surrounding dentin. He covered the pulp stumps with calcium hydroxide and reported a success rate of 96%. Fuks and associates' 1993 report of long-term success confirms these findings and indicates that this conservative removal of tissue is the treatment of choice (Fig. 34-5).

Rubber dam isolation to prevent contamination of the pulp with oral bacteria is essential. The inflamed pulp is gently removed to a level approximately 2 mm below the exposure site with a sterile bur at high speed. Copious irrigation is mandatory to avoid pulp injury. The preparation should provide adequate space for the calcium hydroxide pulp dressing and a zinc oxide and eugenol seal. Because eugenol can interfere with the polymerization of composite restorative materials, the site should be covered with glass ionomer liner before restoration.

PULPECTOMY

A pulpectomy involves complete pulp tissue removal from the crown and root and is indicated when no vital tissue remains. It is also indicated when root maturation is complete and the permanent restoration requires a post build-up. In the absence of inflammatory root resorption, treatment is to obturate the canal with gutta percha. The reader is referred to standard endodontic textbooks for more information on this technique.

One of the greatest challenges facing the clinician is the management of a nonvital immature permanent tooth with an open apex. In this case, an apexification procedure is indicated wherein calcium hydroxide is carried to the root apex to contact vital tissues directly. The calcium hydroxide stimulates the formation of a cementoid bar-

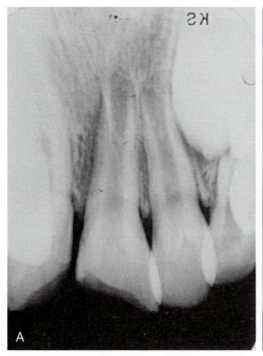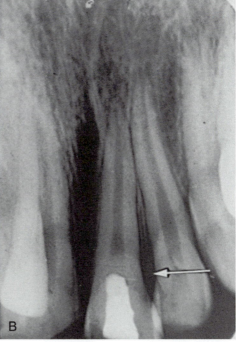

Figure 34–4. *A,* Crown fracture exposing the pulp in an immature permanent incisor. Note the open apex and thin dentinal walls in the root. *B,* A calcium hydroxide pulpotomy stimulated the formation of a calcific barrier *(arrow)* and enabled the root to mature.

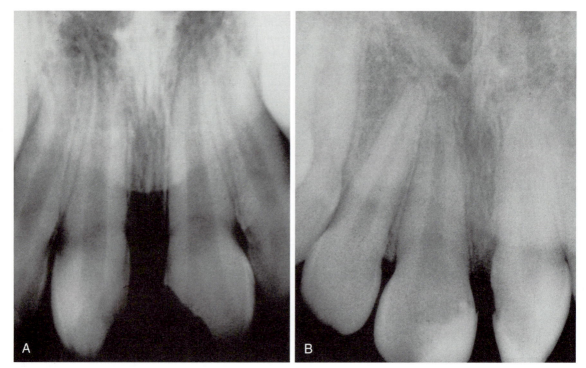

Figure 34–5. *A,* Maxillary right permanent central incisor suffered crown fracture with pulp exposure. *B,* One-year postoperative radiograph of the same tooth successfully treated with a calcium hydroxide partial pulpotomy. Note completion of root development both apically and laterally.

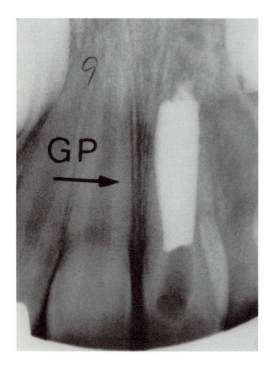

Figure 34–6. An apexification procedure allowed this immature permanent tooth to be obturated successfully with gutta percha (GP). The root, however, remains fragile and at increased risk of future trauma because no further dentinal wall apposition can occur.

rier against which gutta percha can subsequently be condensed. Even though a good apical seal can be achieved in this manner, no dentinal wall deposition will occur in the root and it will remain thin and fragile (Fig. 34-6). Refer to Chapter 33 for more detailed information regarding the apexification technique.

An alternative to the apexification technique for managing devitalized immature incisors is the "apical barrier technique" (Harbert, 1991). This method employs the use of generic tricalcium phosphate (g-TCP) powder, which is condensed through the root canal to the apex. The material is mixed with saline to a wet, sand-like consistency, inserted with an amalgam carrier, and condensed with amalgam or endodontic pluggers. Gutta percha can then be packed against the g-TCP plugs at the same visit, significantly reducing the time and expense associated with the management of these teeth (Fig. 34-7). Other materi-

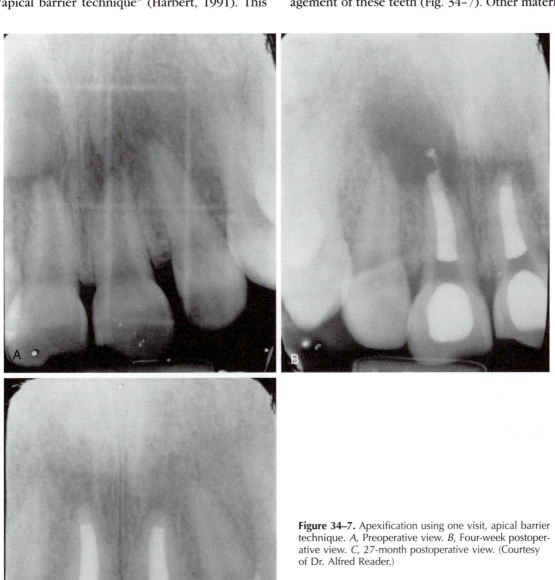

Figure 34–7. Apexification using one visit, apical barrier technique. *A,* Preoperative view. *B,* Four-week postoperative view. *C,* 27-month postoperative view. (Courtesy of Dr. Alfred Reader.)

als recommended for use in the apical barrier technique include synthetic hydroxy apatite, freeze-dried bone, or bioceramic glass.

CRITERIA FOR SUCCESS

Criteria to judge success of the techniques used to manage pulpal insult in fractured teeth include the following:

1. Completion of root development in immature teeth
2. Absence of clinical signs, such as pain, mobility, or fistula
3. Absence of any radiographic signs of pathologic processes, such as periapical radiolucency of bone or root resorption

Posterior Crown Fractures

Posterior crown fractures in the permanent dentition pose a restorative challenge for the clinician. These fractures usually occur secondary to hard blows to the underside of the chin, and vertical crown fractures frequently result (Fig. 34–8). Full coverage with stainless steel or cast metal crowns is frequently the only alternative. The reader is reminded to watch for mandibular fractures and cervical spine injuries in these cases (Bertolami and Kaban, 1982).

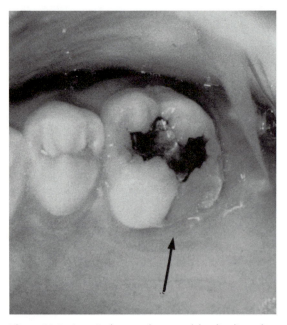

Figure 34–8. A vertical crown fracture of the distolingual cusp *(arrow)* occurred secondary to a blow to the underside of this child's chin.

Root Fractures

The prognosis for teeth with root fractures is best when the fracture occurs in the apical one third of the root. The prognosis worsens progressively with fractures that occur more cervically on the root. Bender and Freedland (1983) reported that over 75% of teeth with intra-alveolar root fractures maintain their vitality.

Appropriate management of root fractures in permanent teeth involves repositioning the coronal portion of the tooth fragment (if it is displaced) and firm immobilization with a splint for 2 to 3 months (Andreasen and Andreasen, 1994). Root canal therapy should not be initiated until clinical and radiographic signs of necrosis or resorption are apparent. Even in those cases, treatment can often be limited to the coronal fragment because, in most instances, the apical fragments maintain their vitality.

Techniques for splinting teeth are discussed later in this chapter.

Managing Sequelae to Dental Trauma

In Chapter 15, common reactions of the teeth to trauma are described. Three of the most challenging sequelae include pulp canal obliteration, inflammatory resorption (both external and internal), and replacement resorption. These pathologic processes can occur after crown fractures or luxation injuries.

PULP CANAL OBLITERATION

Pulp canal obliteration (PCO) is a degenerative pathologic process that ultimately leads to obliteration of the pulp canal (Figs. 34–9 and 34–10B). Andreasen (1989) has shown that its occurrence depends on the type of luxation injury sustained and the stage of root development. Thus, immature teeth with open apices suffering moderate to severe injuries are likely to undergo PCO. It was noted previously that most primary teeth with PCO resorb normally, and thus treatment for them is usually not indicated. Treatment of permanent teeth is controversial, however.

Some clinicians contend that as soon as PCO is diagnosed, a pulpectomy with gutta percha should be performed. This treatment is advocated because of reports of later development of pulpal necrosis and periapical change. Further, difficulty in completing routine endodontic procedures after pulp canals have calcified is noted. Andreasen, however, counters that pulp necrosis is an infrequent sequela of PCO, reportedly as

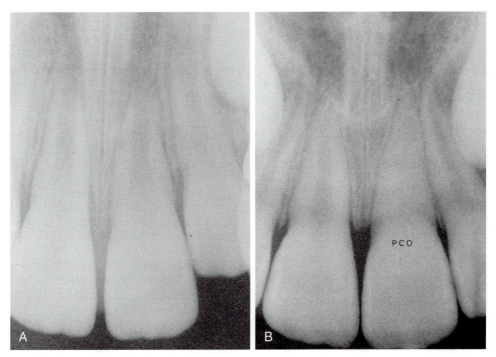

Figure 34–9. *A,* 10-day postoperative view of immature maxillary left central incisor in 7-year-old child that had been extruded and repositioned. *B,* 16-month postoperative view demonstrating pulp canal obliteration (PCO).

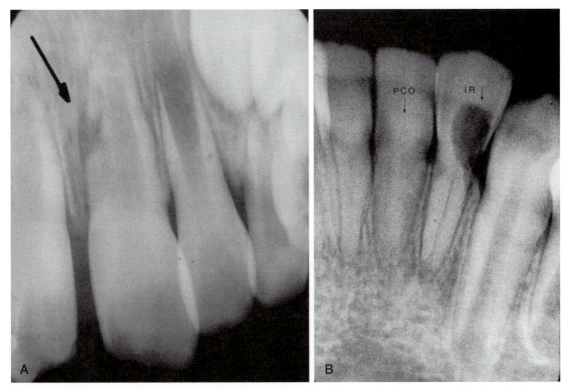

Figure 34–10. *A,* External inflammatory resorption *(arrow).* *B,* Internal inflammatory resorption (IR) of the lateral incisor; pulp canal obliteration (PCO) of the permanent central incisor. (*B* from McTigue DJ: Management of orofacial trauma in children. Pediatr Ann *14*:125, 1985.)

low as 1% (Andreasen, 1989). Further, she states that endodontic procedures can be successfully completed in a great majority of obliterated canals (Andreasen and Andreasen, 1994, p. 566). The dentist, then, is advised to closely monitor PCO in permanent teeth and to initiate endodontic procedures only when periapical changes are noted.

INFLAMMATORY RESORPTION

Inflammatory resorption can occur externally or internally (see Fig. 34-10). It commonly arises after luxation injuries when the periodontal ligament is inflamed and the pulp is necrotic (Tronstad, 1988). Odontoclastic activity can occur so rapidly that the teeth are destroyed in a matter of weeks.

Immediate treatment of inflammatory resorption is essential. As soon as this process is detected radiographically, the pulp tissue in the tooth is thoroughly extirpated. Copious irrigation with sodium hypochlorite aids the dissolution of organic debris in the canal. In permanent teeth, calcium hydroxide is placed in the canal with a technique identical to that used to induce apexification (see Chapter 33). Here the objective is not to induce apical closure but to create an environment unfavorable for the resorptive process. It is theorized that calcium hydroxide has antiseptic properties because of its extremely alkaline pH. This medicament apparently percolates through the dentinal tubules to the areas of resorption at the periodontal ligament and halts its progress.

Depending on the severity of the inflammatory resorption, calcium hydroxide may need to be retained in the tooth for 6 to 24 months. Repeated applications may be necessary if the resorption progresses. When radiographs confirm that the process is not continuing, gutta percha is placed as the final filling material.

REPLACEMENT RESORPTION (ANKYLOSIS)

Replacement resorption occurs most commonly after severe luxation injuries such as avulsions or intrusions in which periodontal ligament cells are destroyed. Alveolar bone directly contacts cementum on the involved tooth and becomes fused with it. Then as the bone undergoes its normal physiologic, osteoclastic, and osteoblastic activity, the root is resorbed or "replaced" with bone (Fig. 34-11).

This type of resorption cannot be treated once the tooth is firmly immobilized by the process. In young children with rapid bone turnover, roots are completely resorbed in 3 to 4 years. In adults, the process may take up to 10 years. Replacement resorption can be prevented only by prompt and appropriate treatment of luxation injuries.

Treating Luxation Injuries in the Permanent Dentition

The reader is referred to Chapter 15 for the definition of the various types of luxation injuries. Luxation injuries damage the supporting structures of the teeth, that is, the periodontal ligament and alveolar bone. Additionally, in mature teeth with closed apices, the pulp frequently becomes necrotic. Pulp necrosis occurs less frequently when immature teeth with open apices are luxated but, as noted earlier, PCO is common in these cases.

Vitality of the periodontal ligament is far more important than pulp vitality in determining the prognosis of luxated teeth. The primary objective of treatment in these injuries is to *maintain periodontal ligament vitality.*

CONCUSSION

Concussion injuries in permanent teeth must be followed closely. Although the prognosis is normally good, pulp necrosis and root resorption have been reported. Involved teeth can be carefully taken out of occlusion if the child complains of pain.

SUBLUXATION

Pulp necrosis occurs far more commonly in subluxated permanent teeth than in primary teeth. These teeth should be monitored closely with radiographs for at least 1 year, and root canal therapy should be instituted at the first sign of pathologic change. Immature teeth with open apices are less likely to undergo pulpal necrosis. Splinting subluxated teeth should be avoided.

INTRUSIVE LUXATION

The prognosis for intruded permanent teeth is not good. These teeth frequently undergo pulpal necrosis, root resorption, and alveolar bone loss.

The treatment of choice is to reposition the intruded teeth orthodontically using light forces (Spalding et al., 1985) (Fig. 34-12). The pulp should be extirpated within 2 weeks after the

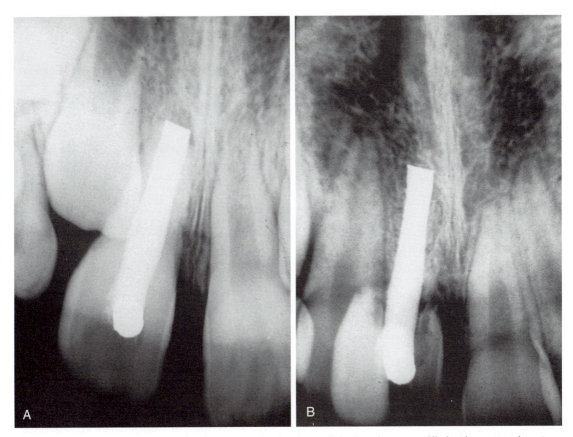

Figure 34–11. *A*, A permanent incisor that had been avulsed and stored dry for 3 hours was filled with gutta percha prior to reimplantation. *B*, Three years later, replacement resorption has completely destroyed the root.

injury, and calcium hydroxide should be placed in the root canal using the same technique as described for apexification in Chapter 33. Radiographic monitoring of the tooth should occur for at least 1 year, and the calcium hydroxide in

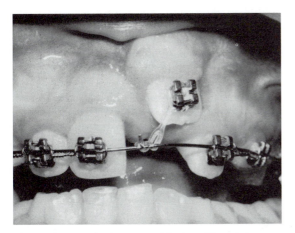

Figure 34–12. Orthodontic repositioning of intruded permanent incisor prevents replacement resorption (ankylosis) and alveolar bone loss.

the canal should be replaced if signs of root resorption persist.

As opposed to my method with the primary dentition, I do not wait for the intruded permanent tooth to re-erupt. Permanent teeth with closed apices re-erupt slowly, if at all, and are likely to undergo replacement resorption (Turley et al., 1984). Those with open apices may re-erupt but the process could take several months, in which time the root could be badly resorbed.

Current evidence indicates that immediate surgical repositioning is only indicated for intruded permanent teeth that are loose and freely mobile. Firmly intruded permanent teeth should not be surgically repositioned because this may enhance both root resorption and alveolar bone loss (Andreasen and Andreasen, 1994, p. 340).

EXTRUSION

Extruded permanent teeth (Fig. 34–13A) should be repositioned and splinted for 2 to 3 weeks. It normally takes the periodontal ligament fibers this period of time to reanastomose. Extruded

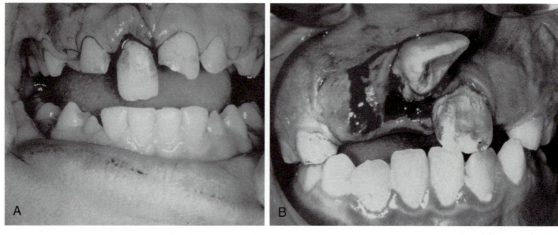

Figure 34–13. *A*, Extrusion injury of maxillary right central incisor and crown fracture of maxillary left central incisor. *B*, Laterally luxated tooth.

permanent teeth with closed apices undergo pulpal necrosis; therefore, root canal therapy should be initiated after the teeth are splinted. Extruded teeth with open apices have a chance at maintaining their vitality, and so the decision to initiate therapy should be delayed until clinical or radiographic signs indicate necrosis.

LATERAL LUXATION

Alveolar bone fractures frequently occur in lateral luxation injuries and can complicate their treatment (Fig. 34-13B). In the most severe cases, periodontal ligament and marginal bone loss occurs. Treatment is to reposition the teeth and alveolar fragments. A splint should then be applied for 3 to 8 weeks, depending on the degree of bone involvement. With good oral hygiene, alveolar bone regeneration can occur in children in approximately 8 weeks. My current protocol includes prescribing a 0.12% chlorhexidine mouth rinse. If the apices are closed, the pulps will likely become necrotic; therefore, endodontic therapy should be instituted soon after the teeth are splinted. Again, teeth with open apices should be monitored until signs of necrosis are evident.

AVULSION

The prognosis for long-term retention of an avulsed permanent tooth worsens the longer the tooth is out of its socket (Andreasen and Hjorting-Hansen, 1966). The primary therapeutic concern is to maintain the vitality of periodontal ligament (PDL) fibers and the longer they are out of the mouth, the worse the prognosis for their

survival. *It is thus imperative that the avulsed tooth be immediately reimplanted by the first capable person,* whether that person be a parent, teacher, or sibling (Fig. 34-14).

Owing to a variety of circumstances, it is sometimes not possible to reimplant a tooth immediately. Research has shown that the best transport medium for avulsed teeth is cell culture media such as Viaspan or Hanks balanced salt solution (HBSS) (Hiltz and Trope, 1991). Viaspan is not readily available for clinical use but HBSS is available in an avulsed tooth preserving system called "Save-A-Tooth" (Smart Practice, Phoenix, AZ). Use of such a system significantly increases the likelihood of periodontal ligament cell survival, even for an extended extraoral period (i.e., several hours) (Krasner and Person, 1992).

The best alternative storage medium if culture medium is not available is milk (Blomlof, 1981; Courts et al., 1983). It is readily available, relatively aseptic, and its osmolality is more favorable to maintaining the vitality of the periodontal ligament cells than is saline solution or tap water. Although some studies have indicated that storing the tooth in the patient's mouth (saliva) may be favorable toward PDL survival, the danger of an alarmed child swallowing, aspirating, or chewing on the tooth eliminates this option in my opinion. Water is not a good transport medium because it is a hypotonic solution and causes PDL cells to swell and rupture. Thus, in these cases, with the tooth stored in milk, the patient should be taken to the dentist as soon as possible.

Because root resorption is so closely correlated with the extraoral period, the dentist should reimplant the tooth in its socket as soon as possible

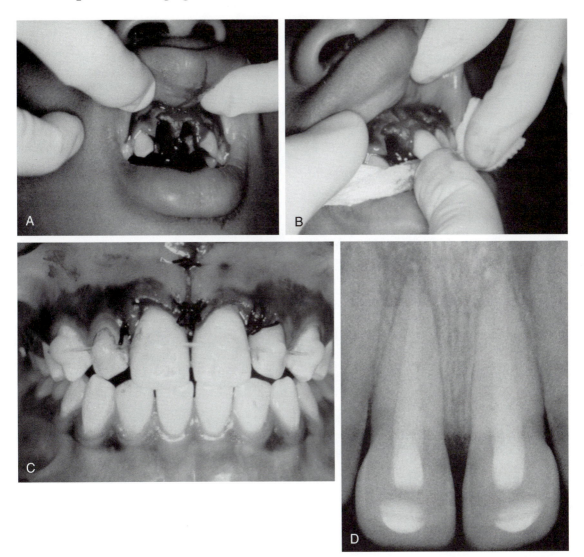

Figure 34–14. *A*, Both maxillary permanent central incisors avulsed. *B*, Reimplanting avulsed teeth with finger pressure. *C*, Esthetic, flexible splint fabricated using 50-pound test monofilament fishing line retained with composite resin. *D*, Calcium hydroxide pulpectomies completed to prevent inflammatory resorption. (Courtesy of Dr. Jeff Hays.)

after the child arrives. Adequate evidence, however, supports the immediate placement of the avulsed tooth into HBSS while the patient is brought to the dental operatory and appropriate informed consent is being obtained from the parent (Trope, 1995). Soaking the tooth may replace depleted PDL cell metabolites (Krasner and Rankow, 1995), reduce ankylosis, and help débride necrotic cells, foreign bodies, and bacteria (Matsson et al., 1982). My current protocol is again to prescribe an oral mouth rinse of 0.12% chlorhexidine used empirically to reduce the likelihood of bacterial invasion of the PDL space. Studies have failed to demonstrate any benefit to pulp or periodontal healing from systemic antibiotics (Andreasen et al., 1995).

When immature teeth with open apices are avulsed, the ideal treatment objective is revascularization of the pulp in addition to maintenance of PDL health. This enables physiologic maturation of the immature root, including apexogenesis and root wall thickening. The tooth should be splinted for approximately 2 weeks. This gives the neurovascular tissues an opportunity to re-anastomose. Success in these cases has been reported, and thus dentists should await clinical or radiographic signs of necrosis prior to initiating root canal therapy. When the splint is removed, the dentist may note that the tooth is mobile. This mobility is preferable to long-term rigid splinting because the latter has been correlated with an increased incidence of replacement resorption. The mobility of the tooth physiologically interrupts areas of incipient resorption/ankylosis on the PDL, allowing it to heal normally.

In mature teeth with closed apices, a splint which affords the tooth functional mobility should be applied for 7 to 10 days. The necrotic pulp should be extirpated and replaced with calcium hydroxide (CaOH) after 1 week to prevent the initiation of inflammatory root resorption (Fig. 34–14D). Importantly, *root canal therapy should not be performed in the hand prior to reimplantation.* This extends the extraoral period and places the PDL at greater risk to injury as a result of the additional manipulation of the tooth. The CaOH can be removed and gutta percha pulpectomy performed after 1 month. In cases in which the pulp was not removed within 2 weeks of the reimplantation or inflammatory resorption is evident radiographically, the CaOH should be maintained in the tooth for a minimum of 6 months.

Periodontal ligament cells on avulsed teeth that have been stored dry for more than 1 hour are necrotic, and these teeth will eventually ankylose and resorb. There is some evidence that the pace of this resorption can be reduced if these teeth are soaked in fluoride for approximately 20 minutes prior to reimplantation (Coccia, 1980). Trope (1995) also recommends thorough débridement of the necrotic PDL cells prior to reimplantation using a 5-minute citric acid soak prior to the fluoride soak.

In summary, the procedure for reimplantation of a mature tooth is as follows:

1. Hold the tooth by the crown to prevent damage to the periodontal ligament.
2. Gently rinse the tooth with tap water. No attempt should be made to scrub or sterilize the tooth.
3. Manually reimplant the tooth in the socket *as soon as possible.*
4. Apply a light, functional splint.
5. Complete CaOH pulpectomy after 1 week and then remove splint.

SPLINTING TECHNIQUE

Various methods of splinting teeth have been advocated, but it is apparent that the ideal splint should possess the following characteristics. It should

1. Be passive and atraumatic
2. Be flexible
3. Allow for vitality testing and endodontic access
4. Be easy to apply and remove

TABLE 34–1. Splinting Periods

Avulsions	1–2 weeks
Extrusions	2–3 weeks
Lateral luxations with bone damage	3–8 weeks
Root fractures	2–3 months

The composite resin-retained arch wire splint has been advocated as the best system to meet these criteria (Kehoe, 1986). To allow for flexibility, a light orthodontic arch wire or a 30- to 60-pound test monofilament fishing line can be used (Fig. 34–14C). See Table 34–1 for a summary of splinting periods.

SUMMARY

Advances in dental research have greatly improved the ability of dentists to ensure long-term retention of traumatized teeth in children. It is the dentist's responsibility to stay abreast of this new information and to be available to his or her patients when they are in need of urgent treatment.

REFERENCES

Andreasen, FM: Pulp healing after luxation injuries and root fractures in the permanent dentition. Endod Dent Traumatol 5:111, 1989.

Andreasen FM, Andreasen JO: Diagnosis of luxation injuries: The importance of standardized clinical, radiographic and photographic techniques in clinical investigations. Endod Dent Traumatol 1:160, 1985.

Andreasen JO, Andreasen FM: Textbook and Color Atlas of Traumatic Injuries to the Teeth, 3rd ed. Copenhagen, Munksgaard, 1994.

Andreasen J, Borum M, Jacobsen H, Andreasen F: Replantation of 400 avulsed permanent incisors. 2: Factors related to pulpal healing. Endod Dent Traumatol 11:59, 1995a.

Andreasen J, Borum M, Jacobsen H, Andreasen F: Replantation of 400 avulsed permanent incisors. 4: Factors related to periodontal ligament healing. Endod Dent Traumatol 11:76, 1995b.

Andreasen JO, Hjorting-Hansen E: Replantation of teeth. I: Radiographic and clinical studies of 110 human teeth replanted after accidental loss. Acta Odont Scand 24:263, 1966.

Bender IB, Freedland JB: Clinical considerations in the diagnosis and treatment of intra-alveolar root fractures. JADA 107:595, 1983.

Bertolami CN, Kaban LB: Chin trauma: A clue to associated mandibular and cervical spine injury. Oral Surg 53:122, 1982.

Blomlof L: Storage of human periodontal ligament cells in a combination of different media. J Dent Res 60:1904, 1981.

Coccia C: A clinical investigation of root resorption rates in reimplanted young permanent incisors: A five-year study. J Endod 6:413, 1980.

Courts FJ, Mueller WA, Tabeling HJ: Milk as an interim storage medium for avulsed teeth. Pediatr Dent 5:183, 1983.

Cvek M: A clinical report on partial pulpotomy and capping with calcium hydroxide in permanent incisors with complicated crown fracture. J Endo 4:232, 1978.

Fuks A, Gavra S, Chosack A: Long-term follow up of traumatized incisors treated by partial pulpotomy. Pediatr Dent 15:334, 1993.

Harbert H: Generic tricalcium phosphate plugs: An adjunct in endodontics. J Endo 17:131, 1991.

Hiltz J, Trope M: Vitality of human lip fibroblasts in milk, Hanks balanced salt solution and Viaspan storage media. Endod Dent Traumatol 7:69, 1991.

Jarvinen S: Incisal overjet and traumatic injuries to upper permanent incisors: A retrospective study. Acta Odontol Scand 36:359, 1978.

Kehoe J: Splinting and replantation after traumatic avulsion. JADA 112:224, 1986.

Krasner P, Person P: Preserving avulsed teeth for replantation. JADA 123:80, 1992.

Krasner P, Rankow H: New philosophy for the treatment of avulsed teeth. Oral Surg Oral Med Oral Pathol Oral Radiol Endod 79:616, 1995.

Matsson L, Andreasen J, Cvek M, Granath L: Ankylosis of experimentally reimplanted teeth related to extra-alveolar period and storage environment. Pediatr Dent 4:327, 1982.

Mesaros S, Trope M: Revascularization of traumatized teeth assessed by laser Doppler flowmetry: Case report. Endod Dent Traumatol 13:24, 1997.

Spalding PM, Fields HW, Torney D, et al: The changing role of endodontics and orthodontics in the management of traumatically intruded permanent incisors. Pediatr Dent 7:104, 1985.

Tecklenburg F, Wright M: Minor head trauma in the pediatric patient. Pediatr Emerg Care 7:40, 1991.

Tronstad L: Root resorption—etiology, terminology and clinical manifestations. Endod Dent Traumatol 4:241, 1988.

Trope M: Clinical management of the avulsed tooth. Dent Clin North Am 39:93, 1995.

Turley PK, Joiner MW, Hellstrom S: The effect of orthodontic extrusion on traumatically intruded teeth. Am J Orthod 85:47, 1984.

Vongsavan N, Matthews B: Experiments on extracted teeth into the validity of using laser doppler techniques for recording pulpal blood flow. Arch Oral Biol 38:431, 1993.

White K, Cox C, Kanka J, et al: Histologic pulpal response of acid etching vital dentin. J Dent Res 71:188, 1992.

Chapter 35

Treatment Planning and Treatment of Orthodontic Problems

John R. Christensen and Henry W. Fields, Jr.

Chapter Outline

By the time orthodontic treatment is considered, the patient's data base has been gathered. A list of orthodontic problems is generated from this data base, and the problems are ranked in order from most to least severe (Proffit et al., 1999). Severity is determined by patient, functional, and esthetic concerns. The clinician is specifically trained to identify functional and esthetic problems but does not always consider the concerns of the parent and child. These concerns should be listened to carefully. This attention often dictates treatment satisfaction outcomes. Often the motivation for treatment can be elicited from these concerns. If the child patient desires to have treatment, cooperation will usually be good during treatment, and little parental support will be necessary. This is called internal motivation. External motivation, motivation supplied by the parent for treatment, will require continuous parental support to successfully complete treat-

ment. It is also possible that the chief complaint or reason for seeking treatment may rank low on the treatment priority list or be addressed later in the treatment plan. An explanation should be provided to the child and parent to justify this situation.

After the problem list has been generated and each problem has been ranked in order of severity, possible solutions to each problem should be listed. The solution list should be comprehensive—that is, all reasonable solutions should be considered for each specific problem without regard for the other problems. After the solution list has been constructed, the clinician should look for similar solutions that are listed for more than one problem. In some cases, the best solution for one problem is the best solution for all problems, and the treatment plan is easily derived. Unfortunately, in most cases, a solution for one problem is not the solution for the others, and, worse, may actually magnify the second problem. Treatment planning is not entirely scientific, and clinical wisdom is needed to decide on a plan in these cases.

SKELETAL PROBLEMS

Orthodontic problems in the preadolescent patient are generally thought of as either dental or skeletal in origin. The complexity of these problems varies tremendously. Many dental problems are well within the treatment domain of the general practitioner. Skeletal problems, as diagnosed from the facial profile analysis and confirmed by supplemental means, are best treated by a specialist. The general practitioner, however, should have an understanding of how skeletal discrepancies are treated.

Three basic alternatives for treating skeletal discrepancies exist: growth modification, camouflage, and orthognathic surgery. Growth modification attempts to change skeletal relationships by using the patient's remaining growth to alter the size or position of the jaws. Camouflage and orthognathic surgery usually are considered only in the nongrowing or adult patient. The camouflage type of orthodontic treatment is aimed at hiding a mild skeletal discrepancy by moving teeth situated on the jaws so that they fit together. The skeletal discrepancy still exists, but it is disguised by a normal occlusion and acceptable facial esthetic appearance. Orthognathic surgery places the jaws and teeth in a normal or near normal position through the use of surgical procedures and pre- and postsurgical orthodontic treatment (Proffit, 1991).

Three assumptions are made when growth modification is undertaken. First and most obvious, the patient must be growing. The normal child in the 6- to 12-year age group is actively growing, and the face is growing. Traditionally, clinicians have thought that it is easiest to correct skeletal problems if the child is undergoing maximum facial growth during treatment. Although the data to support this contention are not voluminous or clear (Hagg et al., 1987), clinicians have long sought to predict maximum somatic growth and maximum facial growth from other indicators. There appears to be wide variation in the amount of facial growth occurring at one time and an equally wide variation in the coordination of facial growth with overall body growth and other indicators that have been chosen (Chertkow, 1980; Pileski et al., 1973; Thompson et al., 1976). Because of this state of inaccuracy,

the clinician should use as many indicators as possible (personal growth history, skeletal growth maturation, presence of secondary sexual characteristics, and onset of menarche) to make an educated decision about whether the child is growing at an acceptable rate. Females tend to enter the adolescent growth spurt at around 10 and males at around 12.

Traditionally, patients have been treated for skeletal and dental problems at the transition from the mixed to permanent dentitions. This has enabled practitioners to treat successfully most problems and deal with a more mature patient who is both reasonably cooperative and compliant. Asynchrony between dental development and rapid facial growth may create a situation in which the patient may be ready for growth modification but not for orthodontic dental treatment, or vice versa. These patients must be handled individually by balancing the dental and skeletal interventions.

The second assumption made when growth modification is undertaken is that the practitioner can accurately diagnose the source of the skeletal discrepancy and then design treatment that will apply the appropriate amount and direction of force to correct the discrepancy. Diagnosis is not an exact science and may be confusing even when using cephalometric measures (Fields et al., 1991), and the discrepancy may be due to a number of small skeletal problems rather than to one easily identified discrepancy. Force delivery to dental and skeletal structures is also inexact, and the clinical impression and treatment response may dictate alteration in the amount and direction of force applied to modify growth.

The third assumption is that growth modification is usually only one portion of a treatment plan. Most appliances used to modify growth—headgears and functional appliances, for example—are designed to alter skeletal structures rather than precisely move teeth. Although the appliances are capable of causing tooth movement, they are not as precise as fixed orthodontic appliances and usually are used prior to or in conjunction with fixed appliances. Therefore, most growth modification treatments are followed immediately or at a later time by traditional fixed orthodontic appliances to move the teeth into an ideal or final position.

Three theories are offered to explain how growth modification works to achieve the desired results. The first theory suggests that growth modification appliances change the absolute size of one or both jaws. For example, a Class II skeletal profile may be treated by making a deficient mandible larger to fit a normal-sized maxilla or by limiting the size of an oversized maxilla. Some investigations on animals have shown that absolute size change is possible, but clinical application in humans has not been as successful. Certain individuals do show dramatic size changes, but there appears to be large variability in patient response to growth-modifying appliances, with moderate changes in various structures being the rule rather than the exception.

Growth modification may work by accelerating the desired growth but not changing the ultimate size or shape of the jaw. A deficient mandible may not end up larger than it ultimately would have been, but it may achieve its final size sooner. This requires the clinician to make some final dentoalveolar changes to establish an ideal occlusion following growth modification. This type of growth modification response also shows large individual variability.

There is support for this interpretation of growth modification based on recent randomized clinical trials that demonstrate little difference between an early and a late treatment group of patients with skeletal Class II malocclusion (Tulloch et al., 1998).

A third possibility is that growth modification may work by changing the spatial relationship of the two jaws. The ultimate size of the jaw and its rate of growth are not changed, but by modifying the orientation of the jaws to each other, a more balanced profile may result. For example, a convex profile and an increased lower facial height could be made more proportional to each other if the vertical growth of the maxilla could be inhibited and the mandible allowed to rotate upward and forward. The profile would then become less convex and the vertical relations more ideal. Jaw reorientation would be successful in a concave Class III patient with a short face if the mandible could be rotated downward and backward (more vertical) to create a more acceptable profile. Reorientation does not work well in Class II short faces or Class III long faces because correcting one problem (e.g., the vertical) makes the other problem (e.g., the anteroposterior) worse.

From the best available data, it appears that if a patient is growing, on average modest changes can be accomplished. These are reasonably comparable if attempted early or late. On the other hand, early treatment may be defensible for young Class II patients with esthetic complaints and those who are trauma-prone and in danger of injuring their maxillary incisors.

Growth Modification Applied to Anteroposterior Problems

Anteroposterior skeletal problems are Class II and Class III in nature. These descriptions are not very informative, however, because the source of the discrepancy may be the maxilla, the mandible, or a combination of the two. Therefore, the first step in patient evaluation is to identify the source of the problem and then design a treatment plan to resolve the problem.

CLASS II MAXILLARY PROTRUSION

Class II maxillary protrusion is best treated by headgear therapy to restrict or redirect maxillary growth on the basis of randomized clinical trials and retrospective studies (Baumrind et al., 1983; Tulloch et al., 1998). Headgear places a distal force on the maxillary dentition and the maxilla (Fig. 35–1). Theoretically, the relative movement of dental and skeletal structures depends on the amount and time of force application. In actual practice, it is probably not possible to move selectively only teeth or bones (Baumrind et al., 1983). Generally, tooth movement is greater with higher forces, but skeletal change can successful occur with either heavy or light forces. The best approach is probably to apply forces ranging

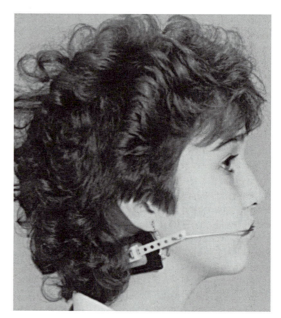

Figure 35–1. The class II maxillary protrusive patient is best treated by headgear therapy to restrict or redirect maxillary growth. This patient is being treated with cervical headgear that places a distal and extrusive force on both maxillary skeletal and dental structures. The force is provided by a neck strap attached to the outer bows of the headgear.

from 12 to 16 ounces per side for 12 to 14 hours and then monitor the skeletal and dental changes and adjust accordingly. Certainly, the skeletal and dental response varies according to the type of headgear chosen and the resultant direction of force exerted by the headgear. The most common varieties, cervical and high-pull, provide predominantly distal and occlusal and distal and superior forces, respectively. Traditionally, one avoids using a headgear that tends to extrude posterior teeth in a long-faced person or one with limited overbite. The same type of headgear would be useful in a patient with a short face and a deep bite, however.

Class II maxillary protrusion may also be treated with a functional appliance. Although a functional appliance is primarily designed to stimulate mandibular growth, studies have indicated that it has some secondary effects of restricting forward maxillary skeletal and dental movement (Bookstein, 1982; Tulloch et al., 1998). This happens because the mandible, which is postured forward, returns to a more distal position because of the distal muscle and soft tissue forces transmitted through the appliance to the maxilla and the maxillary teeth. The maxillary teeth tend to tip lingually rather than to move bodily, and the mandibular teeth tip facially.

CLASS II MANDIBULAR DEFICIENCY

The mandibular-deficient patient is usually treated with a functional appliance that positions the mandible forward in an attempt to stimulate or accelerate mandibular growth (Fig. 35-2). Retrospective clinical studies have shown that these appliances can produce a small average increase in mandibular projection (2-4 mm/year) (McNamara et al., 1985; Remmer et al., 1985). This has been confirmed by randomized clinical trials (Keeling et al., 1998; Tulloch et al., 1998). Patient response varies greatly. In many cases, this increased growth does not totally correct the Class II skeletal problem for several reasons. First, the amount of growth is not enough to overcome the discrepancy. Second, all the available growth would need to be directed to produce anteroposterior change. This is usually not the case because some dental eruption and vertical growth occur. This interaction between anteroposterior and vertical dimensional changes decreases ultimate mandibular projection and Class II correction because the mandible grows downward and forward and not straight forward. The rest of the anteroposterior discrepancy is treated by restricting maxillary growth, tipping the maxillary teeth back, and tipping the mandibular teeth forward. Different appliances can be designed that exaggerate the secondary responses of maxillary restriction and dental movement if desired. Some studies indicate that headgear treatment may cause a small increase in mandibular growth, but it is unlikely that the amount of mandibular stimulation by this method would be of clinical significance (Baumrind and Korn, 1981).

CLASS III MAXILLARY DEFICIENCY

True midface deficiency can be treated by using a reverse-pull headgear or face mask to exert anteriorly directed force on the maxilla (Turley, 1988) (Fig. 35-3). Some authors believe that the ideal time to attempt this treatment is between the ages of 6 and 8 if skeletal change is desired. The face mask applies force to the maxilla through an appliance (either a removable splint or fixed appliance) attached to the teeth; tooth movement also occurs. In fact, after age 8 the theory is that this type of appliance has a tendency to exert a predominantly tooth-moving force. The reason for the greater dental effect with increasing age is assumed to be more complex and integrated maxilla at the sutures. Data (Merwin et al., 1997) indicate that there is little anteroposterior difference in treatment effect whether treatment is applied early or late.

Functional appliances designed to stimulate maxillary growth do not seem to be effective. The improvement in facial profile obtained by using these appliances in patients with very minor Class III problems is usually the result of a downward and backward rotation of the mandible. The occlusion improves as a result of facial tipping of the maxillary incisors and lingual tipping of the lower incisors.

CLASS III MANDIBULAR EXCESS

Class III mandibular protrusion has been historically treated by chin cup therapy (Fig. 35-4). The theory of chin cup therapy is to apply a distal and superior force through the chin that inhibits or redirects growth at the condyle. Again, studies in animals have shown some change in absolute mandibular size, but clinical application in humans routinely has been less successful (Sakamoto et al., 1984; Sugawara et al., 1990). The typical response to chin cup therapy is a distal rotation of the mandible and lingual tipping of the lower incisors. Therefore, chin cup therapy is well tolerated in patients with mild mandibular protrusion and short to

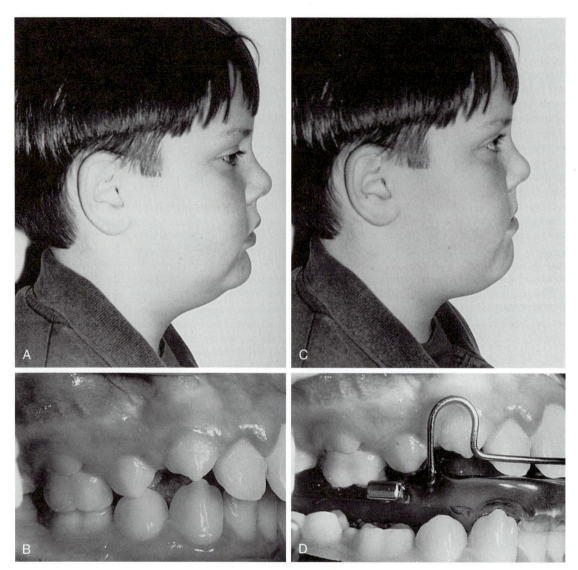

Figure 35–2. The class II mandibular deficient patient is usually treated with a functional appliance that positions the mandible forward in an attempt to stimulate, accelerate, or redirect mandibular growth. *A,* This patient has a class II mandibular deficient profile. *B,* The patient's molar and canine relationships reflect the skeletal class II relationship. *C,* The profile is immediately improved when the functional appliance is in place because the mandible is pushed forward into a class I relationship. *D,* Because functional appliances position the mandible forward using the upper and lower dental arches, there may be movement of the upper and lower teeth. Dental aspects of the malocclusion must be considered during treatment planning.

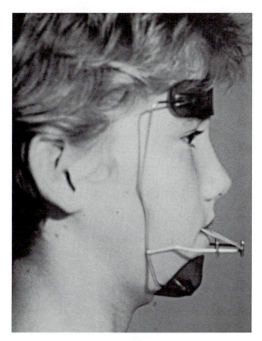

Figure 35–3. The class III maxillary deficient patient is treated by using a reverse pull headgear or face mask to exert anteriorly directed force on the maxilla. The force is provided by rubber bands extending from the face mask to intraoral hooks or wires.

less of philosophy, treatment prior to adolescence and midpalatal suture closure is recommended.

Three basic appliances are used to correct the constriction, but the appliances are not interchangeable. In Chapter 27, the quad helix and the W arch for treatment of maxillary constriction are described. The appliances provide both skeletal and dental movement in the 3- to 6-year-old child (Beil and LeCompte, 1981). As the patient grows older, more dental change and less skeletal change occur. This is true because the midpalatal suture, which was open at an early age, has developed bone interdigitation that makes it difficult to separate. More force is required to separate the suture after initial interdigitation of the suture to obtain true skeletal correction than a quad helix or W arch can deliver.

In the older preadolescent patient, in whom there is a chance that the midpalatal suture is closed, an appliance that can deliver large amounts of force is necessary to correct the skeletal constriction (Haas, 1965). Rapid palatal expansion is the term given to the procedure in which an appliance cemented or bonded to the

normal vertical proportions. It is contraindicated, however, in a person with a long lower face because the anteroposterior correction would come at the expense of an increased vertical dimension. Functional appliances designed to treat Class III mandibular excess show the same minor changes as those occurring in Class III maxillary deficiency.

Growth Modification Applied to Transverse Problems

The most common transverse problem in the preadolescent is maxillary constriction and posterior crossbite. Treatment of maxillary constriction can begin as soon as the problem is discovered if the child is mature enough to accept treatment. Treatment has the potential to eliminate crossbites of the succedaneous teeth, increase arch length, and simplify future diagnostic decisions that can be complicated by functional shifts. Most clinicians agree with the philosophy of early correction if there is a mandibular shift. Generally, it is believed that long-term facial symmetry attributable to soft tissue enlargement can result from untreated mandibular shifts. Regard-

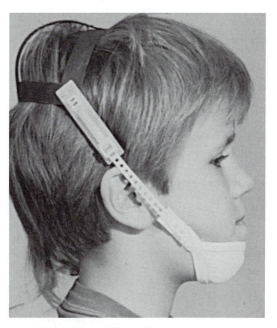

Figure 35–4. The class III mandibular protrusive patient has historically been treated with chin cup therapy. The chin cup was designed to apply a distal and superior force through the chin to inhibit growth at the condyle. In clinical practice, this device has not proved to be routinely successful, although chin cup therapy does cause a distal rotation of the mandible. Therefore, the chin cup may be useful for treating mild mandibular protrusion in which the vertical proportions are short to normal.

teeth is opened 0.5 mm/day to deliver 2000 to 3000 g of force (Fig. 35–5). In the active phase of treatment, there is little dental movement because the periodontal ligament has been hyalinized, which limits dental movement, and the force is transmitted almost entirely to the skeletal structures. During retention, however, the skeletal structures begin to relapse toward the midline. Because the teeth are held rigidly by the appliance, there is some compensatory dental movement to maintain the same width. Depending on the amount of expansion needed, active treatment normally takes 10 to 14 days. Another approach to skeletal expansion is slow rather than rapid palatal expansion (Hicks, 1978). Essentially the same appliance is used, although force levels are calibrated to provide only 900 to 1300 g of force. Coupled with a slower activation rate, slow palatal expansion widens the palate by dental and skeletal movement. Although the final position of the teeth and supporting structures is approximately the same in rapid and slow expansion, proponents of slow expansion maintain that slower expansion is more physiologic and stable. Transverse growth modification also can be accomplished by means of acrylic or wire buccal shields attached to functional appliances or lip bumpers. The buccal shields relieve the teeth and alveolar structures from the resting pressure of the cheek muscles and soft tissues. Transverse expansion of 3 to 5 mm can be achieved, although the changes vary considerably. Whether the movement is dental or skeletal and whether it will remain stable remains in question because there are no controlled experimental studies to provide answers.

Growth Modification Applied to Vertical Problems

Vertical skeletal problems are manifest as long and short facial heights and usually are located

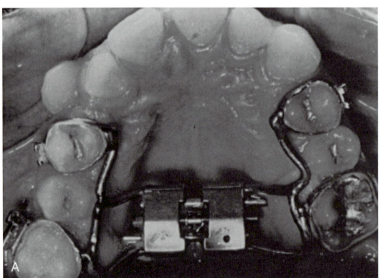

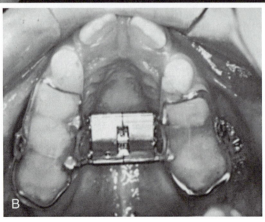

Figure 35–5. Rapid palatal expansion is used to treat maxillary constriction and posterior crossbite when there is a chance that the midpalatal suture is partially closed. The jackscrew in the appliance provides approximately 2000 to 3000 g of force when it is opened 0.5 mm per day. Depending on the amount of expansion needed, the appliance is normally activated two times each day for 10 days to 2 weeks. The appliance can be either *(A)* cemented on the teeth with orthodontic bands or *(B)* bonded to the teeth.

below the palatal plane (Fields et al., 1984). The short-faced person has a reduced mandibular plane angle and under-erupted teeth. In the long-faced patient, the mandibular plane angle, lower facial height, and amount of dental eruption are increased compared with the patient with a normal face. Vertical skeletal problems can be treated with growth modification techniques and some can be treated successfully; however, even when the treatment has been successful, maintaining the correction is extremely difficult. The face grows vertically for a long time, and there is a tendency for the original growth pattern and growth problem to recur.

VERTICAL EXCESS

Vertical skeletal excess may be treated by extraoral force, intraoral force, or a combination of the two. Extraoral force is delivered by means of a high-pull headgear through the maxillary first molars. The force is applied in a superior and distal direction and is designed to inhibit vertical development of the maxilla and eruption of the posterior maxillary teeth (Fig. 35–6). Because no force is applied to the mandibular teeth, they are free to erupt and compensate for the lack of vertical development in the maxilla. In some cases, this compensatory eruption can eliminate

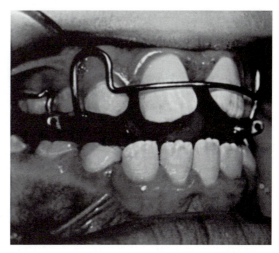

Figure 35–7. Vertical skeletal excess also can be treated with a functional appliance designed to inhibit eruption of the maxillary and mandibular teeth. The appliance is constructed in such a way that the mandible is placed in an open posture in an increased vertical position. The force of the mandible attempting to return to its normal, more closed vertical position is transmitted to the maxilla and to the teeth in both arches.

all the positive effects of the high-pull headgear and lead to downward and backward rotation of the mandible instead of forward mandibular projection.

An alternative method for controlling vertical development is to block the eruption of the maxillary and mandibular teeth. A functional appliance can be designed that will force the mandible open to an increased vertical rest position. The force of the mandible attempting to return to its original vertical rest position is transmitted to the maxilla and the teeth in both arches. This results in mandibular growth being directed forward because no dental eruption has occurred to increase the vertical dimension (Fig. 35–7). To supplement the skeletal treatment effect on the maxilla, headgear can be attached to the functional appliance that allow the headgear and the functional appliance to be worn at the same time (Lagerstrom et al., 1990) (Fig. 35–8). Developments in rare-earth magnets may also prove to be of value in restricting vertical facial development. Magnets placed to repel each other in each arch may provide enough force to restrict vertical eruption and skeletal growth. By whatever means vertical excess is treated, excellent patient cooperation is necessary because treatment must be continued as long as the patient is growing.

VERTICAL DEFICIENCY

Vertical skeletal deficiencies can be treated with either headgear or functional appliances, de-

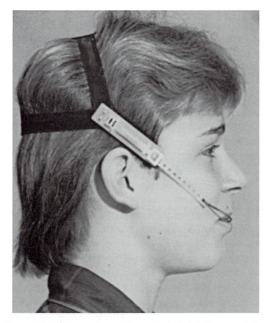

Figure 35–6. The patient with vertical skeletal excess is best treated with high-pull headgear. The force, generated by the strap resting on the head, is applied in a superior and distal direction and is intended to inhibit vertical development of the maxilla and eruption of the maxillary posterior teeth.

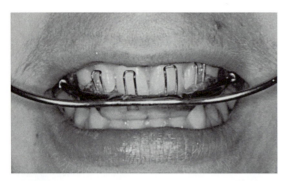

Figure 35–8. In some cases, a headgear tube is added to a functional appliance such as the one described in Figure 35–7. This tube allows the patient to wear the functional appliance and the high-pull headgear at the same time to further restrict vertical skeletal and dental growth.

pending on the accompanying anteroposterior relationships. The force vector from the headgear should direct the maxilla distally and extrude the maxillary posterior teeth, which would require cervical pull headgear. Because functional appliances are typically designed to inhibit eruption of upper and lower anterior teeth and promote eruption of the posterior teeth, they can also increase vertical facial height. As in vertical skeletal excess, the original growth pattern tends to recur, and retention should be designed to prevent this recurrence.

DENTAL PROBLEMS

Space Maintenance

A philosophy for space maintenance and the appliances recommended for the primary dentition are discussed in Chapter 25. The same philosophy and appliances apply to space maintenance in the 6- to 12-year-old age group. Treatment of early loss of primary teeth in the mixed dentition requires some additional thought and consideration, however. Loss of posterior teeth in the primary dentition is a nearly universal indication for space maintenance therapy. In the mixed dentition, the timing of permanent tooth eruption, timing of tooth loss, presence of succedaneous teeth, and extent of crowding must also be accounted for.

Premature loss of a primary molar at a very early age delays the eruption of the permanent tooth. On the other hand, premature loss of a primary molar at a later age may actually accelerate the eruption of the permanent tooth and make space maintenance unnecessary. In general, eruption of the permanent premolar will be

delayed if the primary molar is lost before age 8, whereas the premolar will tend to erupt earlier than normal if the primary molar is lost after age 8. A more accurate method of determining delayed or accelerated eruption of permanent teeth is to examine the amount of root development and alveolar bone overlying the unerupted permanent tooth from panoramic or periapical films. The succedaneous tooth begins to actively erupt when root development is approximately one half to two thirds completed. In terms of alveolar bone coverage, roughly 6 months' time should be anticipated for every millimeter of bone that covers the permanent tooth. If it is apparent that the tooth will be delayed in erupting and the space is adequate, space maintenance is absolutely indicated. Because space loss usually occurs within the first 6 months after the premature loss of a primary molar, space maintenance should be undertaken unless the tooth is expected to erupt within 6 months or unless there is enough space in the arch that a 1- or 2-mm space reduction will not compromise the eruption of the permanent tooth.

A second factor to consider is the amount of time that has elapsed since the primary tooth was lost. At one extreme is the case of a primary molar scheduled for extraction. At the other extreme is a primary molar already missing for 6 months or longer. In the first case, space maintenance is certainly indicated to prevent space loss when the tooth is extracted. In the second case, the majority of space loss has already occurred, and space maintenance may not be indicated. The clinician should complete space and profile analyses and make a decision based on those findings. If there is excess space in the arch or if so much space has been lost that extraction of permanent teeth is inevitable, space maintenance is contraindicated. A space maintainer is indicated to prevent any more space loss if the space remaining is only marginally adequate to allow the permanent tooth to erupt.

The absence of a permanent successor also complicates space maintenance in the mixed dentition. The second premolar is the most commonly missing posterior tooth in the permanent dentition, excluding the third molars. If the primary second molar is lost prematurely, the clinician must make a decision about the space that would have been occupied by the missing second premolar. Two choices can be made. One alternative is to maintain space in the arch and eventually construct a fixed prosthesis or have an implant placed and restored. This is feasible only if the skeletal and dental relationships are Class I, there is no crowding, and there is good interarch occlusion. This is a more inviting alternative if only one of the premolars is missing (i.e., a unilateral missing premolar). The advent of resin-bonded bridges and intraosseous implants has made this option more popular. Another alternative is to allow or encourage the space to close. Factors that favor this solution include crowding within the arch, protrusive incisors and lips, bilateral missing premolars, and possibly other missing teeth.

The amount of crowding in the arch is an important factor in the decision about space maintenance, and it is predicted from the space analysis and put in perspective by the facial form analysis. If the incisor position is normal and there is adequate space or minor crowding in the arch, space maintenance should be initiated. Early loss of a primary molar in an arch with substantial crowding must be considered carefully, however. Space maintainers alone will not solve a problem of this magnitude. Either permanent teeth will need to be extracted or the arches will need to be expanded. Expansion is possible only if the incisor position is normal or retrusive and the periodontal health is good enough to allow the incisors to be moved facially. If expansion is contemplated, space maintainers should be placed. In some cases, however, crowding of this magnitude is treated by extracting two first premolars and closing the remaining space orthodontically.

If no space maintenance is implemented and tooth movement results from drifting prior to first premolar extractions, less space remains to be closed later. Consultation with a specialist is usually desirable before this type of decision is made. If the crowding approaches 10 mm/arch, space maintainers may need to be placed even though permanent tooth extraction is inevitably required. The average width of a premolar is approximately 7 mm; therefore, the extraction of two premolars would effectively result in a gain of 14 mm of arch length. If further space is lost in an arch that is already severely crowded, a two-premolar extraction may not resolve all of the crowding. Space maintainers would ensure that no further decrease in arch length occurs. In some instances, timed extraction (called serial extraction) can alleviate the crowding and relieve the demands of subsequent orthodontic treatment.

Probably the most significant difference between space maintenance strategy in the mixed dentition and that in the primary dentition is bilateral loss of teeth in the mandibular arch. In the primary dentition, two band and loop appliances are indicated; in the mixed dentition,

the lingual arch is preferred if all lower incisors have erupted. Primary second molars or permanent first molars may be used as abutment teeth. If oral hygiene is a problem, it is recommended that primary second molars be banded. This is done so that if decalcification under bands occurs as a result of poor oral hygiene, it occurs on teeth that will eventually exfoliate.

Space maintenance in the mixed dentition requires close supervision as permanent teeth erupt and primary teeth exfoliate. When primary abutment teeth exfoliate, an appliance may need to be remade, using permanent teeth as abutments. Space-maintaining appliances obviously should be removed when the permanent tooth erupts into its proper position.

Potential Alignment and Space Problems

ECTOPIC ERUPTION

Problems associated with ectopic eruption of the permanent first molar have been discussed. A 3- to 6-month observation period usually is the best initial therapy if the resorption is not too severe, because there is a possibility that the molar will self-correct spontaneously or jump distally and erupt into its normal position (Fig. 35-9). Intervention is necessary if the molar is still blocked from erupting at the end of the observation period or if the permanent molar is severely impacted (Kennedy and Turley, 1987). The goal of treatment is to move the ectopically erupting tooth away from the tooth it is resorbing.

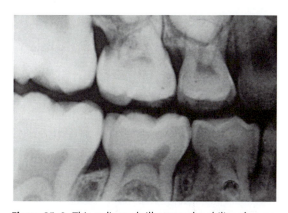

Figure 35-9. This radiograph illustrates the ability of an ectopically erupting permanent first molar to self-correct spontaneously. Note that the distal root of the primary maxillary second molar has been resorbed. Usually this type of resorption is the result of an erupting permanent molar that is caught on the distal aspect of the primary molar. If the resorption does not progress too far, the permanent molar usually "jumps" past the resorptive defect in 3 to 6 months.

If a small amount of movement is needed and little or none of the permanent molar is clinically visible, a piece of 20-mil brass wire can be passed around the contact between the permanent molar and the primary second molar. The brass wire is tightened every 2 weeks. When the wire is tightened, the periodontal ligament space is compressed and the molar is forced distally until it can slip past the primary molar and erupt (Fig. 35–10). In some cases, a steel spring clip separator may be used to dislodge the molar, but only in cases in which there is minimal resorption of the primary molar. It may be difficult to seat the spring if the contact point between the molars is below the cementoenamel junction of the primary molar. Some authors advocate elastomeric separators, but they must be carefully supervised because they may dislodge in an apical direction, causing a periodontal abscess. Some elastomeric separators are not radiopaque and can be difficult to locate.

A second method of moving the permanent molar distally is to band the primary second molar and apply a distal force to the permanent molar through a helical spring or elastomer (Fig. 35–11). This type of tooth movement requires that the occlusal surface of the permanent molar be visible so that force can be applied to move the tooth distally. A small ledge of resin or a metal button can be bonded to the occlusal surface to serve as the point of force application, or the end of the spring can be bonded directly to the impacted tooth. Salivary contamination of the occlusal surface, however, sometimes makes bonding a frustrating and difficult procedure. Such a band and spring appliance should be evaluated every 2 weeks and can work effectively in a short time because of the minimal root development on the permanent molar.

Occasionally, the primary second molar needs to be removed if the permanent molar has caused extensive resorption of the primary root structure. In these cases, loss of arch length is certain, and some plan of treatment for the impending space deficiency should be considered in advance. If there is a congenitally missing second premolar or premolar extraction followed by space closure is being considered, then reduction in arch length by mesial movement of the molars is anticipated and advantageous. To manage the space after extraction of the primary molar, a distal shoe can be placed to guide eruption of the permanent molar. A distal shoe maintains space but does not regain much space lost prior to the primary molar extraction. An alternative plan is to allow the permanent molar to erupt and then regain the space with a space-regaining appliance (described subsequently).

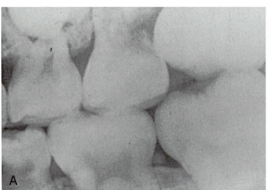

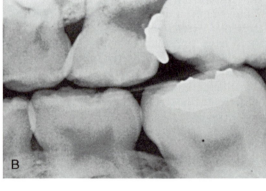

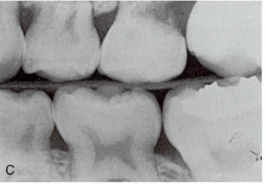

Figure 35–10. *A,* This radiograph shows an ectopically erupting permanent maxillary left first molar. *B,* Because only a small amount of movement is required to correct the ectopic eruption, a piece of 20-mil brass wire is slipped around the contact point between the permanent molar and the primary second molar and is tightened. *C,* After the wire has been tightened three times at 2-week intervals, the molar is dislodged and begins to erupt into a normal position. (From Fields HW, Proffit WR: Orthodontics in general practice. *In* Morris AL, Bohannan HM, Casullo DP [eds]: The Dental Specialties in General Practice. Philadelphia, WB Saunders, 1983.)

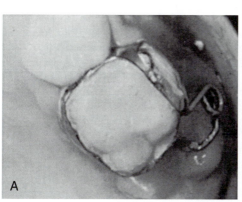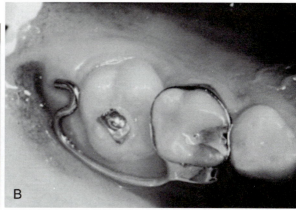

Figure 35–11. *A,* A band and helical spring appliance is used to treat an ectopically erupting permanent molar that requires a large amount of movement. The primary second molar is banded, and a helical spring is soldered to the band. A small ledge of composite resin, a metal button bonded to the occlusal surface of the permanent molar, or a small preparation can serve as a point of force application. The spring is reactivated at monthly intervals until the permanent molar is dislodged. (From Fields HW, Proffit WR: Orthodontics in general practice. *In* Morris AL, Bohannan HM, Casullo DP [eds]: The Dental Specialties in General Practice. Philadelphia, WB Saunders, 1983.) *B,* Another band and spring design with a metal button bonded to the occlusal surface of the erupting permanent molar. Elastomeric chain or thread is attached from the button to the distal hook on the wire and changed monthly to provide the distal force to dislodge the molar.

After the space is regained, a space maintainer should be placed.

Ectopic eruption of lateral incisors is usually an early indication of crowding but may only be the result of aberrant tooth positioning. If a primary canine exfoliates prematurely as a result of ectopic eruption, the lower incisors typically drift to that side of the arch, creating a midline discrepancy. If the laterals cause resorption and exfoliation of both primary canines, the incisors usually tip lingually and decrease arch length. It appears that the space problem is corrected because the incisor alignment usually improves, but this is only temporary, and the space shortage will become apparent again when the permanent canines begin to erupt. Whether the loss of primary canines is unilateral or bilateral, the clinician should determine whether there is an arch length inadequacy and assess anteroposterior lip and incisor position. This information helps determine whether space maintenance, space regaining, or more extensive treatment is needed.

The goal of treatment should be to prevent a midline shift and manage the space according to the long-term plan. This can be accomplished by placing a lingual arch with a soldered spur distal to the lateral incisor to hold the midline if adequate space is present and the incisors are in a good position. If the midline has already shifted, the contralateral primary canine can be removed to promote spontaneous midline correction. If space loss cannot be tolerated, a lingual arch should be placed following extraction. If there is

sufficient crowding, so that space maintenance is contraindicated, or if the incisors are considered too protrusive to be maintained in this position, no lingual arch should be placed following the extraction of the contralateral primary canine. In situations in which both canines exfoliate prematurely because of ectopic eruption, similar treatment decisions should be made, although the clinician does not normally need to worry about a midline shift.

MISSING PERMANENT TEETH

The absence of permanent teeth creates many treatment problems for the clinician, and most treatment decisions of this nature are best made by a specialist. The maxillary lateral incisor and the mandibular second premolar are the most common missing teeth in the permanent dentition. Treatment decisions are based not only on which tooth is missing but also on arch length, incisor position, and lip and profile esthetics.

Treatment of missing maxillary lateral incisors varies depending on whether one or both incisors are absent and on the position of the permanent canine when it erupts into the arch. The canine either erupts into the normal canine position or resorbs the primary lateral incisor and spontaneously substitutes for the missing lateral incisor. If the canine erupts into its proper position, the primary lateral incisor will eventually need to be removed because it does not make an esthetically pleasing substitute for the permanent lateral incisor and because the root will eventually be resorbed. The missing lateral incisor can be replaced with a resin-bonded bridge, a conventional bridge, or an implant. A bridge or an implant is the treatment of choice when the occlusion, incisor position, and profile are nearly ideal and when closing space orthodontically is not appropriate (Fig. 35–12).

If the permanent canine erupts into the lateral incisor position, the primary canine must be extracted and the space closed, or the permanent canine must be moved back into the correct position and a bridge constructed or an implant placed for the missing lateral incisor. Crowding or protrusive incisors usually call for space closure and substitution of canines for lateral incisors. These canines require recontouring by enamel removal and resin addition to improve the esthetic appearance of the teeth. Canine substitution cases are considered difficult to treat well. Normal pretreatment occlusion favors bridge or implant placement (Fig. 35–13).

Arch length, incisor position, and facial appearance must be thoroughly evaluated before a treatment plan is generated when a premolar is congenitally missing. Unlike primary canines and laterals, a primary molar may be a reasonable substitute for a missing premolar. The size, shape, and restorative status of the primary molar

give some indication of the possibility of maintaining the tooth for a period of time. Ankylosis and advanced root resorption indicate that the primary molar should be removed. Most clinicians favor removing the primary molar and closing the space orthodontically, but in certain situations a resin-bonded bridge, conventional bridge, or implant may be a more ideal treatment. These situations occur most likely in Class I skeletal and dental patients with ideal or near ideal occlusions or when a tooth is missing unilaterally.

If the arch is so crowded that teeth need to be extracted, or if the incisors are too protrusive or the profile too full, the retained primary molar should be removed and the case treated in a manner similar to that for a four-premolar extraction case. Typically, first premolars are removed in an extraction case, but the majority of congenitally missing premolars are second premolars. If it can be determined that the second premolar is missing and that extractions are necessary to resolve the arch length inadequacy, the primary molar can be removed early, allowing the space to close by mesial drifting of the permanent first molar and distal drifting of the anterior teeth. Unfortunately, congenital absence of the second premolar may not be definitively determined at an early age, and this delays the extractions. The

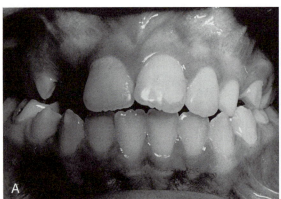

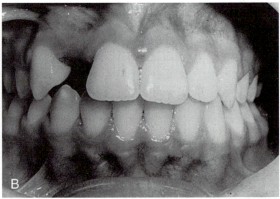

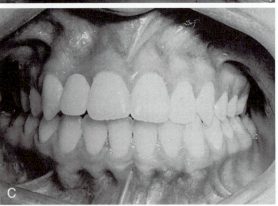

Figure 35–12. *A*, This patient is missing the maxillary right lateral incisor and has a right posterior crossbite. Because the patient has class I molars and relatively good alignment, a decision was made to replace the missing lateral incisor prosthetically. *B*, At the end of treatment, a space identical in size to the left lateral incisor was created to replace the right lateral incisor. *C*, A right lateral incisor pontic was created by shaping a denture tooth to the appropriate width and length. Orthodontic wire is inserted into the pontic on the lingual surface and bent to fit the lingual surface of the canine and central incisor. The wire is bonded with resin to each abutment tooth. This type of restoration does not work with a deep bite because of the shearing force of occlusion on the lingual surface.

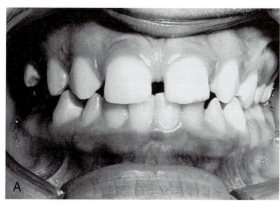
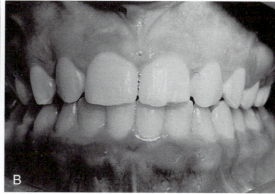

Figure 35–13. *A,* This patient was missing both maxillary lateral incisors. A treatment plan was developed to bring the canines forward to substitute for the missing lateral incisors. *B,* At the end of treatment, the patient had class II molar and canine relationships because of the substitution. The patient elected not to reshape the canines to resemble lateral incisors.

longer the extractions are delayed, the less drifting and spontaneous space closure will occur. Using the space of the missing second premolars to reduce protrusion is much more complicated and requires the teeth to be retracted into the space of the missing teeth. This precludes dental drifting and should be planned by the specialist.

SUPERNUMERARY TEETH

A supernumerary tooth may create space and eruption problems. It can cause permanent teeth to erupt into malalignment or even prevent eruption. Treatment is usually directed at removing the supernumerary before it causes any eruption problems. Management of the supernumerary varies depending on the size, shape, and number of supernumeraries and the dental development

of the patient. Typically, the supernumerary is detected on a panoramic radiograph or an anterior occlusal film unless there is clinical evidence of an extra tooth at an earlier age. If the supernumerary is conical and is not inverted, there is a reasonable chance that it will erupt, at which time it should be removed (Fig. 35-14). If the supernumerary is inverted, is tubercular in shape, or is significantly impeding eruption of the adjacent teeth, it should be surgically removed (Fig. 35-15). Ideally, the surgery is timed so that removal of the supernumerary tooth does not interfere with permanent tooth development. The earlier the supernumerary can be removed, however, the more likely it is that the permanent teeth will erupt normally. Surgery to remove a supernumerary is often complicated, especially if there are multiple supernumerary

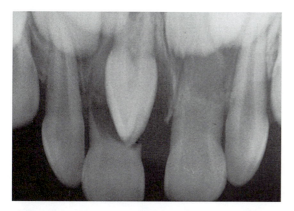

Figure 35–14. A conical supernumerary in the maxillary central incisor region was detected during a radiographic examination after a traumatic injury to the maxillary anterior region. This supernumerary was not interfering with the normal eruption of the permanent incisors and was allowed to erupt before it was removed.

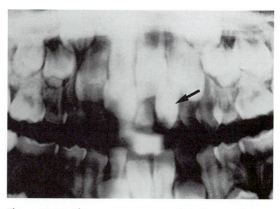

Figure 35–15. This supernumerary tooth in the maxillary anterior region significantly affected the eruption of the permanent maxillary left central incisor. The supernumerary tooth was surgically removed, and the central incisor was moved orthodontically to the correct position.

teeth or if access to the supernumerary is limited. These cases are appropriately referred to a specialist.

TOOTH SIZE DISCREPANCIES

Isolated tooth size discrepancies can cause alignment problems. The maxillary lateral incisor commonly creates this type of problem because it is undersized or pegged in shape. Occasionally the lateral incisor can be restored to its normal size with composite resin and no other treatment. As discussed in the earlier part of the chapter on tooth size analysis, sometimes the pegged lateral requires a combination of tooth movement and restorative dentistry to achieve normal occlusion. Depending on the size of the discrepancy, the pegged lateral can be treated in one of three ways (Fig. 35-16). If the lateral incisor is only slightly smaller than normal, the entire space can be closed.

An alternative method for a marginally small incisor is to move the lateral incisor orthodontically until it contacts the central incisor and leave space distal to the lateral. The canine usually is not brought forward to close the space because this would put the canine in an end-to-end relationship and disrupt the previously normal occlusion. This solution is generally not esthetically pleasing unless only a small space is left distal to the lateral and requires retention to hold the space.

A third solution, usually reserved for incisors that are considerably undersized, is a combination of orthodontic tooth movement and resin bonding to reshape the crown. The lateral incisor needs to be positioned so that the resin addition will be cosmetically pleasing and will restore near-normal crown anatomy. This type of treatment is best performed by a specialist. Fusion and gemination in the permanent dentition are even more difficult to treat and should also be referred to a specialist.

Dens evaginatus and incisor talon cusps provide interesting challenges in securing an ideal occlusion (Fig. 35-17). In most cases of dens evaginatus, a fine, thread-like pulp extends from the main pulp chamber into the evagination, and the location of this pulp tissue extension should be determined radiographically. Most such teeth

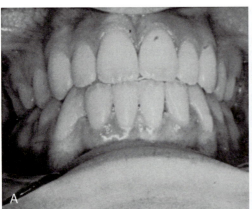

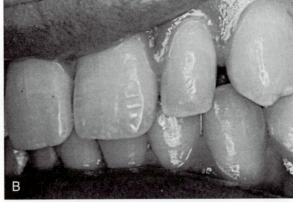

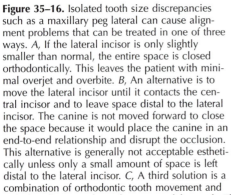

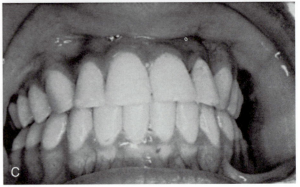

Figure 35-16. Isolated tooth size discrepancies such as a maxillary peg lateral can cause alignment problems that can be treated in one of three ways. *A,* If the lateral incisor is only slightly smaller than normal, the entire space is closed orthodontically. This leaves the patient with minimal overjet and overbite. *B,* An alternative is to move the lateral incisor until it contacts the central incisor and to leave space distal to the lateral incisor. The canine is not moved forward to close the space because it would place the canine in an end-to-end relationship and disrupt the occlusion. This alternative is generally not acceptable esthetically unless only a small amount of space is left distal to the lateral incisor. *C,* A third solution is a combination of orthodontic tooth movement and resin bonding to reshape the crown of the tooth. The lateral incisor is positioned so that the resin addition is esthetically pleasing and restores near-normal crown anatomy. In this patient, two peg laterals were treated with orthodontic tooth movement and resin addition.

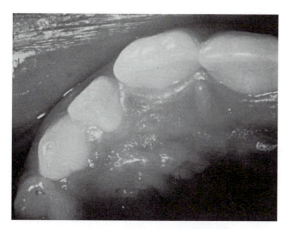

Figure 35–17. Dens evaginatus and incisor talon cusps create problems in the development of good occlusion. The talon cusp on this maxillary right lateral incisor has interfered with the normal positioning of the mandibular right lateral incisor.

in the posterior region do not require treatment because the force of mastication slowly wears the evagination down, and reparative dentin is formed. In the anterior region, however, the attrition must be accomplished mechanically with a hand piece and bur. A small amount of tooth structure is removed at each appointment, and after each session calcium hydroxide paste is applied to the exposed dentin to stimulate the reparative process. Usually the tooth can be treated at monthly appointments without permanent injury to the pulp. When treatment is complete, the exposed dentin is covered with a calcium hydroxide base and a resin restoration is placed.

Alignment Problems

Anterior and posterior tooth irregularities should be regarded as different from anterior and posterior space shortages. Tooth irregularity alone consists simply of rotated and tipped teeth in which there is no shortage of arch length. Arch length discrepancies—that is, a true lack of space—also result in tooth irregularities, but the two conditions are not always related.

Tooth irregularities can be treated with either fixed or removable appliances. If a simple tipping force will align the tooth, a removable appliance with a finger spring is an appropriate appliance choice. A great variety of removable appliances exist; however, several essential components need to be included in the design. The appliance must be retentive so that the force applied to the tooth will not dislodge the appliance. Adams

clasps are often prescribed and are very retentive, although they can be difficult to adjust and may interfere with the occlusion. Other types of clasps, such as ball clasps and c-clasps, are also popular. Multiple clasps should be used to enhance the retention. Additional retention and stability are gained from the palatal acrylic in maxillary appliances. A 22-mil finger spring incorporated into the palatal acrylic delivers a light, continuous force. The spring should be activated 1 to 2 mm to move the tooth approximately 1 mm/month (Fig. 35–18).

Fixed appliances can be used to correct irregularities as well and are indicated when bodily movement of teeth or rotational control is necessary. Orthodontic appliances have evolved to a point where specific brackets are designed for specific teeth. The brackets are constructed to provide proper crown and root positioning when they are precisely placed on the teeth. Before the appliances can be placed, the facial surfaces of the teeth selected for treatment are thoroughly cleaned. Then the teeth are isolated with either cotton rolls or specially designed retractors to provide a field free of salivary contamination with optimal access (Fig. 35–19A).

Via the acid-etch technique, etching solution is painted on the facial surfaces of the teeth. The solution is restricted to the area that will eventually be covered by the bracket (Fig. 35–19B). After the enamel has been etched for 1 minute, the facial surfaces are thoroughly washed with water and dried. If the enamel surfaces appear to be well etched, a bonding agent is applied to the teeth, and the excess is blown

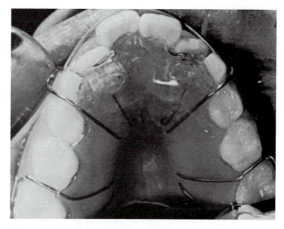

Figure 35–18. Removable appliances can be used to treat alignment problems but are more effective for some problems than for others. Notice that the maxillary right lateral incisor can easily be tipped facially, but it is more difficult to rotate the left lateral incisor and requires use of the lingual finger spring and the labial bow in concert.

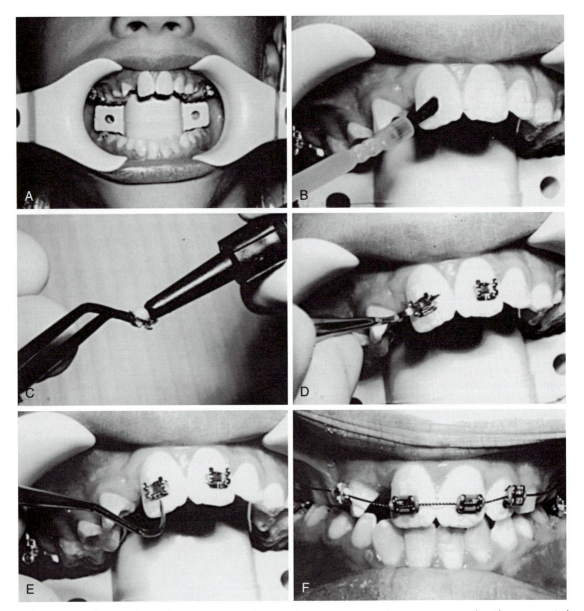

Figure 35–19. *A,* Orthodontic appliances are designed to provide proper crown and root positioning when they are precisely placed on the teeth. Therefore, it is imperative to follow the appropriate sequence when placing the appliances. Before the appliances are placed, the teeth selected for treatment must be thoroughly cleaned. *B,* After the teeth have been cleaned and isolated to provide a field free of salivary contamination, etching solution is painted on the facial surface of the teeth. *C,* A two-paste, autopolymerizing composite resin is mixed, and a small amount is placed on a single bracket pad. *D,* The bracket is placed on the tooth and moved into proper position. Proper position is based on the long axis of the crown, the long axis of the root, or the incisal edge. *E,* After the bracket is positioned properly, it is firmly seated in place. The excess resin expressed from beneath the pad is carefully removed before it is fully polymerized. *F,* This process is repeated until all the brackets have been properly placed. At this point, the arch wire is selected, placed in the brackets, and ligated with steel ligatures or elastomeric ties.

away with an air syringe. A composite resin designed specifically for orthodontic use is placed on a single bracket pad (Fig. 35-19*C*). The resin may be an autopolymerizing two-paste system; a no-mix, one-step system; or a light-cured system. The bracket is placed on the tooth and moved into proper position. Proper position is dictated by the manufacturer's specifications and is based on the long axis of the crown, the long axis of the root, or the incisal edge (Fig. 35-19*D*). After the bracket is in position, it is firmly seated in place with a scaler or explorer. The excess composite resin expressed from beneath the bracket pad is carefully removed before it is fully polymerized (Fig. 35-19*E*). Removal of this excess flash ensures that the bracket slots can be fully engaged and also eliminates a source of plaque retention. This process is repeated until all the brackets have been properly placed.

Finally, an arch wire is selected, placed in the brackets, and ligated with steel ligatures or elastomeric modules (Fig. 35-19*F*). The clinician should understand the physical properties of wires because a wire must be selected that is strong enough to withstand the force of occlusion in the posterior segments yet flexible enough in the anterior region to be deflected into the brackets and deliver a light, continuous force. Small stainless steel wires, some titanium alloys, and braided stainless steel wires usually provide ample strength and flexibility as an initial arch wire. Occasionally, loops must be bent into the arch wire to produce anterior flexibility and posterior strength. Retention is essential after the correction of irregularity because the teeth have a strong propensity to relapse. Gingival fibers reorganize very slowly following these types of movements, and in some cases irregularity returns even if retention is well conceived. Some clinicians have suggested that if the periodontium is healthy, a circumferential supracrestal fiberotomy may be performed to reduce relapse.

When treatment is complete or nearly complete, the supracrestal gingival fibers are cut with a scalpel and a No. 12B blade under local anesthesia. Theoretically, the stretched gingival fibers will not need to reorganize but will reattach in a new position after being cut. Care should be taken if this procedure is used in patients with a thin gingival covering.

Many children have a midline diastema in the mixed dentition, and this is considered a normal stage of development. Occasionally, a large midline diastema is present that is due to a mesiodens or other midline intrabony pathology, protruding incisors, or a tooth size problem. A diastema caused by a midline supernumerary

tooth or abnormality is treated by removing the supernumerary tooth or the abnormality. The supernumerary tooth should be removed as early as possible without causing injury to the adjacent permanent teeth. Early removal of the mesiodens allows the permanent teeth to erupt normally, and the space usually closes spontaneously.

In some cases, a large diastema may be due to faciolingual rather than mesiodistal positioning of the incisors. Flared incisors are cosmetically unappealing and are at greater risk of traumatic injury (Andreasen and Ravn, 1972). If the teeth can be tipped back into an ideal position to close the diastema and if the overbite will not hinder tooth movement, a removable appliance is recommended. The appliance is designed to include at least two clasps for retention, palatal acrylic and a 28-mil labial bow with adjustment loops (Fig. 35-20). The labial bow is activated to tip the incisors lingually by closing the adjustment loops. At the same time, acrylic must be removed from the lingual side of the appliance to permit tooth movement and excess gingival tissue. The labial bow is activated approximately 2.0 mm/month until the diastema is closed and the teeth are in ideal position.

Fixed orthodontic appliances are suggested if the incisors are so protrusive that bodily movement is required to close the diastema or if the teeth are rotated. The molars are banded, and the incisors are bonded with orthodontic brackets. The teeth are aligned initially if necessary with small, round arch wires and then are retracted via a larger rectangular wire with closing

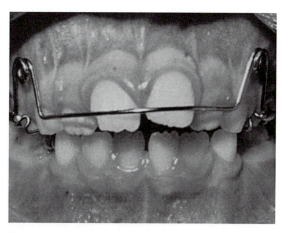

Figure 35-20. A large diastema that is due to excessively protruding incisors is sometimes treated with a removable appliance if the overbite will not interfere with retraction of the incisors. The appliance incorporates a labial bow with adjustment loops that are activated to tip the incisors lingually. By tipping the incisors lingually, both the diastema and the incisor protrusion are corrected.

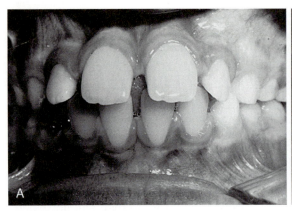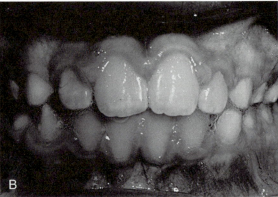

Figure 35–21. *A,* If bodily movement is required to close a diastema, fixed appliances are suggested. Typically, the incisors are bonded with orthodontic brackets and the molars are banded. Space, such as that shown here, is closed with either closing loops or elastomeric chain to retract the teeth. *B,* Retention is necessary to maintain space closure and is usually accomplished with a removable appliance. If the frenal attachment is thought to be the cause of the diastema, frenectomy can be completed at the end of the active appliance phase or during the retention phase.

loops or elastomeric chain (Fig. 35-21). Rectangular arch wires are necessary to provide full control of tooth position during retraction. Headgear may be necessary to reinforce the molar anchorage at the same time because the molars have a strong tendency to come forward while the incisors are retracted. The choice of headgear is based on the vertical dimensions of the face.

If the diastema is due to a relative discrepancy between the upper and lower teeth of mandibular anterior excess tooth size, treatment usually requires the addition of resin to the interproximal surfaces of the maxillary incisors. Closing the space by means of orthodontic procedures only will eventually result in relapse because the occlusion will force the space open again.

Treatment to close a midline diastema not associated with an anteroposterior position or a tooth size problem is usually initiated if the diastema is significantly esthetically objectionable, greater than 3 mm, or if it is still present after the permanent canines have fully erupted. A diastema larger than 3 mm usually inhibits or disturbs eruption of the lateral incisors and should be closed before these teeth emerge. Both of these types of diastema are due to faulty mesiodistal positioning of the incisors, but the choice of appliance is still based on the type of tooth movement required to close the space. If the central incisors can be tipped together to close the diastema, a removable appliance should be used. Finger springs are either incorporated into the palatal acrylic or soldered to the labial bow to engage the distal edge of the incisor crown (Fig. 35-22). The springs are activated 2 mm/month, and closure should not take more than 2 months.

Brackets are bonded on the facial surface of the central incisors if the teeth require bodily mesiodistal movement or rotational control to close the diastema. After initial alignment, a large segmental or full rectangular arch wire is placed in the brackets, and the teeth are moved together via elastomeric chain. The chain is attached only to the mesial wings of each bracket while the distal wings are ligated separately. This prevents the teeth from rotating when the space is closing (Fig. 35-23).

No matter which type of treatment is used to close a midline diastema, retention can be a problem and should be planned. In most cases, a removable appliance maintains the space clo-

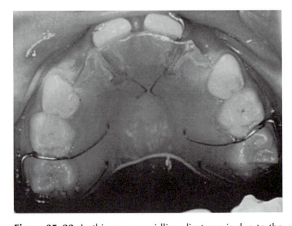

Figure 35–22. In this case, a midline diastema is due to the mesiodistal positioning of the maxillary central incisors. A removable appliance with finger springs incorporated into the palatal acrylic closes the space, tipping the teeth together. (From Fields HW: Treatment of nonskeletal problems in preadolescent children. *In* Proffit WR, et al [eds]: Contemporary Orthodontics. St. Louis, Mosby–Year Book, 1999.)

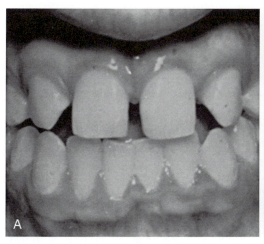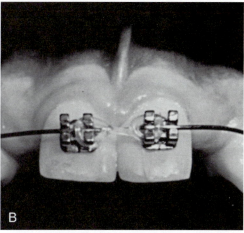

Figure 35–23. *A*, If bodily mesiodistal movement is needed to close a diastema, fixed appliances are placed on the teeth. *B*, After initial alignment, either a segmental or a full arch wire is placed in the brackets, and the teeth are moved together with an elastomeric chain.

sure. The appliance needs to be adjusted periodically if the diastema is closed before the lateral incisors and canines have erupted fully. If the diastema reopens during or following retention, the incisors should be realigned. At that time, a surgical procedure, frenectomy, can be performed if the frenum is thought to be the cause of the diastema reopening. The frenectomy is performed after the space is closed because the scar tissue created by the procedure may actually impede closure if the surgery is accomplished first. If the diastema again reopens following retention and the surgical procedure, a 17.5-mil multistranded wire can be bonded to the lingual surface of the incisors to keep the teeth together. The only contraindications to a bonded wire retainer are an excessively deep bite and poor oral hygiene.

Crowding Problems

The first sign of crowding in the mixed dentition usually coincides with the eruption of the permanent incisors. Arch length insufficiency may manifest in several ways, ranging from slight incisor rotation and irregularity to gross incisor malalignment. The first step should be to perform a space analysis and determine the extent of the arch length inadequacy. This finding is then placed in the context of the facial profile analysis.

MILD CROWDING

A true arch length discrepancy of 0 to 2 mm may not be apparent or may be manifested as a mild irregularity, most likely in the incisor region. Mild irregularity is considered normal in patients who have no arch length discrepancy. Longitudinal studies of persons with ideal occlusions show that there is a period when up to 2 mm of transitional irregularity occurs early in the mixed dentition (Moorrees et al., 1969). Observation is usually the best course. Some patients have little or no overall arch length shortages and demonstrate noticeable crowding during incisor eruption. Treatment may be indicated for these children if the lateral incisors erupt lingual to their proper position or in very irregular positions. If treatment is deemed necessary, interproximal enamel can be removed from the mesial or distal surface of the primary canines (or from both places) to provide space (Fig. 35–24). Disking may be accomplished with a hand-held strip, a sandpaper disk in a slow-speed hand piece, or a tapered bur in a high-speed hand piece. The procedure is performed without anesthesia so that the child can indicate any discomfort. Extreme discomfort usually indicates that sufficient enamel has been removed to cause the pulpal tissues to react. Typically, careful disking yields 2 to 4 mm of space. A professional-strength topical fluoride preparation can be applied to the canines after disking and may reduce postoperative sensitivity.

If it is apparent that disking will not alleviate the anterior irregularity, it may be appropriate to extract the primary canines and place a lingual arch so that the available space can be used by the larger incisors for alignment and later the smaller premolars can erupt in the remaining space. For the most part, this therapy is under-

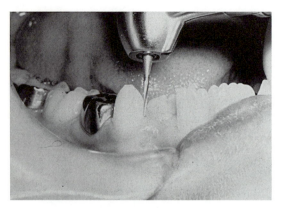

Figure 35–24. When the arch length discrepancy is determined to be 2 mm or less and the lateral incisor is erupting lingual to its proper position, the primary canine can be disked with either a high- or low-speed handpiece or a hand-held strip. In this case, a tapered fissure bur in a high-speed handpiece is being used to disk the mesial surface of the primary canine.

taken in the mandibular arch, although there are a few situations in which it is indicated in the maxilla. A lingual arch is necessary because the lower incisors tend to tip lingually without the support of the primary canines. This results in shortening of arch length. In this situation, the lingual arch is placed in a passive state—that is, the arch exerts no force to move the incisors and increase the space. The clinician should communicate to the parent that this treatment requires close supervision and that the primary first molars may need to be disked or extracted when the permanent canines erupt. The lingual arch remains in place until the second premolars have erupted or until it is evident that there will be sufficient space for all the permanent teeth to erupt. Essentially, one is using the leeway space and controlling all available arch length to achieve alignment of the teeth. In some cases, this means that the molars (those that are end-to-end) will not achieve a Class I relationship because the mandibular mesial molar shift has been prevented. Either headgear or interarch mechanics such as elastics will need to be used to achieve the correct occlusal relationships. In other situations, a Class I molar relationship may have already been present and this is not a concern.

MODERATE CROWDING

Treatment of a moderate arch length discrepancy of less than 5 mm is based on the facial profile, incisor position, crowding, and the amount of facial keratinized tissue. If the profile is straight,

with good anteroposterior or slightly retrusive position of the lips and incisors, a small amount of expansion can be tolerated to accommodate all the teeth. Expansion is not a good treatment option if the incisors are already protrusive. The clinician must always keep in mind the interaction between crowding, incisor position, and profile because they are essentially part of the same problem, expressed in a different way.

Moderate crowding may be either localized or generalized. Localized crowding may be the result of space loss after extraction or premature exfoliation of a primary tooth. If space loss is 3 mm or less, the adjacent tooth usually can be tipped into proper position with either a removable appliance or an active lingual arch. For example, a removable appliance with a finger spring can tip a permanent maxillary first molar distally after removal of a primary second molar compromised by ectopic eruption (Fig. 35–25). Other fixed appliances such as a Nance Lingual Arch supporting segmental arches and compressed coil springs can be used to move posterior teeth distally. Alternatively, headgear can be used if bilateral space regaining is desired. After the space has been regained, arch length should be near ideal and can be maintained. A band and loop appliance or a lingual arch can be placed to maintain the space.

If localized crowding is not due to terminal molars drifting anteriorly but is located in the midportions of the arch, permanent tooth impaction is likely. Orthodontic tooth movement is necessary to increase the space and allow room for eruption. Fixed orthodontic appliances are

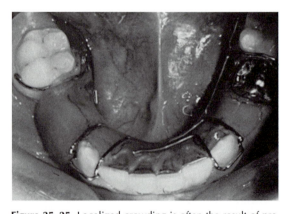

Figure 35–25. Localized crowding is often the result of prematurely exfoliating primary teeth. In this case, the primary mandibular right second molar was lost prematurely, allowing the permanent first molar to drift mesially. A removable appliance has been designed to tip the permanent first molar back with a finger spring. The spring is activated until the molar is correctly positioned. Then a band and loop or lingual arch can be placed.

placed on the entire arch, and the arch is aligned with light, flexible arch wires. After alignment, a heavy arch wire is placed to maintain good arch form during space-regaining movements. A compressed coil spring provides the force necessary to open the space (Fig. 35-26A). After the space has been opened, it may be necessary to expose the crown of the tooth surgically if it does not erupt within a 6-month period. Surgical exposure of the crown requires the elevation and repositioning of soft tissue to provide adequate keratinized tissue around the impacted tooth (Fig. 35-26B). Adequate attached gingiva is essential for good periodontal support and esthetic appearance. If the clinician is not well versed in surgical exposure, the patient is best referred to a specialist. When the crown is exposed, an orthodontic attachment is bonded to the crown, and the tooth is moved with traction into the arch (Fig. 35-26C).

Patients characterized by anterior or generalized crowding of less than 5 mm present difficult treatment decisions. As stated earlier, incisor and lip position provide important guides to whether arch length can be created by expansion. Upright or lingually inclined incisors may be moved facially into correct alignment if the lips are retrusive. The risk associated with generalized arch expansion is instability of the new position, how-

ever (Little et al., 1988, 1990). Movement of teeth facially may upset the existing equilibrium and result in relapse after the appliances are removed. Relapse does not occur in all cases; some patients maintain increased arch dimensions and remain stable after treatment is complete. There does not seem to be a good method of predicting stability, however (Little, 1987). Unfortunately, clinical judgment and long-term retention must be relied on in many cases.

If the clinician elects to alleviate arch length inadequacy by expansion (because the leeway space will not supply enough needed space), several approaches can be taken. An active lower lingual arch can be constructed with adjustment loops to tip the incisors facially if the overbite is not prohibitively deep to prevent movement of the facial incisors (Fig. 35-27) and perhaps to move the molars distally a small amount. The adjustment loops, located mesial to the molars, should not be activated beyond 1 mm because the activation of such a large wire (36 mil) places extremely large forces on the teeth. When the appliance is properly activated, the wire contacts the tooth high on the cingulum of the incisors. The direction of force is apical, but it tips the incisors facially because of the inclination of the lingual surface of the teeth. In 4 to 6 weeks, the appliance can be activated another millimeter.

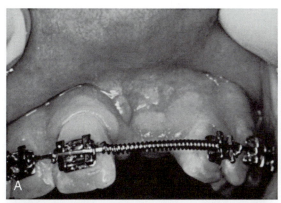
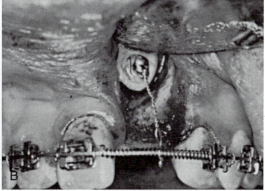
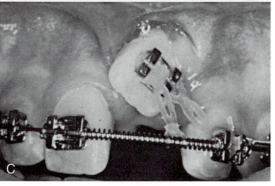

Figure 35–26. *A*, If localized crowding is confined to the anterior or premolar region, tooth impaction is likely. Orthodontic tooth movement is necessary to create space for eruption of the impacted tooth. In this case, the permanent maxillary left central incisor was impacted, and a coil spring was placed to open up space for tooth eruption. *B*, The tooth did not erupt within 6 months; therefore, the crown of the tooth was surgically exposed, bonded, and ligated to the base arch wire. *C*, After the soft tissues have healed sufficiently, orthodontic forces are applied to the tooth to bring it into the arch.

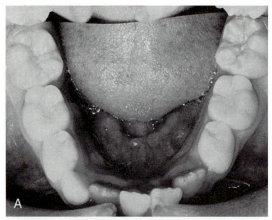

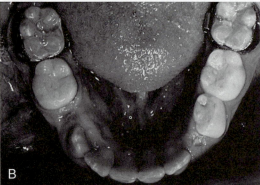

Figure 35–27. *A,* Generalized crowding of less than 5 mm is occasionally treated with an adjustable lingual arch if the overbite is not too deep to prevent facial movement of the mandibular incisors. The appliance is activated by opening the adjustment loops. In this case, a lingual arch was inserted after removal of the mandibular primary right canine. The canine was removed to keep the midline from shifting any further to the left. *B,* The same patient after 3 years of lingual arch therapy. The midline has shifted back to the right. The crowding is being treated by facial movement of the incisors and by use of the leeway space.

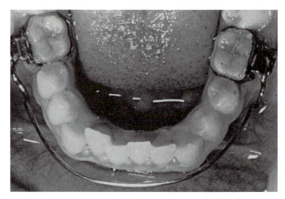

Figure 35–28. A lip bumper is also used to treat generalized crowding of less than 5 mm. The lip bumper is designed to decrease lower lip pressure on the teeth and to allow generalized expansion by facial movement of the teeth.

This process is repeated until arch length is adequate for the permanent dentition. Primary canines may need to be disked or removed as discussed previously if the crowding is in the anterior region.

A lip bumper, a wire appliance inserted in tubes on the lower molars, may be used to decrease lower lip pressure and achieve generalized arch expansion in the incisor, canine, and premolar regions (Fig. 35-28). The location of the expansion depends on the location of the lip bumper. The lip bumper removes resting pressure of the lips and cheeks from these teeth. The teeth move facially as a result of lack of lip pressure and the force of resting tongue pressure. The pressure from the lower lip may tip the molar distally (Nevant et al., 1991). Remem-

ber that ultimately both arches must be coordinated.

Arch expansion may also be accomplished via a functional appliance with buccal shields in the vestibule. The buccal shields disrupt the equilibrium between the tongue and the cheek and allow the teeth to move facially (Fig. 35-29). Some investigators claim that properly constructed buccal shields actually stretch the underlying periosteum of the bone and cause skeletal remodeling in the transverse dimension. Although this claim has not been substantiated by careful investigation, there is no doubt that enough expansion can be created in this manner to relieve minor to moderate crowding.

Like removable appliances, fixed (banded and

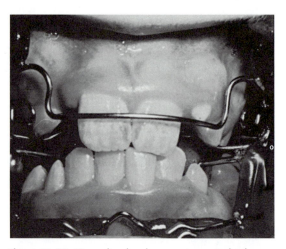

Figure 35–29. Generalized arch expansion can also be accomplished via a functional appliance with buccal shields. The buccal shields disrupt the equilibrium between the facial musculature and the tongue and allow the teeth to move facially.

bonded) appliances can be used to tip teeth. Fixed orthodontic appliances are necessary to increase arch length when bodily movement of teeth is required to alleviate crowding and align the teeth. Banded and bonded appliances also offer the opportunity to efficiently control rotational problems of teeth. A variety of arch wire designs can be used to expand the arch depending on the teeth with attachments. Clearly, any dimension of the arch can be altered with this method. After the expansion has been completed, a lower lingual arch is placed to retain the expansion.

In most cases, further treatment is necessary to align the remaining permanent teeth when they erupt. In addition, distal movement of the maxillary molars may be required if some of the leeway space probably was used to align the mandibular teeth and cannot be used for the mesial molar shift. When a Class I molar relationship is present initially, this is not an issue. Therefore, multibonded appliances should be used sparingly, generally only in cases in which the molars are already Class I and there is some increased overjet, unless one is prepared to complete the case appropriately by adjusting the interarch relationships. Regardless of which appliance is selected, expansion is achieved at the expense of incisor position and profile.

SEVERE CROWDING

Crowding of more than 5 mm is considered severe. This amount of crowding is treated either by generalized arch expansion or by removal of selected permanent teeth. This degree of generalized arch expansion can be accomplished with different appliances but usually requires bodily tooth movement with fixed appliances. Achieving considerable expansion often is difficult. Incisor position, profile, and periodontal status all influence whether the patient should be treated without extraction. This type of patient is most appropriately referred to a specialist.

The decision to extract teeth is based on the factors listed previously and is further influenced by the location of the crowding, the position of the dental midline, and the dental and skeletal relationships of the patient. After careful case analysis, appropriate teeth may be removed to make subsequent tooth movement easier to accomplish and to minimize the effects of extraction on the profile. The permanent first premolar is most often selected for extraction because it is located at a midpoint in the arch and because the space it occupies can be used to correct midline problems, incisor protrusion, molar rela-tionship problems, or crowding. Other teeth can be removed depending on the specifics of the case and the type of therapy used. Extraction cases are best treated by a specialist.

In some children, crowding is so severe in the mixed dentition that expansion is not feasible, and extractions are necessary to obtain a suitable occlusion that is in harmony with the supporting structures and the facial profile. In these cases, a planned sequence of extractions of primary and permanent teeth can benefit the patient by reducing incisor crowding and irregularity in the early mixed dentition, which will make subsequent orthodontic treatment easier and quicker. The extractions also make room for teeth to erupt over the alveolus and through keratinized tissue rather than being forced buccally or lingually into positions that may affect the periodontal health of the teeth. Guidance of eruption and serial extraction are terms used to describe this sequence of extractions (Hotz, 1970; Kjellgren, 1947). Guidance of eruption was originally developed to treat severe crowding without orthodontic appliances but now is viewed as the first step in treatment culminating in fixed orthodontic appliance therapy. For this reason, the clinician should consult with a specialist before embarking on a planned extraction sequence.

Guidance of eruption should be considered an option when crowding is greater than 10 mm/arch, a measurement that should be confirmed by space analysis after the permanent lateral incisors have erupted. In addition, the patient should have a Class I dental and skeletal pattern with good lip and incisor position (unless one is prepared to address these problems) because guidance of eruption does not correct skeletal problems. Guidance of eruption begins in the early mixed dentition with the eruption of the lateral incisors. If a significant arch length discrepancy is predicted, the primary canines should be removed. This allows the incisors ample room to erupt and align. Typically, the incisors also tip lingually and upright, causing the bite to deepen. Faciolingual incisor displacement usually improves, but rotations are more resistant to spontaneous correction.

The child is then observed for 2 years or until it appears that the canines and premolars are ready to erupt. At that time, another space analysis should be completed to ensure that the arch length deficiency is still great enough to warrant permanent tooth extraction, and a radiograph should be obtained to determine the position of the unerupted teeth. The goal of treatment is to encourage the eruption of the permanent first premolar so that it can be extracted before the permanent canine erupts. Unfortunately, the mandibular canine erupts first nearly half the time in the mandibular arch. If it appears that the canine is ahead of the premolar and will erupt facially, the primary first molar should be removed when half to two thirds of the first premolar root is formed. At this stage of root development, premolar eruption will be accelerated, and the premolar will erupt before the canine enters the arch. This makes removal of the first premolar much easier. In the maxillary arch, the first premolar normally erupts before the canine, and this is not a problem. In some cases, the primary first molar is removed but the permanent canine still erupts before the first premolar. This can lead to impaction of the first premolar, requiring surgical removal. Similarly, it may become apparent that the permanent canine will erupt before the first premolar regardless of the extraction sequence. In this situation, the primary first molar and first premolar are both removed at the same time. This procedure is called *enucleation* because the premolar is removed from within the alveolar bone.

Surgical removal of teeth from within the alveolar bone should be avoided if possible because it carries the potential for creating bone and soft tissue defects. These occur if the alveolar bone is fractured or removed. New alveolar bone will not be stimulated to form because no tooth will erupt through this area. Surgical soft tissue defects resolve infrequently.

An alternative extraction sequence has been advocated to prevent lingual tipping of the lower incisors and the subsequent increase in overbite, but this sequence is recommended only when incisor crowding is limited. The primary canine is not removed when the lateral incisor erupts. Instead, the primary canine is retained and the primary first molar is extracted to accelerate the eruption of the permanent first premolar. This allows some anterior crowding to resolve. The premolar is extracted when it erupts into the arch. The primary canine is often extracted at the same time as the premolar or is left to exfoliate when the permanent canine erupts. The drawback of this alternative is that substantial incisor crowding is not readily resolved, which somewhat defeats the goal of selective tooth removal to encourage good dental alignment.

Anteroposterior Dental Problems

ANTERIOR CROSSBITE

Anterior crossbite in the mixed dentition is not an uncommon finding. The clinician should de-

termine whether the crossbite is skeletal or dental in origin from the profile analysis and intraoral findings. Skeletal problems should be referred to a specialist, whereas dental problems can be addressed immediately. The most common cause of nonskeletal crossbite is a lack of space for the permanent maxillary incisors to erupt. A space analysis verifies the space shortage. Anterior crossbite develops because the permanent tooth buds form lingual to the primary teeth. When space is inadequate, the incisors are forced to erupt on the lingual side of the arch. If it is apparent that the permanent incisors are beginning to erupt lingually, the adjacent primary teeth should be disked or removed to provide space for the permanent incisors. If space is provided as the incisors are just beginning to erupt, they will migrate facially out of crossbite, and appliance therapy may not be necessary.

If the incisor fails to erupt facially or if the anterior crossbite is not diagnosed early in the mixed dentition, appliance therapy is needed to correct the crossbite. Space for the incisors is gained by either disking or extracting the adjacent primary teeth. At this point, a decision must be made as to whether the teeth should be tipped into position or bodily moved into place. If tipping will accomplish treatment goals, either a removable appliance or a fixed appliance can be used to correct the crossbite. As described earlier, a removable appliance can be used to tip one or more teeth into proper alignment. The appliance is constructed of palatal acrylic with at least two Adams clasps for retention and a 22-mil finger spring to move the teeth (Fig. 35–30). The spring is a double-helix design that provides a physiologic amount of force over an extended range of action. The spring is activated 2 mm to

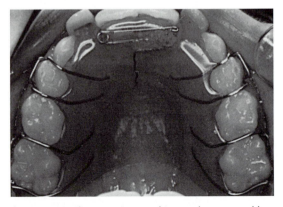

Figure 35–30. If an anterior crossbite can be corrected by tipping the teeth facially, a removable appliance will accomplish this goal. In this case, a single finger spring is tipping both maxillary central incisors out of crossbite.

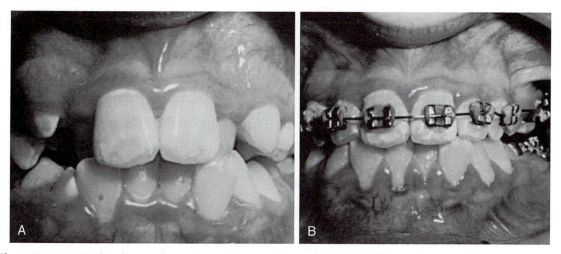

Figure 35–31. *A,* Fixed appliances also can be used to tip teeth out of anterior crossbite. In this patient both maxillary lateral incisors were in anterior crossbite. *B,* After the brackets were placed, progressively larger round wires were used to tip the teeth out of crossbite. A rectangular arch wire will be used to achieve proper crown and root position.

provide 1 mm of tooth movement per month. As with all removable appliances, the child must cooperate by wearing the device full-time to allow the appliance to accomplish the desired tooth movement.

An anterior crossbite with an accompanying deep overbite does not necessarily require a biteplane or bite-opening device during treatment. Most persons habitually keep the mandible open and occlude it only during swallowing and parafunctional movements. If the crossbite has not improved after 3 months of active treatment, it may be necessary to open the bite by adding acrylic to the appliance to cover the occlusal surfaces of the posterior teeth. This limits closure and keeps the anterior teeth apart, which allows uninhibited incisor movement. In most cases, the crossbite will correct quickly and the biteplane can be removed. Extended use of a biteplane is discouraged because the teeth not in contact with the appliance will continue to erupt, creating a vertical occlusal discrepancy.

Fixed appliances also can tip teeth out of crossbite and do not require as much cooperation from the child. A fixed appliance also provides precise control of tooth movement in all three planes of space by using rectangular wires (Fig. 35–31). The disadvantage of either a labial or a lingual fixed appliance is the patient's inability to clean around the teeth and appliance thoroughly, which can result in marginal gingivitis and caries. A maxillary lingual arch is a suitable appliance to correct an anterior crossbite if the teeth require tipping. The maxillary arch is constructed of 36-mil wire and has adjustment loops similar to those used in a lower lingual arch.

Finger springs made of 22-mil wire provide the tooth-moving force. The springs are usually soldered on the opposite side of the arch from the tooth being moved, to increase the length and range of the spring (Fig. 35–32). The springs are activated approximately 3 mm before the appliance is cemented into place. During cementation, the springs are tied with steel ligatures to the lingual arch so that they will not interfere with the seating of the appliance. After the excess cement has been cleaned away, the ligature is cut away to activate the springs. In some cases, the spring slips over the incisal edge of an incisor that is not fully erupted. In these cases, a stainless steel guide wire is soldered to the lingual arch at the midline to prevent the spring from

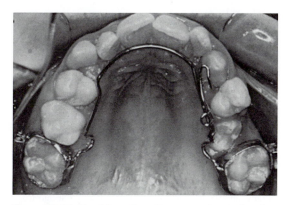

Figure 35–32. Fixed lingual appliances can be used to tip the teeth out of anterior crossbite. This patient required facial movement of the maxillary left canine to correct the crossbite. A small finger spring was soldered to the base lingual arch and was activated to provide the force necessary to move the tooth.

slipping incisally. Three millimeters of activation provide 1 mm of tooth movement per month. The appliance should be removed, reactivated, and recemented at 4- to 6-week intervals until the crossbite is corrected.

In older patients, space may need to be created for crossbite correction by arch expansion because there are no primary teeth to disk or extract. In this situation, the permanent molars should be banded and the incisors bonded with orthodontic brackets.

An anterior crossbite that requires bodily movement of teeth to correct the problem is best treated with bonded brackets and a planned sequence of arch wires. Initially, teeth can be tipped out of crossbite. Usually an arch wire is selected that is strong enough to withstand the force of occlusion in the posterior segments yet flexible enough in the anterior region to engage the brackets of the malaligned teeth. This generally requires a stainless steel arch wire with loops bent mesial and distal to the tooth in crossbite (Fig. 35–33). Loops in the anterior region are designed to provide horizontal or vertical tooth movement and exert optimal force to move the teeth out of crossbite while stabilizing those that are in the correct position. Alternatively, a flexible titanium alloy wire can be used for alignment. This requires no wire bending or loop forming but moves both the teeth in crossbite and those not in crossbite.

After alignment is completed by either method, an arch wire is inserted into the brackets that is capable of delivering a root-positioning

force to the tooth previously in crossbite. The purpose of such a force is to move the root into proper position so that the entire tooth essentially moves forward out of crossbite.

Retention must be planned in all cases, regardless of the appliance selected. Active tooth movement is usually continued until the crossbite is slightly overcorrected. The correction should be retained with a passive fixed or removable appliance for 2 months if there is a positive overbite. If there is not adequate overbite, retention should be continued until adequate overbite develops. Circumferential supracrestal fiberotomy should also be considered if rotational movement was made during treatment. In a small number of cases, the anterior crossbite is caused by excessive spacing and flaring of the mandibular incisors. A removable appliance can be constructed with an adjustable 28-mil labial bow to retract the lower incisors and close the space. The appliance should be activated 2 mm/month, and treatment should be continued until the space is closed and there is positive overbite and overjet. The tooth movement can be retained with the same removable appliance, which is made passive.

INCISOR PROTRUSION

Incisor protrusion in the mixed dentition is a serious esthetic problem for the preadolescent patient. Protrusive incisors not only are unattractive but also are more prone to dental injury than incisors with a normal angulation. For these reasons, treatment is usually undertaken to move the incisors lingually into a more suitable position if the overbite is not prohibitively deep. This treatment is used for a dental problem, not a skeletal problem. Skeletal problems should be referred to a specialist for growth modification.

Treatment of incisor protrusion has already been discussed in the earlier section on treatment of diastemas in the mixed dentition. To summarize, teeth that can be tipped back into ideal alignment should be treated with a removable appliance that incorporates an active labial bow. The bow is activated by means of an adjustment loop to provide a lingual tipping force to the flared incisors. One to two millimeters of palatal acrylic is removed from the appliance to allow the crown to move lingually and to accommodate the palatal tissue that tends to bunch up behind the tooth being moved. The retention schedule should be full-time wear for 3 months.

In some cases, bodily movement of teeth is necessary to correct incisor protrusion. The max-

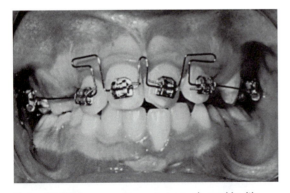

Figure 35–33. In some cases anterior teeth need bodily movement to correct a crossbite. To meet this need, fixed appliances must be placed to position the teeth properly. Initially, an arch wire is selected that is strong enough to withstand the force of occlusion in the posterior segments and flexible enough to engage the brackets of the malaligned teeth. Often it is necessary to place loops in the arch wire to provide enough flexibility to engage the brackets properly. After the teeth have been tipped out of crossbite, a rectangular wire is used to position the roots.

illary first molars should be banded, and brackets should be bonded to the anterior permanent teeth. A small, round, flexible arch wire is placed in the brackets to align the teeth initially. Anterior tooth retraction is accomplished by means of a rectangular arch wire with a closing loop or elastomeric chain. A headgear device or a transpalatal arch is usually used during retraction to supplement anchorage. The choice between cervical, combination, or high-pull headgear is based on the patient's vertical facial dimensions. Cervical headgear is generally used when the patient has normal vertical facial proportions, whereas high-pull headgear is indicated when the patient has increased lower facial height. The clinician should follow the progress of a patient undergoing incisor retraction carefully to prevent problems associated with retraction. A complication encountered during incisor retraction is movement of the root of the permanent lateral incisor into the path of the unerupted permanent canine. The lateral incisor root either impedes eruption of the canine or may be resorbed. The wire should be bent or the bracket placed so that the lateral incisor root is upright or even tipped slightly mesially.

Transverse Dental Problems

Posterior crossbite correction in the mixed dentition can be difficult and confusing. The clinician must rely on a well-documented data base to determine whether skeletal or dental correction is necessary. The presence of a mandibular shift also is an important finding. A posterior crossbite with an associated mandibular shift should be treated as soon as possible to prevent soft tissue and dental compensation. Crossbites can be corrected with a W arch or a quad helix in the primary and early mixed dentitions. Both skeletal and dental movements occur with these appliances, and it is difficult to effect only one or the other. In the late mixed dentition, the midpalatal suture may be more interdigitated, and the clinician can make primarily dental or skeletal changes depending on the appliance selected to treat the case. Skeletal problems should be referred to a specialist, but dental problems can be treated without referral.

Posterior dental crossbites are either generalized or localized. Generalized crossbites of dental origin are usually bilateral and are corrected with a W arch or a quad helix (Fig. 35–34). If the crossbite is due to a unilateral dental constriction, an unequal W arch (made of 36-mil wire) or a quad helix (made of 38-mil wire) can be

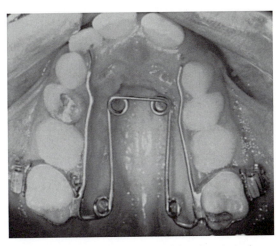

Figure 35–34. Posterior crossbites of dental origin in the mixed dentition can be treated with either a W arch or a quad helix. In this patient, a quad helix is being used to correct a bilateral posterior crossbite.

used to expand the arch. Alternatively, a lower lingual arch can be used to stabilize the lower teeth, and cross elastics can be worn to the maxillary arch to correct the crossbite unilaterally. These appliances have been discussed in previous sections. Localized crossbites are usually due to displacement of single teeth in one or both arches. For example, a maxillary lingual crossbite involving the permanent first molars is usually the result of lingual displacement of the maxillary molar or the facial displacement of the mandibular molar. If only one tooth is causing the problem, a removable appliance with a finger spring can be used (Fig. 35–35). If teeth in opposing arches are at fault, it is easy to correct the problem using a simple crossbite elastic. The offending teeth are fitted with orthodontic bands without attachments. After the bands are fitted, they are removed, and a button is welded to the opposite surface of the band from the direction in which the tooth is to be moved.

In the example just noted, a button is welded to the lingual surface of the maxillary band and to the buccal surface of the mandibular band. After the bands have been welded and cemented, a medium weight (3/16-inch, 6-ounce elastic) is attached from button to button through the occlusion (Fig. 35–36). The elastic should be worn full-time, except when the patient is eating, and should be changed at least once per day. The elastic should be worn until the crossbite is slightly overcorrected. It may be prudent to leave the bands in place and discontinue the use of elastic for 1 month to ensure that the teeth do not relapse into crossbite. When the occlusion is

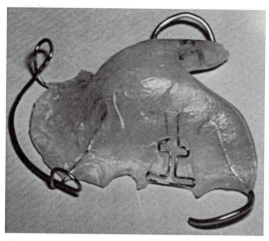

Figure 35–35. Localized posterior crossbites are usually caused by malalignment of a single tooth in one or both arches. This removable appliance is designed to correct a lingually displaced primary second molar with a T spring. The spring tips the displaced tooth facially.

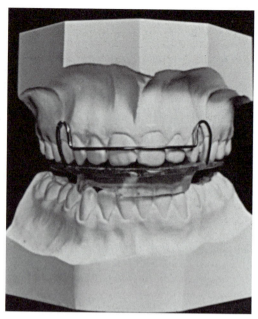

Figure 35–37. In the 6- to 12-year age group, a deep overbite can be treated with a removable appliance designed to inhibit anterior eruption and allow posterior eruption. This appliance is blocking maxillary and mandibular anterior eruption and maxillary posterior eruption. The mandibular posterior teeth are free to erupt, decreasing the overbite. This type of treatment is infrequently prescribed alone for deep overbite.

stable after 4 to 6 weeks without elastic force, the bands can be removed. Buttons are now available that can be bonded directly to the tooth, making bands unnecessary, but there is a risk of bond failure and appliance aspiration.

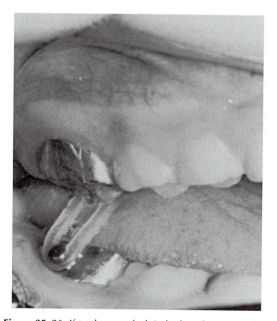

Figure 35–36. If teeth are at fault in both arches, a simple crossbite elastic is used to correct the crossbite. Bands can be placed on both permanent right first molars, and buttons can be welded to the lingual side of the maxillary band and to the facial side of the mandibular band. A medium weight elastic (4- to 6-ounce) is attached from one button to the other to provide the force required to correct the crossbite.

Vertical Dental Problems

Vertical problems in the mixed dentition are primarily open bite or deep bite malocclusions. Dental open bite is most often the result of an active digit habit that has impeded eruption of the anterior teeth. In some cases, the digit habit has been discontinued, but the open bite has been maintained because the tongue rests between the teeth and prevents eruption. Treatment is essentially the same as that described for digit habits in the late primary and early mixed dentitions. If therapy without an appliance is unsuccessful, a palatal crib (see Fig. 26-6) is effective if the patient desires to stop the habit. The crib reminds the child to refrain from the habit and blocks the tongue from being placed forward. Therapy is successful in the majority of cases unless the child is unwilling to abandon the habit. Skeletal open bite treatment has been described, and these patients should be referred to a specialist.

Dental deep bite is caused by over-eruption of the anterior teeth or under-eruption of the posterior teeth. It should be distinguished from skeletal deep bite, which is characterized by a

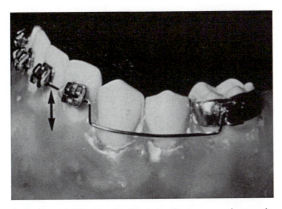

Figure 35–38. Fixed orthodontic appliances are also used to treat deep overbite in the mixed dentition. In this example, the mandibular curve of Spee is reduced by intruding the mandibular incisors. A utility arch wire is bent so that it rests passively in the mandibular or buccal vestibule. The arch wire is activated by lifting the wire up and placing it in the incisor brackets *(arrow)*. This creates a light intrusive force on the anterior teeth and a light extrusive force on the molars.

flat mandibular plane angle and a short vertical dimension as well as by over- and under-erupted teeth. In a normal incisor-to-lip relationship, 2 mm of the maxillary central incisor is exposed when the lip is at rest. If more than 2 mm of incisor is exposed, maxillary anterior over-eruption must be considered. In the mandibular arch, over-eruption is difficult to diagnose; however, the curve of Spee may provide some clue. An excessive curve of Spee (2 mm or more) suggests mandibular incisor over-eruption.

Treatment of deep bite in a growing patient can usually be incorporated into comprehensive orthodontic treatment. Occasionally, treatment in a mixed dentition is aimed at preventing further anterior eruption and encouraging or allowing posterior eruption. In these cases, the incisor teeth are blocked from erupting with a removable appliance. The appliance is constructed so that acrylic touches the upper and lower incisors but allows the posterior teeth to erupt (Fig. 35–37). The appliance must be worn full-time to enable correction to take place and then must be worn as a retainer to maintain the correction until the patient stops growing vertically.

If the deep bite is deemed to be the result of maxillary incisor over-eruption or a combination of maxillary and mandibular over-eruption, fixed orthodontic appliances are placed on the teeth. A utility arch or intrusion arch, a wire that connects the permanent first molars to the incisors, is constructed to exert a light intrusive force on the incisors (Fig. 35–38). Because there is an equal and opposite reaction to every force

placed on the teeth, the molars experience an extrusive force. Specifically, the molar erupts and tips distally and facially. Facial movement of the molars can be counteracted by a transpalatal arch or a lower lingual arch, but neither will prevent the distal tipping. In the maxillary arch, headgear that delivers distal root tip to the molars can offset the extrusive and distal crown tipping forces of utility and intrusion arches. The utility arch is a deceptively simple appliance, but it may create more orthodontic problems than it remedies unless it is used with thought and care. Often overbite reduction is the first phase of comprehensive orthodontic treatment, and consultation with a specialist is appropriate.

REFERENCES

Andreason JO, Ravn JJ: Epidemiology of traumatic dental injuries to primary and permanent teeth in a Danish population sample. Int J Oral Surg *1*:235–239, 1972.

Baumrind S, Korn EL: Patterns of change in mandibular and facial shape associated with the use of forces to retract the maxilla. Am J Orthod *80*:31–47, 1981.

Baumrind S, Korn EL, Isaacson RJ, et al: Quantitative analysis of the orthodontics and orthopedic effects of maxillary traction. Am J Orthod *84*:383, 1983.

Bell R, LeCompte E: The effects of maxillary expansion using a quad helix appliance during the deciduous and mixed detentions. Am J Orthod *79*:152–161, 1981.

Bookstein FL: On the cephalometrics of skeletal change. Am J Orthod *82*:177–198, 1982.

Chertkow S: Tooth mineralization as an indicator of the pubertal growth. Am J Orthod *77*:79–91, 1980.

Fields HW, Proffit WR, Nixon WL, et al: Facial pattern differences in long-faced children and adults. Am J Orthod *85*:217–223, 1984.

Fields HW, Lowe BF, Phillips C, et al: Evaluation of Anteroposterior Skeletal Classification Methods in Children and Adults. AAO Annual Meeting Program, Seattle, WA, 1991.

Haas AJ: The treatment of maxillary deficiency by opening the mid-palatal suture. Angle Orthod *35*:200, 1965.

Hagg U, Pancherz H, and Taranger J: Pubertal growth and orthodontic treatment. *In* Carlson DS, Ribbens KA (eds): Craniofacial Growth During Adolescence, Monograph 20, Craniofacial Growth Series, Center for Human Growth and Development, The University of Michigan, Ann Arbor, MI, 1987.

Hicks E: Slow maxillary expansion: A clinical study of the skeletal versus the dental response to low magnitude force. Am J Orthod *73*:121–141, 1978.

Hotz RP: Guidance of eruption versus serial extraction. Am J Orthod *58*:1–20, 1970.

Keeling SD, Wheeler TT, King GJ, et al: Anteroposterior skeletal and dental changes after early Class II treatment with bionators and headgear. Am J Orthod *113*:40–50, 1998.

Kennedy DB, Turley PK: The clinical management of ectopically erupting first permanent molars. Am J Orthod *92*:336–345, 1987.

Kjellgren B: Serial extraction as a corrective procedure in dental orthopedic therapy. Trans Eur Orthod Soc, pp 134–160, 1947.

Lagerstrom LO, Nielsen IL, Lee R, et al: Dental and skeletal contributions to occlusal correction in patients treated with the high-pull headgear/activator combination. Am J Orthod 97:495–504, 1990.

Little R: The effects of eruption guidance and serial extraction on the developing dentition. Pediatr Dent 9:65–69, 1987.

Little RM, Riedel RA, Artun J: An evaluation of changes in mandibular anterior alignment from 10 to 20 years postretention. Am J Orthod 93:423–428, 1988.

Little RM, Riedel RA, Stein A: Mandibular arch length increase during the mixed dentition: Postretention evaluation of stability and relapse. Am J Orthod 97:393–404, 1990.

McNamara JA, Bookstein FL, Shaughnessy TG: Skeletal and dental changes following functional regulator therapy on Class II patients. Am J Orthod 88:91–110, 1985.

Merwin D, Ngan P, Hagg U, et al: Timing for effective application of anteriorly directed orthopedic force to the maxilla. Am J Orthod 112:292–299, 1997.

Moorrees CFA, Gron AM, Lebret LML, et al: Growth studies of the dentition: A review. Am J Orthod 55:600–616, 1969.

Nevant CT, Buschang PH, Alexander RG, et al: Lip bumper therapy for gaining arch length. Am J Orthod 100:330–336, 1991.

Pileski RCA, Woodside DG, Gavin JA: Relationship of the ulnar sesamoid bone and maximum mandibular growth velocity. Angle Orthod 43:162–170, 1973.

Proffit WR: The need for surgical-orthodontic treatment. In Proffit WR, White RP (eds): Surgical Orthodontic Treatment. St. Louis, Mosby–Year Book, 1991.

Proffit WR, et al: Contemporary Orthodontics, 3rd ed. St. Louis, Mosby–Year Book, 1999.

Remmer HR, Manandras AN, Hunter WS, et al: Cephalometric changes associated with treatment using the activator, the Frankel appliance, and the fixed appliance. Am J Orthod 88:363–372, 1985.

Sakamoto T, Iwase I, Uka A, et al: A roentgenocephalometric study of skeletal changes during and after chin cap treatment. Am J Orthod 85:341–350, 1984.

Sugawara J, Asano T, Endo N, et al: Long-term effects of chincup therapy on skeletal profile in mandibular prognathism. Am J Orthod 98:127–133, 1990.

Thompson, GW, Popovich, F, Anderson DL: Maximum growth changes in mandibular length, stature, and weight. Hum Biol 48:285–293, 1976.

Tulloch JFC, Phillips C, Proffit WR: Benefit of early Class II treatment: Progress report of a two-phase randomized clinical trial. Am J Orthod 113:62–72, 1998.

Turley PK: Orthopedic correction of Class III malocclusion with palatal expansion and custom protraction headgear. J Clin Orthod 22:314–325, 1988.

Summary for Section III

The dentist who follows a child from age 6 to age 12 will have had the opportunity to see many changes in the child. The physical changes will be dramatic, and those that have to do with facial form, occlusion, the advent of the permanent teeth, and the esthetic appearance of these permanent teeth are the professional responsibility of the dentist. He or she must supervise the exfoliation of the 20 primary teeth in the 6-year-old and supervise through the next 6 years the eruption of the 28 permanent teeth that are found in most 12-year-olds. The dentist must provide answers to parents concerned about the appearance of their child, intercept those developing malocclusions that are within his or her treatment talents and, when appropriate, refer those malocclusions that need specialist care.

As in previous age groups, the prevention of both hard and soft tissue diseases is important. The repair of trauma and pulpal therapy and the effective restoration of carious teeth, both primary and permanent, are also important in children 6 to 12 years of age. One thing significantly different during the transitional years is the increase of information about the ultimate occlusion of the child. The dentist is responsible for making sure that in the later stages of the transitional dentition and in the early permanent dentition, the dental and facial appearance of the child has been anticipated, any apparent problems have been diagnosed correctly, and, in problem cases, treatment has been planned and performed according to the most desirable timing and techniques. Another demand of this age group is pulpal and restorative care of the young permanent teeth.

As is true for children between ages 3 and 6, children between the ages of 6 and 12 are generally fun to treat. Obviously, the management modalities and type of conversation one would have with a 6-year-old necessarily are refined and sophisticated over the years because the mental functioning of a 12-year-old is for all practical purposes the same as that of an adult. The only thing his or her mind lacks is the continuing education and experience that school and life will bestow.

The dentist who can deliver the child from age 6 to adolescence with no amount or just a modest amount of hard tissue disease, no remarkable soft tissue diseases, allegiance to prevention and developed home care habits, and harmonious dentofacial relationships has indeed mastered the ultimate obligations in treating this age group.

Adolescence

Adolescence represents an extremely important time in the dental care of the child patient. Certainly, prevention of dental diseases is one of the pivotal concerns of the dentist who cares for adolescents. Adolescence marks a time in which the role of the parent in the child's dental home care needs to be minimized, and the responsibility of the adolescent for managing his or her own oral health program must be emphasized. Some adolescents are able to do this easily and seem to be inherently motivated to practice proper oral hygiene on a day-by-day basis. However, there are certainly exceptions, and some of these exceptions can be extremely stubborn. The dentist must play a role in educating and motivating such patients, for not only is caries a problem but also periodontal disease and its unfortunate implications become increasingly important as the child proceeds to the later years of adolescence.

Another preventive concern is the fact that adolescents, particularly older adolescents who have their own transportation, sources of money, and freedom to choose their own diet, may stray away from the diet that was maintained in their home and adopt a regimen containing many more snacks and a possibility of much more sugar ingestion. This can predict increased dental disease.

Adolescence is also a time very likely to impose on a child stressful life situations and anxieties regarding social circumstances. These, paired with fatigue, a poor diet, and increasing responsibilities at school and in life in general, may create enough stress to bring about the onset of certain stress-related oral diseases, such as necrotizing ulcerative gingivitis.

Another concern of the dentist who treats adolescents is their dentofacial appearance. More so than at any other age, the adolescent wants a dentition that is attractive. Previous irregularities in the dentition or in the color of the teeth that are visible during conversation or smiling may become of deep concern to the child, and demands may be put upon the dentist to make sure that these problems are corrected. However, crown and bridge procedures in the adolescent as well as other restorative techniques may be more difficult than at later ages because of the height of the gingiva on the clinical crown and the relatively large size of the pulpal tissues. Although acid-etch techniques have revolutionized the way that dentists can handle anterior esthetic problems, the crown and bridge are still needed to resolve certain problems. In certain cases, the dentist may need to employ an interim treatment plan until there has been sufficient reduction of the pulpal chamber.

A certain percentage of adolescents are athletically involved, and this, paired with their larger bodies and the greater velocity exerted when they play their sport, predicts that dental trauma for certain sports is very high. A dentist who has athletes among his or her child patient population must be aware of the prevention concerns and needs that this group presents.

Third molar extractions may become needed in late adolescence. The dentist needs to follow the development of these molars and assess their position in the jaw to determine if and when extraction is needed.

Last, adolescence represents a relatively long period of life in our society. The dentist must be well versed in understanding the different characteristics of adolescents as they relate to age. Obviously, the conversation of a dentist with a 13-year-old will be substantially different from that with an 18-year-old. The dentist needs to be acutely aware of these differences and must be versatile in his or her communication style with this age group.

36

The Dynamics of Change

Chapter Outline

Physical Changes

Body

J. R. Pinkham

Adolescence in some societies is a very short transitional period that marks the arrival of a child to full citizenship within his or her respective tribe and culture. In a technologic society such as Europe or North America today, adolescence is a time of enormous transition and is certainly not of short duration. Hence, the term *teenager* has become synonymous with the term *adolescent* in our society. Literature describing the adolescent may portray the adolescent as an old child or a young adult. Certainly, it is an in-between age in our society and needs to be understood as something independent of either childhood or adulthood.

Critical to the definition of adolescence regardless of culture and to the understanding of the adolescent physically is the concept of puberty. Puberty is the landmark in physical development when an individual becomes capable of sexual reproduction. In common law, this has been established historically in our society as age 14 for boys and age 12 for girls. The advent of puberty is paralleled by the development of genital tissue and secondary sexual characteristics, such as the development of hair in the area of the genitals.

It is also a time when there is an increase in the mass of muscles, a redistribution of body fat, and an increase in the rate of skeletal growth. A growth spurt is associated with this time of life. This growth spurt follows two different forms, depending on gender. In females it appears early compared with males. The average onset in males is 2 years later than that in females. The fact that males experience their growth spurt later than females and therefore have a longer maturation period before the growth period is one of the reasons why the height of males generally exceeds the height of females. The earlier growth spurt of females also accounts for the period of time during which mean height of a group of young female adolescents may exceed that of males. It is important to realize also that in females menarche serves as a signal that growth is ending, but for males there is no such marker. The magnitude of the velocity of change during the growth spurt also differs between the sexes. In 1975, Tanner and colleagues concluded that the growth spurt in females peaks at 9 cm change per year at age 12, and that in males it peaks at just over 10 cm at age 14.

REFERENCE

Tanner JM, Whitehouse RH, Marshall WA, et al: Assessment of Skeletal Maturity and Prediction of Adult Height: TW 2 Method. New York, Academic Press, 1975.

Craniofacial Changes

Jerry Walker

During and following adolescence, continued changes in the skeletal growth of the face and skull take place because the facial sutures are still open and viable (Kokich, 1976) and mandibular growth has the potential to continue. These changes not only cause variation and individuality in facial appearance (Enlow, 1990) but affect the dental structures as well. The continued changes make a final and nonchanging dentition and occlusion a difficult concept to imagine, much less attain. There is a slow increase in

facial height accompanied by an increase in prognathism in males (Bjork, 1947; Behrents, 1985).

Profile changes occur as changes in specific locations take place. The brow area becomes larger as a result of pneumatization of the frontal sinuses and apposition on the glabella (Ranly, 1980). Also, appositional changes during adolescence and early adult life in the frontal bone area and brow result in this area becoming more prominent (Behrents, 1985). In adolescence the nose and chin also become more prominent. The tip of the nasal bone lies well ahead of the basal bone of the premaxilla. Soft tissue changes also contribute to the growth in the length of the nose and can affect the harmony existing between the nose, lips, and chin. The mandible shows a greater prognathism than the maxilla because of the circumpubertal growth spurt, which has more effect on the mandible than on the maxilla, especially in males. The chin also becomes more prominent owing to local bone deposition. Lip prominence is reduced by these changes in adjacent structures.

Underlying maxillary changes also occur. The maxillary sinuses, which have since birth expanded laterally and vertically, occupy the space left by the permanent teeth as they erupt. By puberty, the sinuses are usually fully developed, although they may continue to enlarge. There is considerable individual variation in the size of the maxillary sinuses, and they often lack symmetry. Lowering of the palatal vault continues because of remodeling. In 1966 Bjork concluded that sutural growth as well as appositional

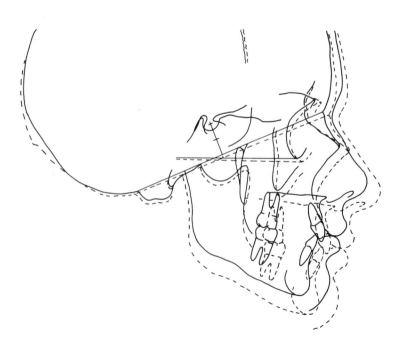

Figure 36–1. This anterior cranial base superimposition of the Bolton Standard 12- and 18-year-olds (*solid line* and *broken line,* respectively) demonstrates the magnitude of anteroposterior and vertical skeletal growth during this period as well as the soft tissue change. (Redrawn from Broadbent BH Sr, Broadbent BH Jr, Golden WH: Bolton Standards of Developmental Growth. St. Louis, CV Mosby, 1975.)

TABLE 36–1. Growth of the Aging Skeleton: Sexual Dimorphism in Craniofacial Growth

	Females	Males
Circumpubertal growth spurt	10–12 years	12–14 years
Mature size	Growth plateaus at 14 with increases to 16 years	Active growth to 18 years
Supraorbital ridges	Absent	Well developed
Frontal sinuses	Small	Large
Nose	Small	Large
Zygomatic prominences	Small	Large
Mandibular symphysis	Rounded	Prominent
Mandibular angle	Rounded	Prominent lipping
Occipital condyles	Small	Large
Mastoid processes	Small	Large
Occipital protuberance	Insignificant	Prominent

From Behrents RG: Growth in the Aging Craniofacial Skeleton. Ann Arbor, MI, Center for Human Growth and Development, University of Michigan, 1985.

growth of the maxilla contributed significantly to the increase in the height of the maxillary body (Fig. 36–1). This can be an example of sexual dimorphism in skeletal growth (Table 36–1). Vertical maxillary facial growth is often greater in females. Because the mandible does not continue to grow as much in females, marked vertical changes in the maxilla can result in downward and backward positioning of the mandible and an increase in facial convexity (Fig. 36–2) (Behrents, 1985).

Mandibular growth contributes more than pro-

file changes. This growth may be sufficient to develop room for the third molars. In many cases, growth is inadequate, and these molars become impacted (Fig. 36–3). The marked mesial inclination of the posterior permanent teeth diminishes somewhat as the mandible completes its growth from under the maxilla and the lower incisors tend to become upright. Often this is accompanied by crowding of the lower incisors (Ranly, 1980).

Late mandibular growth imparts an increase in the vertical height of the mandibular ramus,

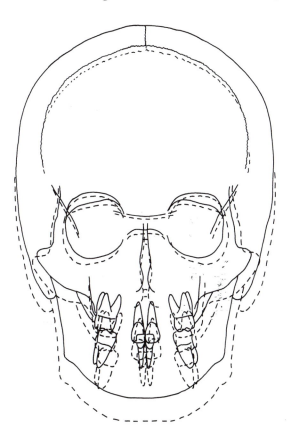

Figure 36–2. This anterior cranial base superimposition of the Bolton Standard 12- and 18-year-olds (*solid line* and *broken line*, respectively) demonstrates the magnitude of transverse and vertical skeletal growth during this period. (Redrawn from Broadbent BH Sr, Broadbent BH Jr, Golden WH: Bolton Standards of Developmental Growth. St. Louis, CV Mosby, 1975.)

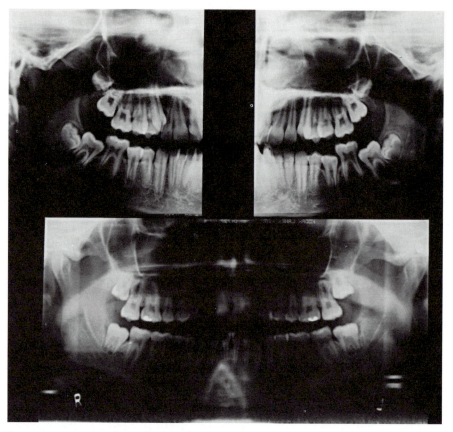

Figure 36–3. These two panoramic radiographs show the changes that occur during adolescence. Some eruptive and mesial drift is expected, combined with distal incisor movement. Third molar eruption often occurs at the end of this age period.

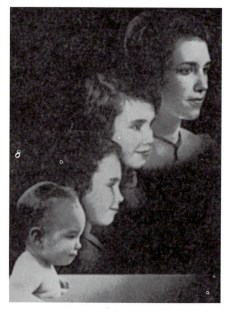

Figure 36–4. Changes in the skull from infancy to the completion of adolescence. (Courtesy of William L. Briedon. From Enlow DH: Handbook of Facial Growth. Philadelphia, WB Saunders, 1990.)

which becomes more upright. The elongation of the ramus accommodates the massive vertical expansion of the nasal region and the lowering of the palate, which is accompanied by dental eruption. Usually the maxillary and mandibular growth are compatible and coordinated (Fig. 36–4). If they are not, significant orthodontic problems can result. Particularly in males, there can be late anterior growth that is undesirable (Behrents, 1985).

REFERENCES

Behrents RG: Growth in the Aging Craniofacial Skeleton. Monograph 17, Craniofacial Growth Series. Ann Arbor, Center for Human Growth and Development, 1985.

Bjork A: The face in profile. Sven Tanalak Tidskr *40*:Suppl 5B, 1947.

Bjork A: Sutural growth of the upper face studied by the implant method. Acta Odontol Scand *24*:109-127, 1966.

Broadbent BH Sr, Broadbent BH Jr, Golden WH: Bolton Standards of Developmental Growth. St. Louis, CV Mosby, 1975.

Enlow DH: Handbook of Facial Growth. Philadelphia, WB Saunders, 1990.

Kokich VG: Age changes in the human frontozygomatic sutures from 20 to 95 years. Am J Orthod *60*:411-430, 1976.
Ranly DM: A Synopsis of Craniofacial Growth. New York, Appleton-Century-Crofts, 1980.

Dental Changes

C. A. Full

All of the permanent teeth generally have erupted by age 12, except possibly the four second molars, which may erupt as late as age 13, and the third molars, which usually erupt between the ages of 17 and 21.

Except for the third molars, the dentist should be concerned about any unerupted permanent tooth after age 13 and should examine the area in question radiographically.

The roots of all teeth are considered to have been completed by age 16 except for those of the third molars, which can achieve completion as late as age 25.

Cognitive Changes

J. R. Pinkham

The adolescent continues his or her cognitive development and by middle to late adolescence is capable of extremely sophisticated intellectual tasks. High ability at abstract thinking allows the adolescent to deal with complex and difficult vocational and educational challenges. Formal operational thinking and the ability to store information in the memory after perceiving it are hallmarks of the maturation of cognitive ability in adolescents.

The new information available to the adolescent, along with more sophisticated ways of analyzing this information, often makes him or her appear to be a rebel, a complainer, or an accuser. Persons of this age often ascertain the possible and become discontented, even angry, with the real. Kiell pointed out in 1967 that Aristotle, more than 2000 years ago, concluded that adolescents "are passionate, irascible, and apt to be carried away by their impulses." It has been noted that the thoughts of adolescents are both *introspective* and *analytical*. They are also *egocentric*. This dwelling upon one's self may make an individual overly self-conscious. Clothes, cars, hair style, tastes in music, and identity with certain people or groups probably reflect the adolescent's involvement in self-consciousness.

In summary, by mid- to late adolescence, most young people are capable of formal operational thinking and can, both in and out of school, master subject material that is extensive, difficult, and abstract. Many have matured into skillful, enthusiastic communicators and conversationalists. Many are also opinionated and perhaps argumentative. These last two characteristics may make for some trying times for parents, teachers, and dentists.

REFERENCE

Kiell N: The Universal Experience of Adolescence. Boston, Beacon, 1967.

Emotional Changes

J. R. Pinkham

The very rapid and dramatic changes that occur in adolescents may be paralleled by many emotional circumstances. The self-confidence and personal identity of the adolescent may be compromised if his or her feelings about body image are negative. In 1984, Mussen and colleagues noted that the following issues create the possibility of misinterpretation and anxiety for this age group:

- Being attractive or unattractive
- Being loved or unloved
- Being strong or weak
- Being masculine or feminine

For females, the onset of menstruation may also present circumstances that can be anxiety-provoking. This is not necessarily true, but the chances of anxiety rise if there is a prevailing negative reaction to the menstrual process by family and peers, if the child is showered with sympathy, or if there is considerable pain before and during menses. Anyone who works with postmenarchal females should be aware that some of them will display irritability or depression at times.

The advent of puberty and the hormones associated with puberty lead to sexual feelings and urges. The timing of this process, its nature and magnitude, and the choice of what to do about these feelings and urges are handled differently from one adolescent to another. Family guidance, the adolescent's own values, the values of peers, and the value system of the person that the adolescent first loves are just a few of the factors that ultimately predict how he or she will deal with these new feelings.

One last emotion is critical to understanding adolescents. This is the emotion of love. Adolescents are capable of great commitment to one another, and some of these relationships can become long-term commitments. Unfortunately, many such relationships do not last, as one partner becomes uninterested. This can lead to genuine depression for the abandoned partner. The term "puppy love" is a terrible misnomer and belies exactly how painful these broken relationships can be.

REFERENCE

Mussen PH, Conger JJ, Kagan J, et al: Child Development and Personality, 6th ed. New York, Harper & Row, 1984.

Social Changes

J. R. Pinkham

Adolescence represents the final transition socially from childhood to adulthood. When it is over, if everything proceeded as it should, the emerging young adult will be able to establish and maintain loving and sexual relationships with a partner, be independent of the parents, be capable of working with peers, and be self-directed. These are formidable social challenges, and some adolescents cannot master them. Delinquency, attempted or successful suicide, alcohol and drug use and abuse, running away from home, teenage prostitution, and dropping out of school are some of the frequently cited instances of adolescent failure to socialize properly.

Peers are important social agents in large technologic societies, in which children of the same age group are often kept together. It can be argued that as relationships and dependencies on parents start to decline, the importance of peers escalates. Increasingly, the adolescent may find that it is difficult to share secrets, thoughts, and fantasies with his or her parents. In these situations, the close friend becomes the adolescent's confidant(e), and the peer is a valuable and useful audience.

Despite the obvious value of peers, there are peer relationships that are not so fortunate for the involved adolescent. For example, to avoid rejection or ridicule from peers an adolescent may try drugs, participate in criminal acts, or defy authority.

Another important social change in the adolescent is an increase in the size and range of acquaintances. Children younger than adolescence tend to limit their friends to those of their neighborhood, school, and perhaps church. Adolescents, on the other hand, may have individual friends, belong to a clique of friends, and can identify with larger groups such as an Explorer troop or a football team. An adolescent's ability to sustain relationships with all three of these groups indicates good social skills and is a sign that the socialization process is going well.

Popularity is an important desire in adolescents. There are few adolescents who are not preoccupied with acceptance by peers. The following qualities in an adolescent seem to correlate with social acceptance by peers:

- Friendly, likes other people
- Energetic and enthusiastic
- Flexible and forgiving
- Laughs, good sense of humor

- Outgoing
- Self-confident but not conceited
- Appears natural
- Tolerant of the shortcomings of others
- Shows leadership qualities
- Others feel good when this person is around

The adolescent who gets along with his or her peer group seems to relate successfully to adults. Those who do not achieve peer acceptance seem to have more difficulty with adults and grow up to have a variety of social and emotional difficulties (Hartup, 1983).

REFERENCE

Hartup WW: The peer system. *In* Mussen PH (ed): Handbook of Child Psychology, 4th ed. Vol. 4. Personality and Social Development (EM Hetherington, ed). New York, John Wiley, 1983.

Epidemiology and Mechanisms of Dental Disease

Steven M. Adair

Adolescents have benefited from the dramatic progress in the reduction of the prevalence of dental caries in this country. Over 15% of 17-year-olds were found to be caries-free in a large-scale survey in 1987–86 (Epidemiology and Oral Disease Prevention Program, 1989). This was a 46% improvement over a 1979–80 survey that found 10.7% free of decay (National Caries Program, 1981). This chapter explores recent data on caries prevalence in teenagers. The reasons for the significant reductions in caries prevalence are discussed in Chapter 29, but this chapter also discusses the major basis for the control of caries in the United States in the latter half of this century—water fluoridation.

EPIDEMIOLOGY OF CARIES IN THE ADOLESCENT YEARS

The most recent, comprehensive data on the caries experience of school children in the United States were compiled by the Epidemiology and Oral Disease Prevention Program of the National Institute of Dental Research (NIDR) in a nationwide study conducted in 1986-87. Over 39,000 children, ages 5 to 17, were examined. Only visual-tactile criteria were used for caries determinations. No radiographs were taken. Thus, the findings are probably conservative compared with what would have been determined had routine office examination criteria been applied. The 48 contiguous states were divided into seven geographic regions. Each region was further subdivided into urban and rural areas.

Figure 36-5 demonstrates the mean number of decayed, missing, and filled permanent tooth surfaces (DMFS) for adolescent children by age and sex. The DMFS for 12-year-olds, who may not have erupted all permanent teeth, was 2.66. For 14-year-olds, who would generally have all permanent teeth erupted with the exception of third molars, the DMFS was 4.68, about 75% higher. At the time of the survey, 17-year-olds demonstrated a mean DMFS of slightly over 8. These increases reflect the effects of time on a somewhat increasing number of permanent tooth surfaces susceptible to decay during adolescence (Table 36-2). As was true in the transi-

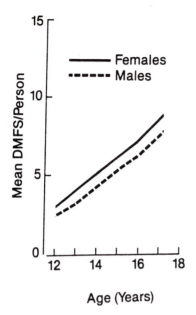

Figure 36–5. Mean decayed, missing, filled tooth surfaces (DMFS) for children aged 12 to 17 in the United States by age and sex. (Redrawn from National Institute of Dental Research, Epidemiology and Oral Disease Prevention Program: Oral Health of United States Children. The National Survey of Dental Caries in U.S. Schoolchildren, 1986–87. NIH Publication No. 89-2247, 1989.)

tional dentition, females had slightly higher DMFS scores than males.

The 1986-87 survey found that the DMFS of whites was somewhat lower than that of nonwhites. This difference was about 17% for children ages 5 to 13. For 12- to 17-year-olds, the difference was maintained, but for 17-year-olds alone it was over 22%. A more telling statistic is the percentage of the DMFS score that is attributable to decay. For whites ages 5 to 17, that figure was 10.6%. For nonwhites, 23.8% of the DMFS was represented by decayed surfaces. Clearly,

nonwhites suffer more dental disease and, as a group, present higher treatment needs than whites do. Adolescents from urban areas demonstrated slightly less dental disease than their counterparts from rural areas. This difference is not as great as might be expected on the basis of water fluoridation alone. The percentage of decayed surfaces for the rural children, 14.8, was slightly higher than that of urban children, 12.7.

On a geographic basis, adolescents from the Southwest had the lowest DMFS scores (Fig. 36-6). This was true for all ages 5 to 17 as well. Adolescents from the Pacific region had the highest DMFS scores. For ages 5 to 17, the highest DMFS scores were found in New England.

COMPARISONS

The magnitude of the caries reductions in the United States can best be appreciated by comparison with previous similar surveys. The most complete surveys for comparison are those conducted by the National Center for Health Statistics (NCHS) in 1966-70 and 1971-74, and by the NIDR in 1979-80, as illustrated in Table 36-3. Data for the NCHS studies were collected on subjects ages 12 to 17 and are compared to NIDR subjects of the same age. The data in Table 36-3 are for decayed, missing, and filled *teeth*, not surfaces, because of the manner in which data were collected in the two earlier NCHS studies. The diagnostic criteria used were practically identical in all studies. As the table demonstrates, the mean DMFT for 12- to 17-year-old children has declined by 46% since 1966-70. The reduction in DMFT was 26% from 1971-74 to 1979-80; an additional 27% reduction occurred between the 1979-80 and the 1986-87 surveys. These differences would be more striking if comparisons of DMFS could be made.

TABLE 36–2. DMFS of U.S. Children Aged 12–17

	DMFS*				
Age	Whites	Nonwhites	Rural	Urban	Total
12	2.48	3.35	2.82	2.60	2.66
13	3.62	4.23	3.88	3.71	3.76
14	4.48	5.31	4.92	4.59	4.68
15	5.53	6.27	6.19	5.54	5.71
16	6.54	7.19	6.81	6.63	6.68
17	7.63	9.63	7.75	8.15	8.04
All ages	5.06	5.93	5.38	5.21	5.26

*Decayed, missing, and filled permanent tooth surfaces only
  Data from National Institute of Dental Research, Epidemiology and Oral Disease Prevention Program: Oral Health of United States Children. The National Survey of Dental Caries in U.S. Schoolchildren, 1986-87. NIH Pub. No. 89-2247. Bethesda, MD, National Institutes of Health, 1989.

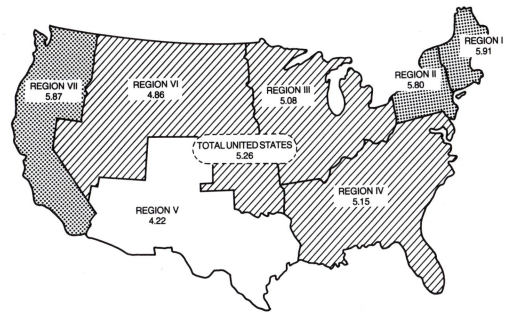

Figure 36–6. Mean decayed, missing, filled tooth surfaces (DMFS) of 12- to 17-year-old children by geographic region, 1986–1987. (Modified from National Institute of Dental Research, Epidemiology and Oral Disease Prevention Program: Oral Health of United States Children. The National Survey of Dental Caries in U.S. Schoolchildren, 1986–87. NIH Publication No. 89-2247, 1989.)

A similar comparison can be made for the percentage of caries-free 12- to 17-year-old children from each survey. As illustrated in Table 36–4, that percentage has increased markedly since the surveys began.

BASIS FOR CARIES REDUCTIONS

The basis for the striking reductions in caries prevalence in children in the United States has been explored in more detail in Chapter 29. There seems to be no change in the disease process itself, and per capita consumption of sugars in this country has not changed appreciably since the 1960s. The best explanation appears to be the more widespread exposure to fluoride in various forms. In addition to optimally fluoridated water supplies, exposure to fluoride has increased through therapeutic products (dentifrices, mouthrinses, and other topical and systemic agents), some of which are ingested by younger children. Residents of fluoride-deficient communities also ingest foods processed in fluoridated communities. This increased fluoride ingestion in fluoride-deficient communities has been called the *halo effect* and has led to lower caries rates and higher enamel fluorosis prevalence than would have been expected from the original studies of artificial fluoridation. The best example of this phenomenon was demonstrated in the 1986–87 NIDR survey. The mean DMFS of 5- to 17-year-old children residing in fluoridated communities was 2.79, compared with 3.39 for

TABLE 36–3. Mean DMFT of 12- to 17-Year-Old Children in Four National Caries Surveys, 1966–1987

NCHS 1966–1970	NCHS 1971–1974	NIDR 1979–1980	NIDR 1986–1987
6.2	6.2	4.6	3.35

NCHS = National Center for Health Statistics; NIDR = National Institute of Dental Health

Modified from Brunelle JA, Carlos JP: J Dent Res *61*(Special Issue):1346-1351, 1982.

TABLE 36–4. Percentage of Caries-Free 12- to 17-Year-Old Children in Four National Caries Surveys

NCHS 1963–1965	NCHS 1971–1974	NIDR 1979–1980	NIDR 1986–1987
10.4	9.7	17.2	29.5

NCHS = National Center for Health Statistics; NIDR = National Institute of Dental Health

Modified from Brunelle JA, Carlos JP: J Dent Res *61*(Special Issue):1346-1351, 1982.

children from fluoride-deficient communities. This is a difference of 17.7%.

WATER FLUORIDATION

No single preventive dentistry measure has had the impact and success in reducing disease than the adjustment of the fluoride concentration in community drinking water supplies. In addition to providing caries reductions in the range of 50% to 70%, water fluoridation is the most cost-effective means of caries prevention. It has been estimated that the annual per capita cost of water fluoridation in the United States is between $0.12 and $5.41, depending on the size of the community, with the annual mean cost being $0.51 (Report of the Workshop on Changing Patterns of Fluoride Intake, 1992).

HISTORY

According to Sognnaes (1979), the first observation of dental mottling was probably that reported by Kuhns in 1888. He described a dark enamel discoloration in a family that had resided in Durango, Mexico. Better known, however, is the 1901 publication by Eager describing the various enamel imperfections in the teeth of Italian emigrants bound for the United States from Naples. He described a wide range of clinical features, from minor imperfections, to "browning" of the teeth, to a lack of enamel accompanied by extreme darkening. Eager speculated that the cause might be volcanic fumes or subterranean fires that contaminated the air or entered the drinking water. The condition was called *denti di Chiaie* after a Professor Stefano Chiaie, who was credited with first describing it. Other terms applied to the various forms of the mottling were *denti neri* (black teeth) and *denti scritti* (teeth written upon). Most importantly, Eager realized that the condition seemed to occur in certain locations and that the incidence among children greatly diminished when the water supply was changed.

That same year, Dr. Frederick S. McKay began practicing in Colorado Springs and noticed staining in the enamel of many of his patients. Further investigation led him to the conclusion that this "Colorado brown stain," as it came to be known, followed a distinct geographic pattern. McKay invited G.V. Black to join in the investigation. The result was a full report of their clinical and histologic findings, published in 1916. The term *mottled enamel* was used to describe an en-

demic condition affecting 87.5% of the population in specific regions. McKay and Black advanced the idea that the causative factor, still undetermined at that time, was present during the development of the enamel, and furthermore, that in children who resided in these locations for specific periods of time, only certain groups of teeth were affected.

Black and McKay described the appearance of affected teeth as ranging from paper-white, to brown, to black, with every conceivable intermediate degree represented. They noted that the general morphology of the teeth was normal. Perhaps their most important observation was that these teeth seemed remarkably resistant to decay.

The histologic analysis of the teeth showed that the abnormal enamel was generally confined to the outer one third, with less involvement of the inner layers and dentin. Both the enamel interprismatic substance and the enamel rods were found to be affected. Some dentin involvement was noted.

Although both Eager and McKay had speculated on the possible causative factors, it was not until 1926 that McKay openly implicated drinking water supplies. He was unsure, however, as to what substances (or the absence of them) might contribute to mottling. It is interesting to note that in 1925, a study was published by McCollum and colleagues in which it was found that rats on high-fluoride diets developed staining in their incisors. This fact was not related to human enamel mottling for years.

In 1930, Kempf and McKay demonstrated that enamel mottling in people living in Bauxite, Arkansas, disappeared only after the town changed its community water supply. There followed several studies in the 1930s conclusively linking water-borne fluoride with both enamel mottling and resistance to decay. The character of the studies of mottling, which now was called *dental fluorosis*, began to change, emphasizing whether a fluoride concentration could be found that would balance the benefits of caries protection with the risk of enamel discoloration.

By employing a system of fluorosis classification, Dean (1934) and others were able to determine that in communities with about 1.0 part per million (ppm) fluoride in the drinking water, fluorosis was not an esthetic problem. Moreover, these communities had a lower caries prevalence than similar communities without fluoride. The relationship between fluoride content of the drinking water, caries prevalence (DMFT), and dental fluorosis is demonstrated in Figure 36–7.

At this point, fluoride research took a logical

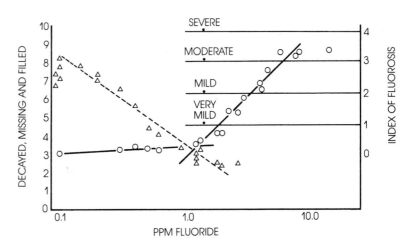

Figure 36–7. Relationship between the fluoride content of the drinking water, caries prevalence, and the index of dental fluorosis. (Redrawn from Hodge HC, Smith FA: Some public health aspects of water fluoridation. *In* Shaw JH [ed]: Fluoridation as a Public Health Measure. Washington, DC, © AAAS, Pub. No. 38, 1954, p. 88. Used by permission of SCIENCE.)

but dramatic turn. The emphasis now was placed on whether fluoride could be added to community water supplies to effect caries reductions. Between 1945 and 1947, large independent clinical studies were undertaken in four pairs of North American cities to test the results of fluoridation. These studies constitute some of the best-designed and -controlled public health trials ever undertaken. In most cases, each city was paired with a neighboring city, similar in almost all respects except for the lack of fluoride in the water supply. Table 36–5 illustrates the results of follow-up examinations of children 12 to 14 years of age conducted about 15 years after fluoridation was begun. Children residing in the trial cities had DMFT scores 50% to 70% lower than their counterparts in the control cities.

Further studies of water consumption led to the recognition that fluid intake is directly proportional to the average maximum daily air temperature of the community. Thus, a range of water fluoride concentrations from 0.7 to 1.2 ppm was developed by the Public Health Service

to reflect the climate of various communities. The water fluoride concentration should vary inversely with the population water consumption.

CURRENT STATUS

Today, over 132 million people in the United States live in areas served by fluoridated water supplies (Report of the Workshop on Changing Patterns of Fluoride Intake, 1992). Thus, over 50% of the U.S. population benefits from drinking water with sufficient fluoride to provide significant caries protection.

COST-EFFECTIVENESS

Although the cost of labor, equipment, and chemicals involved in fluoridation may rise, it is still the most cost-effective caries-preventive measure available. As stated before, the mean

TABLE 36–5. Comparison of Caries Scores and Percent Reduction in 12- to 14-Year-Old Children in Communities With and Without Water Fluoridation

City	Fluoride Status	Year	DMFT per Child	Percent Caries Reduction
Kingston	No F	1960	12.46	
Newburgh	F	1960	3.73	−70.1
Sarnia	No F	1959	7.46	
Brantford	F	1959	3.23	−56.7
Grand Rapids	No F	1945	9.50	
	F	1959	4.26	−55.2
Evanston	No F	1946	9.03	
	F	1959	4.66	−48.4

From Newbrun E (ed): Fluorides and Dental Caries, 3rd ed., 1986. Courtesy of Charles C Thomas, Publisher, Springfield, Illinois.

annual per capita cost of fluoridation is about $0.51. Using a simple formula for determining the cost/benefit ratio (cost of preventive program divided by savings in cost of treatment) and assuming an expected caries reduction of 55% to 65%, water fluoridation has been estimated to have a 1:60 cost/benefit ratio. Another informal calculation indicates that in a 75-year lifespan, the mean total individual cost of fluoridation is roughly equivalent to the cost of a single one-surface dental restoration at 1991 fees (Report of the Workshop on Changing Patterns of Fluoride Intake, 1992). These calculations do not even consider such intangibles as less pain and discomfort from disease or treatment, less time lost from work or school, improved function and appearance, and potential reductions in the prevalence of periodontal disease or certain types of malocclusion. This 1:60 cost/benefit ratio can be contrasted with ratios of 1:18 for fluoride mouthrinsing, 1:3.4 for daily use of supplemental fluoride tablets, and 1:1 for professionally applied topical fluoride (Davies, 1973; Silverstein et al., 1975).

FUTURE OF FLUORIDATION

A generation ago it was optimistically predicted that fluoridation of almost all communal water supplies could be accomplished in as little as 5 years. Obviously, this was not the case. Such predictions were based on unrealistic expectations of the public's and the profession's understanding of the scientific, political, and social issues involved. In the United States, the public referendum has been the most common means of introducing water fluoridation. This has undoubtedly contributed to delays in its implementation because the referendum opens the way for public debate and gives a forum to those opposed to fluoridation on emotional or political grounds. Opponents of fluoridation have used a variety of quasi-scientific and factually deficient arguments with some measure of success when the issue has been open to public debate. Until local boards of health are empowered to make decisions regarding fluoridation, it is likely to continue to be a political issue.

Further fluoridation of public water supplies requires more effort to achieve than in the past. Most water supplies of the major metropolitan areas in the United States have been fluoridated, so there are few large populations remaining that could benefit from fluoridation of large cities. Certainly, these efforts are worth pursuing, and the goal of 75% of the population consuming optimally fluoridated water by the year 2000 may be gaining renewed momentum (Report of the Workshop on Changing Patterns of Fluoride Intake, 1992). There will always remain, however, large segments of the population using private well water supplies, and these supplies cannot be economically fluoridated. One possible solution to this is school water fluoridation, which has been shown to be effective in reducing the caries experience of children in predominantly rural areas not served by a fluoridated community water system.

EFFECT OF DISCONTINUING FLUORIDATION

A disturbing trend toward discontinuing water fluoridation became evident in the 1960s and 1970s. Perhaps the most widely publicized case was that of Antigo, Wisconsin, which discontinued fluoridation in 1960 after 11 years of protection. Fluoridation was resumed in 1965. The caries experience of kindergarten children rose 92% from 1960 to 1964, and by 1966 the mean number of primary teeth decayed or treated for decay (def) increased by 112%. The caries experience of the older children, who had consumed fluoridated water during a period of tooth formation, also began to rise. This is not surprising because it is known today that fluoride exerts a major effect through a frequent, low-dose contact with teeth.

SUMMARY

Caries prevalence among adolescents in the United States has declined dramatically since the 1960s. The initial reductions brought about by water fluoridation have been improved further by the widespread availability of fluoride in other forms—dentifrices, mouthrinses, systemic supplements, and professionally applied topical agents. In addition to this, the halo effect of exposure to foods and beverages processed in fluoridated communities has substantially improved the dental health of persons residing in fluoride-deficient areas. Caries has not yet disappeared, and attempts at further reductions may reach a point of diminishing returns. Nevertheless, the goal of maintaining an individual patient free of caries into young adulthood is certainly achievable for those with access to dental care.

REFERENCES

Black GV, McKay FS: Mottled teeth: An endemic developmental imperfection of the enamel of teeth heretofore unknown in the literature of dentistry. Dent Cosmos *58* (Part I):477-484, (Part II):627-644, (Part III):781-792, (Part IV):894-904, 1916.

Davies GN: Fluoride in the prevention of dental caries. Br Dent J *135*:79-83, 131-134, 233-235, 293-297, 333-335, 1973.

Dean HT: Classification of mottled enamel diagnosis. JADA *21*:1421-1426, 1934.

Eager JM: Denti di chiaie teeth (chaie teeth). US Public Health Rep *16*:2576, 1901.

Epidemiology and Oral Disease Prevention Program, National Institute of Dental Research: Oral health of United States children: The national survey of dental caries in U.S. school children: 1986-87. NIH publication No. 89-2247, 1989.

Kempf GA, McKay FS: Mottled enamel in a segregated population. Public Health Rep *45*:2923-2940, 1930.

McCollum EV, Simmonds N, Becker JE, Bunting RW: The effect of additions of fluoride to the diet of the rat on the quality of the teeth. J Biol Chem *63*:553-562, 1925.

McKay FS: Water supplies charged with disfiguring teeth. Water Works J *79*:72-772, 79-80, 1926.

National Caries Program, NIDR: The prevalence of dental caries in United States Schoolchildren, 1979-80. NIH publication No. 82-2245, 1981.

National Center for Health Statistics: Decayed, missing and filled teeth among youths 12-17 years: United States: Vital and Health Statistics, Series 11, No. 144, DHHS Pub No. (HRA) 75-1626. Washington, D.C., US Government Printing Office, 1974.

National Center for Health Statistics: Decayed, missing and filled teeth among persons 1-74 years: United States: Vital and Health Statistics, Series 11, No. 223, DHHS Pub No. (PHS) 81-1673. Washington, D.C., US Government Printing Office, 1981.

Report of the Workshop on Changing Patterns of Fluoride Intake: Workshop Report—Group I. Bawden JW, Conference Editor. J Dent Res *71*:1218-1220, 1992.

Silverstein SJ, Wycoff SJ, Newbrun E: Sociological, economical and legal aspects of fluoridation. *In* Newbrun E (ed): Fluorides and Dental Caries, 2nd ed. Springfield, IL, Charles C Thomas, 1975.

Sognnaes RF: Historical perspectives. *In* Johansen E, Taves D, Olsen TO (eds): Continuing Evaluation of the Use of Fluorides. Boulder, CO, Westview Press, 1979.

37

Examination, Diagnosis, and Treatment Planning for General and Orthodontic Problems

Paul S. Casamassimo, John R. Christensen, and Henry W. Fields, Jr.

Chapter Outline

The classic portrayal of adolescence as a time of rising hormones, rebelliousness, and fads contrasts vividly with the way dentistry has viewed adolescent oral health. Dentistry for children ends abruptly with eruption of the permanent premolars and canines. Adult dentistry begins at the earliest with consideration of what to do with the third molars. For many dental professionals, the intervention that comes first to mind for the adolescent is orthodontic care, which is often begun during the preadolescent transitional period.

Entirely opposite to the prevailing beliefs about the quiescence of the teenage years is the reality of a rapidly changing patient challenging his or her environment head-on and learning to cope in the process. The implications of these changes for dentistry (Casamassimo, 1991) are summarized as follows:

1. *Rapid, unpredictable, and irregular skeletal and dental growth.* The adolescent growth spurt is associated with accompanying facial growth of up to 35% of total height of the face. More than a dozen teeth, primary and permanent, erupt and exfoliate between the ages of 10 and 13 years. Immunologic changes, hormonal shifts, and other subtle and not so subtle physical developments alter the oral cavity.

2. *The environmental challenges, with their obstacles and pitfalls.* Few adults would choose to return to adolescence. Drugs, smoking, sexually transmitted diseases, peer pressure, acne,

more competitive education, career decisions, alcohol, and family pressure make up some of the challenges facing today's adolescent. Perhaps the most poignant statement on this aspect of the teenage years is that accidental death is the leading cause of mortality. Dental professionals see trauma, oral manifestations of sexual activity, hormonal gingivitis, smokeless tobacco–induced hyperkeratosis, noncompliance with dental recommendations, and drug-related behaviors, to mention a few examples.

3. *The need to learn to cope, make decisions, and become independent.* It isn't surprising that primitive cultures associated emerging adulthood with rituals and great significance. Adolescence has always been a time to make decisions, seek independence from families, deal with sexuality, and choose a career. The dentist often sees this turmoil in poor compliance with oral hygiene or refusal to accept treatment. The missed appointment is just one of many ways to say, "I am too involved in my search for self, my changing values, and handling my environment to worry about my teeth."

THE PATIENT HISTORY

The health history of the adolescent is constantly changing and must be kept current. An adult history format captures both of these elements. More important, perhaps, from the standpoint of accuracy is the process of obtaining information from the teenager. The following are some of the topics that need consideration when the history is taken from the adolescent patient.

The health history should address the issues of smoking, recreational drugs and alcohol, birth control, pregnancy, and sexually transmitted diseases. The controversy over inclusion of these issues is easily quieted by the simple realities of adolescent life in the United States. Consider the facts:

- Every day, approximately 3000 teenagers start smoking.
- Out-of-wedlock births have increased by 50% in recent years.
- Radiation and medications used in dentistry can be dangerous to a fetus.
- The majority of adolescents now try drugs or alcohol before leaving high school. Untoward interactions between prescribed and illicit medications can be fatal.
- Sexually transmitted diseases are epidemic in the adolescent age group. Dentists have con-

tracted a variety of infectious diseases from these patients.

Inadequate surveying of these elements of the health history puts both dentist and patient at risk. These issues can be addressed forthrightly by including them as choices interspersed with others on a health history form. Another less threatening approach is to word these questions in the past tense or to associate a risk with them to alert the patient to their importance.

The history-taking process should allow privacy and encourage disclosure. Taking an accurate history may mean allowing the adolescent to assume greater participation in the process. The desired yield on the adolescent history from this perspective is information that might not be available from or known to a parent, such as those items described previously. The dentist may be caught in a double bind by providing an environment that fosters disclosure if pregnancy or illicit drug use is uncovered and the parents are unaware of it. This is a risk that requires counseling and resolution prior to dental treatment, and the dentist's responsibility is to help direct the family to address the issue. Unfortunately, the adolescent may see this as betrayal or breach of confidence, and the relationship between the dentist and patient may be jeopardized. No easy way exists to deal with this type of problem, but the dentist who treats adolescents should be aware of the responsibilities of the situation. It also may mean delaying treatment until the problem is resolved.

The dentist can do some things that both facilitate an accurate history and deal consistently with identified problems of a serious nature:

- Encourage parents to complete histories with adolescents, not for them.
- Allow the adolescent the opportunity to contribute to the history alone, which can be done in the context of a final check prior to treatment at chairside.
- Never treat an adolescent without a consenting parent available.
- Explain suspicions or concerns to both parent and adolescent.
- Establish a policy on deferring treatment and dealing with identified problems of a serious nature that is medicolegally consistent and sound.
- Have resources available in case consultation with a specialist is needed. It is far better to have an established professional relationship than to seek help from a stranger.

Oral Dangers of Smokeless Tobacco

Georgia K. Johnson

Christopher A. Squier

[Revisions arranged by J.R. Pinkham at UIowa]

The Problem

The recent decades have seen marked changes in patterns of tobacco use in the United States. Although the number of cigarette smokers has remained unchanged, there has been an increase in smokeless tobacco users, largely due to increased consumption of moist snuff by adolescents and children. Smokeless tobacco use usually begins during adolescence, but in certain parts of the country regular use may start among preschoolers. Use is more common among males than females, with an average of 20% of U.S. high school males reporting smokeless tobacco use in the past month (Morbidity and Mortality Weekly Report, 1995).

Acquisition of the Habit

Peer pressure probably plays an important role in smokeless tobacco use among adolescents. Other teens reportedly begin using smokeless tobacco because their fathers and grandfathers have done so. To some adolescents the use of these products by sports figures has made this a socially acceptable habit that projects a "machismo" image. Although smoking is usually banned by high school athletic programs, there are often no restrictions on smokeless tobacco use. This perpetuates the misconception that smokeless tobacco is a safe and acceptable alternative to cigarette smoking. These considerations, coupled with the fact that snuff use does not restrict athletes' activities and can be used fairly discretely, make it a convenient form of tobacco use. The plasma nicotine levels attained by smokeless tobacco users are similar to those of smokers, and as a result, users often become addicted to nicotine. In our experience, this addiction is even stronger than that of smokers, which is probably because there is a constant plasma nicotine level, unlike the variable levels associated with cigarette smoking.

Health Concerns

Frequent users of smokeless tobacco have an increased risk of developing localized gingival recession, white lesions (leukoplakia), and oral cancer. Although long-term exposure is usually necessary to produce malignancy, white lesions and, to a lesser degree, gingival recession are common in teenage users. Current data are insufficient to support a statistically significant association between smokeless tobacco use and prevalence of gingivitis, periodontitis, or dental caries (DHHS, 1986).

Public Health Implications and Prevention

The popularity of smokeless tobacco among adolescent males raises serious long-term public health concerns. Early initiation of the habit, the markedly addictive nature of smokeless tobacco, and the strong link between prolonged use and an increased relative risk of oral cancer set the stage for what could be a greatly increased prevalence of malignant oral disease in the future. Because it is so difficult to break this habit, public health efforts have been largely directed toward prevention. Federal legislation has been enacted banning radio and television advertising of smokeless tobacco products, and warning labels are required on smokeless tobacco products. Another preventive measure has been the inclusion of smokeless tobacco units in school-based health education programs. In comparison with the number of smoking cessation programs, there are relatively few smokeless tobacco cessation programs, and the success rates of such programs have been lower than those for smoking.

Role of the Dentist

In many cases, the only manifestations of smokeless tobacco use are oral changes, and therefore, dentists in general and pediatric dentists in particular can play an important role in early detection of use and in patient education. Questions should be included in the health history about the use of all forms of tobacco. The presence of soft tissue changes, including gingival recession and leukoplakia, should be documented and monitored. Any ulcerative or exophytic mucosal lesions at the site of tobacco placement should be referred to a specialist for evaluation and possible biopsy. Patients with oral lesions should be advised to discontinue the habit and referred to a tobacco cessation program if one is available. Once use is discontinued, leukoplakic lesions usually disappear within a week or two. If lesions persist as long as a month after discontinuation of the tobacco habit, a biopsy should be performed. Smokeless tobacco–induced gingival recession is best treated with soft tissue grafting once the cause has been eliminated. If attempts at cessation fail, the patient should be encouraged to place the tobacco at a different oral site while the lesion is monitored.

REFERENCES

Department of Health and Human Services (DHHS): The Health Consequences of Using Smokeless Tobacco. A Report of the Advisory Committee to the Surgeon General. DHHS (NIH) Pub. No. 86-2874. Bethesda, MD, National Cancer Institute, 1986.
Department of Health and Human Services (DHHS): Youth risk behavior surveillance—United States, 1993 Morbidity and Mortality Weekly Report *44*:No. SS-1, 1995.
Acknowledgments: This work was supported in part by PHS Grants R01 DE07930 and R29 DE10153-01.

THE EXAMINATION

The techniques of clinical examination remain the same for the adolescent, but closer attention is paid to identification of problems specific to this group, such as occlusal disharmonies, periodontal conditions, and temporomandibular joint disorders. Table 37–1 lists some of the clinical findings peculiar to adolescent patients.

Behavioral Assessment

The access to dental care available to most healthy Americans has made it unlikely that a teenager will present for a first visit at that period in life, although first visits during adolescence are possible. Most people have made at least one visit to a dentist before they reach adolescence. Personality changes and other behavioral aberrations can suggest problems for the adolescent. Extremes in behavior, such as depression or overt flirting, may indicate sexual abuse in the adolescent female, especially if the child demonstrates a reluctance to allow oral examination. Depression, manifested by severe introversion, can also be a sign of suicidal tendency, family dysfunction, or even drug use. It is not the dentist's responsibility to diagnose or manage these kinds of problems, but the dentist should be aware of the impact of the problem on the child and comment to parents about noticeable changes in behavior. Few behavioral problems should be encountered that will preclude delivery of care, yet exceptions do occur. The follow-

TABLE 37–1. Possible Clinical Findings in Examination of the Adolescent

Structure	Finding	Comment
Extraoral Evaluation		
Skin	Acne	May be painful locally
		Adolescent may take antibiotics
		Can show up as radiopacity on some radiographs if calcification occurs
	Cosmetic use	Can complicate evaluation of skin
		Can cause local allergic response
Neck	Hematoma	From suction; indicates sexual activity
Ears	Healing or scarred punctures	Multiple ear piercing common in both sexes
Hair	Coloring and preparation	Can complicate examination of scalp
Intraoral Examination		
Mucosa	Generalized erythema	Effect of smoking
		Sexually transmitted disease
Buccal mucosa	Erythema, hyperkeratosis	Use of smokeless tobacco
Tongue	Coating, odor	Smoking; poor hygiene; fungal overgrowth from medication
Breath	Acetone; alcohol	Excessive dieting; alcohol abuse; metabolic disorders (e.g., diabetes)
Gingiva	Inflammation	Hormonal change
	Pregnancy tumor	Use of oral contraceptives
		Pregnancy
Teeth	Erosion	Bulimia
	Wear facets	Temporomandibular joint disorders/bruxism
	Excessive stain	Tobacco use
	Discoloration	Existing pulpal pathosis from trauma

ing are situations that may require behavioral management:

1. *Sexual abuse.* The young adolescent female or male who has been sexually abused with oral penetration may be reluctant to accept dental care from a dentist of the same sex as the perpetrator. Aids in uncovering this situation are a good history of previous compliance, behavioral cues such as depression, and overt refusal of care when oral contact is made. Nonetheless, confirmation is difficult because the abuse may be unknown to the parents. It may be the limit of the dentist's role to recommend counseling for such a child in the hope that intervention may uncover the cause.

2. *Rampant caries.* Clinicians have noted that rampant caries, a condition of rapid onset and progression of decay in an adolescent (more often a female), is often associated with personality problems (Fig. 37-1). The typical pattern is a shy, reluctant, introverted person who is passive about treatment. The behavioral manifestations can be varied, with the girl crying silently or not saying a word during the appointment. In some

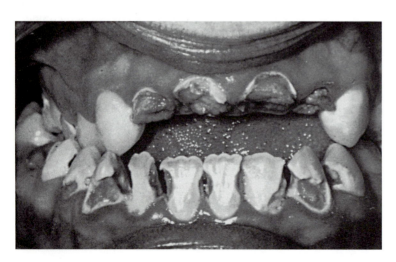

Figure 37–1. This 14-year-old girl has rampant caries, which is a distinct clinical entity with rapidly progressing decay, multiple pulpally involved teeth, and short onset. Patients may give a history of minimal caries prior to development of overt signs of decay.

cases, appointments can degenerate as the child whimpers and finally loses her composure. Time and engagement in conversation are often the most successful behavioral management keys in dealing with these adolescents. Dramatic changes in behavior can occur with the dentist's verbal reinforcement of improved hygiene and provision of even temporary esthetic anterior restorations that allow the patient to smile and experience a more positive self-image.

3. *Extreme anxiety.* Pinkham and Schroeder (1975) described the behavioral management of the child who shows extreme anxiety at the prospect of dental treatment. Desensitization by psychological intervention may hold the key to development of acceptable clinical behavior in such children. Tools available to the dentist are the use of noninvasive therapies at first, reinforcement of positive accomplishments, positive peer interaction, and involvement with a psychologist. The poorly managed or unmanaged adolescent phobic may become the adult dental phobic.

4. *Anorexia nervosa.* Treatment of the child with an eating disorder can be difficult. Experience indicates that these patients, mostly females, tend to develop dependency on a male authority figure. They also require a dentist's full attention during office visits and, unless counseled, may demand time outside scheduled appointments.

5. *Illicit drug use.* Clinicians have noted bizarre behavior on the part of adolescents and young adults who present for treatment after taking unprescribed medications. A number of untoward reactions to dentist-administered medications have been associated with prior ingestion of drugs or alcohol by a young patient. Manifestations of drug ingestion may vary from a slight mental dissociation or drifting to outright verbal aberrations or extreme changes in personality.

Management of behavioral problems in the adolescent can be complex and often involves parents and other professionals. On the other hand, a number of adolescents show age-appropriate behavior that may be disruptive to delivery of care. Most practitioners treating adolescents try to treat these patients alone rather than in a setting in which other peers are present. This one-on-one relationship provides the necessary attention to the patient and prevents disruptive interactions. Any dentist who has worked with a group of seventh- or eighth-grade students will appreciate this recommendation. The teenager who is acting up but simply expressing healthy emotions should respond to reason and provide compliance.

An important part of behavior management in this age group involves the simple transfer of information. A good communicator is aware of the characteristics of adolescence, which enhances his or her ability to relate to teenagers. These characteristics are as follows:

1. *Peers are important.* The adolescent's relationship to those outside the nuclear and extended family becomes important. Friends, classmates, teammates, and popular persons of similar age are all involved in the life of the teenager. A dentist can enhance his or her ability to communicate with adolescents by asking about peer interaction and by knowing who is involved in the teen's life.

2. *Fads and experimentation are part of adolescence.* Successful adolescent practitioners are those who are aware of the trends, popular fads, and celebrities that are of interest to teens. A clear demonstration of this to teens is the presence of posters or contemporary music in the operatory. The dentist who knows the trends and interests of the adolescent has an edge in establishing communication and in reaching the teen at a level that is nonauthoritarian. These are an entree into the teen's world that can be fostered and can lead to discussion of more significant issues with a sense of relationship. Contrast that access to the barrier that arises when both teen and dentist see themselves as worlds apart.

3. *Teens are trying to establish independence, searching for identity, making educational or career choices, and experimenting with sexuality.* All of these involve a certain degree of stress. Within that stressful period are times of anxiety, satisfaction, anger, excitement, and a host of other emotions. The dentist is a small part of the adolescent's world but is a mirror of it. How the practitioner fosters the healthy development of personality in a child and counsels him or her toward independence and career may be important in terms of both the teen's life and his or her dental health. In talking with teens, it is helpful to remember their "problem list" and to empathize with the stress of their lives, which is real to them. The office visit should be a mirror of life. It should provide a respite from pressures and be a cameo of the role that the adolescent plays as an adult patient. The relationship that the dentist would like to have with the adolescent as an adult should be fostered.

4. *The basis of success in adolescent-adult interactions is a good relationship.* The most significant factor in successful compliance and communication is the quality of the relationship between the dentist and the adolescent. In earlier periods of life, the child could be successfully

motivated with reason, praise, or other approaches. The changing values and their short-term intensity in adolescence belie the use of these approaches in fostering long-term motivation. A feeling of trust, good communication, and a perception by the teenager of the dentist's sincere interest provide a strong motivation for compliance.

General Appraisal

The general appraisal of the adolescent is confounded by the timing of physical growth changes, especially in the early teenage years. Within a group of young teenagers, girls can tower over boys and look far more like adults than their male peers. Similarly, within a group of boys, variations in voice tone, skin condition, amount and distribution of fat, and skeletal proportion are often remarkable. Differentiation of growth disorders is difficult at best.

DETERMINATION OF DEVELOPMENTAL STATUS

Patients in early adolescence are clearly growing, but in the later stages growth slows dramatically and at some point nearly ceases. Extremely slow growth proceeds after that into early adulthood. The same is true for facial growth. When patients are clearly growing, growth modification can be attempted. The question does arise in late adolescence regarding whether growth is continuing. At that point, growth modification should not be attempted and camouflage or surgical intervention should be considered.

This judgment on treatment method would be much easier if a biologic marker could be identified that provided definitive information about the developmental status of the patient. Growth modification could be started if the marker indicated that sufficient growth remained to alter skeletal relationships. To be clinically useful, this biologic marker would need to be reliable, easily identified, recognized in both sexes, and closely correlated with the growth of the facial bones. Unfortunately, a single biologic marker of this description is not available. A number of clinical markers have been identified. Studies have indicated, however, that the relationship between the markers and facial growth, although statistically significant, is not so precise that growth can be predicted accurately. Because of the limited predictive value of the markers, one marker or another may be used to determine whether there is remaining growth, but it is extremely difficult

to determine the extent of any remaining growth.

Height and weight measurements are often used to determine the patient's growth status. Measurements are plotted on standardized growth charts, which indicate the relative size of the patient. An average-size child is located near the 50th percentile, and a large child is somewhere near the 90th percentile. A single measurement does not provide the clinician with all pertinent growth information, but it does give some idea about where the patient is developmentally compared with other children at this age.

A series of measurements, which may be available from the patient's physician or school nurse, provides much more information. The measurements can be plotted in one of two ways. The first way is to plot the measurements on a cumulative growth chart (Fig. 37-2). This provides information about the patient's total amount of growth up to the last measurement. The normal growth curve is sigmoidal, and the pubertal growth spurt corresponds to the steepest portion of the slope. Because growth charts are based on mean growth rates, the individual patient may show an accelerated or delayed growth spurt if the individual's growth rate is not coincident with the mean growth rate. More important, some concern should be expressed if the patient is not following the percentiles—for example, dropping from the 50th to the 40th to the 30th percentile over time. This suggests there may be a physical or psychological problem requiring medical attention.

Height and weight measurements can also be plotted as yearly growth increments rather than as total growth achieved up to that point (Fig. 37-3). By plotting measurements this way, changes in the growth rate can be easily identified. A sharp rise in height usually signals the start of the pubertal growth spurt, and growth modification treatment should be initiated immediately if it is required.

Height and weight measurements also can be compared with the height and weight of the patient's natural parents and siblings. Although the interaction between environment and heredity is not clearly understood, there is some familial influence on ultimate size, and it may be possible to glean useful information from the comparison.

Hand-wrist radiographs are used by some investigators to judge the skeletal age and development of the patient (Fig. 37-4). The size and maturational stage of certain hand and wrist bones are compared with published standards

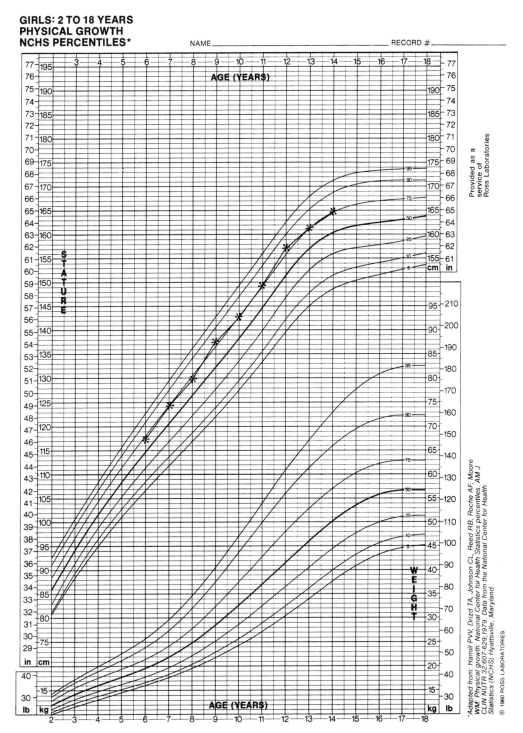

Figure 37–2. A standardized growth chart is used to indicate the relative size of the patient. A single measurement does not provide the clinician with all pertinent growth information, but it does give some idea of the developmental level of the patient compared with other children at a particular time. A series of measurements plotted on a standardized growth chart provides much more information than a single measurement. The measurements may be plotted in two ways. In the cumulative growth chart method, illustrated here, asterisks plot the measurements. This chart shows the patient's total amount of growth up to the last measurement. This female patient has been measured yearly, starting at age 6, and is roughly following the 75th percentile line. (Adapted from Hamill PVV, Drizd TA, Johnson CL, et al: Physical growth: National Center for Health Statistics percentiles. Am J Clin Nutr *32*:607–629, 1979. Data from the National Center for Health Statistics [NCHS], Hyattsville, MD. Courtesy of Ross Laboratories.)

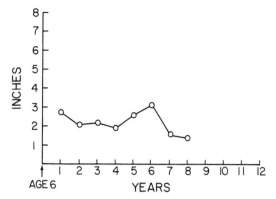

Figure 37–3. Growth information also can be plotted as yearly growth increments rather than as total growth achieved to a certain point. The growth data for the female patient described in Figure 37–2 are plotted here incrementally, beginning at age 6. By plotting measurements this way, changes in the growth rate can be easily identified. A sharp rise usually signals the start of the pubertal growth spurt, and growth modification should be initiated immediately if it is required.

of normal bone development and skeletal age (Greulich and Pyle, 1959). Unfortunately, the correlation between the appearance of reliable bone markers (skeletal growth status) and mean maximum mandibular growth velocity is not perfect and should not serve as the only index of facial growth. The ability to reliably read hand-wrist radiographs requires consistent practice. These radiographs should be used when growth is clearly a significant question. A hand-wrist radiograph for an 8-year-old invariably indicates future growth potential. But these radiographs are appropriate to determine the potential for remaining growth when skeletal problems remain to be corrected or are becoming a significant problem.

Secondary sexual characteristics provide some information about the amount of growth the patient has yet to experience. In females, breast stage development and menarche are markers that can be used to assess developmental status. Breast development determination is obviously not practical in the dental office and is of little clinical use. Menarche, however, can be determined from the health history questionnaire or from an interview at the initial patient examination. Unfortunately, the pubertal growth spurt precedes menarche by more than 1 year (Tanner, 1978). Therefore, menarche is basically used to decide whether growth modification is still feasible.

In the male, there is no single indicator such as menarche by which to judge developmental status. The amount and texture of facial hair and

the patient's general physical appearance are two highly variable indicators of male developmental status and maturity. Facial hair usually appears near or following peak statural growth.

For a person with an obvious skeletal problem, more than one cephalometric head film of the patient may be available. These head films can be superimposed on each other to provide information about the amount and direction of growth that has occurred over time (Fig. 37–5). Although past growth tendencies do not guarantee that the patient will continue to grow or will grow in the same pattern, comparing head films provides a great deal of information about the patient. It is unlikely, however, for the average patient to have a series of head films available for pretreatment review.

The patient's developmental status can also be judged from the developmental stage of the dentition. Panoramic or periapical radiographs can be used to determine the stage of development of individual permanent teeth. The results can then be compared with standards relating dental development to chronologic age (Moorrees et al., 1963). Studies, however, indicate that the relationship between dental age and skeletal

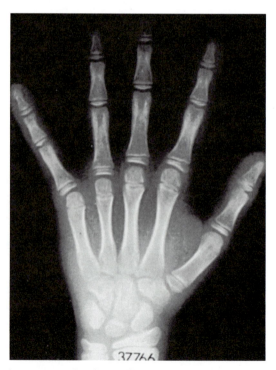

Figure 37–4. A hand-wrist film is used occasionally to judge the skeletal age and skeletal development of a patient. The size and stage of certain bones are compared with published standards for known normal bone development and skeletal age.

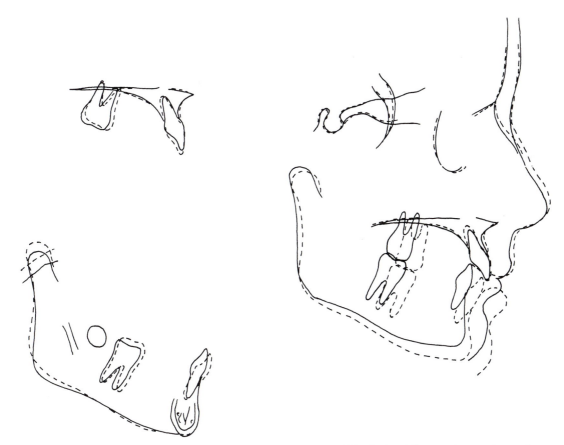

Figure 37–5. If more than one cephalometric head film of a patient is available, the head films can be superimposed on each other to provide information about the amount and direction of growth that have occurred over time. Although past growth tendencies do not guarantee that growth will continue in the same amount or in the same pattern, superimposed films provide substantial information about facial growth.

maturation is weak and clinically useless (Chertkow, 1980).

In summary, a number of biologic markers are available by which the clinician can assess the developmental status of the patient. Unfortunately, no one marker by itself provides definitive information about the patient's growth potential. The most logical approach is to gather all available information and make an educated guess about the patient's growth potential and suitability for growth modification.

Head and Neck Examination

The principles of the head and neck examination of the teenager are similar to those applied to the adult or child. Variations from normal can be caused by a variety of factors, the most notable of which are growth and developmental changes and the effects of the adolescent's environment.

The physical changes and habits in the teen

require modification of the procedures used in children. On the positive side, the loss or redistribution of body fat and the elongation of the neck allow one to perform a better lymph node evaluation. These changes facilitate a thorough head and neck and cancer examination.

Facial Examination

In the facial examination the dentist analyzes the soft tissue profile and the frontal face. During adolescence the face is beginning to assume adult-like features, and treatment decisions can be based more on current rather than on projected facial appearance. This does not mean that growth is complete, only that it has slowed considerably from its previous pace during the early adolescent growth spurt. The adult profile tends to be straighter than the adolescent's because of continued mandibular skeletal growth. In addition, the soft tissue of the chin increases slightly in thickness. The nose also continues to grow, both horizontally and vertically. Most of this growth is horizontal, but the nasal tip tends to drop down a small amount. The lips are less protrusive in the adult because of these nasal and chin changes combined with a slight thinning of the soft tissue thickness of the lips.

For patients with Class I skeletal and dental characteristics, the facial profile examination should provide an adequate basis for analysis when minor orthodontic treatment is considered. For the patient with a skeletal problem, a cephalometric radiograph and analysis are required to diagnose the problem definitively and prescribe treatment. When physical growth is occurring, facial growth usually is also occurring.

Treatment of skeletal orthodontic problems during preadolescence or early adolescence, when the adolescent growth spurt is still active, can result in growth modification. The preadolescent patient is assumed to be growing and is expected to experience a pubertal growth spurt. The early adolescent, especially the male, still has enough growth remaining to allow significant skeletal changes to occur with treatment. The adolescent, by definition, has experienced the pubertal growth spurt and is on the down side of the growth rate curve. Adults, on the other hand, have such limited facial growth that it is of little therapeutic potential.

These differences in growth potential have a large impact on how skeletal malocclusion is treated in the adolescent. The point is that as the individual becomes more skeletally mature, less skeletal growth modification can be accomplished. Therefore, as noted earlier, it is essential to establish the growth or developmental status of the patient in order to plan sensible treatment.

INTRAORAL EXAMINATION

The larger oral cavity of the adolescent permits good visualization. Also, normal intellectual status and reasonable behavior provide cooperation in functional assessment of the occlusion and the temporomanibular joint. On the negative side, there are more teeth to evaluate, gingival and periodontal issues are present that were not critical in early childhood, and unpredictable growth changes can occur. The clinician should approach the adolescent as an adult, especially in the later teen years. For the first visit, the dentist may choose to "walk" the adolescent through the examination, using a hand mirror to explain procedures and normal findings.

PERIODONTAL EVALUATION

In the adolescent more emphasis is placed on the periodontal examination. The prevalence of periodontal disease begins to increase in this age group (Poulsen, 1981). The reason for this increase in periodontal disease is unknown at this time. Therefore, a thorough evaluation of the supporting structures is an absolute necessity. A periodontal probe is used to measure pocket depths, the width of keratinized gingiva, and the amount of attached gingiva, and to establish a bleeding index (Fig. 37-6). Periodontal probing should be confined to fully erupted teeth. Mobility tests may reveal slightly increased mobility in erupted teeth without complete root formation. The use of disclosing agents to reveal plaque, although helpful, may be discontinued at the patient's request. If a panoramic radiograph is used for diagnosis, selected periapical films may be needed if the clinical examination detects any unusual periodontal findings. Referral to a specialist is suggested if significant periodontal disease is evident. During orthodontic treatment, gingival, plaque, and bleeding indices should be established at regular intervals to detect newly active periodontal disease.

RELATED HARD AND SOFT TISSUE PROBLEMS

A number of pathologic conditions may occur in adolescence and may be first noticed in this period. One is temporomandibular joint dysfunction (TMD), described in more detail later in this chapter. Anorexia nervosa often shows up in enamel erosion of all teeth if vomiting is a regular component of this psychiatric disorder (Brady, 1980). Bulimia is the term given to those who vomit regularly to purge themselves of food in a misdirected attempt to control their weight. Bulimia affects far more girls than boys, but boys can exhibit similar behavior. The regurgitated stomach contents, which are highly acidic, erode the enamel of teeth in a process called perimyolysis (Fig. 37-7). Dentin is exposed, making teeth sensitive and encouraging decay. Enamel flakes off, leaving sharp edges. Restorations may appear to have grown out of their preparations as enamel and dentin dissolve around them. During clinical examination, these problems speak for themselves; however, in the early bulimic, they may be absent. It may help to air-dry the teeth to look for etching of surfaces.

Treatment of bulimia is a psychiatric problem. Treatment of the teeth is equally difficult and expensive. Pulpal pathosis, elongated clinical

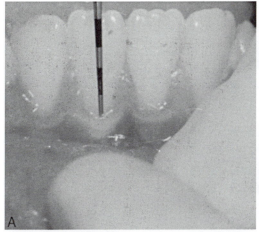
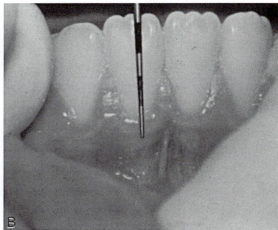
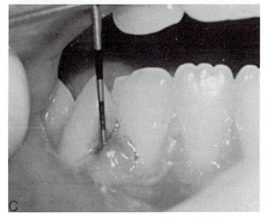

Figure 37–6. The prevalence of periodontal disease begins to increase in the adolescent patient; therefore, a thorough evaluation of the periodontium is absolutely necessary. A periodontal probe is used to measure pocket depth *(A)* and the width of the keratinized gingiva *(B)* and to probe to establish a bleeding index *(C)*. The amount of attached gingiva is determined by subtracting the pocket depth from the width of the keratinized gingiva.

crowns, gingival recession, and loss of vertical dimension are a few of the treatment issues noted in bulimia. Unless the vomiting is stopped, extensive treatment may be futile. The dentist should work with a psychotherapist to deal with this problem.

Another pathologic problem is dental trauma. The clinical and radiographic examination should address tooth crazing, chips, or discoloration with adjunctive radiographs to clarify the status of teeth. Not all teeth that appear sound clinically are healthy (Fig. 37-8), and not all trauma is to hard tissues. The effects of smoking and oral sexual activity (Fig. 37-9) may be identified during the examination.

Evaluation of third molars is usually completed during the mid- to late-adolescent period. Parents commonly ask about treating these teeth. The reasons for extraction of third molars include impaction or failure to erupt; potential or existing pathosis, such as cysts or ameloblastoma; decay; posteruption malposition; nonfunction as a result of an absent opposing tooth; difficulty with hygiene; and recurrent pericoronitis. If any

of these are considerations, third molars should be removed during adolescence.

The concept of anterior crowding as the result of forward pressure from third molars is currently unproved and is not a reason to extract. Surgical access and root development are important issues in determining when to extract. Some root development is desired to stabilize teeth, but complete root development can make extraction more difficult and may increase the likelihood of root fractures. Females using oral contraceptives and smokers also run a high risk of postsurgical dry socket.

OCCLUSAL EVALUATION

Evaluation of the occlusion in three spatial planes is similar to the intraoral examination described in previous chapters. The major difference is that arch length deficiencies are no longer predicted from space analyses but are measured directly from the casts because all permanent teeth usually have erupted by this age. The first step is to measure the arch circumference by dividing the

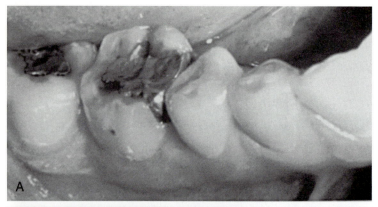

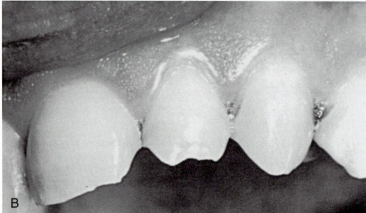

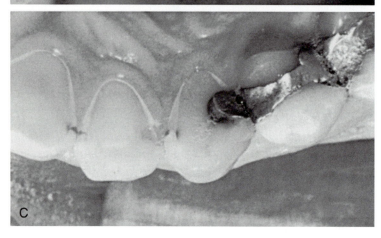

Figure 37–7. Common intraoral findings for a bulemic patient are as follows: *A,* Loss of occlusal enamel with exposure of dentin; *B,* Ragged incisal edges as a result of fracturing of enamel; and *C,* Lingual exposure of dentin highlighted by outlines of remaining enamel and exposed surfaces of restorations. (From Casamassimo P, Castaldi C: Considerations in the dental management of the adolescent. Pediatr Clin North Am *29*:648, 1982.)

arch into segments extending from the mesial of the permanent first molar to the mesial of the contralateral first molar (Fig. 37-10*A*). Each segment is measured over the contact points and incisal edges of the teeth. The segments are added together to yield the total arch circumference. Next, the mesiodistal width of each individual permanent tooth is measured, and the widths are added together (Fig. 37-10*B*). The difference between the arch circumference and the sum of the mesiodistal widths indicates the amount of

crowding or spacing within the arch. If one or two primary teeth have not exfoliated, the width of the contralateral erupted permanent tooth can be substituted for the unerupted permanent tooth.

Careful attention should be paid to teeth adjacent to edentulous areas because these teeth may need to be repositioned orthodontically prior to restorative treatment. The pulpal and restorative status of these teeth helps to determine the direction of treatment.

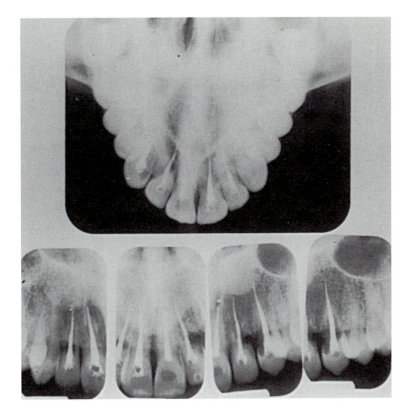

Figure 37–8. Severe resorption of roots secondary to trauma is evident on radiographic examination. These teeth were remarkably stable clinically despite the amount of root resorption.

Once again, the interaction between the facial profile and dental crowding should be considered. Committing the patient to treatment based solely on dental characteristics can have a disastrous effect on the facial profile.

The anteroposterior, transverse, and vertical occlusal components should be evaluated as described in Chapter 30.

Radiographic Evaluation

The adolescent radiographic examination ranges from a transitional to an adult multifilm survey, depending on the child's dentition.

The issues surrounding radiographic examination in the adolescent are related to the type and frequency of exposure. The types of films used

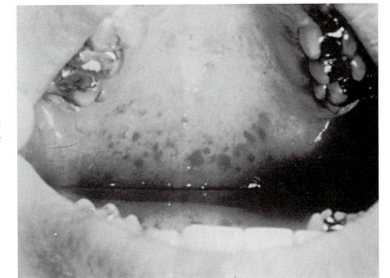

Figure 37–9. This patient exhibits palatal hematomas secondary to oral sex. Negative intraoral pressures cause blood to be pulled to the surface of the palatal tissue.

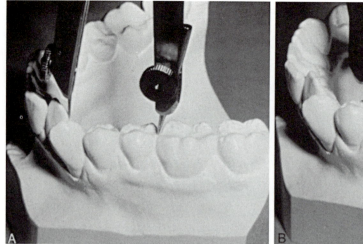
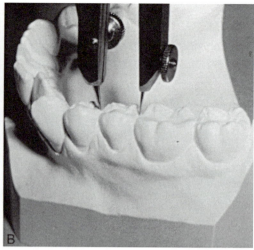

Figure 37–10. *A,* Arch length analysis in the adolescent patient is measured directly from casts rather than by using prediction tables of mixed dentition space analysis because all permanent teeth usually have erupted by this age. The first step is to measure the arch circumference by dividing the arch into segments extending from the mesial of the permanent first molar to the mesial of the contralateral first molar. *B,* Next, the mesiodistal width of each individual permanent tooth is measured, and the widths are added together. The difference between the arch circumference and the sum of the mesiodistal width indicates the amount of crowding or spacing within the arch.

in adolescent radiography should be determined by the number of teeth present and the reason for radiographic examination. For the new adolescent patient with major dental care needs, a survey should include, at the minimum, three to five anterior maxillary periapical films, three mandibular anterior films, a periapical film of each posterior quadrant, and right and left bitewing films. The anterior films should be adult size No. 1, whereas posterior films should be No. 2 size films. It is also recommended that all tooth-bearing areas be surveyed within 2 years of the eruption of the permanent second molars. This can be achieved with a full-mouth survey or a panoramic radiograph combined with bite-wing radiographs.

The radiographic examination in this age group should address mainly growth and development issues: the eruption status of unerupted premolars and canines. Later in adolescence, a final issue is third molar development. The development of these teeth can be evaluated by using periapical radiographs or a third molar panoramic radiograph (Fig. 37–11).

The adolescent should be able to tolerate size 2 intraoral films. For the child with a small oral cavity, techniques to aid in positioning are described in the radiographic section of Chapter 30.

Multiple or serial periapical radiographs are required for diagnosis of pathosis or for management of conditions that require significant follow-up such as endodontic therapy for traumatized incisors.

Bite-wing radiography during early adolescence is affected by the developing occlusion and lack of contacts. It may be that most if not all posterior surfaces can be adequately visualized until the premolars have fully erupted. The benefit of exposing bite-wing films to examine two or four interproximal surfaces should be

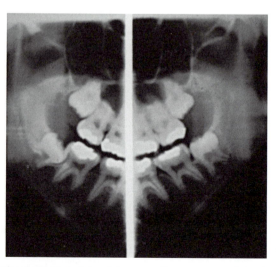

Figure 37–11. In late adolescence, the presence and developmental status of unerupted third molars are evaluated by using periapical radiographs, a conventional panoramic radiograph, or a "third molar" panoramic radiograph as shown here.

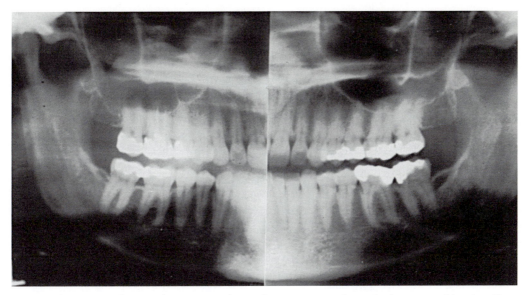

Figure 37–12. A large mucosal cyst in the sinus is evident in this panoramic radiograph of a 21-year-old patient. The cyst is possibly a reaction to pulpal pathosis in the permanent maxillary first and second molars.

weighed against the risk. In these cases, the history of decay and a thorough clinical examination help to determine whether films are necessary.

The panoramic film has a role in adolescent dentistry as a full mouth radiographic survey for a new patient who does not have major treatment needs. For this adolescent, who is essentially clinically disease-free, the panoramic film and bite-wing survey may be adequate to determine dental health. The panoramic film reveals bone pathosis and orients the examiner to the presence and position of third molars. The panoramic film also grossly displays sinuses and the temporomandibular joint (Fig. 37–12), which may be less well displayed on a multifilm intraoral survey. Table 37–2 summarizes the issues that apply to radiography of the adolescent patient.

TREATMENT PLANNING FOR NONORTHODONTIC PROBLEMS

In the adolescent patient, attention must be paid to the long-term consequences of immediate treatment. Although the transitional dentition is considered in terms of its effect on the adult, the adolescent dentition must be considered as being that of the adult. In other words, there are no teeth to follow, only substitutes.

All phases of treatment planning should be addressed. The adolescent depicted in Figure 37–13 illustrates the complexity of problems re-

quiring preventive, periodontal, restorative, and endodontic management.

All adolescents should receive the benefit of a preventive plan that addresses the particular needs of the adult dentition such as flossing. In addition, the preventive plan should address environmental concerns such as smoking, diet, trauma prevention, and the effect of medications on the periodontium and teeth.

Periodontal and gingival concerns are now solidly tied to restorative care. In the child, the minor inflammation around a stainless steel crown on a primary tooth that is due to grossly adjusted margins is tolerated. In the adolescent, with a cast crown, the tissues must be completely healthy.

Restorative treatment planning for the teen is characterized by a number of issues (Castaldi and Brass, 1980):

1. Pulp size is large, affecting choice of coronal coverage.

2. Anterior teeth continue to erupt, requiring consideration of various types of esthetic restorations for traumatized or defective teeth to prevent exposure of margins.

3. Esthetic awareness by the patient may force the dentist to undertake treatment of congenital or acquired discoloration or may require repeated treatment of teeth if transitional procedures are used.

4. Partially erupted posterior teeth may not serve as good abutments for protheses.

5. Decreased chewing efficiency resulting from

TABLE 37–2. Radiographic Issues in the Adolescent

Aspect	Recommendation
Frequency	
Full mouth survey	No suggested frequency or interval
Bite-wing radiographs	No suggested frequency or interval:
	Should be taken if clinical caries noted
	Should be taken if multiple interproximal restorations present and are being followed
	Should be taken if incipiencies noted on previous films and are being followed
	Interval for these situations should be individualized and reevaluated at each periodic examination
Periapical radiographs	No suggested frequency or interval:
	Pathosis or treatment needs should dictate frequency
	To determine developmental status of third molars
Panoramic radiographs	Possible component of a full mouth survey for a disease-free new patient
	"Third molar" panoramic radiograph to determine developmental status of third molars
Type	
Full mouth survey	Number of films included to be based on tissue coverage needed
	Early adolescence (12–14 years):
	Maxillary and mandibular periapicals (No. 1 size)
	Canine periapicals (No. 1 or 2)
	Bite-wings (two films, No. 2 size)
	Four posterior quadrant periapicals (No. 2 size) to include premolars and erupted molars
	Late adolescence (16–21 years):
	Complete set (21-film) survey
Bite-wing radiographs	Size determined by oral access, but No. 2 size used if possible
	One film sufficient until eruption of second molars
	Position varies with the location and number of posterior contacts
Periapical radiographs	Should be adult No. 1 size films rather than No. 2 size, used as occlusal film as in primary tooth survey. An exception to this would be use of No. 2 film as initial trauma screen.
Panoramic radiographs	Can be used with bite-wings for a full mouth survey and is desirable in caries-free and pathosis-free patients after a clinical examination
	"Third molar" panoramic radiograph can be used to determine developmental status of third molars

loss of a posterior tooth may force interim replacement with a removable appliance, although this may not be the treatment of choice.

6. Planned or active orthodontic treatment may delay restoration of missing teeth.

7. Active athletic involvement may require interim replacement of teeth.

The use of acid-etch composite resins and porcelain veneers has greatly improved the treatment of adolescent restorative problems by providing esthetically acceptable, reasonably priced, conservative, and interim and permanent restorations. Their consideration as treatment options in restorative treatment planning is a must.

The two remaining elements of importance in adolescent treatment planning are inter-related. They are consent and compliance. The adolescent under the age of majority requires the consent of the parents for treatment. Payment for services also demands clarification of consent.

The proposed treatment is best explained with both parent and adolescent present, although the actual delivery of care can occur with the adolescent alone in the operatory. Good one-on-one dialogue during active treatment helps to ensure compliance. Some general guidelines for communication to maximize success include the following:

1. Show the adolescent the same respect and interest as you would an adult.

2. Be sincere.

3. Treat the adolescent in privacy as an adult, separate from younger children.

4. Outline procedures and explain reasons for them.

5. Minimize or eliminate authoritarian posturing, using your knowledge rather than age as a reason for your role as a dentist.

6. Be flexible enough to adapt to a changing relationship.

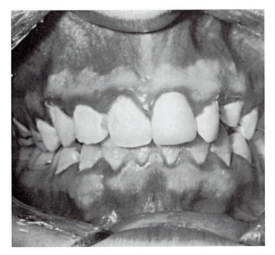

Figure 37–13. The dentition of a 19-year-old male. The final treatment problems included caries, bone loss, defective crowns, and pulpal involvement of two anterior maxillary teeth.

TREATMENT PLANNING AND TREATMENT FOR ORTHODONTIC PROBLEMS

Adolescent orthodontic problems create difficult treatment decisions for the general practitioner and the specialist. The nature of the malocclusion heavily influences how the problem will be treated.

Skeletal Problems

If the malocclusion is skeletal, treatment is aimed at altering the relationship or orientation of the jaws and teeth. This can be accomplished by growth modification, camouflage, or orthognathic surgery. Because the physical maturity of the adolescent patient varies among persons of the same age, any one of three treatments may be appropriate. If the developmental assessment of the patient suggests that the patient is actively growing, growth modification is a viable treatment alternative. Growth modification, previously discussed, attempts to change the actual size, shape, or orientation of the jaws to obtain an acceptable occlusion. Functional appliances and extraoral traction are used to secure these changes.

In the nongrowing, physically mature person, skeletal malocclusion is appropriately treated by camouflage or orthognathic surgery. Camouflage is the orthodontic movement of teeth without changing the underlying skeletal malocclusion.

Camouflage should be considered only when the soft tissue profile is acceptable and when tooth movement will not change or compromise the profile. Teeth are tipped or bodily moved on the denture base to positions considered less than ideal but acceptable for normal occlusion. For example, a mild Class II mandibular deficiency with a relatively prominent bony pogonion can be treated by camouflage (Fig. 37-14). To camouflage this type of problem, the upper teeth are tipped backward and the lower teeth are tipped forward to bring the teeth together and disguise the skeletal problem. In conjunction with the tipping of teeth for camouflage, teeth in the maxillary arch can be extracted to provide more space in which to tip the upper teeth backward. Although a small amount of soft tissue change may occur and the final position of the mandibular incisors may be less than ideal, functional occlusion can be achieved without surgery. Camouflage of Class II skeletal problems is more acceptable in women and camouflage of Class III problems is more acceptable in men because the respective convex and straight profiles are more acceptable for these groups. Camouflage of Class III problems usually is addressed with lingual tipping of mandibular anterior teeth to obtain an acceptable overbite and overjet while at the same time moving the upper dentition anteriorly. The mandibular tipping is often more easily accomplished when extractions are performed in the lower arch.

Skeletal malocclusion in the nongrowing patient can also be treated with orthognathic surgery (Proffit, 1991). The specialist works with an oral and maxillofacial surgeon to reposition one or both jaws into proper alignment surgically. Typically, the orthodontic treatment plan calls for a presurgical period of orthodontic tooth movement to align teeth in both arches and position the teeth over the bony bases so that they will fit together following the surgery. Orthognathic surgery is performed under general anesthesia, and the maxilla, mandible, or both jaws are repositioned. It is possible to move the entire jaw or individual segments of the jaw in nearly any direction within the constraints of the soft tissue covering. There is some restriction on the amount of change that can be achieved, and some types of change are more stable than others. Following the surgical procedure, the jaws are immobilized with wires or bone plates and screws and are then allowed to heal in the new position for several weeks. After healing is demonstrated, a short period of postsurgical orthodontic procedures is necessary to settle the teeth into the final occlusion.

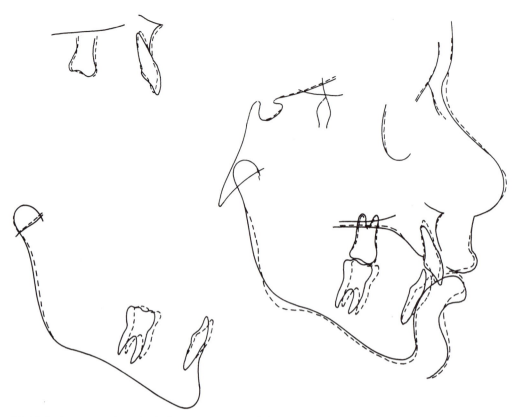

Figure 37–14. In the nongrowing, physically mature patient, skeletal malocclusion is appropriately treated by camouflage or orthognathic surgery. Camouflage is the orthodontic movement of teeth without changing the underlying skeletal malocclusion. The patient represented in these diagrams had a mild class II mandibular deficiency with a relatively prominent bony chin prior to treatment *(solid line)*. The skeletal problem was camouflaged by tipping the maxillary incisors backward and the mandibular incisors forward. Although a small amount of soft tissue change may occur and the final position of the mandibular incisors may be less than ideal, a functional occlusion can usually be achieved without surgery *(broken line)*.

Dental Problems

If the orthodontic problem in the adolescent is strictly dental, conventional orthodontic treatment can be used to treat the malocclusion. Identification and treatment of dental orthodontic problems have already been discussed and basically do not change with the age of the patient. There is one aspect of dental orthodontic treatment that has not been discussed and should be mentioned in this section, however. Despite the preventive efforts of the dental profession, some persons continue to lose permanent teeth to either decay or trauma. When this occurs, a combination of orthodontic tooth movement and restorative dentistry is recommended to obtain an optimal esthetic and functional result.

In the anterior region, orthodontic treatment is often designed to move teeth to simplify prosthetic treatment. To provide precise control of tooth movement, orthodontic brackets should be bonded to all the anterior teeth and bands should be placed on the permanent first molars. Treatment must be carefully planned so that only the teeth that require movement are affected and the other teeth remain stationary. This means that molar, canine, and midline relationships should be carefully studied and controlled during treatment. For example, if one lateral incisor is missing or if the lateral incisor is peg-shaped, the space between the central incisor and the canine on that side should equal the distance between these two teeth on the other side. This ensures that the restored width of the lateral incisor matches that of the contralateral lateral incisor.

Elastomeric chain, arch wire loops, and coil springs can be used to open, close, and stabilize space (Fig. 37–15). Once the space has been opened and is nearly ideal, a closed coil spring or loops bent into the arch wire are used to hold or maintain the space until the restorative or prosthetic treatment is completed. Although this type of treatment sounds simple, close attention to detail is necessary. Uncontrolled tooth move-

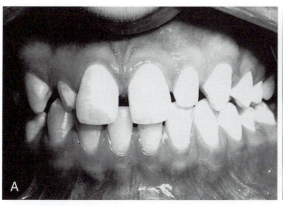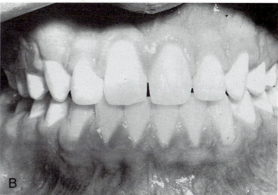

Figure 37–15. Orthodontic treatment is often necessary to move teeth to simplify prosthetic treatment. *A,* In this patient, the anterior space was closed and the lateral incisors were positioned to allow proper mesiodistal crown dimensions. *B,* Resin crown build-ups were placed following orthodontic treatment. Retention is important to keep the space completely closed.

ment can result in unanticipated changes in the midline, overjet, and overbite.

In the posterior region, orthodontic treatment may be necessary to upright teeth that have tipped into extraction sites after loss of permanent teeth. Typically, the permanent first molar is lost as a result of carious or periodontal involvement, and the second molar tips mesially into the extraction site while the second premolar tips distally. Both teeth next to the edentulous area may need to be uprighted to improve the periodontal and restorative potential. Orthodontically, uprighting of teeth will (1) facilitate more conservative, ideal restorations, (2) eliminate plaque-forming areas, (3) improve the alveolar ridge contour, (4) improve the crown-to-root ratio, and (5) re-establish long axis force loading of the teeth. This is best accomplished with limited single-arch, fixed appliance treatment. Bonded brackets or bands are placed on the canine and first and second premolars. The second molar is banded. In addition, a 32-mil wire is bonded to the lingual surface of both canines to provide additional anchorage and stability during molar uprighting. There is a possibility that the arch form could change or that other teeth could move inadvertently if the lingual wire is not in place.

After the appliance has been placed, either segmental or continuous arch wire mechanics can be used to upright the teeth. Selection of mechanics depends on the severity of the tipping. If the tooth is not severely tipped, a light, round, continuous arch wire can be placed from the molar to the canine. Next, the occlusion on the molar should be adjusted by reducing the length of the crown with a bur to allow the molar to erupt and upright. Finally, any periodontal defects around the tipped teeth should be

thoroughly curetted to reduce inflammation and loss of attachment during treatment. Occlusal adjustments and curettage should be performed at each appointment. At subsequent appointments, the size of the arch wire is progressively increased until it is of sufficient size and strength to upright and position the teeth ideally. Sometimes a coil spring placed between the premolar and molar is required to tip the molar distally and increase the edentulous space.

If the molar is too tipped for a continuous arch wire to be placed, segmental mechanics are employed. The canine-premolar segment is aligned independent of the molar via a progression of arch wires similar to that just described. When initial alignment of this segment is completed, an uprighting spring is bent from 19.5- to 25-mil stainless steel wire (Fig. 37–16*A*). A helix is bent in the spring to provide more flexibility and a greater range of activation. In addition, a hook is bent into the end of the uprighting spring to allow the spring to be attached to the segmental wire just distal to the canine bracket; this allows the uprighting spring room to move distally along the segmental wire as the molar becomes upright (Fig. 37–16*B*). The force of activation should provide approximately 75 to 100 g of force to "upright" the molar.

After the molar has been ideally positioned, tooth movement must be retained until a prosthetic replacement can be fabricated. The clinician can use either a fixed or a removable retainer. A fixed retainer is simply a 21- to 25-mil rectangular wire that rests on the occlusal surfaces of the abutment teeth. The wire should be bent down in the edentulous area to remain out of occlusion. Small rests can be placed in the occlusal surfaces of the abutment teeth with a high-speed hand piece, especially if the abutment

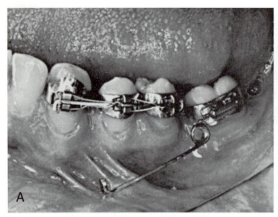
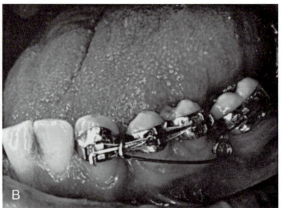

Figure 37–16. Occasionally, a permanent first molar is missing in adolescents and young adults, and molar uprighting is necessary before prosthetic treatment can begin. The canine and premolar teeth are stabilized independently with a large segmental rectangular wire. The canines are usually stabilized further, using a bonded or banded lingual wire. After the anterior teeth are stabilized, the molar can be uprighted using a 19.5 × 25-mil helical spring placed in a bonded or banded tube on the tipped molar. *A*, The spring is passive prior to engagement of the arch wire. *B*, The spring engaged on the arch wire delivers the uprighting and extrusive forces to the tipped molar. Reduction of occlusal interference is necessary to allow the molar to move freely. (From Fields HW, Proffit WF: Orthodontics in general practice. *In* Morris AL, Bohannan HM, Casullo DP [eds]: The Dental Specialties in General Practice. Philadelphia, WB Saunders, 1983, p 327.)

teeth are scheduled for full-coverage restorations. The wire can be retained with either composite resin or amalgam. The major problem with wire retainers is bond and wire breakage under the stress of occlusion. If the patient does not return to have the wire repaired, relapse occurs rapidly. A removable appliance also can be used as a retainer. The edentulous area is filled with acrylic, and clasps are placed on either molars or premolars, depending on retention needs. Again, the removable appliance must be worn faithfully until the restorative treatment is completed.

Adolescent orthodontic treatment is a challenging exercise in problem solving. A good data base and growth assessment are necessary to allow the proper decisions about treatment alternatives. Unless the orthodontic problem is obviously the result of dental malalignment, the patient should be referred to a specialist because of the difficulty in managing skeletal discrepancies in patients of this age.

TEMPOROMANDIBULAR JOINT DISORDERS IN CHILDREN AND ADOLESCENTS

In 1982, the term temporomandibular joint disorder (TMD) was adopted to encompass a range of conditions related to the masticatory system, including the temporomandibular joint, dentition, musculature, and supporting bone. Chil-

dren and adolescents are susceptible to the range of conditions included under the term TMD, but the prevalence in this population is unknown. Certain afflictions of the temporomandibular joint (TMJ) are clearly identifiable, such as degeneration of the joint from arthritis or agenesis of the condyle in inherited conditions such as Goldenhar's syndrome. These conditions usually have obvious clinical signs and can be supported with imaging and history. A more difficult diagnostic problem is idiopathic TMD, a constellation of pain and joint signs without conclusive historical or imaging support.

Most authorities agree that the prevalence of TMD in children is unknown. An international conference on pediatric TMD held in 1989 (American Academy of Pediatric Dentistry, 1990) identified many of the problems involved in trying to characterize TMD in childhood. These include the lack of a consistent definition of TMD and lack of meaningful historical and clinical criteria in studies of the condition.

A number of studies have attempted to identify the occurrence of subjective and objective indicators of TMD in children. In spite of the shortcomings of these studies, they suggest several characteristics of TMD in the pediatric population.

1. *Objective signs are common in the child population, but many have no clinical significance.* Several studies identify a high prevalence of the following clinically observable findings:

Occlusal wear or interferences (Heikinheimo et al., 1990)

Joint sounds (Dahl et al., 1988)
Limitation of opening and mandibular deviation on opening (Nielsen et al., 1988)

These signs are common in asymptomatic children who have no complaints of pain. They may reflect normal variations in the child population or transient changes consistent with normal growth.

2. *Symptoms such as pain are less frequently associated with clinical signs.* A difficulty associated with both clinical diagnosis of TMD in individual children and determination of the prevalence of the condition in the pediatric population is the subjectivity of symptoms. Children often have difficulty in describing pain, localizing it, or understanding questions related to it (Riolo et al., 1988). At the clinical level, the younger the child, the more difficult are the localization of pain and an accurate history. Toothache, headache, ear pain, and muscle soreness are easily confused. Because children rarely seek care unilaterally, true TMD may not be addressed if parents are not concerned or can see no outward signs of illness.

3. *The relationship between signs and symptoms remains unclear.* Studies do not point to a clear etiologic factor for TMD in children. The occurrence of signs or symptoms in studies of children range to well over 50% of subjects (American Academy of Pediatric Dentistry). Children with both symptoms and signs who need treatment, however, account for only about 2% of subjects. The absence of a clear relationship between signs and symptoms probably relates to the quality of diagnostic tests and imaging as well as to study limitations. Most diagnostic techniques used in research are noninvasive, nonspecific clinical examinations during function. TMJ imaging also has limitations of cost and quality representation of anatomic and pathologic findings. The role of psychological factors in TMD is difficult to determine in the study setting and often in practice.

The clinician needs to be aware of the poor correlation between TMD and a number of clinical and historical variables. Occlusal interferences, although significant in the adult, have little consistency in predicting TMD in children. A history of trauma has a much stronger relationship with TMD in the adult than in the child, for reasons made clear later in this chapter. Malocclusion, parafunctional habits, and orthodontic treatment have been implicated as precursors of TMD, but none of these has shown a clear and consistent relationship to TMD when scrutinized closely. The clinician is warned not to grasp

these signs to support a diagnosis of TMD. None has consistently proved valuable in predicting TMD in either group or individual situations. To date, many causes have been established for TMD, but most of these have a clear and obvious relationship to their clinical manifestations. Degenerative disease, developmental abnormalities, and other conditions usually are obvious from historical and clinical evaluation. TMD in children is most commonly idiopathic, however. Table 37-3 suggests some causes of TMD in children.

4. *The efficacy of treatment for pediatric TMD remains controversial, and many techniques are unproved.* The lack of agreement on what constitutes TMD in children and the lack of well-designed studies testing various treatment methods using randomization and clear success criteria hamper development of a reliable armamentarium. Authorities agree that irreversible removal of occlusal interferences in children is contraindicated. Preventive orthodontic therapy to eliminate risk factors has not withstood the test of time, nor has orthodontic therapy to treat existing TMD. Use of occlusal splints, which is not an invasive technique and is often the initial intervention, also has produced mixed results. Early identification of a clear cause is often a mixed blessing because these causes tend often to be irreversible and have significant effects on the joint or masticatory system. Treatment often involves surgery and significant orthodontic and physical therapy.

The clinician interested in TMD management should recognize that overdiagnosis and overtreatment are perhaps the most consistent aspects of dealing with this disorder in children.

Diagnosis of TMD in Children

Every dentist who treats children should include a TMD screening examination to establish a base-

TABLE 37–3. Some Established Causes of TMD in Children and Adolescents

Inherited
  Hemifacial microsomia
  Hemifacial atrophy
  Juvenile rheumatoid arthritis
  Ankylosis
  Cleft-related
Acquired
  Infectious (septic arthritis)
  Traumatic (sports injury)
  Iatrogenic (cortisone-damaged, surgical displacement, irradiation)
  Factitial (habits, hobbies)
  Neoplastic (tumors)
  Idiopathic

line. The patient history must include a thorough medical history to rule out inherited or acquired conditions (see Table 37–3). Trauma needs to be addressed.

The clinical examination should include a series of muscle palpations. The muscles are palpated bilaterally and simultaneously by the clinician, who is directly in front of or behind the patient. The patient is asked whether it feels the same on both sides, if one side feels different, or if either side feels sore. The muscles palpated should include the following at a minimum: temporalis, lateral pterygoid, masseter, and medial pterygoid. The lateral and medial pterygoid muscles are palpated intraorally, and the others are palpated extraorally.

The age at which the full list of palpations is usually done begins at about age 6, and selected palpations are done at a younger age, such as palpation of the temporomandibular joints while the patient opens wide and closes. This can help to detect any irregular movement of the condyles as well as clicks or pain. Sore or tense muscles usually indicate overuse. For example, a clencher or bruxer may have sore masseters. Sore lateral pterygoids may indicate a shift or slide, which requires excessive use of these muscles.

The range of motion and deviation on opening the mouth should be recorded. The maximum opening is measured with a millimeter gauge placed between the right maxillary and mandibular incisors. The amount of overbite is added because that is actually the distance the mandible opens. If there is an open bite, the amount is subtracted from the maximum measurement. The child should be able to open approximately 35 to 45 mm. Opening in the 20- to 35-mm range may indicate a possible muscular problem, and a width of under 20 mm may indicate a problem in the joint such as a displaced disk. Any deviation on opening should be noted, including the path of the deviation and the approximate opening at which it occurred. This is done for patients beginning at 3 to 4 years of age. Clicks or sounds during opening should also be noted at this time. Clicks are usually the result of an incoordination of the disk and condyle on movement.

Lateral movement of the mandible is not routinely recorded for children under 7 years of age because many of them have difficulty in following the directions, but over age 7 most children are able to comply. They are asked to "move the bottom jaw towards the shoulder I'm touching." The amount of lateral movement is measured in millimeters of change in the maxillary and mandibular dental midlines. The child should be able to move approximately 8 to 12 mm on each

side. The amount of protrusive movement is also recorded. Severely decreased movement may indicate a permanently dislocated disk or severe muscle problems, whereas excessive movement may indicate an unstable joint due to damaged or loose ligaments.

Shifts should be carefully noted. A shift is the change from the first point of contact in centric relation to maximum intercuspation in all three planes of space.

Imaging and TMD

The role of imaging in TMD diagnosis has changed in recent years, but basic principles of radiographic diagnosis and test selection criteria apply. For example, joint sounds noted on routine clinical examination do not merit radiographic examination in the absence of symptoms. Examination or history should indicate that a recent change has occurred to justify any radiographs in the absence of symptoms.

A panoramic radiograph or a selected cranial view is considered a basic radiographic evaluation. More complex imaging needs to be performed by those specializing in TMD views. Arthrograms and tomography are examples of diagnostic imaging that can demonstrate disk relationships. Magnetic resonance imaging (MRI) and computed tomography (CT) are more sophisticated techniques that can be helpful but are clearly beyond the skills of most practitioners. The selection criteria for initial TMD imaging include the following (AAPD, 1990):

1. Recent trauma or history of progressive pathologic joint condition
2. Significant dysfunction and alteration in range of motion
3. Significant occlusal changes (open bite, mandibular shift)

Okeson (1989) has outlined a thorough examination procedure for TMD patients, and the reader is referred to this source for a more thorough coverage of this topic, which is beyond the scope of this chapter.

Treatment of TMD in Children

Basic principles of TMD management also apply to the care of children. The clinician should first determine whether he or she wants to address the problem or seek further assistance from clinicians actively involved in TMD therapy. Dentists should have established referral sources that include medical and psychological professionals as well as other dentists. Reversible techniques should be employed first, and splint therapy using custom-designed appliances is often a starting point in therapy. Because medication, counseling, and physical therapy may be indicated concurrently, a dentist may determine that referral to another case-managing dental specialist skilled in TMD treatment is in the patient's best interest.

Management of children is complicated by a host of variables not commonly encountered in adults. Compliance can be a major issue, especially with exercises or splint wear. Adolescent adjustment problems may trigger TMD, and these issues may not be readily discussed with parents or dentists. Growth, loss of teeth, and eruption of succedaneous teeth are clinical problems to be dealt with in treating the child at several stages in this period of life.

Currently, adjunctive diagnostic and treatment therapies, such as kinesiology, thermography, jaw tracking, and others, have no established efficacy in management of TMD in children and should be avoided.

REFERENCES

American Academy of Pediatric Dentistry (AAPD): Treatment of temporomandibular disorders in children: Summary statements and recommendations. JADA *120*(3): 265-269, 1990.

Brady WF: The anorexia nervosa syndrome. Oral Surg *50*:509-513, 1980.

Casamassimo PS: Dental and oral health problems: Prevention and services. *In* Congress of the United States, Office of Technology Assessment: Adolescent Health, Vol. 11. Background and the effectiveness of selected prevention and treatment services, OTA-H-466. Washington, D.C., U.S. Government Printing Office, 1991.

Castaldi CR, Brass GA: Dentistry for the Adolescent. Philadelphia, WB Saunders, 1980.

Chertkow S: Tooth mineralisation as an indicator of the pubertal growth spurt. Am J Orthod 77:79-91, 1980.

Dahl B, Krogstad B, Ogaard B, et al: Signs and symptoms of craniomandibular disorders in two groups of 19-year-old individuals, one treated orthodontically and the other not. Acta Odontol Scand *46*:89-93, 1988.

Greulich WW, Pyle SI: Radiographic Atlas of Skeletal Development of the Hand and Wrist. Palo Alto, Stanford University Press, 1959.

Heikinheimo K, Salmi K, Myllarniemi S, et al: A longitudinal study of occlusal interferences and signs of craniomandibular disorder at the ages of 12 and 15 years. Eur J Orthodont *12*:190-197, 1990.

Moorrees CA, Fanning EA, Hunt EE Jr: Age variation of formation stages for ten permanent teeth. J Dent Res *42*:1490-1502, 1963.

Nielsen L, Melsen B, Terp S: Clinical classification of 14- -16-year-old Danish children according to functional status of the masticatory system. Commun Dent Oral Epidemiol *16*:47-51, 1988.

Okeson JP: Management of Temporomandibular Disorders and Occlusion, 2nd ed. St. Louis, CV Mosby, 1989.

Pinkham JR, Schroeder CS: Dentist and psychologist: Practical considerations for a team approach to the intensely anxious dental patient. JADA *90*:1022-1026, 1975.

Poulsen S: Epidemiology and indices of gingival and periodontal disease. Pediatr Dent *3*:82-88, 1981.

Proffit WR: The need for surgical-orthodontic treatment. *In* Proffit WR, White PR (eds): Surgical-Orthodontic Treatment. St. Louis, Mosby–Year Book, 1991.

Riolo ML, ten Have TR, Brandt D: Clinical validity of the relationship between TMJ signs and symptoms in children and youth. J Dent Child *55*:110-113, 1988.

Tanner JM: Foetus into Man. London, Open Books, 1978.

Chapter 38

Prevention of Dental Disease

Arthur Nowak and James Crall

Chapter Outline

The time of adolescence has been described as the period between childhood and adulthood. It has also been described as a period of change, rebellion, friction, and problems. It is a period when the patient progresses from junior high school to senior high school and then goes off to college, the military, or the work force. It is a period of preference for peer group relationships and avoidance of all other associations, either social or familial.

The period witnesses the completion of growth and development in both females and males. All permanent teeth have erupted except for the congenitally missing or impacted third permanent molars. The occlusion has stabilized either on its own or with orthodontic intervention. Most studies show a gradual but general increase in the incidence of dental caries during this period. Periodontal disease becomes clinically evident because there are fewer routine and supervised home care sessions and because professional intervention occurs less frequently.

Dietary habits undergo dramatic changes during this period. As adolescent girls complete their maximum growth and development and begin the long process of "figure development," they begin many dietary experiments and modifications. Some of these modifications can lead to serious pathologic conditions such as anorexia nervosa and bulimia. In adolescent boys, similar modifications in dietary habits occur. During this period the male's skeletal growth and body weight usually undergo dramatic changes, peaking at around age 16 to 18. Caloric requirements increase dramatically, and large amounts of protein and carbohydrates are consumed. In both groups, irregular meals, fast food meals, frequent snacking, and unusual eating patterns are all common.

How do these adolescent characteristics, which have been so frequently described and routinely observed, affect the dentist in providing professional dental care? Fortunately, because this population has had the advantages of both systemic and topical fluorides, the problem of caries is usually confined to the occlusal surfaces of the posterior teeth. Nevertheless, with the eruption of the posterior teeth in an environment of increased plaque secondary to reduced cleansing and frequent snacking, usually of foods high in carbohydrates and retentive to the teeth, the immature enamel of the smooth surfaces is at high risk for caries.

Therefore, periodic professional visits, combined with an emphasis on continuing home care, optimal use of topical fluorides, and assistance in dietary management, are the goals and challenges of the dentist who treats adolescent patients.

DIETARY MANAGEMENT

As with younger age groups, the overall recommendations on dietary management for adolescents should concentrate on balanced intake, reduction of the frequency of snacking, and selection of foods that are not retentive to the teeth and soft tissues. Unfortunately, these recommendations conflict with the lifestyles of adolescents. With their newly gained independence; rebellious attitude toward established social systems; acceptance of recommendations from television, radio, and movie idols; and peer group pressure, it is a difficult task for the dentist and his or her staff to convey this recommendation and expect compliance.

Fortunately, owing to the increasing social development that occurs in the mid years of adolescence, there is a strong desire to look attractive, and the mouth, being the center of the face, takes on importance. The challenge we have as dentists is to somehow make the daily care of teeth, including dietary regulations, attractive to this group.

For the patient who has been at high risk for dental disease during the early years and has had caries in the primary dentition, dietary management is recommended again. Depending on the patient's present oral status, emotional and psychological maturity, and parental influences, counseling can be performed with the patient only or, if indicated, with the parents. At this age the adolescent may enjoy independence from the involvement of the parents. The dentist must decide whether or not to include the parents and to inform the parents about the results of the counseling.

For the patient who has active lesions in the developing permanent dentition, dietary management and modifications are definitely indicated along with a comprehensive program of oral cleaning and topical daily fluoride use. It is best to arrive at a complete understanding with the patient about the importance of this information and his or her willingness to cooperate. If not, it will be only a paper exercise and a waste of time for both parties involved. If the patient is interested and is willing to cooperate, a dietary history is indicated.

Initially, a 24-hour dietary history will probably be sufficient. Based on the information provided by the history as well as from the patient about the usual daily schedules and the patient's academic, athletic, and social obligations, the dentist or staff responsible for counseling can assist in devising a plan of care with the patient.

Having the patient recognize the problem and agree either orally or in writing to a solution improves compliance. During the periodic examination, the patient's progress or lack of progress can be evaluated. Plans may have to be modified frequently depending on the patient's changing needs. Because food preferences, social pressures, and growth changes occur frequently, this plan must allow for flexibility.

Although a 24-hour dietary history will be helpful, more information will be provided by a 5- or 7-day history including the weekend days. For the history to be accurate, the patient should complete the first day's record with the dentist, paying particular attention to all liquid and solid foods consumed both at meals and between meals. Information about how much of the food was consumed and where the food was eaten will be helpful.

Once the dietary history has been received, a staff person assigned to counseling responsibilities should carefully review it with the patient. Foods high in refined carbohydrates or retentive to the oral tissues should be circled. Intake of fresh fruits and vegetables should be noted. Overall balance of the diet should be evaluated. Unusual foods or dietary patterns should be listed.

The patient should then be asked to list the problem areas and categorize them according to the ease with which they can be changed. With the problems identified and written in a sequence most acceptable to modification, the patient then develops a plan. It is important that it be his or her plan and not the dentist's. It is the dentist's role to guide the patient to develop a realistic plan that will be built on successes. Periodic review determines the status of the dietary modifications. Reinforcements and rewards are helpful, but the patient's own perception of success are the most rewarding aspect for both dentist and patient. Computerized programs are also available that facilitate the analysis and provide appropriate recommendations.

For the patient with a developmental disability, the challenge is great. Depending on the severity of the disability, dietary habits may or may not be affected. For the patient with a severe neuromuscular involvement, diet and eating methods will already have been modified. Parents or caretakers must be made aware of potential problems—holding the food in the mouth, slow passage of food from the mouth to the digestive tract, and rumination are all potentially devastating to the mouth and teeth. If regulation of the diet is not possible, efforts should be made to ensure more frequent and thorough cleansing as well as daily use of topical fluorides.

HOME CARE

Personal hygiene, like any established societal activity, is met with varying responses during adolescence. Nagging by the parent or dentist will probably lead to a negative response. When the patient understands the importance of oral hygiene and is ready to make a daily commitment, the dentist can assist him or her in developing a routine of oral hygiene that will be acceptable to the patient as well as maintaining a healthy oral environment.

During this period, dental flossing should become a part of the daily oral hygiene routine. Adolescents should have well-developed eye-hand coordination and fine motor activity. For those who still have difficulty with the traditional method of flossing, a floss holder may be helpful.

The goal of the patient should be to perform one thorough cleansing each day, ideally before bed. The patient should be informed of the importance of thoroughness; therefore, a period before bed should be set aside for the routine of brushing and flossing. After meals a vigorous rinse with water should be encouraged. If orthodontic appliances are present, additional time as well as modifications of the routine will be necessary to remove not only the plaque but also the debris caught around the brackets and wires. Additional massaging of the marginal gingiva is also important.

For the adolescent patient with a developmental disability, daily home care is equally important. Again, depending on the severity of the disability, either the patient, the parent, or an aide is responsible for the care. If patients are unable to keep the mouth open, a mouth prop may be helpful.

Chemical plaque control agents have become popular adjuncts to daily oral hygiene. It has been reported that a number of patients may profit from their daily use, especially patients with special health care needs or patients with orthodontic applicances. Studies have confirmed the improvement that results from the use of

these agents in reducing plaque, gingivitis, and gingival bleeding sites (Beiswanger et al., 1991; Brightman et al., 1991; Grossman et al., 1986). Adolescents frequently experience marginal gingivitis secondary to plaque deposits. Consideration should be given to prescribing the addition of antimicrobial mouth rinses to daily oral hygiene practices (Bhat, 1991).

For a patient with a developmental disability or an acute or chronic medical condition and who may be unable to rinse and spit, an alternative method is to apply the antimicrobial rinse with a brush and then remove the excess rinse with a suction device or catch the dribble in a pan.

FLUORIDE ADMINISTRATION

Approach to the Adolescent Patient

Although most adolescents have the ability to carry out effective oral hygiene procedures, many neglect to perform these activities regularly. The key to promoting effective caries prevention during what can be a hectic and trying stage of life often depends on recognizing the predominant motivational factors operating in this age group and adopting an approach that is based on less than ideal compliance. The focus on personal appearance and hygiene in this age group can be used as a powerful motivator for developing preventive activities. Another strategy involves appealing to the adolescent's desire to be viewed as autonomous and capable of taking care of himself or herself.

Regardless of the psychological basis for the motivation, time should be taken to ensure that adolescents understand the nature of the disease processes that the preventive programs are addressing and the general mechanisms by which the prescribed measures are thought to counteract these processes. This emphasis on education is more likely to be accepted and will produce better long-term outcomes than a more authoritarian or condescending approach.

Caries Activity During Adolescence

In spite of a well-documented decline in caries levels in children in the United States and other Western countries, adolescence still marks a period of significant caries activity for many persons. Cross-sectional data from the 1988–1991 survey of caries prevalence in schoolchildren in the United States (Kaste et al., 1996) showed that the mean number of decayed, missing, and filled permanent tooth surfaces (DMFS) increased from 0.9 for 12-year-olds to 4.4 for 17-year-olds. The results of that study indicated that, on average, the DMFS index increased by 1.3 on buccal-lingual surfaces, 0.5 on interproximal surfaces, and 2.4 on occlusal surfaces between the ages of 12 and 17. Thus, fluoride administration should continue to be an important concern during this stage of continuing caries susceptibility.

Topical fluorides (along with occlusal sealants) are the primary preventive agents during adolescence because the entire permanent dentition except for the third molars normally has erupted by age 13 (Bell et al., 1982). Most studies have shown that fluorides reduce the incidence of smooth-surface caries to a greater extent than that of occlusal caries (Backer-Dirks et al., 1961; Clarkson, 1991). Therefore, the combination of fluoride therapy and occlusal sealants can be used to provide optimal protection for all surfaces of the teeth.

High-Frequency/Low-Concentration Applications

As with younger children, the daily use of a fluoride dentifrice should form the basis of a sound personal preventive dentistry program, regardless of whether the person lives in a fluoridated or a nonfluoridated community. Additional protection can be provided daily by the use of a 0.05% sodium fluoride rinse. Frequent rinsing seems particularly advisable for those "on-the-go" teenagers who do not take the time to practice thorough plaque removal. Frequent exposures to fluoride may help to suppress the cariogenic potential of the oral flora and can help to establish an environment that may inhibit demineralization or promote remineralization (DePaola, 1980). As noted previously, fluoride mouth rinses also are indicated for persons who have difficulty removing plaque because of the presence of orthodontic appliances or for those with predisposing medical conditions.

Applications of More Concentrated Fluoride Agents

Daily applications of more concentrated fluoride gels may be indicated for some teenagers who exhibit poor oral hygiene or who continue to exhibit high levels of caries between recall examinations. These gels can be applied by brushing or by means of customized plastic trays. Custom trays are easily fabricated using vacuum-forming devices to adapt the plastic tray material over stone models of the patient's maxillary and mandibular arches. The best time to apply the gels is just before bedtime to allow the fluoride to remain in contact with the teeth for a longer time. Professional applied topical fluorides should be applied every 6 months during adolescence for those with a history of caries activity or who are assessed to be at greater risk for developing caries.

Adolescence is a time of heightened caries activity for many persons as a result of increased intake of cariogenic substances and inattention to oral hygiene procedures. Because fluorides have been shown to exert a greater anticaries effect in patients with higher baseline levels of caries activity and because the concurrent use of various forms of fluoride often produces greater caries reductions than when the agents are used separately, multiple exposures to a variety of fluoride sources should be encouraged during this period in an attempt to control the caries process.

REFERENCES

Backer-Dirks O, Houwink B, Kwant GW: The results of 6½ years of artificial drinking water in the Netherlands: The Tiel-Culemborg experiment. Arch Oral Biol 5:284-300, 1961.

Beiswanger BB, Mallat ME, Mau MS, et al: 0.12% Chlorhexidine rinse as an adjunct to scaling and root planing. J Dent Res 70 (Special Issue):458, 1991.

Bell RM, Klein SP, Bohannan HM, et al: Characteristics of the data analysis population. In Results of Baseline Dental Exams in the National Preventive Dentistry Demonstration Program. Santa Monica, Rand Corporation, 1982, p 26.

Bhat M: Periodontal health of 14- to 17-year-old U.S. school children. J Public Health Dent 51:5-11, 1991.

Brightman LJ, Terezhalmy GT, Greenwald H, et al: The effects of a 0.12% chlorhexidine gluconate mouthrinse on orthodontic patients aged 11 through 17 with established gingivitis. Am J Ortho Dentofac Orthop 100:324-329; 1991.

Clarkson BH: Fluoride: Biological implications and dietary supplementation. In Pinkham JR (ed): Pediatric Dental Care: An Update for the 90's. Evansville, IN, Bristol-Myers, Squibb Co, 1991, pp 23-24.

DePaola PF: The anticaries effect of single and combined topical fluoride systems in school children. Arch Oral Biol 25:649-653, 1980.

Grossman F, Reiter G, Sturzenberger OP, et al: Six-month study of the effects of a chlorhexidine mouthrinse on gingivitis in adults. J Periodont Res Suppl 16:33-43, 1986.

Kaste LM, Selwitz RH, Oldakowski JA, et al: Coronal caries in the primary and permanent dentition of children and adolescents 1-17 years of age: United States, 1988-1991. J Dent Res 75 (Special Issue):631-641, 1996.

National Institute of Dental Research: Oral Health of United States Children: The National Survey of Dental Caries in U.S. School Children: 1986-1987. NIH Pub. No. 89-2247. Bethesda, MD, National Institutes of Health, 1989, pp 14-17.

39

Esthetic Restorative Dentistry for the Adolescent

John W. Reinhardt and Marcos A. Vargas

Chapter Outline

A pleasing, attractive appearance is the dream of most adolescents in our society. Great effort and expense are invested in gaining or maintaining that appearance through means such as dieting, use of cosmetics, and selection of apparel. An important component of the idealized physical appearance is a radiant smile displaying teeth that are attractive in shape and color and do not distract during speaking and smiling.

The use of dental techniques and materials to help young people obtain the most attractive appearance possible is a clinical challenge requiring knowledge, disciplined attention to detail, and skill. In return for their efforts, dentists receive the satisfaction of seeing a young person develop a healthy self-image that can have a positive effect on his or her maturation into adulthood.

Newly developed and improved composite resins along with the acid-etch technique have made it possible to restore esthetic defects with conservative treatment. The use of visible light–cured composite resins has made the job easier.

A multitude of composite resins are available and offer a choice of physical properties such as viscosity, opacity and translucency, and surface smoothness.

FUNDAMENTALS OF MATERIAL SELECTION

Choice of materials is an important consideration for dental esthetic factors. The clinical success of composite restorations depends on adhesive systems that provide durable bonding of composite to dentin and enamel, effectively sealing the margins of restorations and preventing postoperative sensitivity and microleakage.

In order to achieve this, a current-generation adhesive system should be used (Fig. 39-1). Most of these systems work by demineralizing the dentin-enamel surface with an acid, which is usually 37% phosphoric. After etching, a primer resin is applied that facilitates the penetration of an adhesive resin into the demineralized dentin and

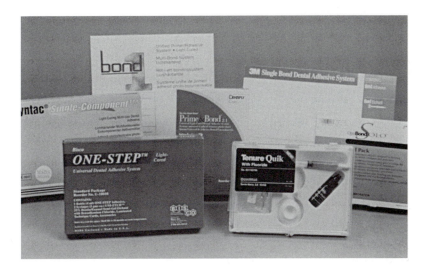

Figure 39–1. Representative dentin-enamel adhesive products.

enamel to form a hybridized layer of resin/tooth (Nakabayashi et al., 1982; Van Meerbeek et al., 1992) as shown in Figure 39-2. Manufacturers have introduced single-bottle primer/adhesive systems. These agents combine the primer resin with the adhesive resin into a single component (bottle), thus simplifying the bonding procedure.

Choice of composite resins for esthetic restorations can be confusing because a variety of products are available with slightly different physical properties. Basically, the two types of composite resins that can be used are *microfilled*—those with filler particles averaging 0.04 μm in diameter—and *hybrid*—a blend of different particle sizes, including submicron (0.04 μm) and small particle (1 to 4 μm). The particle size difference between microfilled and hybrid composite resins is readily apparent under magnification (Fig. 39-3).

The mechanical and physical properties of hybrid composite resins are superior to those of microfilled resins because they contain a higher proportion of filler particles. Because of their particle size, however, microfilled resins can be polished to an enamel-like luster. Microfills are primarily indicated when esthetic restorations are required, such as Class V and direct resin veneers. In Class IV restorations, a hybrid material may be used as a substrate that can be veneered by a microfilled composite resin.

Regardless of whether a microfilled or hybrid composite resin is chosen, the use of visible light–curing products is recommended. In addition to the convenience of extended working

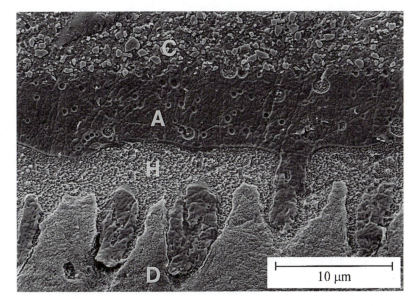

Figure 39–2. Scanning electron microscopic view of the resin-to-dentin bond, showing composite resin (C), adhesive (A), hybrid layer (H), and dentin (D).

10 μm

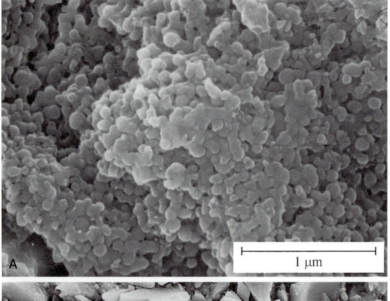

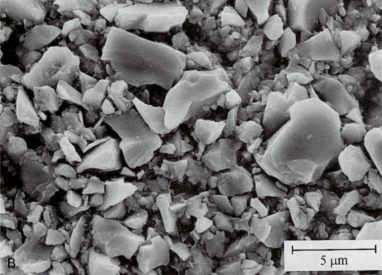

Figure 39–3. Scanning electron microscopic views demonstrating the difference between typical microfilled *(A)* and hybrid *(B)* composite resins.

time and rapid polymerization, these materials also have lower porosity and are less likely to become discolored than the chemically cured (spatulated two-paste) systems.

Polymerization of light-cured composite resins is accomplished by using an intense blue light with a peak wavelength of approximately 470 nm. A typical light-curing polymerization unit uses a gun-type handpiece that contains the bulb and cooling fan (Fig. 39-4). This instrument offers interchangeable light transmission tubes to gain access to various areas of the mouth. Light intensity should be periodically checked (via a radiometer) so that a minimal output of 300 mW/cm^2 can be maintained. Several modern light-curing units incorporate light meter devices into their bases, so curing radiometers are not needed (Fig. 39-5).

Eye protection is important when using the curing lights because direct viewing of the light is detrimental to vision (Ham, 1983). Amber filters, which block the intense blue component of the light, are commercially available and can be hand held or worn as eyeglasses (Fig. 39-6). In the absence of specific protective devices, one should avoid looking directly at the light.

FUNDAMENTALS OF CLINICAL TECHNIQUE

Shade selection is the first step in a successful esthetically pleasing restorative procedure. The teeth to be matched should be cleaned with a rubber prophylaxis cup and flour of pumice. Moistened shade tabs should be held near the

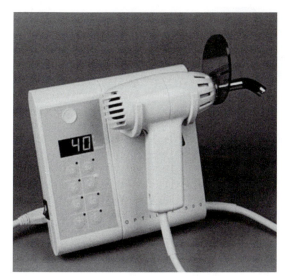

Figure 39–4. A typical dental composite resin light-curing unit.

tooth to be matched, using only room light or indirect sunlight. One should not use the high-intensity operatory light when selecting shades. The proper value (Munsell "whiteness") may be better determined by squinting. If shade selection takes more than a few seconds, one may need to resensitize the eyes by staring momentarily at a dark blue or gray object.

Many clinicians allow the patient to choose between two similar shades. The composite resin shade guide may vary from the actual shade of the composite paste. One way to verify the actual shade is to place a small portion of composite resin on the tooth surface and polymerize it, observe the appropriateness of that shade, and then remove it with a hand instrument. One

should not etch the tooth prior to doing this or removal will be difficult. It is generally best not to combine shades of composite resin by mixing because porosity may be introduced into the paste.

It is extremely important to maintain an uncontaminated field during the insertion of composite resins. The most reliable way to control moisture is through the use of a well-adapted rubber dam. If not using a rubber dam, one should place cotton rolls and 2 × 2 inch gauze sponges to prevent moisture contamination. Another technique for maintaining a dry field is to use a commercially available lip and cheek retractor (Fig. 39-7). This plastic device, when used in conjunction with gauze sponges, provides excellent access and good field control.

Use of a base or liner to protect pulp tissue in deep preparations is generally believed to be important, although some practitioners are now questioning that long-held belief. Many believe that a glass ionomer liner should be used in deep areas of a cavity preparation that are thought to be within 0.5 to 1.0 mm of pulpal tissue (Fig. 39-8). The liner provides chemical adherence to tooth structure and slow release of fluoride.

After etching (15 seconds of etch and 5–10 seconds of rinse), an appropriate dentin-enamel bonding agent should be placed. Next, the light-cured composite resin should be inserted in layers no greater than 2.0 mm in thickness, using at least 40 seconds of light exposure per layer. Thin layers and adequate length of time for light exposure help ensure the maximum degree of polymerization. Maximum polymerization provides optimal strength and color stability of the restoration. It is important to cover the light-curing composite resin on the mixing pad so that room light does not initiate the polymerization process. In addition, it may be necessary to lessen the intensity of the operating light.

Plastic or metal instruments are useful for ma-

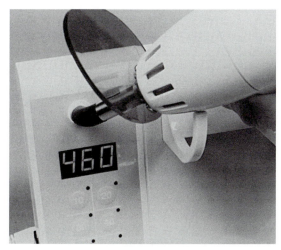

Figure 39–5. Light-curing unit showing power output via an incorporated curing radiometer.

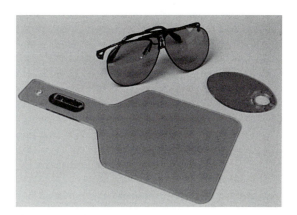

Figure 39–6. Filtering devices designed to protect eyes when using light-curing techniques.

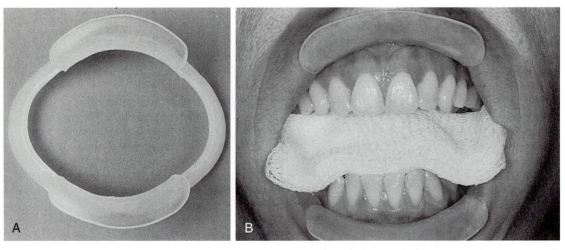

Figure 39–7. *A* and *B,* Isolation of teeth may be enhanced through the use of a lip-retracting device.

terial placement and contouring. Fine sable or camel-hair brushes allow easy contouring and blending of composite resin into the proper form. To prevent composite from adhering to the brushes and instruments, they should be lightly lubricated via gauze sponges moistened with bathing alcohol.

After the polymerization process, one may contour and finish the restoration using carbide finishing burs, ultrafine diamond burs, or finishing disks. Fine-pointed burs are helpful to contour areas that are difficult to reach such as embrasures. Rounded burs may be used on concave surfaces, and disks may be used on flat or convex surfaces. After contouring and finishing, the restoration should be polished with a series of polishing disks or rubber abrasive instruments. The final finish and polish of interproximal areas is best done with abrasive strips.

FUNDAMENTALS OF TOOTH COLOR AND FORM

The ideal esthetic restoration appears so natural it is difficult to discern from the surrounding tooth surface or adjacent teeth. Color and translucency must be considered together to achieve

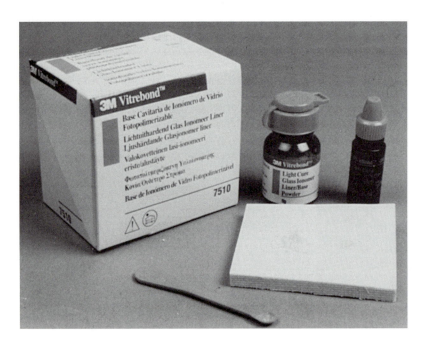

Figure 39–8. A light-curable glass ionomer liner.

an optimal result. One may alter areas of discoloration on a tooth by applying color modifiers or opaquing agents to improve the appearance, then covering those areas with composite resin.

Composite resins with greater opacity, such as hybrid and microfilled opaque pastes, should be used in most situations. The purpose of selecting an opaque material is to prevent excessive translucency, which can allow intraoral darkness to show through a restoration and cause a dark, unappealing result.

Highly translucent materials such as nonopaque microfilled pastes should be used only for Class III restorations and small Class IV restorations on highly translucent teeth. In many cases, use of a hybrid composite as a foundation under a microfilled composite improves both the strength and the appearance of the restoration.

Form and anatomy of anterior esthetic restorations can also be controlled to make the restoration appear natural-looking. In general, embrasure spaces should be symmetrical whenever possible, and contours should match those of the adjacent teeth. Adolescent anterior teeth usually show little evidence of wear and display prominent incisal embrasure spaces, rounded incisal point angles, and developmental characteristics such as mamelons on incisal edges. These characteristics are especially noticeable in young women and should be used whenever possible to enhance a feminine smile.

RESTORATIONS FOR FRACTURED ANTERIOR TEETH

Trauma to the anterior dentition can often result in tooth fractures involving incisal edges. Injuries such as these can cause pulpal as well as esthetic problems and should be carefully evaluated through clinical and radiographic means. Clinical findings may range from little or no dentin exposure with minimal thermal and pressure sensitivity to the acute distress of a pulp exposure. Radiographs help in diagnosing the presence or absence of root fractures. Treatment must begin with pulpal therapy as a first consideration, and if pulpectomy or pulpotomy is necessary, it should begin simultaneously with the restorative procedures.

Some clinicians consider the Class IV composite resin restoration an interim restoration for adolescents until a more permanent ceramic crown can be fabricated. With modern materials and techniques, however, the strength and color stability of composite resin Class IV restorations are such that they can be considered "final" res-

torations that will provide relatively long service. For early adolescents with severely fractured anterior teeth, these restorations can provide years of service, allowing the teeth to mature so that pulpal injury during crown preparation is less likely.

Clinical Technique

Acid-etching techniques have lessened the need for extensive mechanical retentive features in Class IV restorations. The primary retentive feature is a beveled enamel cavosurface margin, a minimum of 1.0 to 2.0 mm in length. Beveling allows maximal bond strength and minimizes leakage by exposing the ends of the enamel rods to etching. Because anterior restorations are sometimes subject to strong shearing forces that can be greater than the bond strength of the restoration to the tooth, features such as grooves, retentive points, or pins may be used to gain additional retentive strength. Supplemental retentive features are usually unnecessary, however.

After administering anesthesia, placing the rubber dam, and preparing the bevel (using a medium grit diamond bur), a base or liner may be applied to exposed dentin. When one is conditioning the tooth, the etchant should be applied to enamel and then to dentin. In order to avoid overetching, it is important that dentin not be etched for more than 15 seconds. After rinsing (for at least 5 seconds), the surface should be left slightly moist to avoid collapsing the exposed collagen network. The primer resin (or in some cases, a single-component primer/adhesive) is then applied to the dentin and should be in contact with dentin for at least 15 seconds for most adhesive systems. No problem should occur if this primer contacts the enamel. After 15 seconds, the primer should be dried with a gentle stream of air in order to evaporate the solvent without displacing the primer. It is imperative that a shiny surface be obtained after this step; if not, most adhesive systems require additional application of primer. After priming, when using two-component systems, the adhesive resin is applied with a brush and light cured for 10 seconds. Care should be taken to avoid pooling or overthinning. As a final step, composite resin is applied as described previously. A wedged celluloid matrix strip can prevent etching and bonding an adjacent tooth. After placing, finishing, and polishing the composite resin, one carefully checks the restoration for interferences in all excursive movements (Figs. 39-9 and 39-10).

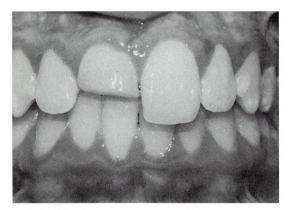

Figure 39–9. The incisal edge of tooth No. 8 was fractured as the result of an accident.

Occlusal stresses on the restoration should be minimized.

RESTORATION OF DIASTEMAS

Many adolescents, as well as adults, consider spaces between anterior teeth (diastemas) unattractive. Historically, the only restorative treatment to fill these spaces has been the construction of crowns larger than the original teeth. Even though many patients disliked their appearance with diastemas, most were unwilling to undergo the trauma and expense of crowning sound teeth simply to gain an esthetic improvement. Improved composite resin materials and acid-etching technology now allow restoration of diastemas using a method that is nondestructive, reversible, and relatively inexpensive. Patients should be forewarned, however, that fracture and staining are possible drawbacks of composite resin diastema closures and that replacement is likely to be needed after 5 to 10 years.

When an adolescent patient wants a diastema closure, whether the spaces are the result of natural development or postorthodontic discrepancies, careful evaluation and planning are necessary prior to treatment. If the patient is nearing completion of orthodontic therapy but is still undergoing treatment, the restorative dentist may advise the orthodontist about the optimal arrangement of anterior teeth for diastema closure. The orthodontist may then complete active treatment and place the patient into a retention phase prior to closing the diastema. It is best to allow a minimum of a few months between the end of active orthodontic treatment and diastema closure therapy so that anterior teeth will be more stable and will settle into their final position. The

use of diagnostic study casts is highly recommended for evaluation and treatment planning. A diagnostic wax-up of the proposed restorative treatment can aid both the patient and clinician in envisioning the result.

Important pretreatment considerations include the size and location of the space or spaces and the size (length and width) and shape of the teeth to be restored. Normally, composite resin is added to the teeth on both sides of the space. For patients who are undergoing orthodontic treatment, one should determine if the remaining space would best be left in one place, such as the midline between teeth Nos. 8 and 9, or distributed over interproximal areas throughout the anterior segment. One must also consider the length and width of the teeth to be restored. If the width becomes greater than the length, those teeth appear more "square," causing an unattractive result that may be as displeasing as the original diastema. Because of occlusal patterns and chewing stresses, teeth usually cannot be lengthened with composite resin without creating a high probability of resin fracture. Light reflections, however, can be used to create the illusion of a longer and narrower tooth when the composite resin is extended to cover most or all of the facial surface of a tooth. To create the illusion of a narrower tooth, one should form mesial and distal line angles in composite resin that are positioned slightly nearer the middle of the tooth and add definite vertical anatomic highlights (developmental depressions). In some situations periodontal crown lengthening may be considered to obtain a favorable width-to-length ratio. For some patients, the best treatment is partial diastema closure, in which an existing space is made smaller by enlarging the teeth with composite resin but not making the teeth so

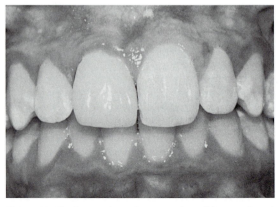

Figure 39–10. Composite resin restoration of fractured tooth shown in Figure 39–9.

large that they become displeasing. In summary, esthetic possibilities must be carefully evaluated and explained to the patient before treatment is begun.

Clinical Technique

After cleaning, shade selection, and isolation (as described previously), treatment should begin on one tooth at a time. The space to be eliminated should be carefully measured via a periodontal probe, calipers, or Boley gauge, because after one tooth is restored in an effort to eliminate half the space, it is usually difficult to determine how much of the space has actually been restored. The entire labial surface of the tooth should be etched and bonding agent applied because most of the labial surface will be covered with a thin layer of composite to allow a subtle color transition from composite to tooth. In addition, covering most of the labial surface allows the use of visual illusions that cause the tooth to look narrower or longer, as described previously.

Composite resin (preferably a resin that is viscous and opaque) should be applied, beginning at the gingival margin of the interproximal area. Using instruments and brushes, one should shape the material to allow a smooth-flowing gingival embrasure without creating an overhanging ledge. The entire proximal surface as well as the labial surface can be built up and polymerized at once or incrementally. After this build-up, one should finish the interproximal area to the proper contour and polish it. Next, the second tooth is restored similarly. A celluloid matrix and wedge are usually inserted after the gingival increment is polymerized to retain the composite resin and to prevent the restorations from bonding together. Some clinicians prefer to build the

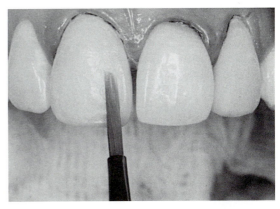

Figure 39–12. The initial increment of composite resin being contoured with a sable brush prior to polymerization (see Fig. 39–11).

second restoration without using a matrix. In that case, the two restorations must be gently separated with a thin metal instrument using a torquing motion. Upon completion, the matrix is removed and contouring and polishing are completed (Figs. 39–11 to 39–14).

Anterior teeth that are unusually small, such as peg lateral incisors, may be restored in the same manner as teeth requiring both mesial and distal diastema closure restorations. Again, careful treatment planning is advised to determine whether the restorations should be done only on the smaller tooth or on both the small and adjacent teeth for maximal cosmetic benefit. Preoperative diagnosis is again necessary to determine whether lengthening is feasible. One should forewarn patients that the possibility of fracturing increases as length increases. In situations where fracturing is a concern, a hybrid resin should be used as a substrate and a microfilled resin placed

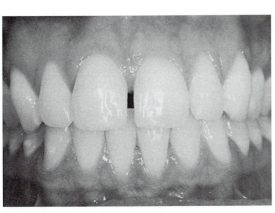

Figure 39–11. A preoperative view of a maxillary midline diastema, which the patient found unattractive.

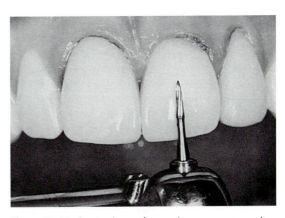

Figure 39–13. Contouring and removing excess composite resin following build-up of the second tooth (see Figs. 39–11 and 39–12).

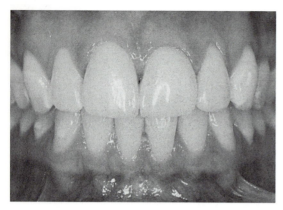

Figure 39–14. A postoperative view of the completed case (see Figs. 39–11 to 39–13).

on the surface. This technique increases the strength and esthetics of the restoration.

RESTORATION OF DISCOLORED TEETH

Although there are many causes of tooth discoloration in adolescents, the most common discolorations result from trauma, enamel hypoplasia (often caused by fluorosis), and the administration of tetracycline antibiotics during childhood. These lesions vary from small white or yellowish flecking of the surface enamel, called enamel "dysmineralization" (Croll, 1991), to the deep intrinsic bluish-gray color often visible in tetracycline staining.

Treatment of Hypoplastic Spots

Discrete hypoplastic white or yellow-brown spots can be improved by enamel microabrasion (Croll, 1989a, 1989b, 1990, 1991) or by making shallow saucer-shaped preparations in enamel to remove the intensely colored tooth structure and then restoring the enamel with composite resin. Microabrasion is the preferred technique whenever possible because it is a treatment that requires less enamel removal and does not necessitate placement of a restoration. The technique for enamel microabrasion involves application of an acidic abrasive paste via a reduced-speed dental handpiece. Microabrasion is sometimes used in combination with vital bleaching (which is described later in this chapter).

Veneers

Composite resin or porcelain veneers provide a treatment option for patients who have moderate to severe staining of one or more teeth. Patients are most concerned about the appearance of their maxillary teeth, especially the anteriors, because they are more visible in speaking and smiling. In addition, mandibular teeth are often less likely to be successfully veneered because of limited space (insufficient overjet) and unfavorable forces at the junction of tooth and veneer during normal chewing. For veneer treatment to be successful, the patient must have excellent periodontal health because the placement of veneers will result in contours and margins that require good oral hygiene to maintain gingival health. In addition, patients should be warned

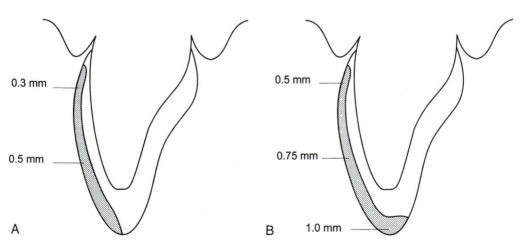

Figure 39–15. Cross-sectional views of a laboratory-processed veneer of ideal thickness without incisal coverage *(A)* and a veneer of greater thickness with incisal coverage *(B)*.

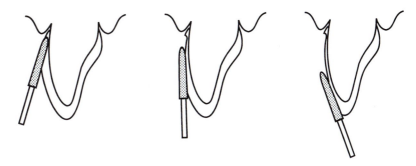

Figure 39–16. Cross-sectional view of the steps in diamond bur placement needed for preparing the facial surface of a maxillary anterior tooth.

that biting on hard objects, such as raw carrots or pencils, may dislodge or break veneers.

Although the anticipated longevity of an esthetic veneer restoration might be less than that of a porcelain-fused-to-metal crown, the cost is also less. In addition, veneers can be placed with minimal tooth preparation, thus preserving the natural dentition. Veneers may be made by direct build-up of composite resin in the mouth or by indirect procedures (constructed on laboratory models) using composite resin or porcelain.

LABORATORY-CONSTRUCTED VENEERS

The indirect veneer technique has the advantage of requiring less total chair time because the veneers are constructed in the laboratory. Excellent esthetically pleasing contours can be achieved using porcelain or composite resin laboratory techniques. Disadvantages include the necessity of two appointments, laboratory expense, and the possibility of creating an excess bulk of restorative material.

The indirect technique usually requires the removal of some enamel (ideally 0.3-0.5 mm but occasionally more in severely stained teeth) from the facial surface to provide space for the veneer (Fig. 39-15). Tooth preparation is best accomplished with a medium grit diamond bur (Fig. 39-16), with the goal of producing a Chamfer finish line throughout the surfaces to be covered. This preparation extends to the proximal surfaces just to include the contact points (Fig. 39-17). Gingivally, the preparation must extend far enough to cover the stained enamel sufficiently to improve the color. For better periodontal health, the finish line should be kept supragingival whenever possible. Following the preparation, an accurate impression of the teeth should be made using standard techniques and an elastomeric impression material such as polysulfide or silicone.

At the second appointment, one should isolate the teeth and clean them with pumice. After trying on (using water, glycerin, or a try-in paste

to help hold the veneers in place) and adjusting the veneers, they should be cleaned with the etching gel and silanated. The preparations should be acid-etched individually or in pairs and the veneers bonded in place, beginning with the central incisors. Celluloid matrices help protect adjacent teeth. Light-cured or dual-cured resins of moderate viscosity are preferred for bonding. Excess resin should be removed from margins with brushes prior to polymerization. Adequate polymerization time (40-60 seconds in each area) should be used because the veneers will shield some light transmission. Finishing and polishing are usually necessary only at the margins and may be done with abrasive strips and rubber cups (Figs. 39-18 to 39-20).

DIRECT VENEERS

Veneers made of light-cured composite resins can be constructed directly in the mouth. Compared with the indirect type, direct veneers offer the advantages of improved marginal adaptation, placement in one appointment, greater operator control, and no laboratory fee. The disadvantages include the fact that direct veneers require more time, greater skill, and more patience on the part

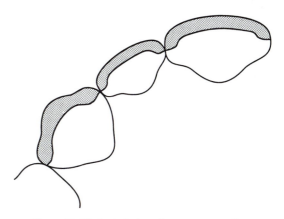

Figure 39-17. Incisal view of veneer preparations.

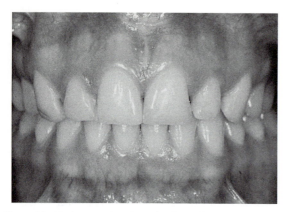

Figure 39–18. Preoperative view of esthetically unpleasing maxillary anterior teeth.

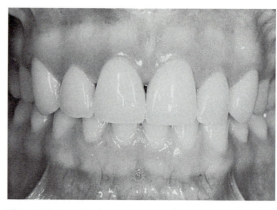

Figure 39–20. Porcelain veneers in place on teeth 6 to 11 (see Figs. 39–18 and 39–19).

of the clinician. Also, results are more difficult to predict.

The clinical direct technique may be performed with or without any enamel removal. Darkly stained teeth usually require some enamel removal because more composite resin is needed to mask the underlying enamel. The teeth are then pumiced and individually etched, and bonding agent is applied. Again, celluloid matrices are used between adjacent teeth. Opaquing agents may then be painted on to cover more intensely stained areas or entire surfaces, although the use of these agents can cause an unesthetic flat appearance in the color of the final restoration. For the best appearance, opaquing agents should be used minimally and with care. When dark banding is present, an alternative approach is to remove the band with a round bur and then replace the tooth structure with an opaque hybrid composite resin. Next, the composite resin (microfilled) should be applied in a layer 1.0 to 1.5 mm in thickness and contoured via brushes. The

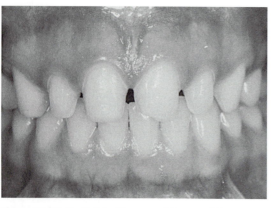

Figure 39–19. Teeth 6 to 11 prepared for porcelain veneers (see Fig. 39–18).

gingival third of the restoration should usually be an opaque yellow shade, and the remaining enamel should be covered with opaque gray or universal composite, overlapping and blending the shades to create a natural-looking, gentle color transition. In many cases, a nonopaque shade can be used on the incisal one fourth to allow a natural, translucent appearance (Fig. 39–21). After all composite resin has been added to a single tooth and contouring with brushes is complete, the material should be polymerized by exposing each area to the curing light for 40 to 60 seconds. The curing light should overlap areas for each period of exposure because narrow-tipped lights may require four or five separate exposures to cure the entire labial surface. A wider light-curing tip (e.g., 11 mm diameter) is recommended to minimize the need for overlapping exposure. Finishing and polishing are best done with burs and disks, as described previously.

Vital Bleaching

Vital bleaching techniques involve the application of peroxide solutions to increase the value (whiteness) of teeth that are unusually dark. Two basic methods have been reported in the literature, "power bleaching" (Cohen and Parkins, 1970) and "night guard (or mouthguard) vital bleaching" (Haywood and Heymann, 1989).

Power bleaching is an in-office procedure in which a concentrated hydrogen peroxide solution is applied to rubber dam–isolated teeth while heating the teeth, usually with an electric lamp. This method of bleaching usually requires numerous (three or more) office visits and often causes temporary tooth sensitivity to thermal

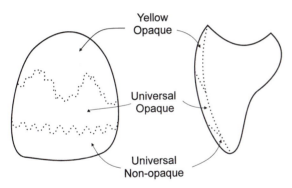

Figure 39–21. The use of overlapping shades of composite resin to create a natural-looking, directly placed veneer.

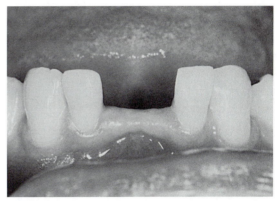

Figure 39–22. Preoperative view of a patient missing teeth 24 and 25.

changes. Typically, patients who have had this treatment require periodic retreatment to maintain the desired color.

Night guard vital bleaching is a dentist-directed, "at home" treatment. This method of vital bleaching involves a custom mouthguard and a milder peroxide solution (usually 10% carbamide peroxide) that the patient applies and wears outside the dental office, often at night during sleep, for about 2 to 3 weeks. Night guard vital bleaching appears to work as well as power bleaching and causes less thermal sensitivity. Concerns were initially raised about the potentially hazardous soft tissue effects of applying peroxide solutions in this manner, but long-term studies of the safety and efficacy are demonstrating no harmful effects.

Peroxide bleaching methods appear to work best on teeth that are mildly discolored, predominantly yellow, and from which the discoloration originates in enamel, rather than dentin.

BONDED BRIDGES AND SPLINTS

Cast metal appliances can be bonded to enamel, using composite resin cements. This procedure, in which the inner surfaces of metal are micro-abraded with aluminum oxide in the laboratory to create micromechanical retentive areas, is useful for attaching bridges and splints. Bridges constructed by this technique offer two advantages over conventional bridgework: greater conservation of tooth structure and lower cost. Splints can be made using the same technique for patients requiring fixed postorthodontic stabilization.

Diagnosis and treatment planning should include careful evaluation of occlusion. Ideally, the retainers would cover 80% to 90% of the lingual enamel surfaces of those teeth in order to pro-

vide maximal retention. Anterior teeth with markedly translucent incisal edges may not allow coverage to extend near those edges because metallic or resin coverage can cause an unnaturally opaque appearance. Diagnostic study models are helpful. The teeth must have adequate enamel for bonding, because the presence of exposed dentin or restorations can significantly decrease retentive strength. Enamel may be reduced (0.5 mm) to provide space for the metal retainer, and occasionally opposing teeth may also be reduced slightly. For anterior bridges and splints, lingual enamel can be slightly reduced with diamond burs, ending in a supragingival chamfer. Small proximal grooves aid resistance, retention, seating, and longevity of the restoration. Shade selection for pontics should be made prior to preparation.

An impression of the prepared arch should be made with an accurate elastomeric impression material such as polysulfide or silicone rubber. Using a sharp red pencil, the extensions of the preparations should be outlined on the working

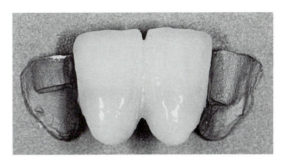

Figure 39–23. Facial view of porcelain-fused-to-cast-metal appliance that will replace teeth 24 and 25 (see Fig. 39–22).

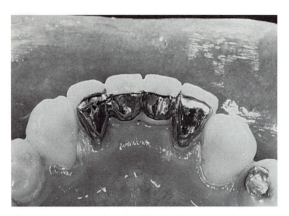

Figure 39–24. Incisal view of bonded bridge in place (see Figs. 39–22 and 39–23).

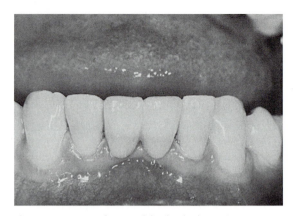

Figure 39–25. Facial view of the finished case (see Figs. 39–22 to 39–24).

model. If preparation grooves are not used, it is helpful to request from the laboratory technician incisal rests that serve as guides for accurate seating of the appliance. These guides can be removed with carbide burs after cementation of the appliance.

The appliance should be seated to make any adjustments of shade, contour, or occlusion. It is advisable to air-abrade (with aluminum oxide) the interior of the retainers. Teeth should be isolated with a rubber dam while the appliance is cleaned in an ultrasonic water bath. After pumicing and etching the abutment teeth, composite resin luting cement (autopolymerizing) is mixed and applied to the appliance. The appliance must be seated and held with firm pressure for several minutes while the resin cement hardens; otherwise, the rubber dam may push the appliance incisally, resulting in incomplete seating. It is helpful to remove excess cement with a soft brush or cotton pellet whenever access allows. Following cementation, one should carefully cut the rubber dam with a scissors and remove it. Remaining excess cement may be removed with a diamond or carbide bur (Figs. 39–22 to 39–25).

In the unlikely and unfortunate event of a retainer loosening from an abutment tooth, the appliance should be removed and returned to the laboratory for re-etching or abrasion roughening. It may then be reattached via the same procedure.

REFERENCES

Cohen S, Parkins FM: Bleaching tetracycline-stained vital teeth. Oral Surg Oral Med Oral Pathol 29:465-471, 1970.

Croll TP: Enamel microabrasion for removal of superficial discoloration. J Esthetic Dent 1:14-20, 1989a.

Croll TP: Enamel microabrasion: The technique. Quint Int 20:385-400, 1989b.

Croll TP: Enamel microabrasion for removal of superficial dysmineralization and decalcification defects. JADA 120:411-415, 1990.

Croll TP: Enamel dysmineralization and decalcification. In Enamel Microabrasion. Chicago, Quintessence Publishing, 1991, pp 1-102.

Ham WT: Ocular hazards of light sources: Review of current knowledge. J Occup Med 25:101-103, 1983.

Haywood VB, Heymann HO: Nightguard vital bleaching. Quint Int 20:173-176, 1989.

Nakabayashi N, Kojima K, Masuhara E: The promotion of adhesion by the infiltration of monomers into tooth substrates. J Biomed Mater Res 16:265-273, 1982.

Van Meerbeek B, Inokoshi S, Braem M, et al: Morphological aspects of the resin-dentin interdiffusion zone with different dentin adhesive systems. J Dent Res 71:1530-1540, 1992.

40

Sports Dentistry and Mouth Protection

Dennis N. Ranalli

Chapter Outline

DEVELOPMENTAL EVALUATION OF CHILD AND ADOLESCENT ATHLETES

Medical Assessment

Participation in athletic activities at both the recreational and organized sports levels continues to attract growing numbers of developing children and adolescents. Many dentists who are involved in the treatment of pediatric dental patients are unaware of the patients' involvement in sports simply because standard medical and dental history forms do not usually include questions that elicit this type of information and parents are often unaware of the dentists' need to know. It is advisable, then, as part of a thorough medical history, to ask parents routinely about their child's athletic activities (Ranalli, 1997).

A complete medical examination by a physician is a necessity because several medical conditions in children and adolescents have been identified as causes for limitation or disqualification from participation in athletics. These conditions include hepatitis, infectious mononucleosis, tu-berculosis, diabetes mellitus, loss of a paired organ such as a kidney, hypertension (greater than 140/90 mm Hg), and cardiac conditions (Adamkin, 1978).

Growth Assessment

Another important aspect in the overall evaluation of pediatric dental patients who have identified themselves as participants in sports is the assessment of the developmental and behavioral characteristics of the individual patient. This information, together with an evaluation of the child's physical growth, can be a valuable guide to the dentist in offering sound advice to the patient and parents for selecting age-appropriate athletic activities because a prediction of the nature of athletic injuries can often be based on the child's stage of psychosocial development and physical maturity. Young children are often not ready to cope psychologically with the complex rules or physical demands associated with some team sports (Pinkham and Kohn, 1991).

Participation in sports involves many health hazards for growing children and adolescents. Parents who permit their children to engage in athletic pursuits run a calculated risk to enable the child or adolescent to achieve beneficial goals. The physical and mental health benefits that are gained, such as improving overall physical function, relieving anxiety, and improving school performance, must be evaluated by informed parents and judged to outweigh the risks of injury to the child or adolescent athlete (Adamkin, 1978).

An Athlete's Bill of Rights suggests several factors that are necessary to improve the risk-benefit ratio in safeguarding the health of high school athletes (Hein, 1962): "Proper conditioning helps to prevent injuries by hardening the body and increasing resistance to fatigue. Careful coaching leads to skillful performance, which lowers the incidence of injuries. Good officiating promotes enjoyment of the game as well as the protection of players. Right equipment and facilities serve a unique purpose in protection of players. Adequate medical (and dental) care is a necessity in the prevention and control of athletic injuries."

Intraoral Assessment

The overall developmental evaluation of child or adolescent athletes must include a thorough oral and dental examination for accurate diagnosis and proper treatment of dental caries, juvenile periodontal diseases, hard and soft tissue pathology, congenital anomalies, and developmental occlusion.

Just as the long bones in young children are not yet fully formed and are more prone to fracture and dislocation during athletic activities, so too is the alveolar bone surrounding the primary teeth less dense, often resulting in traumatic dislocation injuries such as avulsion or intrusive luxation. Intrusive luxation of a primary incisor is potentially one of the most serious traumatic injuries to the underlying developing permanent tooth bud. In addition to the possibility of ankylosis of the traumatized primary incisor, causing delayed or ectopic eruption of the permanent tooth, the underlying developing permanent tooth bud may also be displaced in the crypt. If this displacement occurs during the morphodifferentiation stage of tooth development, an abnormal curvature in the root or crown of the formed permanent tooth may result in a dilacerated tooth. If the traumatic insult occurs later during the apposition stage, when the deposition of dentin and enamel matrix takes place, a local-

ized enamel hypoplasia of the crown of the permanent tooth may result in Turner's tooth (Fig. 40-1).

Young athletes in the early mixed dentition phase should be evaluated radiographically and clinically for the natural processes of root resorption, exfoliation of the primary teeth, and eruption of the permanent successors. Particular attention should be given to space loss associated with the premature loss of primary teeth. In the late mixed dentition phase, the presence of a Class II, Division I malocclusion is indicative of an accident-prone dental profile. The clinical presence of an inadequate lip seal and excessive overjet place the protruding maxillary permanent incisors at greater risk for traumatic injury, especially in young athletes who participate in contact sports (Fig. 40-2). The dentist should keep in mind that the large pulp chambers close to the surface in immature permanent teeth are highly susceptible to pulpal exposures in the event of a traumatic tooth fracture.

The evaluation of developing third molars in adolescent athletes is of particular importance. Not only can an athletic season suddenly be interrupted by the annoying and often painful eruption of third molars with associated acute pericoronitis, but mandibular fractures in the gonial angle region of developing third molars can also occur in adolescent athletes (McCarthy, 1990).

The labial mucosa, specifically that in the mandibular anterior region of adolescent athletes, should be evaluated for the presence of soft tissue changes such as leukoplakia associated with the habitual use of smokeless tobacco. Snuff-dipping is a common habit among athletes, and

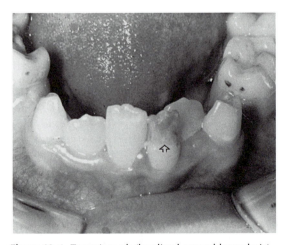

Figure 40–1. Turner's tooth (localized enamel hypoplasia) of the mandibular left permanent central incisor as the result of a traumatic injury during the apposition stage of tooth development.

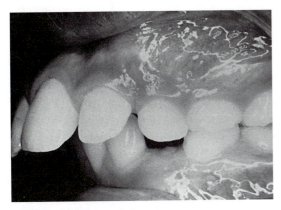

Figure 40–2. Excessive overjet and lack of lip protection place these maxillary permanent incisors at risk for traumatic injury during athletic activities.

unfortunately, it is occurring at an increasing rate, even among young children (National Institutes of Health, 1986). Child and adolescent athletes should be warned at every opportunity about the serious intraoral and systemic dangers of this addictive habit. The use of smokeless tobacco has been associated most frequently with baseball; however, amateur wrestlers and male athletes who compete in sports that are organized according to weight classifications sometimes dip snuff to suppress appetite and control body weight (Guggenheimer, 1991). Thus, an evaluation by the dentist should also include a sports-specific dietary history.

Dietary Assessment

The dentist can choose from a variety of accepted dietary assessment methods to evaluate child and adolescent athletes. These include the dietary history approach, the 24-hour recall method, the 7-day recall method, or the 7-day record of actual intake, either weighing, measuring, or estimating of portion sizes (Block, 1982). Whichever method the dentist selects, the special concerns related to specific sports must be kept in mind during the evaluation process.

Amateur boxers and wrestlers often practice aberrant eating behaviors and intentionally become dehydrated to meet weight classification requirements. These practices can have a negative impact not only on strength and performance but also on the cardiovascular system. On exertion in such situations, hyperthermia and even death can result. Female athletes who participate in sports such as gymnastics or ballet and engage in similar aberrant eating behaviors are subject to the same systemic manifestations.

Unhealthy nutritional practices may also predispose these young athletes to the possibility of injuries such as tibial stress fractures and shin splints (Loosli and Benson, 1990).

Adolescent athletes who attempt to control weight through dehydration and fasting are vulnerable to hypoglycemic syncope, caused by inadequate glucose reaching the brain. Such a pathophysiologic event can be precipitated in conjunction with a stressful dental appointment. Even if observable symptoms are not present, hypoglycemia by definition is a venous blood glucose level below 50 mg/100 ml (Malamed, 1978).

The dentist should be alert for the following clinical manifestations of hypoglycemia: palpations, sweating, confusion, irritability, headache, seizure, and unconsciousness. To prevent such episodes, the dentist should recommend that the dieting athlete eat a light meal or snack before the dental appointment. Additionally, a ready source of carbohydrate, such as orange juice, candy, or a container of cake frosting, should be available in the dental office emergency kit. Should an episode of hypoglycemic syncope occur during a dental appointment, a small amount of the cake frosting can be placed in the mucobuccal fold area for rapid systemic glucose absorption.

Especially with female adolescent athletes, the dentist should be alert for signs of the severe eating disorders of anorexia nervosa and bulimia. Enamel erosion on the lingual surfaces of the teeth, known as perimylolysis, is associated with the binge-purge cycle and persistent vomiting. An accompanying clinical feature can be enlargement of the parotid glands (Hasler, 1982). These severe eating disorders are often associated with psychological problems. In such instances, the dentist is obliged to recommend an appropriate referral for counseling.

At the other end of the spectrum are athletes such as football players, who desire to add bulk for increased size. This can present a dilemma for the dentist because one method of accomplishing this goal is to increase carbohydrate intake substantially. Dietary guidelines that minimize the effects on the teeth of highly cariogenic diets should be recommended. For example, it should be emphasized that the quantity of carbohydrates ingested is less critical for the dentition than the frequency of exposure or the type of carbohydrates consumed (Weiss and Trithart, 1960). Fruit, pretzels, and diet soda can be recommended as substitutes for sticky candy and sugar-containing soft drinks. Furthermore, these alternative foods can be consumed in greater quantities one or two times a day by those athletes desiring weight gain rather than bathing the teeth continuously with cariogenic sugars (Bibby, 1975).

One popular method of replacing fluids lost during athletic competition is ingesting sports drinks. The use of these electrolyte- and carbohydrate-containing drinks has not been shown conclusively to produce an advantage greater than water in maintaining electrolyte concentration or plasma volume or in improving intestinal absorption (Squire, 1990). For the great majority of young athletes, cold water remains the ideal replacement beverage.

Athletes of all ages are susceptible to misinformation regarding the exaggerated benefits of "supernutrition." In particular, athletic-minded adolescents are easily convinced that miracle supplements and fad diets will give them that "competitive edge" in their selected event. Although it is true that athletes have higher-than-average needs for energy and water, their requirements for vitamins, protein, fats, and most minerals do not exceed those of the nonathlete. Adopting a fad diet of selected foods over a long period of time may predispose a person to deficiencies of selected nutrients that unknowingly may be lacking in the diet. Excessive supplementation may interfere with absorption and utilization of other essential nutrients that are equally important to the athlete. When one considers the nutritional requirements of the child and adolescent athlete, the developmental consequences of major deviations from a well-balanced diet cannot be overlooked.

After this thorough developmental evaluation of the child or adolescent athlete has been concluded, appropriate advice and recommendations may then be given about the prevention of specific sports-related traumatic injuries to the craniofacial and intraoral structures.

MOUTH PROTECTION FOR CHILD AND ADOLESCENT ATHLETES

The single most important device for protecting the teeth and mouth as well as for reducing the likelihood of jaw fractures, neck injuries, concussions, or brain damage during athletic activities is the use of an intraoral mouth guard (Heintz, 1968; Hickey et al., 1967; Stenger et al., 1964). Unfortunately, only a very few organized amateur sports require mouth guards during practice sessions and in game situations. Amateur sports that mandate the use of mouth guards at the present time are boxing, football, ice hockey,

men's lacrosse, and women's field hockey. In 1990 the National Collegiate Athletic Association (NCAA) began to require that football players use brightly colored mouth guards instead of the more conventional clear variety. This new rule was enacted so that coaches and referees could better determine whether players were actually wearing this required piece of athletic equipment. At the professional sports level, only boxing mandates the use of a mouth guard, but increasing numbers of professional athletes in other sports seem to be using mouth guards voluntarily.

Although the use of mouth guards in conjunction with helmets and face masks has proved to be effective in reducing both the frequency and severity of traumatic craniofacial and intraoral injuries in athletes who participate in organized sports that require their use, acceptance of mouth guards in most other amateur sports has been minimal at best. For example, young athletes who participate in popular team sports such as baseball, basketball, and soccer and even in school physical education classes where mouth guards are not required continue to experience a high incidence of intraoral injuries, concussions, and even death (Mueller et al., 1989; U. S. Consumer Product Safety Commission, 1981).

One important aspect of dental professional responsibility to our athletic child and adolescent patients is to act as an advocate with local athletic associations, school boards, and sports regulatory agencies to promote the enactment of rules requiring the use of mouth guards in these and other sports in which they are not mandatory, to prevent future traumatic sports-related injuries and protect these young athletes.

Types of Mouth Guards

The American Society for Testing and Materials (ASTM, 100 Barr Harbor Drive, W. Conshohocken, PA 19428) uses the following classification to categorize mouth guards (Fig. 40–3):

Type I: Stock
Type II: Mouth-formed
Type III: Custom-fabricated (over a model)

ASTM Standard Practice for Care and Use of Mouthguards (1986) also lists several design considerations and special limitations. A mouth guard is best fitted by a dentist. The mouth guard should cover all remaining teeth in the maxillary arch except in athletes with mandibular prognathism. In these instances, all teeth in the mandibular arch should be covered instead. The imprint

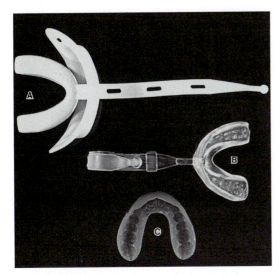

Figure 40–3. The three categories of athletic mouth guards include: *A*, Type I, stock; *B*, Type II, mouth-formed; and *C*, Type III, custom-fabricated.

of the opposing arch is not recommended because proper position is difficult to achieve and is unnecessary. The imprint does not improve protection, adds bulk, and can be uncomfortable for the athlete. A properly fitted mouth guard also reduces breathing interference.

For children in the developmental dentition phases, in which occlusal changes occur frequently, Type II thermally moldable mouth guards are recommended because they can be repeatedly reformed (ASTM, 1986). Adolescent athletes wearing fixed orthodontic appliances or those with congenital abnormalities such as cleft palate should be provided with mouth guards only under the supervision of a dentist.

Type I stock mouth guards are popular because they are inexpensive and are readily available in most sporting goods stores. Because they are preformed and are worn directly as manufactured, however, they are the least retentive, most bulky, and interfere most with breathing and speech. They must be held in place by clenching the teeth together. Because they offer the least amount of protection, stock mouth guards are not recommended (Ranalli, 1991). Unfortunately, because the overall costs of stock mouth guards are extremely low, especially when purchased in large quantities, and because they do not require the services of a dentist, some junior leagues and high school athletic departments opt for this type of mouth protector. Nevertheless, in these instances, some consolation can be taken from the fact that any mouth protection is better than none at all.

Type II mouth-formed mouth guards are priced reasonably, and good retention can be achieved if proper fitting is performed by a dentist. Results are often unsatisfactory, however, when athletes attempt to fit this type of mouth guard themselves (Ranalli, 1991).

Two varieties of mouth-formed mouth guards are available. The thermoplastic variety is placed in boiling water until it becomes softened. After insertion into the mouth, it is molded to the oral and dental structures. To avoid burning the oral soft tissues or possible damage to the dental pulp in immature permanent teeth, care should be exercised in regard to the temperature prior to inserting the softened protector. The mouth guard should be less than 132°F when inserted wet and should not be inserted in a dry mouth. If a tighter fit is desired, this type of mouth guard can be resoftened and remolded. This procedure is commonly known as the boil-and-bite technique. The Type II thermoplastic variety is the most commonly used athletic mouth guard.

The soft-lined variety of Type II mouth guards offers good retention. The more rigid mouth guard shell is lined with ethyl methacrylate soft lining material. For best results, the liner should be changed before every game, although some athletes object to the taste of the freshly mixed ethyl methacrylate material (Guevara and Ranalli, 1991).

Type III custom-fabricated mouth guards are far superior to Types I and II in terms of adaptation, retention, and protection. They are the most comfortable and interfere least with breathing and speech. Type III mouth guards are fabricated over a dental model using vacuum-formed thermoplastic material. Because this technique requires the services of a dentist and the final product is more expensive to the consumer than the other types of mouth guards, custom-fabricated mouth guards are unfortunately the least-used type of mouth guard.

When information about the advantages of custom-fabricated mouth guards is presented to the parents in a consultation session, the practitioner may consider several approaches. The first and most compelling reason is the superior quality of custom-fabricated mouth guards in terms of comfort and player safety. The concept of maximum protection for maximum prevention should be emphasized. In these terms, a custom-fabricated mouth guard is in fact a cost-effective alternative. Even though the actual cost is higher compared with the other types of mouth guards available, the relative cost is low compared with other equipment such as athletic shoes. Furthermore, the actual cost is far more conservative than the fees associated with emergency and long-term treatment of a traumatic athletic injury. Additionally, the dental model used to fabricate the original mouth guard should be preserved so that in the event of damage or loss of the mouth guard, a new replacement can be made quickly and easily (Ranalli, 1997).

The increasing demands of the marketplace have resulted in the introduction of a variety of new mouth guard products. Three of these new products deserve mention. One is the boil-and-bite, bimaxillary jaw joint positioner. This device increases the distance between the head of the condyle and the glenoid fossa and is designed to decrease the likelihood of repeated damage to the temporomandibular joint region as well as concussions caused from a traumatic force to the mandible. Another is an anatomically molded boil-and-bite mouthguard made of ethylene vinyl acetate. This product includes a vertical dimension control system. The third is a custom-fabricated, heat-pressure–laminated mouth guard. This mouth guard is constructed using multiple layers of material and is designed for greater adaptation (retention) as well as resistance to distortion over time.

Regardless of the type of mouth guard finally selected, all mouth guards should be stored in a plastic container when not in use to avoid damage due to excessive heat and cold (ASTM, 1986). Mouth guards should be washed daily in cold or lukewarm water because the use of hot water may result in distortion. Prior to insertion, the mouth guard can be rinsed with any commercially available mouthwash to freshen the taste (Guevara and Ranalli, 1991). Mouth guards should be inspected regularly during the course of an athletic season to detect distortions, splits, or bite-through problems (Fig. 40–4). When such deficiencies are detected, fabrication of a new mouth guard should be recommended (Ranalli, 1991).

Vacuum-Formed Technique for Custom-Fabricated Mouth Guards

As with all dental procedures, universal precautions for infection control must be followed precisely. After a thorough diagnosis has been made and all necessary restorations have been completed, dental prophylaxis should be performed immediately prior to making the impression to ensure the best possible adaptation (Guevara and Ranalli, 1991).

An alginate impression of the entire maxillary arch is taken in a muscle-molded rim-lock tray.

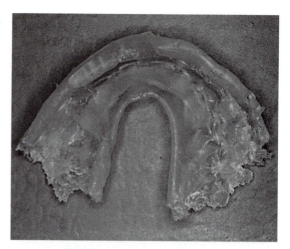

Figure 40–4. Distortions, splits, and bite-through problems indicate the need to fabricate a new mouth guard for proper retention, comfort, and maximum protection of the athlete.

After the impression material is set fully and the tray is removed from the mouth, the impression should be washed under cold running water and then disinfected by immersing or spraying it with an EPA-registered, ADA-approved disinfectant such as sodium hypochlorite. Before pouring the model, excess water and disinfecting solution should be removed with a gentle stream of air.

Following removal of these excess liquids, the dental model is poured immediately via a thick mix of dental stone. After proper setting, the impression is separated gently from the dental model. The model is trimmed, stone bubbles are removed, and voids are filled in. For athletes who wear fixed orthodontic appliances, the dental model should be relieved with plaster over the area of the appliance and prior to vacuum-forming the mouth guard. The dental model should also be modified so that the finished mouth guard will not interfere with anticipated orthodontic tooth movements (Croll and Castaldi, 1989; Dukes, 1962).

The cold, wet dental model is centered on the vacuum former. A 5.5-inch square sheet of polyvinyl acetate-polyethylene is positioned on the vacuum machine and heated until the sheet shows a 1- to 2-inch sag (Fig. 40–5A). The heat is switched off as the vacuum is switched on while the softened material is compressed over the dental model (Fig. 40–5B). The vacuum should be kept on for approximately 2 minutes, during which time the softened material can be hand-adapted via a wet paper towel.

When the model is completely cool, excess material is trimmed with scissors and peeled

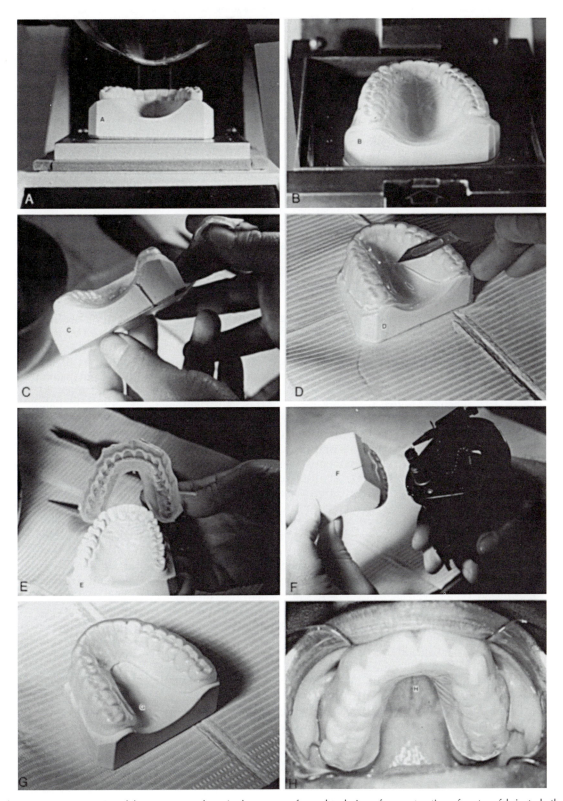

Figure 40–5. *A–H,* Various laboratory procedures in the vacuum-formed technique for construction of custom-fabricated athletic mouth guards. (See text for descriptive details.)

Why Sports Dentistry?

William Chambers

It's a beautiful fall afternoon. You are enjoying a great football game on television when the phone rings. It's your neighbor. His daughter, a patient of yours, was involved in a great game of her own—a soccer match. It seems she made a game-winning block to save a goal. Unfortunately, she blocked the kick at close range with her face. You now spend the next 2 hours of your nice fall afternoon in the office trying to restore a smashed smile for a beautiful young girl.

You may ask what is the point of this story. The point is that you do not have to seek out sports dentistry—sports dentistry will seek you out! With present trends, children (at younger and younger ages) and adults are becoming more and more involved in sports activities. Soccer, basketball, baseball, and softball are just a few sports that include participants with a wide range of ages and skill levels and that all too often involve frequent incidents of orofacial trauma.

Sports dentistry has two major components. The first is the treatment of orofacial injuries, and the second is the prevention of sports-related orofacial injuries. The treatment of orofacial sports injuries calls into play many different dental skills. To provide comprehensive care, a dentist must be knowledgeable and adept in the areas of oral surgery, endodontics, operative dentistry, orthodontics, hospital dentistry, and patient behavior management. The care of sports-related orofacial injuries can be satisfying, especially when a positive treatment result occurs. What automatically comes to mind when treating these injuries, however, is the question, Why did this have to happen? Why do so many young athletes have to suffer such preventable injuries—injuries that can negatively affect the patient's oral health for a lifetime? This realization brings into focus the second aspect of sports dentistry—prevention through sports safety.

My personal interest in sports dentistry evolved through a series of experiences. In college I played basketball at the University of North Carolina at Chapel Hill. Fortunately, I did not suffer any orofacial injuries, but I did witness several injuries to a number of other players. This experience sensitized me to the effect of such injuries on people I know. During dental school, while playing intramural basketball, I was intentionally elbowed in the mouth by a former tight end on the football team. Although my injury was not serious, I took this episode as a personal wake-up call to wear a mouth guard whenever I played basketball. From that day on, I have always worn a mouth guard.

Once I established a private practice in pediatric dentistry, I made many efforts to expand my practice. One effort was to inform the pediatricians I knew that I would be available, through a beeper, to cover their after-hours dental trauma cases. I soon was amazed at the number of orofacial trauma cases I treated during certain seasons of the year (i.e., basketball and baseball seasons). My initial exhilaration in treating these trauma cases eventually led to some real introspective thinking. How could I help prevent some of these injuries? My concern about the number of trauma cases I was seeing, coupled with the fact that both my daughters were now beginning to participate in sports, certainly personalized my interest in prevention.

My initial efforts at prevention were undertaken merely in the leagues in which my children played. As a coach and league official, I urged all players to wear mouth guards. I did this though personal discussions and by sending letters to parents and coaches. Also, my own children set the example by wearing mouth guards. I also urged every patient in my practice to wear mouth guards. This was done during recall visits and in the office newsletter.

Although encouraged by the sudden large numbers of children I saw wearing mouth guards, I realized that this message had to have a broader base to truly make a difference. I then gathered all the information I could on sports dentistry and preventive programs across the country. By presenting this information and a plan of action to the North Carolina Dental Society, we have now begun a statewide program to educate our profession and the public on the need for prevention of orofacial trauma through mouth protectors and other protective safety gear.

What has my interest in sports dentistry meant to me professionally and personally? In my community my practice is recognized for the quality of care we deliver in treating orofacial trauma. But I have received much more personal satisfaction through my efforts to improve children's dental health by helping to prevent serious dental injuries.

Dentistry has always been proud of its efforts in preventive care. We have always been advocates for any issues that represent the best interests of the public's oral health and well-being. Therefore, we have to take the lead in educating ourselves and the public about the measures necessary to prevent and treat sports-related orofacial trauma. On the local level, this effort should take the form of encouraging coaches to recommend and players to wear mouth guards or other protective devices such as batting helmets with face shields. Effectiveness requires direct involvement of the dentist with teams, coaches, parents, and sponsors. On the national level, we can act as advocates before the governing bodies of the various sports organizations to mandate the wearing of such safety equipment.

If as a dental professional you are on a quest to be the best, the bottom line is that you must get involved; you can make a difference—learn and do sports dentistry.

away (Fig. 40-5*C*). The palatal region is cut out in a U shape with a utility knife (Fig. 40-5*D*). After soaking in water, the mouth guard is then removed carefully from the model (Fig. 40-5*E*). The peripheral areas should be trimmed short of the mucobuccal fold, and care should be taken to relieve the frenum areas to avoid the development of sore spots.

Final finishing of rough edges can be accomplished by using polishing stones or rubber wheels and then flaming the mouth guard lightly with an alcohol torch (Fig. 40-5*F*). The completed custom-fabricated mouth guard is now ready for delivery (Fig. 40-5*G*). Following a try-in in the mouth, the mouth guard is adjusted if necessary and then given to the athlete (Fig. 40-5*H*).

PROFESSIONAL ACTIVITIES IN SPORTS DENTISTRY

Because of the ever-increasing number of children and adolescents participating in sports, many dentists already are treating these young athletes in their practices, and many more are likely to be doing so in the future. In addition to the clinical aspects of sports dentistry, a number of other professional activities are available to

dentists interested in enhancing their knowledge or expanding their involvement in this exciting field (Elliott, 1991).

These activities include volunteering for local mouth guard days, becoming a consultant to an athletic department, serving as a sports team dentist, or becoming a member of the Academy for Sports Dentistry.* Some dentists may present seminars in their local communities on topics related to sports dentistry, provide information to governing agencies advocating the enactment of more stringent mouth guard regulations, or become involved in research projects studying various aspects of sports dentistry (Ranalli, 1991, 1997).

Castaldi (1986) suggests that possibly the most effective role that can be played is in our dental schools, where faculty should develop a curriculum and teach the subject of sports dentistry and mouth protection for young athletes to dental students and residents in specialty training programs. Although various elements of sports dentistry, such as suturing techniques, restorations for the treatment of fractured incisors, and endodontic procedures, among others, do exist in the curriculum already, few dental schools have

*Academy for Sports Dentistry, Ms. Susan Ferry, Executive Secretary, 875 N. Michigan Avenue, Suite #4040, Chicago, IL 60611-1901.

an interdisciplinary learning experience in sports dentistry (Kumamoto and DiOrio, 1989). Such experiences are strongly recommended in future curriculum planning.

Whichever of these choices the interested dental professional chooses to make, one fact seems certain. The field of sports dentistry will continue to expand as participation in sports in our society continues to grow. The question remains, to what extent are dentists prepared to participate in the arena of sports dentistry? We as dentists must prepare ourselves now to meet this exciting future challenge.

REFERENCES

Adamkin DH: Medical care of the athlete. Am J Dis Child *132:*181-187, 1978.

American Society for Testing and Materials: Standard practice for care and use of mouthguards. Designation: F 697-80. Philadelphia, American Society for Testing and Materials, 1986, p 323.

Bibby BG: The cariogenicity of snack foods and confections. JADA *90:*121-132, 1975.

Block G: A review of validations of dietary assessment methods. Am J Epidemiol *115:*492-505, 1982.

Castaldi CR: Sports-related oral and facial injuries in the young athlete: A new challenge for the pediatric dentist. Pediatr Dent *8:*311-316, 1986.

Croll TP, Castaldi CR: The custom-fitted athletic mouthguard for the orthodontic patient and for the child with a mixed dentition. Quint Int *20:*571-575, 1989.

Dukes HH: Football mouthpiece for the orthodontic patient. Am J Orthodont *48:*609-611, 1962.

Elliott MA: Professional responsibility in sports dentistry. Dent Clin North Am *35:*831-840, 1991.

Guevara PA, Ranalli DN: Techniques for mouthguard fabrication. Dent Clin North Am *35:*667-682, 1991.

Guggenheimer J: Implications of smokeless tobacco use in athletes. Dent Clin North Am *35:*797-808, 1991.

Hasler JF: Parotid enlargement: A presenting sign in anorexia nervosa. Oral Surg Oral Med Oral Pathol *53:*567-573, 1982.

Hein F: Safeguarding the health of the high school athlete. *In* Ryan A (ed): Medical Care of the Athlete. New York, McGraw-Hill, 1962, pp 16-17.

Heintz WD: Mouth protectors: A progress report. JADA *77:*632-636, 1968.

Hickey JC, Morris AL, Carlson LD, et al: The relation of mouth protectors to cranial pressure and deformation. JADA *74:*735-740, 1967.

Kumamoto DP, DiOrio LP: An interdisciplinary learning experience in sports dentistry. J Dent Educ *53:*491-494, 1989.

Loosli AR, Benson J: Nutritional intake in adolescent athletes. Pediatr Clin North Am *37:*1143-1152, 1990.

Malamed SF: Handbook of Medical Emergencies in the Dental Office. St. Louis, CV Mosby, 1978, pp 164-176.

McCarthy MF: Sports and mouth protection. Genl Dent *38:*343-346, 1990.

Mueller FO, et al: National Centers for Catastrophic Sports Injury Research, Chapel Hill, NC: Seventh Annual Report. Fall 1982-Spring 1989, pp 1-59.

National Institutes of Health, Consensus Conference Statement: Health implications of smokeless tobacco use. Bethesda, MD, National Institutes of Health, U.S. Government Printing Office: 0-153-019:QL3, 1986, pp 1-6.

Pinkham JR, Kohn DW: Epidemiology and prediction of sports related traumatic injuries. Dent Clin North Am *35:*609-626, 1991.

Ranalli DN: Prevention of craniofacial injuries in football. Dent Clin North Am *35:*627-645, 1991.

Ranalli DN: Strategies for the prevention of sports-related oral injuries: A practical guide for the pediatric dentist. J Southeast Soc Pediatr Dent *3:*18-19, 1997.

Squire DL: Heat illness: Fluid and electrolyte issues for pediatric and adolescent athletes. Pediatr Clin North Am *37:*1085-1109, 1990.

Stenger JM, Lawson EA, Wright JM, et al: Mouthguards: Protection against shock to the head, neck, and teeth. JADA *69:*273-281, 1964.

U.S. Consumer Product Safety Commission: Overview of Sports-Related Injuries in Persons 5-14 Years of Age. Washington, DC, 1981, pp 1-47.

Weiss RL, Trithart AH: Between-meal eating habits and dental caries experience in preschool children. Am J Public Health *50:*1097-1104, 1960.

Index
....

Note: Page numbers in *italics* refer to illustrations; page numbers followed by a t refer to tables.

Q

U

V

ISBN 0-7216-8238-3

90038